Library Use Only

613.2 N976j
Nutrition and well—being A
to Z
59778

Nutrition and Well-Being A to Z

EDITORIAL BOARD

Editor in Chief

Delores C. S. James, Ph.D., RD, LD/N
University of Florida
Department of Health Science Education
Gainesville, Florida

Associate Editors

Catherine Christie, Ph.D., RD, LD/N, FADA
University of North Florida
Jacksonville, Florida

Ranjita Misra, Ph.D., CHES
Texas A&M University
Department of Health and Kinesiology
College Station, Texas

EDITORIAL AND PRODUCTION STAFF

Ray Abruzzi, Mark Drouillard, *Project Editors*
Peter Jaskowiak, *Copyeditor*
Dorothy Bauhoff, Jessica Hornik Evans, *Proofreaders*
Wendy Allex, *Indexer*
Marc Borbely, Justin Crawford, Tom Crippen, Victor Inzunza, Paula Kepos, Richard Robinson, *Editorial Support*
Michelle Dimercurio, *Senior Art Director*
Wendy Blurton, *Senior Manufacturing Specialist*
Shalice Shah-Caldwell, *Permissions Specialist*
Denay Wilding, *Image Acquisition Editor, Imaging and Multimedia Content*
Lezlie Light, *Imaging Coordinator, Imaging and Multimedia Content*
Randy Bassett, *Imaging Supervisor, Imaging and Multimedia Content*

Macmillan Reference USA

Frank Menchaca, *Vice President and Publisher*
Hélène Potter, *Director, New Product Development*

Nutrition and Well-Being A to Z

Volume 2 I–Z

Delores C. S. James, Editor in Chief

MACMILLAN REFERENCE USA
An imprint of Thomson Gale, a part of The Thomson Corporation

THOMSON
GALE

Detroit • New York • San Francisco • San Diego • New Haven, Conn. • Waterville, Maine • London • Munich

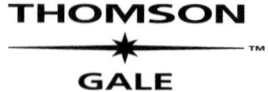

Nutrition and Well-Being A to Z

Delores C. S. James, Editor in Chief

© 2004 Thomson Gale, a part of the Thomson Corporation.

Thomson and Star Logo are trademarks and Gale and Macmillan Reference USA are registered trademarks used herein under license.

For more information contact
The Gale Group, Inc.
27500 Drake Rd.
Farmington Hills, MI 48331-3535
Or you can visit our Internet site at
http://www.gale.com

ALL RIGHTS RESERVED
No part of this work covered by the copyright hereon may be reproduced or used in any form or by any means—graphic, electronic, or mechanical, including photocopying, recording, taping, Web distribution, or information storage retrieval systems—without the written permission of the publisher.

For permission to use material from this product, submit your request via Web at http://www.gale-edit.com/permissions, or you may download our Permissions Request form and submit your request by fax or mail to:

Permissions Department
The Gale Group, Inc.
27500 Drake Rd.
Farmington Hills, MI 48331-3535
Permissions Hotline:
248-699-8006 or 800-877-4253, ext. 8006
Fax: 248-699-8074 or 800-762-4058

Since this page cannot legibly accommodate all copyright notices, the acknowledgements constitute an extension of the copyright notice.

LIBRARY OF CONGRESS CATALOGING-IN-PUBLICATION DATA

Nutrition and well being A to Z / Delores C.S. James, editor in chief.
  p. cm.
    Includes bibliographical references and index.
    ISBN 0-02-865707-1 (set hardcover)—ISBN 0-02-865708-X (volume 1)—
    ISBN 0-02-865709-8 (volume 2)
    1. Nutrition—Encyclopedias.   2. Health—Encyclopedias.
    I. James, Delores C.S., 1961–

RA784.N838 2004
613.2'03—dc22   2004006088

This title is also available as an e-book
ISBN 0-02-865990-2 (set)
Contact your Gale sales representative for ordering information

Printed in the United States of America
10 9 8 7 6 5 4 3

Table of Contents

Volume 1

TABLE OF CONTENTS	v
PREFACE	ix
TOPICAL OUTLINE	xi
FOR YOUR REFERENCE	xv
CONTRIBUTORS	xxi
Addiction, Food	1
Additives and Preservatives	1
Adolescent Nutrition	4
Adult Nutrition	7
African Americans, Diet of	10
Africans, Diets of	15
Aging and Nutrition	20
Alcohol and Health	23
Allergies and Intolerances	26
Alternative Medicines and Therapies	30
American Dietetic Association	34
American Public Health Association	35
American School Food Service Association	35
American School Health Association	35
Amino Acids	36
Anemia	38
Anorexia Nervosa	41
Anthropometric Measurements	42
Antioxidants	42
Appetite	44
Arteriosclerosis	45
Artificial Sweeteners	46
Asian Americans, Diets of	48
Asians, Diets of	52
Atherosclerosis	59
Baby Bottle Tooth Decay	59
Battle Creek Sanitarium, Early Health Spa	60
Beikost	62
Beriberi	62
Beta-Carotene	62
Bezoars	63
Binge Eating	63
Bioavailability	64
Biotechnology	64
Body Fat Distribution	68
Body Image	69
Body Mass Index	71
Breastfeeding	74
Brillat-Savarin, Jean Anthelme	78
Bulimia Nervosa	79
Caffeine	80
Calcium	83
Calorie	87
Cancer	87
Carbohydrates	93
Cardiovascular Diseases	99
Careers in Dietetics	104
Caribbean Islanders, Diet of	107
Carotenoids	112
Central Americans and Mexicans, Diets of	113
Central Europeans and Russians, Diets of	117
Childhood Obesity	121
College Students, Diets of	123
Commodity Foods	127
Comprehensive School Health Program	130
Convenience Foods	132
Corn- or Maize-based Diets	133
Cravings	136
Cultural Competence	139
Dehydration	142

v

Diabetes Mellitus	143
Diarrhea	149
Diet	151
Dietary Assessment	152
Dietary Guidelines	153
Dietary Reference Intakes	155
Dietary Supplements	155
Dietary Trends, American	159
Dietary Trends, International	162
Dietetic Technician, Registered (DTR)	166
Dietetics	166
Dieting	167
Dietitian	168
Digestion and Absorption	169
Disaster Relief Organizations	173
Eating Disorders	176
Eating Disturbances	182
Eating Habits	186
Emergency Nutrition Network	189
Ergogenic Aids	189
Exchange System	193
Exercise	198
Exercise Addiction	201
Expanded Food and Nutrition Education Program	202
Fad Diets	203
Failure to Thrive	206
Famine	207
Fast Foods	209
Fasting	210
Fat Substitutes	211
Fats	214
Female Athlete Triad	219
Fetal Alcohol Syndrome	220
Fiber	221
Food Aid for Development and the World Food Programme	223
Food and Agriculture Organization (FAO)	224
Food Guide Pyramid	225
Food Insecurity	228
Food Labels	231
Food Safety	235
Fortification	239
French Paradox	239
Functional Foods	240
Funk, Casimir	244
Generally Recognized as Safe (GRAS)	245

Genetically Modified Foods	245
Glisson, Francis	249
Global Database on National Nutrition Policies and Programs	249
Glycemic Index	250
Goiter	252
Goldberger, Joseph	253
Graham, Sylvester	254
Grazing	256
Greeks and Middle Easterners, Diet of	256
Green Revolution	261
Growth Charts	262
Growth Hormone	262
Health	263
Health Claims	263
Health Communication	266
Health Education	266
Health Promotion	267
Healthy Eating Index	267
Healthy People 2010 Report	269
Heart Disease	271
Hispanics and Latinos, Diet of	275
HIV/AIDS	279
Homelessness	282
Hunger	287
Hyperglycemia	287
Hypertension	288
Hypoglycemia	292
Glossary	293
Index	309

Volume 2

Table of Contents	v
Preface	ix
Topical Outline	xi
For Your Reference	xv
Contributors	xxi
Illnesses, Food-Borne	1
Immune System	4
Inborn Errors of Metabolism	4
Infant Mortality Rate	7
Infant Nutrition	8
Infection	12
Insulin	12
Irradiation	13
Isoflavones	14

Entry	Page
Johnson, Howard	14
Kellogg, John Harvey	16
Kroc, Ray	18
Kwashiorkor	20
Lactose Intolerance	21
Lay Health Advisor	23
Lead Poisoning	23
Legumes	27
Life Expectancy	28
Lipid Profile	28
Low Birth Weight Infant	31
Macrobiotic Diet	31
Malnutrition	33
Marasmus	36
Marketing Strategies	37
Mastitis	41
Maternal Mortality Rate	42
Meals On Wheels	42
Meat Analogs	42
Medical Nutrition Therapy	43
Mellanby, Edward	46
Menopause	47
Men's Nutritional Issues	51
Metabolism	54
Minerals	58
Mood-Food Relationships	64
National Academy of Sciences (NAS)	67
National Health and Nutrition Examination Survey (NHANES)	68
National Institutes of Health (NIH)	73
Native Americans, Diet of	78
Nongovernmental Organization (NGO)	82
Northern Europeans, Diet of	83
Nutrient Density	87
Nutrient-Drug Interactions	88
Nutrients	90
Nutrition	95
Nutrition Education	96
Nutrition Programs in the Community	96
Nutritional Assessment	99
Nutritional Deficiency	102
Nutritionist	104
Obesity	105
Omega-3 and Omega-6 Fatty Acids	108
Oral Health	110
Oral Rehydration Therapy	113
Organic Foods	113
Organisms, Food-Borne	117
Osteomalacia	122
Osteopenia	122
Osteoporosis	123
Overweight	125
Pacific Islander Americans, Diet of	126
Pacific Islanders, Diet of	128
Pasteur, Louis	132
Pasteurization	133
Pauling, Linus	133
Pellagra	135
Pemberton, John S.	135
Pesticides	137
Phenylketonuria (PKU)	137
Phytochemicals	138
Pica	138
Plant-Based Diets	138
Popular Culture, Food and	139
Pregnancy	142
Premenstrual Syndrome	147
Preschoolers and Toddlers, Diet of	150
Probiotics	154
Protein	155
Quackery	160
Recommended Dietary Allowances	164
Refugee Nutrition Information System (RNIS)	164
Regional Diets, American	166
Regulatory Agencies	170
Religion and Dietary Practices	174
Rice-based Diets	179
Rickets	183
Rosenstein, Nils Rosén von	
Satiety	187
Scandinavians, Diet of	187
School-Aged Children, Diet of	190
School Food Service	194
Scurvy	197
Small for Gestational Age	197
Smoking	198
Society for Nutrition Education	200
South Americans, Diet of	200
Southern Europeans, Diet of	204
Soy	207
Space Travel and Nutrition	210
Sports Nutrition	215
Stark, William	219
Sustainable Food Systems	220
Toxemia	223

Tulp, Nicholaas	223
Underweight	225
United Nations Children's Fund (UNICEF)	225
Vegan	229
Vegetarianism	229
Vitamins, Fat-soluble	232
Vitamins, Water-soluble	238
Waist-to-Hip Ratio	245
Water	245
Weight Loss Diets	248
Weight Management	250
Wellness	253
White, Ellen G.	254
Whole Foods Diet	255
WIC Program	255
Wilson, Owen	258
Women's Nutritional Issues	259
World Health Organization (WHO)	262
Xerophthalmia	264
Yo-Yo Dieting	264
GLOSSARY	267
INDEX	283

Preface

Nutrition is one of the most important factors that impact health in all areas of the lifecycle. Pregnant women need adequate food and health care to deliver a healthy baby who has a good birth weight and a fighting chance for survival. In many regions of the world, the infant mortality rate is very high, meaning that many infants will not live to see their first birthday. Breastfeeding is the ideal method of feeding and nurturing infants, because breast milk contains many immunologic agents that protect the infant against bacteria, viruses, and parasites. Yet, less than 40 percent of infants worldwide are exclusively breastfed (no other food or drink, not even water) for the first four months of life. Children need adequate nutrition to develop and grow to their full potential.

Malnutrition, both undernutrition and overnutrition, is at an all time high, with close to one-third of the world's children suffering from it. The number of undernourished people in the world continues to increase because of little or no progress to reduce poverty. Thousands of children die daily from hunger and its effects, even in technologically advanced countries. Without adequate nutrition, a person's cognitive ability is diminished, which adversely affects their ability to get a good paying job and contribute to their local economy. Paradoxically, childhood and adult obesity in many parts of the developed world are also near epidemic proportions. There are 300 million obese people in the world. In the United States, about 34 percent of Americans are overweight and 30.5 percent are obese.

Life expectancy has increased in many countries and the population of older adults is growing at an unprecedented rate in the United States and other technologically advanced countries. In the United States the average life expectancy is 70, while globally, the average rose to 67 years in 1998, up from 61 in 1980. These countries are unsure of how they will provide adequate health care for this growing segment of the population. Cardiovascular disease (coronary heart disease, hypertension, stroke) and cancer are top killers in many countries and HIV/AIDS continue to ravage our societies, taking individuals in the productive years of their lives.

Arrangement of the Material

Nutrition and Well-Being A to Z is a two-volume set that provides timely information on the personal, cultural, and global issues that affect (or have an impact on) health and nutritional status. Users will find detailed coverage of topics covered in general nutrition, food science, and personal and family courses. This encyclopedia explains fundamental concepts such as amino acids, cutting-edge ideas such as functional foods, social issues such as food insecurity, and political issues such as bioterrorism.

The set was also designed to meet consumer needs. Users will be able to spot a quack health-care provider, discriminate between reliable and unreliable health claims, as well as understand the role of government in keeping food safe. The set also profiles individuals who have made a social, historical, or scientific impact on health, nutrition, and food trends. Most entries are written from a global perspective, and dietary patterns from different regions of the world are discussed. Many professional health organizations are described.

The information in *Nutrition and Well-Being A to Z* is clearly presented and easy to find. Professionals in the field of nutrition, dietetics, food science, agriculture, medicine, health education, and public health wrote with the student in mind. Students and teachers can use the set to reinforce classroom topics on food, nutrition, and health, and to expand discussions on special or new topics. The extensive use of illustrations enhances the learning of the material. Entries are arranged alphabetically and an extensive cross-referencing system encourages the user to further explore other entries. All topics in a volume can be found in the index at the back of the book.

Acknowledgements and Thanks

A project of this magnitude would not be possible without the dedication and hard work of many people. I wish to thank the associate editors, Dr. Catherine Christie and Dr. Ranjita Misra, for the many hours they spent recruiting authors and editing entries. Thank you for your timely turnaround of the materials. The project would not have been possible without the many authors who wrote, and sometimes rewrote, the entries. Thank you for sharing your expertise and time. Amanda Foote, Senior Secretary in the Department of Health Science Education, was extremely valuable in copying and mailing the edited materials to the publishers. I wish to thank the many people at Macmillan Reference USA and the Gale Group for conceiving the project and providing direction throughout the entire project, especially the copyeditors and illustrators. I also send special thanks to Mr. Raymond Abruzzi.

Delores C. S. James

Topical Outline

American Dietary Habits

African Americans, Diet of
Asian Americans, Diets of
Dietary Trends, American
Hispanics and Latinos, Diet of
Native Americans, Diet of
Pacific Islander Americans, Diet of
Regional Diets, American

Biographies

Battle Creek Sanitarium
Brillat-Savarin, Jean Anthelme
Funk, Casimir
Glisson, Francis
Goldberger, Joseph
Graham, Sylvester
Johnson, Howard
Kellogg, John Harvey
Krock, Ray
Mellanby, Edward
Pasteur, Louis
Pauling, Linus
Pemberton, John S.
Rosenstein, Nils Rosén von
Stark, William
Tulp, Nicholaas
White, Ellen G.
Wilson, Owen

Body Function and Processes

Digestion and Absorption
Immune System
Insulin
Metabolism

Dieting, Weight Management, Exercise, Eating Disorders

Addiction, Food
Anorexia Nervosa
Appetite
Binge Eating
Body Image
Bulimia Nervosa
Cravings
Diet
Dieting
Eating Disorders
Eating Disturbances
Eating Habits
Ergogenic Aids
Exercise
Exercise Addiction
Fad Diets
Female Athlete Triad
Grazing
Mood-Food Relationships
Pica
Satiety
Sports Nutrition
Weight Loss Diets
Weight Management
Yo-Yo Dieting

Diseases and Disorders

Arteriosclerosis
Atherosclerosis
Bezoars
Cancer
Cardiovascular Disease
Diabetes Mellitus
Heart Disease
HIV/AIDS
Hyperglycemia
Hypertension
Hypoglycemia
Obesity

Food Habits, Trends, and Alternative Choices

Alternative Medicines and Therapies
Fat Substitutes
Legumes
Macrobiotic Diet
Plant-Based Diets
Popular Culture, Food and
Quackery
Soy
Vegan
Vegetarianism
Whole Foods Diet

Food Industry, Technology, and Food Safety

Additives and Preservatives
Artificial Sweeteners
Biotechnology
Commodity Foods
Convenience Foods
Fast Foods
Fat Substitutes
Food Safety
Fortification
Generally Recognized as Safe
Genetically Modified Foods
Green Revolution
Illnesses, Food-Borne
Irradiation
Marketing Strategies
Meat Analogs
Organic Foods
Organisms, Food-Borne
Pasteurization
Pesticides
Probiotics
Regulatory Agencies

Space Travel and Nutrition
Sustainable Food Systems

Health Programs and Organizations

American Dietetic Association
American Public Health Association
American School Food Service Association
American School Health Association
Comprehensive School Health Program
Disaster Relief Organizations
Emergency Nutrition Network
Expanded Food and Nutrition Education Program (EFNEP)
Food Aid for Development and the World Food Programme
Food and Agriculture Organization (FAO)
Global Database on National Nutrition Policies and Programmes
Meals On Wheels
National Academy of Sciences (NAS)
National Institutes of Health (NIH)
Nongovernmental Organization (NGO)
Nutrition Programs in the Community
Refugee Nutrition Information System (RNIS)
School Food Service
Society for Nutrition Education
United Nations Children's Fund (UNICEF)
WIC Program
World Health Organization (WHO)

Health Risks and Health Assessment

Alcohol and Health
Allergies and Intolerances
Anthropometric Measurement
Body Fat Distribution
Body Mass Index
Caffeine
Dehydration
Diarrhea
Dietary Assessment
Fasting
Food Insecurity
Growth Charts
Homelessness
Hunger
Infection
Lead Poisoning
Lipid Profile
Malnutrition
Nutrient-Drug Interactions
Nutritional Assessment
Nutrient Density
Nutritional Deficiency
Oral Rehydration Therapy
Overweight
Smoking
Underweight
Waist-to-Hip Ratio

International Dietary Habits

Africans, Diets of
Asians, Diets of
Caribbean Islanders, Diets of
Central Americans and Mexicans, Diets of
Central Europeans and Russians, Diets of
Corn- or Maize-based Diets
Dietary Trends, International
Famine
French Paradox
Greeks and Middle Easterners, Diet of
Northern Europeans, Diet of
Pacific Islanders, Diet of
Religion and Dietary Practices
Rice-based Diets
Scandinavians, Diet of
South Americans, Diet of
Southern Europeans, Diet of

Nutrients and Chemical Properties of Food

Amino acids
Antioxidants
Beta-Carotene
Bioavailability
Carbohydrates
Calcium
Calorie
Carotenoids
Fats
Fiber
Functional foods
Glycemic Index
Isoflavones
Minerals
Nutrients
Omega-3 and Omega-6 Fatty Acids
Phytochemicals
Protein
Vitamins, Fat-Soluble
Vitamins, Water-Soluble
Water

Nutritional Deficiencies

Anemia
Beriberi
Goiter
Kwashiorkor
Lactose Intolerance
Marasmus
Osteoporosis
Osteomalacia
Osteopenia
Pellagra
Rickets
Scurvy
Xerophthalmia

Nutrition and the Life Cycle

Adolescent Nutrition
Adult Nutrition
Aging and Nutrition
Baby Bottle Tooth Decay
Beikost
Breastfeeding
Childhood Obesity
College Students, Diets of
Failure to Thrive
Fetal Alcohol Syndrome
Growth Hormone
Inborn Errors of Metabolism
Infant Mortality Rate
Infant Nutrition
Life Expectancy
Low Birth Weight Infant
Mastitis
Maternal Mortality Rate
Menopause
Men's Nutritional Issues
Phenylketonuria (PKU)
Pregnancy
Premenstrual Syndrome
Preschoolers and Toddlers, Diet of
School-Aged Children, Diet of
Small for Gestational Age
Toxemia
Women's Nutritional Issues

Nutrition, Health, and Professional Issues

Careers in Dietetic
Cultural Competence
Dietetics

Dietetic Technician, Registered (DTR)
Dietitian
Health
Health Communication
Health Education
Health Promotion
Lay Health Advisor
Medical Nutrition Therapy
Nutrition
Nutrition Education
Nutritionist
Oral Health
Wellness

Nutrition Standards, Guidelines, Reports

Dietary Guidelines
Dietary Reference Intakes
Dietary Supplements
Exchange System
Food Guide Pyramid
Food Labels
Health Claims
Healthy Eating Index
Healthy People 2010 Report
National Health and Nutrition Examination Survey (NHANES)
Recommended Dietary Allowances (RDA)

For Your Reference

TABLE 1. SELECTED METRIC CONVERSIONS

WHEN YOU KNOW	MULTIPLY BY	TO FIND
Temperature		
Celsius (°C)	1.8 (°C) +32	Fahrenheit (°F)
Celsius (°C)	°C +273.15	Kelvin (K)
degree change (Celsius)	1.8	degree change (Fahrenheit)
Fahrenheit (°F)	[(°F) −32] / 1.8	Celsius (°C)
Fahrenheit (°F)	[(°F −32) / 1.8] +273.15	Kelvin (K)
Kelvin (K)	K −273.15	Celsius (°C)
Kelvin (K)	1.8(K −273.15) +32	Fahrenheit (°F)

WHEN YOU KNOW	MULTIPLY BY	TO FIND
Distance/Length		
centimeters	0.3937	inches
kilometers	0.6214	miles
meters	3.281	feet
meters	39.37	inches
meters	0.0006214	miles
microns	0.000001	meters
millimeters	0.03937	inches

WHEN YOU KNOW	MULTIPLY BY	TO FIND
Capacity/Volume		
cubic kilometers	0.2399	cubic miles
cubic meters	35.31	cubic feet
cubic meters	1.308	cubic yards
cubic meters	8.107×10^{-4}	acre-feet
liters	0.2642	gallons
liters	33.81	fluid ounces

WHEN YOU KNOW	MULTIPLY BY	TO FIND
Area		
hectares (10,000 square meters)	2.471	acres
hectares (10,000 square meters)	107,600	square feet
square meters	10.76	square feet
square kilometers	247.1	acres
square kilometers	0.3861	square miles

WHEN YOU KNOW	MULTIPLY BY	TO FIND
Weight/Mass		
kilograms	2.205	pounds
metric tons	2205	pounds
micrograms (µg)	10^{-6}	grams
milligrams (mg)	10^{-3}	grams
nanograms (ng)	10^{-9}	grams

For Your Reference

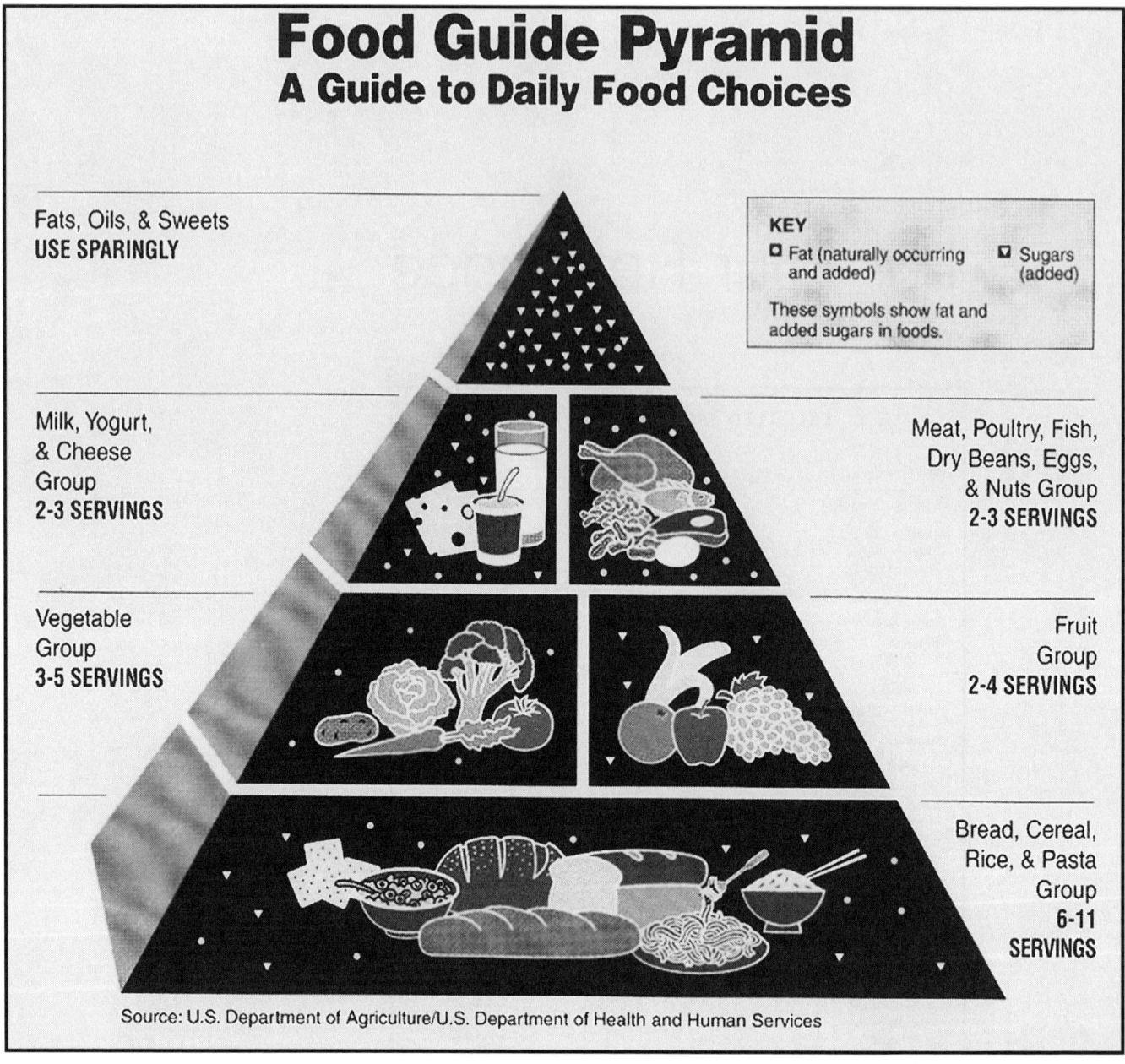

VITAMINS IN FOODS

Vitamin A	liver, carrots, kale, red peppers, milk, spinach, eggs, butter
Vitamin B_6	meat, whole grains, cabbage, peanuts, potatoes, soybeans, liver, fish, beans, milk
Vitamin B_{12}	liver, fish, eggs, milk
Vitamin B_9 (Folate)	tomatoes, spinach, beets, asparagus, potatoes, liver, wheat germ, soybeans, cabbage, whole grains, eggs, milk, meats
Vitamin C	tomatoes, potatoes, most fruits and vegetables
Vitamin D	milk, liver, fatty fish like herring, chicken skin, egg yolks
Vitamin E	most vegetable oils
Vitamin K	broccoli, turnip greens, lettuce, liver, cauliflower, spinach, cabbage, asparagus, Brussels sprouts
Thiamin	meats, whole grains, potatoes, fish, liver, legumes (like beans and peas)
Biotin	liver, soybeans, egg yolks, peanuts, cauliflower, carrots, oatmeal
Riboflavin	eggs, asparagus, liver, milk, fish, meat, whole grains
Pantothenic Acid	liver, fish, eggs, milk, whole grains, meats, legumes (like beans and peas)
Niacin	meats, whole grains, eggs, fish, milk, legumes (like beans and peas)

SOURCE: Adapted from "The Vitamins" by G. F. Coombs Jr.

For Your Reference

RECOMMENDED PYRAMID SERVINGS FOR INDIVIDUALS

Children 2 to 6, most women, some older adults (about 1,600 calories)
- Fats, Oils, & Sweets — Use sparingly
- Milk Group — 2 or 3* servings
- Meat and Beans Group — 5 ounces
- Vegetable Group — 3 servings
- Fruit Group — 2 servings
- Grains Group — 6 servings

Older children, teen girls, active women, most men (about 2,200 calories)
- Fats, Oils, & Sweets — Use sparingly
- Milk Group — 2 or 3* servings
- Meat and Beans Group — 6 ounces
- Vegetable Group — 4 servings
- Fruit Group — 3 servings
- Grains Group — 9 servings

Teen boys, active men (about 2,800 calories)
- Fats, Oils, & Sweets — Use sparingly
- Milk Group — 2 or 3* servings
- Meat and Beans Group — 7 ounces
- Vegetable Group — 5 servings
- Fruit Group — 4 servings
- Grains Group — 11 servings

◆ = 1 serving   ⬠ = 1 ounce

*Older children and teens 9 to 18 and adults over 50 need 3 servings from the Milk group. Others need 2 servings daily.

WHAT COUNTS AS A PYRAMID SERVING?

Grains Group
- 1 slice of bread
- About 1 cup of ready to eat cereal flakes
- ½ cup of cooked cereal, rice, or pasta

Vegetable Group
- 1 cup of raw leafy vegetables
- ½ cup of other vegetables—cooked or raw*
- ¾ cup of vegetable juice

Fruit Group
- 1 medium apple, banana, orange, pear
- ½ cup of chopped, cooked or canned fruit
- ¾ cup of fruit juice

Milk Group
- 1 cup of milk of yogurt
- 1½ ounces of natural cheese (such as Cheddar)
- 2 ounces of processed cheese (such as American)

Meat and Beans Group
The Pyramid recommends 2 to 3 servings for a total of 5 to 7 ounces. The following all count as 1 ounce equivalent:
- 1 ounce of cooked lean meat, poultry, or fish
- ½ cup of cooked, dry beans*
- ½ cup of tofu or 2½-ounce soyburger
- 1 egg
- 2 tablespoons of peanut butter
- ⅓ cup of nuts

*Dry beans, peas, and lentils can be counted as servings in either the Meat and Beans group of the Vegetable group. As a vegetable, ½ cup of cooked, dry beans counts as 1 serving. As a meat substitute, ½ cup of cooked, dry beans counts as 1 ounce of meat.

SOURCE: Adapted from *Home and Garden Bulletin* 267-3. USDA.

BODY MASS INDEX TABLE

	Normal							Overweight						Obese											Extreme Obesity													
BMI	19	20	21	22	23	24	25	26	27	28	29	30	31	32	33	34	35	36	37	38	39	40	41	42	43	44	45	46	47	48	49	50	51	52	53	54
Height (inches)												Body Weight (pounds)																								
58	91	96	100	105	110	115	119	124	129	134	138	143	148	153	158	162	167	172	177	181	186	191	196	201	205	210	215	220	224	229	234	239	244	248	253	258
59	94	99	104	109	114	119	124	128	133	138	143	148	153	158	163	168	173	178	183	188	193	198	203	208	212	217	222	227	232	237	242	247	252	257	262	267
60	97	102	107	112	118	123	128	133	138	143	148	153	158	163	168	174	179	184	189	194	199	204	209	215	220	225	230	235	240	245	250	255	261	266	271	276
61	100	106	111	116	122	127	132	137	143	148	153	158	164	169	174	180	185	190	195	201	206	211	217	222	227	232	238	243	248	254	259	264	269	275	280	285
62	104	109	115	120	126	131	136	142	147	153	158	164	169	175	180	186	191	196	202	207	213	218	224	229	235	240	246	251	256	262	267	273	278	284	289	295
63	107	113	118	124	130	135	141	146	152	158	163	169	175	180	186	191	197	203	208	214	220	225	231	237	242	248	254	259	265	270	278	282	287	293	299	304
64	110	116	122	128	134	140	145	151	157	163	169	174	180	186	192	197	204	209	215	221	227	232	238	244	250	256	262	267	273	279	285	291	296	302	308	314
65	114	120	126	132	138	144	150	156	162	168	174	180	186	192	198	204	210	216	222	228	234	240	246	252	258	264	270	276	282	288	294	300	306	312	318	324
66	118	124	130	136	142	148	155	161	167	173	179	186	192	198	204	210	216	223	229	235	241	247	253	260	266	272	278	284	291	297	303	309	315	322	328	334
67	121	127	134	140	146	153	159	166	172	178	185	191	198	204	211	217	223	230	236	242	249	255	261	268	274	280	287	293	299	306	312	319	325	331	338	344
68	125	131	138	144	151	158	164	171	177	184	190	197	203	210	216	223	230	236	243	249	256	262	269	276	282	289	295	302	308	315	322	328	335	341	348	354
69	128	135	142	149	155	162	169	176	182	189	196	203	209	216	223	230	236	243	250	257	263	270	277	284	291	297	304	311	318	324	331	338	345	351	358	365
70	132	139	146	153	160	167	174	181	188	195	202	209	216	222	229	236	243	250	257	264	271	278	285	292	299	306	313	320	327	334	341	348	355	362	369	376
71	136	143	150	157	165	172	179	186	193	200	208	215	222	229	236	243	250	257	265	272	279	286	293	301	308	315	322	329	338	343	351	358	365	372	379	386
72	140	147	154	162	169	177	184	191	199	206	213	221	228	235	242	250	258	265	272	279	287	294	302	309	316	324	331	338	346	353	361	368	375	383	390	397
73	144	151	159	166	174	182	189	197	204	212	219	227	235	242	250	257	265	272	280	288	295	302	310	318	325	333	340	348	355	363	371	378	386	393	401	408
74	148	155	163	171	179	186	194	202	210	218	225	233	241	249	256	264	272	280	287	295	303	311	319	326	334	342	350	358	365	373	381	389	396	404	412	420
75	152	160	168	176	184	192	200	208	216	224	232	240	248	256	264	272	279	287	295	303	311	319	327	335	343	351	359	367	375	383	381	399	407	415	423	431
76	156	164	172	180	189	197	205	213	221	230	238	246	254	263	271	279	287	295	304	312	320	328	336	344	353	361	369	377	385	394	402	410	418	426	435	443

SOURCE: Adapted from *Clinical Guidelines on the Identification, Evaluation, and Treatment of Overweight and Obesity in Adults: The Evidence Report.*

Contributors

Karen Ansel
Walnut Creek, California

Katherine Beals
Ball State University
Muncie, Indiana

Mindy Benedict
Ponte Vedra Beach, Florida

Frances Berg
Healthy Weight Network and University of North Dakota School of Medicine
Hellinger, North Dakota

Linda B. Bobroff
University of Florida
Gainesville, Florida

Leslie Bonci
University of Pittsburgh Medical Center
Pittsburgh, Pennsylvania

Susan T. Borra
International Food Information Council Foundation
Washington, DC

Karen Bryla
University of Kentucky
Lexington, Kentucky

Lori Keeling Buhi
Bryan-College Station Community Health Center
Bryan, Texas

Slande Celeste
University of Florida
Gainesville, Florida

Nilesh Chatterjee
Texas A&M University
College Station, Texas

Sara Chelland
Department of Nutrition, Food and Exercise Science
Tallahassee, Florida

Catherine Christie
University of North Florida
Jacksonville, Florida

Sonja Connor
Portland, Oregon

William Connor
Oregon Health Sciences University
Portland, Oregon

Marilyn Dahl
Preferred Nutrition Services
Jacksonville Beach, Florida

Raju Das
University of Dundee
Dundee, UK

Ruth DeBusk
Private Practice
Tallahassee, Florida

Sharon Doughten
Cuyahoga Community College
Cleveland, Ohio

Karen Drummond
Yardley, Pennsylvania

M. Cristina Flaminiano Garces
University of North Carolina at Chapel Hill

Beth Fontenot
McNeese State University
Lake Charles, Louisiana

John P. Foreyt
Baylor College of Medicine
Houston, Texas

Mohammed Forouzesh
California State University at Long Beach
Long Beach, California

Marion J. Franz
Nutrition Concepts by Franz, Inc.
Minneapolis, Minnesota

Marjorie Freedman
San Jose, California

Keri M. Gans
New York, New York

Chandak Ghosh
Harvard Medical School
Boston, Massachusetts

Gita C. Gidwani
Johns Hopkins University
Baltimore, Maryland

Emil Ginter
Institute of Preventive and Clinical Medicine
Bratislava, Slovak Republic

Diane Golzynski
California State University
Fresno, California

Leslene E. Gordon
Pasco County Health Department Nutrition Division
New Port Ritchey, Florida

Marcus Harding
International Medical Volunteers Association
Woodville, Massachusetts

Karen Hare
Nutrition Services, Inc.
Fort Collins, Colorado

Beth Hensleigh
Texas A&M University
College Station, Texas

Kirsten Herbes
University of Florida
Gainesville, Florida

Susan Himburg
Florida International University
Miami, Florida

Lenore S. Hodges
Florida Hospital
Orlando, Florida

Steve Hohman
Ohio University
Athens, Ohio

Elissa M. Howard-Barr
Coastal Carolina University
Conway, South Carolina

Delores C. S. James
University of Florida
Gainesville, Florida

Sunitha Jasti
University of North Carolina,
Chapel Hill, North Carolina

Warren B. Karp
The Medical College of Georgia
Augusta, Georgia

xxi

Susan Kim
Williams College
Williamstown, Massachusetts

Seema Pania Kumar
Alexandria Primary Care Associates
Alexandria, Virginia

M. Elizabeth Kunkel
Clemson University
Clemson, South Carolina

Julie Lager
Texas A&M University
College Station, Texas

Jens Levy
University of North Carolina
Chapel Hill, North Carolina

Kheng Lim
University of Medicine and Dentistry of New Jersey
Camden, New Jersey

Nadia Lugo
University of Florida
Gainesville, Florida

Teresa Lyles
University of Florida
Gainesville, Florida

Carole Mackey
Agency for Health Care Administration
St. Petersburg, Florida

Amy N. Marlow
New York, New York

Cindy Martin
Texas A&M University
College Station, Texas

Toni Martin
Duval County Health Department
Jacksonville, Florida

Kiran Misra
Texas A&M University
College Station, Texas

Ranjita Misra
San Diego State University
San Diego, California

Braxton D. Mitchell
University of Maryland
Baltimore, Maryland

Susan Mitchell
Practicalories, Inc.
Winter Park, Florida

Robert J. Moffatt
Florida State University
Tallahassee, Florida

Melissa Morris
University of Florida
Gainesville, Florida

Kweethai C. Neill
University of North Texas
Denton, Texas

Laura Nelson
Texas A&M University
College Station, Texas

Virginia Noland
University of Florida
Gainesville, Florida

Neelima Pania
New York University Hospital
New York, New York

Mary Parke
Duval County Health Department, UIC and Nutrition Program
Jacksonville, Florida

Isabel Parraga
Case Western Reserve University
Cleveland, Ohio

Gita Patel
Nutrition Consultant
Etna, New Hampshire

Nadine Pazder
Morton Plant Hospital
Clearwater, Florida

Judy E. Perkin
University of North Florida
Jacksonville, Florida

Jeffrey Radecki
Robert Wood Johnson Medical School
Piscataway, New Jersey

Sheah Rarback
University of Miami School Medicine
Miami, Florida

Catherine Rasberry
Texas A&M University
College Station, Texas

Barbara L. Rice
Enterprise Advisory Services, Inc.
Houston, Texas

Carlos Robles
University of the Virgin Islands

Judy Rodriguez
University of North Florida
Jacksonville, Florida

Kim Schenck
Colorado Springs, Colorado

Claire D. Schmelzer
Virginia Polytechnic Institute and State University
Blacksburg, Virginia
University of Kentucky
Lexington, Kentucky

Louise Schneider
Lorna Linda University
Lorna Linda, California

Jessica Schulman
University of Florida
Gainesville, Florida

Kyle Shadix
Art Institute of New York City

Jackie Shank
Southeast Nutrition Consultants
St. Augustine, Florida

Heidi J. Silver
National Policy and Resource Center on Nutrition and Aging
Miami, Florida

Donna Staton
International Medical Volunteers Association

Tanya Sterling
Duval County Health Department
Jacksonville, Florida

Milton Stokes
New York, New York

Lisa A. Sutherland
University of North Carolina
Chapel Hill, North Carolina

Marie Boyle Struble
College of Saint Elizabeth
Morristown, New Jersey

D. Michelle Swords
Gainesville, Florida

Patricia Thomas
San Antonio, Texas

Delores Truesdell
Florida State University
Tallahassee, Florida

Katherine Tucker
USDA/HNRCA at Tufts University
Boston, Massachusetts

Simin Vaghefi
University of North Florida
Jacksonville, Florida

Pauline Vickery
Suwannee River Area Health Education Center

Ruth Waibel
Ohio University
Athens, Ohio

Daphne C. Watkins
Texas A&M University
College Station, Texas

Sally Weerts
University of North Florida
Jacksonville, Florida

Paulette Weir
Elmont, New York

Katherine Will
Ohio University
Athens, Ohio

Heidi Williams
Gainesville, Florida

Illnesses, Food-Borne

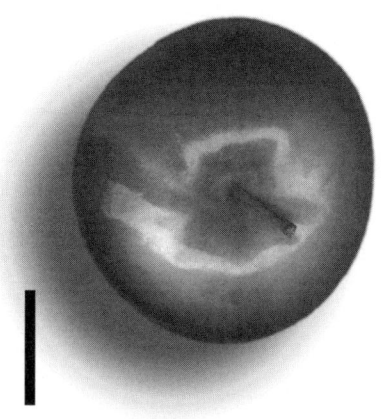

Food-borne illness, often called **food poisoning**, is caused by **pathogens** or certain chemicals present in ingested food. **Bacteria, viruses**, molds, worms, and protozoa that cause disease are all pathogens, though there are also harmless and beneficial bacteria that are used to make yogurt and cheese. Some chemicals that cause food-borne illness are natural components of foods, while others may be accidentally added during production and processing, either through carelessness or pollution. The main causes of food-borne illness are bacterial (66%), chemical (26%), viral (4%) and **parasitic** (4%).

food poisoning: illness caused by consumption of spoiled food, usually containing bacteria

pathogen: organism that causes disease

bacteria: single-celled organisms without nuclei, some of which are infectious

virus: noncellular infectious agent that requires a host cell to reproduce

parasitic: feeding off another organism

toxins: poison

Intoxication and Infection

The two most common types of food-borne illness are intoxication and infection. Intoxication occurs when **toxins** produced by the pathogen cause food poisoning. Infection is caused by the ingestion of food containing pathogens. Some people develop symptoms after ingesting a pathogen, while others never know that they are suffering from food-borne illness. The people that are most at risk are those with compromised immune systems. For these individuals, an incident of food-borne illness can be life threatening. Sanitation procedures, such as hand washing, separating at-risk foods (such as raw meat) from fresh vegetables, cooking foods, and chilling prepared foods, can help prevent food poisoning.

Causes

The following organisms can cause food-borne illness: *Campylobacter jejuni*, *Clostridium botulinum*, *Clostridium perfringens*, *Cyclospora cayetanensis*, **Escherichia coli**, (*E. coli* 0157:H7), *Listeria monocytogenes*, *Salmonella*, *Shigella*, and *Staphylococcus aureus*. *Campylobacter jejuni* is caused by the ingestion of live bacteria and can be transmitted to humans via unpasteurized milk, contaminated water, and raw or undercooked meats, poultry, and shellfish. *Clostridium botulinum*, which causes **botulism**, is the most deadly of all food pathogens. It is transmitted by improperly canned food, whether it is home-canned or commercially prepared. *Clostridium perfringens* is transmitted by eating heavily contaminated food, and it tends to infect those who eat food that has been left standing on buffets or steam tables for long periods. Feces-contaminated food or water transmits *Cyclospora cayetanensis*. Foods such

Escherichia coli: common bacterium found in human large intestine

botulism: poisoning from the bacterium Clostridium botulinum

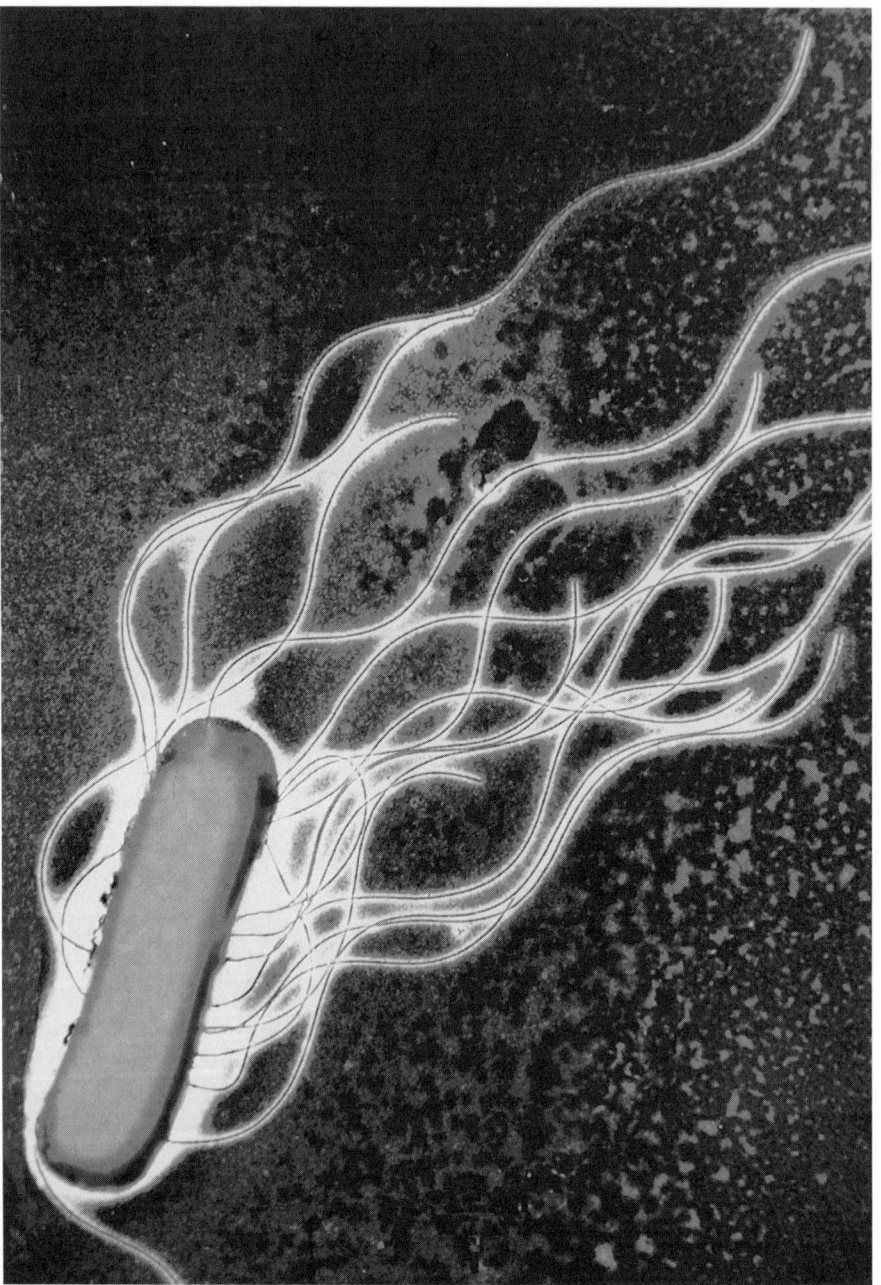

A transmission electron micrograph (TEM) shows a Salmonella sp. bacterium. The bacterium is transmitted through contact with a carrier or by ingestion of contaminated meat or dairy products. [USDA/Science Source/Photo Researchers, Inc. Reproduced by permission.]

as undercooked hamburger or ground poultry and unpasteurized milk or apple juice can transmit *E. coli* 0157:H7. *Listeria monocytogenes* can be transmitted to humans via unpasteurized dairy foods, such as milk, soft cheeses, and ice creams, and via leafy vegetables and processed meats. *Salmonella* is transmitted by eating contaminated food or by contact with a carrier (a human or animal capable of transmitting infectious organisms). Salmonella poisoning may also occur through cross-contamination of uncontaminated foods that have come into contact with uncooked foods. This may occur when one uses the same cutting board to cut both raw chicken and fresh vegetables.

Shigella is a contamination of food by infected food handlers; it is primarily transmitted in cold salads such as tuna, chicken, or potato salad.

Staphylococcus aureus is transmitted by carriers and by eating foods that contain the toxin.

Other substances that cause food poisoning include: mold, *Trichinella spiralis*, and dysentery. Mold is a type of fungus. Some molds produce a **mycotoxin** called aflatoxin that can develop in spoiled peanuts and peanut butter, soybeans, grains, nuts, and spices. *Trichinella spiralis* is a parasitic worm that can be present in undercooked pork. Dysentery is a disease caused by **microorganisms** (protozoa) that are introduced to food by carriers or contaminated water.

Symptoms

Symptoms of food-borne illness often resemble intestinal flu, and they may last a few hours or several days. Serious complications may include bloody diarrhea, severe abdominal cramps, severe illness, or death. Typical symptoms include diarrhea, vomiting, abdominal cramps, headaches, **nausea**, dry mouth, double vision, difficulty swallowing, and flu-like symptoms (such as fever, chills, and backache). Older adults, pregnant women, infants, and people with compromised immune systems (such as those with **diabetes**, AIDS, or **cancer**) may face greater risks and have a higher **incidence** of food-borne illness.

Prevention

It is important to prevent food-borne illness by cleaning, separating, cooking, and chilling foods appropriately. Hands and surface areas should be cleaned with hot soapy water, and food handlers must practice good personal **hygiene** and sanitary food preparation. Raw fruits and vegetables should be washed thoroughly, and unpasteurized milk, bulging cans, and foods showing signs of mold should always be avoided. In order to avoid cross-contamination, raw foods should be kept separate from cooked foods.

Hot foods should be kept hot (at or above 140 degrees Fahrenheit), and cold foods cold (at or below 40 degrees Fahrenheit). Leftovers should be heated to at least 165 degrees before serving.

Ground meats should be cooked at or above 165 degrees. Cooking to proper temperatures and time will kill harmful bacteria that cause food-borne illness. Bacteria multiply rapidly between 40 and 140 degrees. However, the danger zone is between 60 and 125 degrees Fahrenheit. Temperatures in this zone allow rapid growth of bacteria and production of toxins by some bacteria. Therefore, foods should be refrigerated, since cold temperatures keep most harmful bacteria from growing and multiplying. It is recommended that refrigerators be kept between 34 and 38 degrees, while freezers should be kept at 0 degrees. Most food-borne illnesses occur because of the ignorance or carelessness of people who handle food, and such illnesses can be easily prevented.

Treatment

Persons suffering from a food-borne illness should consult a physician if the following symptoms persist for more than two or three days: a fever of 102 degrees or higher, presence of blood in the stool, or **dehydration** (as indicated by dizziness upon standing). Medical help should also be sought if

---

Fight Disease: Wash Your Hands

Amid the technological marvels of the twenty-first century, health care specialists agree that the single most effective way to prevent the transmission of disease is by washing your hands. Unwashed hands are thought to be responsible for one-quarter of food-borne illnesses, including *E. coli* and salmonella, and are a major means of transmission for SARS, meningitis, hepatitis, and the common cold. Studies have shown that infection rates in schools and day-care centers plummet after the launch of hand-washing campaigns. The most important times to wash your hands are after using the toilet or handling a diaper, handling raw food such as chicken, sneezing or coughing into your hand, or being out in public. While anitbacterial soaps are considered no more effective than regular soaps, alcohol gels in "hand sanitizers" have received high praise for their ability to eliminate germs.

—*Paula Kepos*

---

mycotoxin: poison produced by a fungus

microorganisms: bacteria and protists; single-celled organisms

nausea: unpleasant sensation in the gut that precedes vomiting

diabetes: inability to regulate level of sugar in the blood

cancer: uncontrolled cell growth

incidence: number of new cases reported each year

hygiene: cleanliness

dehydration: loss of water

botulism is suspected. Dehydration caused by diarrhea and vomiting should be treated promptly with increased fluid intake or oral rehydration solutions. Sports beverages with **electrolytes** may be helpful. Bed rest can speed recovery, and while ill, any food consumed should be clean, easy to digest, and consumed in small amounts.

The treating physician should notify the local health department, who will then notify the Centers for Disease Control and Prevention (CDC). To minimize risks for food poisoning to others, the local health department should be contacted if the food was consumed at a large gathering; if the food came from a restaurant, deli, vendor, or kitchen that serves a large number of people, or if the food was a commercial product. SEE ALSO FOOD SAFETY; ORGANISMS, FOOD-BORNE.

Tanya Sterling
Toni Martin

electrolyte: salt dissolved in fluid

Bibliography

Mahan, L. Kathleen, and Escott-Stump, Sylvia (2000). *Krause's Food, Nutrition, and Diet Therapy*, 10th edition. Philadelphia, PA: W. B. Saunders.

Townsend, Carolyn E., and Roth, Ruth A. (2000). *Nutrition and Diet Therapy*, 7th edition. Albany, NY: Delmar.

Internet Resources

Clemson Extension, Home and Garden Information Center. "Foodborne Illness: Prevention Strategies." Available from <http://hgic.clemson.edu/factsheets/HGIC3620.htm>

HIVpositive.com. "Foodborne Illness." Available from <http://www.hivpositive.com/f-Nutrition/Foodborne/Foodill.html>

Immune System

immune system: the set of organs and cells, including white blood cells, that protect the body from infection

white blood cell: immune system cell that fights infection

mucosa: moist exchange surface within the body

bacteria: single-celled organisms without nuclei, some of which are infectious

enzyme: protein responsible for carrying out reactions in a cell

protein: complex molecule composed of amino acids that performs vital functions in the cell; necessary part of the diet

stress: heightened state of nervousness or unease

malnutrition: chronic lack of sufficient nutrients to maintain health

nutrition: the maintenance of health through proper eating, or the study of same

calorie: unit of food energy

antioxidant: substance that prevents oxidation, a damaging reaction with oxygen

metabolism: the sum total of reactions in a cell or an organism

metabolize: processing of a nutrient

carbohydrate: food molecule made of carbon, hydrogen, and oxygen, including sugars and starches

protein: complex molecule composed of amino acids that performs vital functions in the cell; necessary part of the diet

The **immune system** is made up of cells, tissues, organs, and processes that identify a substance as abnormal or foreign and prevent it from harming the body. Primary defenses include the **white blood cells**, but skin, **mucosa**, normal **bacteria**, **enzymes**, and **proteins** also provide protection. During times of **stress** and **malnutrition**, immune function may be decreased, meaning that susceptibility to illness is increased. Proper **nutrition**, including adequate protein, **calories**, and **antioxidants** (such as vitamin C, vitamin E, and beta-carotene, which are all found in fruits and vegetables) may help to improve immune response and reduce the risk of illness. SEE ALSO INFECTION.

Catherine Christie

Bibliography

Shils, Maurice, et al. (1999). *Modern Nutrition in Health and Disease*, 9th edition. Baltimore, MD: Williams & Wilkins.

Inborn Errors of Metabolism

Inborn errors of **metabolism** are inherited disorders in which the body cannot **metabolize** the components of food (**carbohydrates, proteins,** and

Inborn Errors of Metabolism

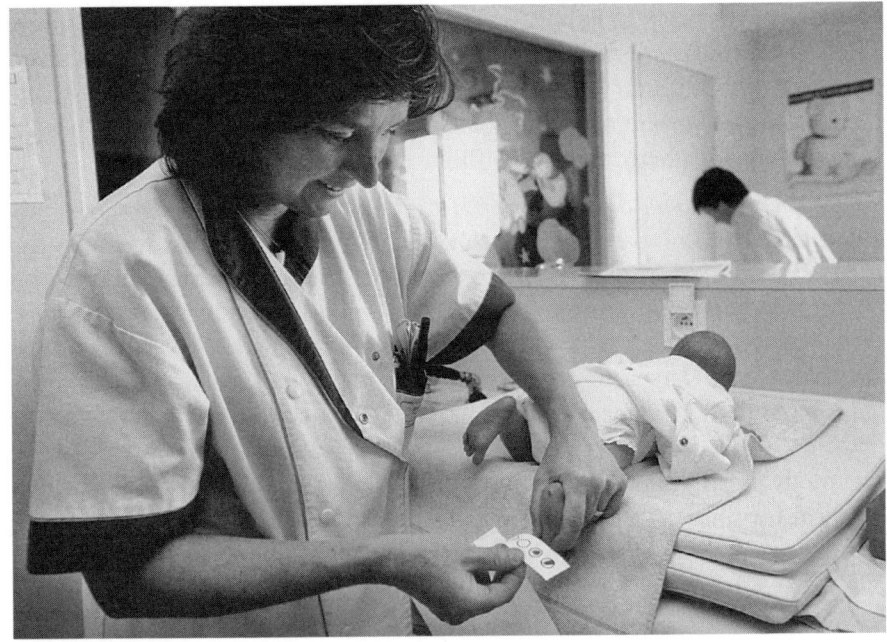

The Guthrie test, given to newborns, helps doctors diagnose some inborn errors of metabolism before they cause permanent damage. The test requires a small sample of blood, usually taken from the heel. [Garo/Photo Researchers, Inc. Reproduced by permission.]

fats). Metabolism is the **biochemical** process that changes food components into **energy** and other required **molecules**. These disorders may be caused by the altered activity of essential **enzymes**, deficiencies of the substances that activate the enzymes, or faulty transport compounds. **Metabolic** disorders can be devastating if appropriate treatment is not initiated promptly and monitored frequently.

Inborn errors of metabolism often require **diet** changes, with the type and extent of the changes dependant on the specific metabolic disorder. The particular enzyme absence or inactivity for each inborn error of metabolism dictates which components are restricted and which are supplemented. Registered dietitians and physicians can help an individual assess the diet changes needed for each disease. The goals of **nutrition** therapy are to correct the metabolic imbalance and promote growth and **development** by providing adequate nutrition, while also restricting (or supplementing) one or more **nutrients** or dietary components. Additional goals in some disorders include reducing the risk of brain damage, other organ damage, episodes of metabolic crisis and coma, and even death. These restrictions and supplementations are specific for each disorder, and they may include the restriction of total fats, simple sugars, or total carbohydrates.

Listed below are several of the metabolic disorders that respond to nutrition therapy. The appropriate dietary restrictions and modifications that are necessary for treatment are also listed.

Disorders of Amino Acid Metabolism

Phenylketonuria (PKU) is the most common disorder of amino acid metabolism. In this disorder the body cannot use the amino acid phenylalanine normally, and excess amounts build up in the blood. If untreated, PKU can cause mental retardation, seizures, behavior problems, and **eczema**. With treatment, persons with PKU have normal development and intelligence. The treatment for PKU consists of a special phenylalanine-restricted diet

biochemical: related to chemical processes within cells

energy: technically, the ability to perform work; the content of a substance that allows it to be useful as a fuel

molecule: combination of atoms that form stable particles

enzyme: protein responsible for carrying out reactions in a cell

metabolic: related to processing of nutrients and building of necessary molecules within the cell

diet: the total daily food intake, or the types of foods eaten

nutrition: the maintenance of health through proper eating, or the study of same

development: the process of change by which an organism becomes more complex

nutrient: dietary substance necessary for health

phenylketonuria: inherited disease marked by the inability to process the amino acid phenylalanine, causing mental retardation

eczema: skin disease causing itching and flaking

5

designed to maintain blood phenylalanine levels within an acceptable range. Medical formulas and foods, which do not contain phenylalanine, are used to provide the necessary intake of protein and other nutrients. Foods containing natural protein are prescribed in limited amounts to meet the body's requirement for phenylalanine, without providing too much.

Maple syrup urine disease (MSUD) is a disorder in which the body is unable to use the amino acids isoleucine, leucine, and valine in a normal way. Excessive amounts of these amino acids and their **metabolites** will build up in the blood and spill into the urine and perspiration, giving them the odor of maple syrup (which is how this disorder got its name). An untreated infant with MSUD may have some or all of the following symptoms: difficulty breathing, sleepiness, vomiting, irregular muscle movement, seizures, or coma, and the disease can cause death. Basic treatment involves restricting foods and infant formula that contain leucine, isoleucine, and valine. Medical formulas and foods, which contain very small amounts of leucine, isoleucine, and valine, are used to provide the necessary intake of protein and other nutrients.

metabolite: the product of metabolism, or nutrient processing within the cell

Disorders of Carbohydrate Metabolism

Galactosemia is a disorder in which the body cannot break down the sugar called galactose. Galactose can be found in food, and the body can break down lactose (milk sugar) to galactose and **glucose**. The body uses glucose for energy. People with galactosemia lack the enzyme to break down galactose, so it builds up and becomes toxic. In reaction to this buildup of galactose the body makes some abnormal chemicals. The buildup of galactose and these chemicals can cause liver damage, kidney failure, stunted growth, mental retardation, and **cataracts** in the eyes.

glucose: a simple sugar; the most commonly used fuel in cells

cataract: clouding of the lens of the eye

If not treated, galactosemia can cause death. Over time, children and young adults with galactosemia can have problems with speech, language, hearing, stunted growth, and certain learning disabilities. Children who do not follow a strict diet have an increased risk of having one or more of the problems listed above. Even when a strict diet is followed, some children do not do as well as others. Most girls with galactosemia have ovarian failure. The treatment for galactosemia is to restrict galactose and lactose from the diet for life. Since galactose is a part of lactose, all milk and all foods that contain milk must be eliminated from the diet, including foods that contain small amounts of milk products such as whey and casein. In addition, organ meats should not be eaten because they contain stored galactose.

Glycogen storage diseases require different treatments depending on the specific enzyme alteration. The most common type of glycogen storage disease is classified as type 1A. In this disorder the body is missing the enzyme that coverts the storage form of sugar (glycogen) into energy (glucose). If food is not eaten for two to four hours, blood glucose levels drop to a low level, leading to serious health problems such as seizures, poor growth, enlarged liver, high levels of some fats circulating in the blood, and high levels of **uric** and lactic acids in the blood. Dietary management of GSD-1A eliminates table sugar (sucrose) and fruit sugar (fructose) and limits milk sugar (lactose), as the body cannot use some sugars in these foods. Frequent meals and snacks that are high in complex carbohydrates are recommended. In addition, often supplements of uncooked cornstarch are often eaten

uric: from urine

between meals to keep blood sugar levels stable. Eating a diet that prevents low blood sugar will promote normal growth, decrease liver enlargement, and the high blood levels of uric and lactic acids.

Disorders of fatty acid metabolism occur when the body is not able to break down **fat** to use as energy. The body's main source of energy is glucose, but when the body runs out of glucose, fats are used for energy. If untreated, these disorders can lead to serious complications affecting the liver, heart, eyes, and muscles. Treatment includes altering the kind and the amount of fat in the diet and frequent feedings of carbohydrate-containing foods.

Urea cycle disorders are inherited disorders of **nitrogen** metabolism. When protein is digested it breaks down into amino acids, and nitrogen is found in all the amino acids. Those who have these disorders cannot use nitrogen in a normal way. Dietary treatment for these disorders is to provide only the amount of protein that the body can safely use. The diet consists mostly of fruits, grains, and vegetables that contain low amounts of protein and, therefore, low amounts of nitrogen.

There are more than nineteen metabolic disorders that respond to nutrition therapy. The role of proper nutrition in the treatment of these disorders is crucial. Because these disorders are rare and require careful monitoring, affected individuals are best served by clinics specializing in metabolic disorders. SEE ALSO PHENYLKETONURIA (PKU).

Patricia D. Thomas

fat: type of food molecule rich in carbon and hydrogen, with high energy content

nitrogen: essential element for plant growth

Bibliography

Acosta, P. B., and Yannicelli, S. (1993). "Energy and Protein Requirements of Infants and Children with Inherited Metabolic Disorders." *Metabolic Currents* 6:1–8.

Acosta, P. B., and Yannicelli, S. (2001). *Ross Metabolic Formula System: Nutrition Support Protocols*, 4th edition. Columbus, OH: Ross Laboratories.

Scriver, C. R.; Beaudet, A. L.; Sly, W. S.; and Valle, D., eds. (2001). *The Metabolic and Molecular Bases of Inherited Disease*, 8th edition. New York: McGraw-Hill.

Infant Mortality Rate

The infant mortality rate is the number of infant deaths (during the first twelve months of life) per 1,000 live births. Before birth, a fetus faces major health risks from **undernutrition** during pregnancy, particularly from inadequate, absent, or delayed prenatal care. A mother's **nutritional deficiencies** may result in a premature birth, which substantially increases the likelihood of infant death.

A poor **diet** inhibits development at critical stages in an infant's life, sometimes causing irreversible effects. This can be the case when a mother stops breastfeeding her child too soon. **Calories, protein, calcium, iron,** and **zinc** are especially crucial for developing infants.

High infant mortality rates are often associated with poverty and poor access to health care. Some international issues include extreme imbalances in the food–population ratio in different regions of a country, rapid depletion of natural resources, cultural attitudes towards certain foods, and AIDS (acquired immunodeficiency syndrome). SEE ALSO MATERNAL MORTALITY RATE; PREGNANCY.

Kim Schenck

undernutrition: food intake too low to maintain adequate energy expenditure without weight loss

nutritional deficiency: lack of adequate nutrients in the diet

diet: the total daily food intake, or the types of foods eaten

calorie: unit of food energy

protein: complex molecule composed of amino acids that performs vital functions in the cell; necessary part of the diet

calcium: mineral essential for bones and teeth

iron: nutrient needed for red blood cell formation

zinc: mineral necessary for many enzyme processes

Bibliography

Wardlaw, Gordon; Hampl, Jeffrey; and DiSilvestro, Robert (2004). *Perspectives in Nutrition.* New York: McGraw-Hill.

Infant Nutrition

The first year of life is a period of very rapid growth. An infant's birth weight doubles after about five months and triples by the first birthday, by which time the infant's length increases by half. Adequate and appropriate **nutrition** is essential during this period, for infants that do not receive sufficient **calories**, **vitamins**, and **minerals** will not reach their expected growth.

Nutrient Requirements

An infant's requirement for calories is determined by size, rate of growth, activity, and **energy** needed for **metabolic** activities. Calorie needs per pound of body weight are higher during the first year of life than at any other time. Since there is variation among infants, a range of recommended calorie intakes have been developed. For the first four to six months of life, breast or formula feeding can provide sufficient calories. Measuring weight and length, and plotting it on a standardized growth grid, can determine the adequacy of an infant's calorie intake.

The calories in an infant's **diet** are provided by **protein**, **fat**, and **carbohydrates**. Protein is a basic part of every cell. Of the protein requirement, 50 percent is used for growth in the first two months of life, a figure that declines to 11 percent by two to three years of age. Fat provides 40 to 50 percent of the calories supplied during infancy and is a source of **essential fatty acids**. Carbohydrates, primarily lactose, are the principal source of dietary energy. Water requirements for the first six months are met when adequate amounts of breast milk or infant formula are consumed.

Breast milk from a well-nourished mother will supply adequate amounts of most vitamins and minerals, as will an **iron-fortified** formula. **Vitamin D** is also recommended for the breastfed infant, particularly infants who live in northern urban areas who are dark-skinned, who are kept covered due to cultural practices, or whose mothers have an inadequate intake of vitamin D. In places where the water supply is severely low in fluoride (less than 3 parts per million), fluoride supplementation might be considered for breastfed infants over six months of age.

Breastfeeding

All professional and international health organizations are in agreement that breastfeeding is the recommended method of infant feeding. Although breastfeeding is clearly essential for infants born in less industrialized countries, benefits are substantial in industrialized countries as well. In less industrialized countries, breastfeeding reduces infant mortality and **morbidity**.

Breast milk is nutritionally superior to formula, and it contains **antibodies** that reduce the risk of infection for the newborn baby. Breastfed infants have a decreased **incidence** of respiratory, **gastrointestinal**, and ear infections. The cost of feeding the infant is reduced, and the very nature of

---

nutrition: the maintenance of health through proper eating, or the study of same

calorie: unit of food energy

vitamin: necessary complex nutrient used to aid enzymes or other metabolic processes in the cell

mineral: an inorganic (non-carbon-containing) element, ion or compound

energy: technically, the ability to perform work; the content of a substance that allows it to be useful as a fuel

metabolic: related to processing of nutrients and building of necessary molecules within the cell

diet: the total daily food intake, or the types of foods eaten

protein: complex molecule composed of amino acids that performs vital functions in the cell; necessary part of the diet

fat: type of food molecule rich in carbon and hydrogen, with high energy content

carbohydrate: food molecule made of carbon, hydrogen, and oxygen, including sugars and starches

essential fatty acids: particular molecules made of carbon, hydrogen, and oxygen that the human body must have but cannot make itself

iron: nutrient needed for red blood cell formation

fortified: altered by addition of vitamins or minerals

vitamin D: nutrient needed for calcium uptake and therefore proper bone formation

morbidity: illness or accident

antibody: immune system protein that protects against infection

incidence: number of new cases reported each year

gastrointestinal: related to the stomach and intestines

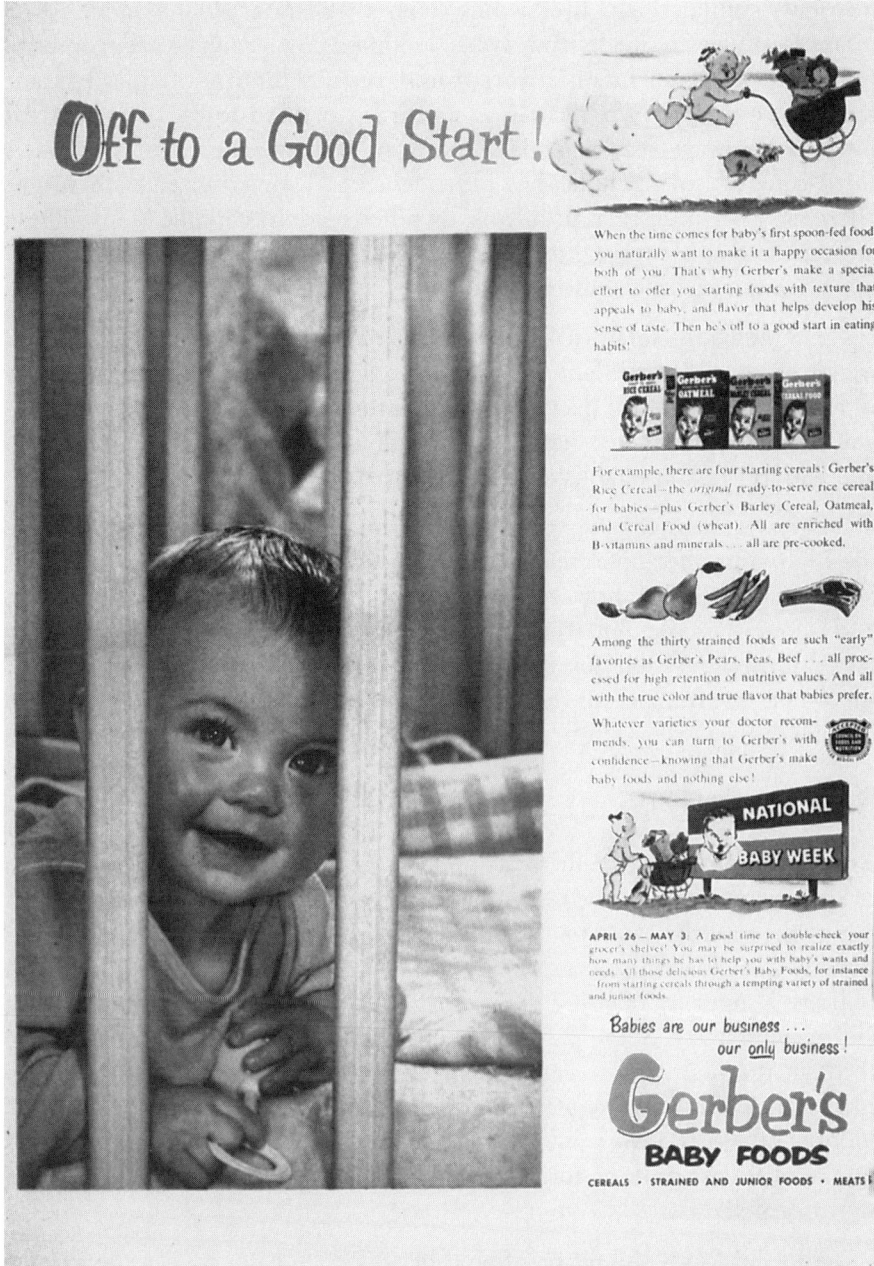

A proper diet can lower the risk of infant disease and mortality. Between four and six months of age, infants are ready for semi-solid foods. Such foods can be purchased, such as the Gerber's product advertised here, or made at home from simple ingredients such as rice, fresh vegetables and fruits, nuts, and juice.
[John H. Hartman Center for Sales, Advertising and Marketing History, Duke University. Reproduced by permission.]

breastfeeding supports the mother-infant bond. There is also evidence that breastfed infants develop fewer **allergies**, and when tested at eighteen months of age they score higher on intelligence tests.

It is not advisable for an infant to receive whole cow's milk before one year of age. Feeding cow's milk before one year has been associated with the development of iron deficiency. If breastfeeding is discontinued before one year of age, an iron-fortified, commercially prepared infant formula is recommended.

Formula Feeding

The governments of most countries have developed nutrient standards for commercial infant formulas. These guidelines ensure that a formula has

allergy: immune system reaction against substances that are otherwise harmless

nutritional requirements: the set of substances needed in the diet to maintain health

elemental: made from predigested nutrients

nutrients similar to the breast milk from a well-nourished woman. Most infant formulas are made from either modified cow's milk or soy, and both types will meet an infant's **nutritional requirements**. Standard infant formula comes in both a low-iron and iron-fortified form. Iron-fortified formula is always recommended, except in very specific circumstances. A third category of formulas has been developed for children with severe allergies, gastrointestinal problems, or other medical complications. These are classified as **elemental** formulas, and are prescribed when an infant cannot tolerate any other type of formula.

The newborn infant will feed between eight to twelve times a day. As weight is gained, the infant will take more at each feeding and the number of feedings per day will decrease. An infant who is receiving adequate feeds will have at least six wet diapers a day, will appear satisfied after a feeding, and will follow the established growth curve.

In less industrialized countries, or in situations where formula costs are too high, infant formulas made from evaporated milk have been used. This is not recommended, however, since an infant would require more vitamin and mineral supplementation, and there is also a risk of incorrectly prepared formula. When any type of formula is prepared, it is essential that the water, bottles, and all the equipment used are sanitized, that hands are washed during preparation, and that the formula is kept refrigerated.

Beikost (Solid Food)

An infant is physically ready for semi-solid foods between four to six months of age. Before this age the reflex that allows babies to suckle will push foods out of the mouth. At around six months infants begin to sit independently, draw in their lower lip as a spoon is removed from the mouth, and they can indicate hunger by opening the mouth—and refusal by closing the mouth and turning away. Some parents believe that solid foods help a baby sleep through the night. However, sleeping through the night is not related to food, but is a developmental milestone that occurs between one to three months of age. To eat solid foods at an early age might reduce an infant's intake of breast milk or formula, which could have a negative impact on nutritional status.

All solid foods should be offered by spoon, not put in a bottle. A new food might initially be rejected, but with repeated offerings acceptance increases. Baby rice cereal is often recommended as the first food for an infant, since it rarely provokes allergic reactions and is iron fortified. The cereal should be mixed with breast milk or formula until it has a semi-liquid consistency. The next foods offered can be single strained fruits, strained vegetables, and at seven to eight months, strained meats. New foods are added one at a time, for two to three days, while the infant is watched for a negative reaction. Reactions would include rashes, vomiting, or diarrhea. Commercially prepared baby foods are convenient, and the first-stage foods are prepared without added sugar and starches. Home-prepared baby foods can be more economical, however.

The American Dental Association recommends juice be given to an infant with a cup rather than a bottle. This decreases the risk of both baby bottle tooth decay and overfeeding. Baby bottle tooth decay, also known as nursing bottle mouth syndrome, is a disorder of extreme dental decay of the upper teeth, caused by infants or toddlers falling asleep while sucking a bottle filled with juice, milk, or any other fermentable liquid.

Self-Feeding

Self-feeding begins when an infant is able to sit up straight, grasp food with the hands or fingertips, and move the food from the hands to the mouth. This usually develops between six to seven months of age. Suitable foods are arrowroot biscuits, teething biscuits, and small pieces of soft fruit or soft cooked vegetables. To prevent choking when an infant is self-feeding, an adult caretaker should always be present.

Between seven and eight months, infants are able to move their shoulders and arms while seated. A more mature up-and-down chewing pattern is developing at this time, making it an appropriate time to begin introducing soft, mashed table foods. Well-cooked vegetables and meats and soft mashed fruits are usually well tolerated. Between ten and twelve months of age infants are becoming more aware of what others are eating, and they will want to imitate other people's eating habits. At this age it is appropriate to offer soft, chopped table foods in a meal pattern similar to the rest of the family. The one year old begins to clumsily self-feed with a spoon and sip from a cup. All these self-feeding skills will be continually refined during the toddler years.

Infancy is a time of tremendous growth that can be best met through breastfeeding. If this is not possible, commercial, iron-fortified infant formulas will provide adequate nutrition. Semi-solid foods are added to prepare the infant for more mature chewing and feeding. Throughout the first year it is important for parents to learn to recognize and accept an infant's cues regarding their feelings of hunger and fullness. Responsiveness to an infant's appetite will prevent overfeeding. Observing an infant's readiness to chew, and providing appropriate foods, will help them develop self-feeding skills and independent eating. SEE ALSO BABY BOTTLE TOOTH DECAY; BEIKOST; BREASTFEEDING.

Sheah Rarback

Bibliography

American Dietetic Association (1997). "Promotion of Breastfeeding." Journal of the American Dietetic Association 97:662–666.

Duyff, Roberta L. (1996). *The American Dietetic Association's Complete Food and Nutrition Guide.* Minneapolis, MN: Chronimed.

Fomon, Samuel J. (2001). "Feeding Normal Infants: Rationale for Recommendations." *Journal of the American Dietetic Association* 101:1002–1005.

Mitchell, Mary K. (1997). *Nutrition across the Life Span.* New York: W. B. Saunders.

Pipes, Peggy L., and Trahms, Cristine M. (1993). *Nutrition in Infancy and Childhood.* St. Louis, MO: Mosby.

Queen Samour, Patricia M.; King Helm, Kathy; and Lang, Carol E. (1993). *Handbook of Pediatric Nutrition*, 2nd edition. Gaithersburg: MD: Aspen.

Roberts, Susan B.; Heyman, Dennis M.; and Tracy, Lisa (1999). *Feeding Your Child for Lifelong Health: Birth through Age Six.* New York: Bantam.

Satter, Ellyn (2000). *Child of Mine: Feeding with Love and Good Sense.* Palo Alto, CA: Bull Publishing.

Williamson, Carol P., ed. (1998). *Pediatric Manual of Clinical Dietetics.* Chicago: American Dietetic Association.

The Benefits of Breastfeeding

Mother's milk, designed as it is to nurture babies, contains the ideal amount and proportion of nutrients an infant needs, and the makeup of breast milk changes as the baby grows to satisfy its developing nutritional requirements. Breast milk contains antibodies that protect infants from many common diseases, including ear infections, diarrhea, and pneumonia, and helps develop the baby's immune system. Babies from families with allergies receive a particular benefit, as breast feeding has been shown to reduce allergies, asthma, and eczema. Unlike most formula, mother's milk contains docosohexaenoic acid and arachidonic acid, which contribute to brain and retinal development, and some studies have suggested that breastfed infants learn more effectively. In addition, they show a lower rate of obesity as adults. Mothers also benefit from breastfeeding in many ways. Of great psychological value, milk production burns 200 to 500 calories a day, speeding the mother's return to pre-pregnancy proportions.

—*Paula Kepos*

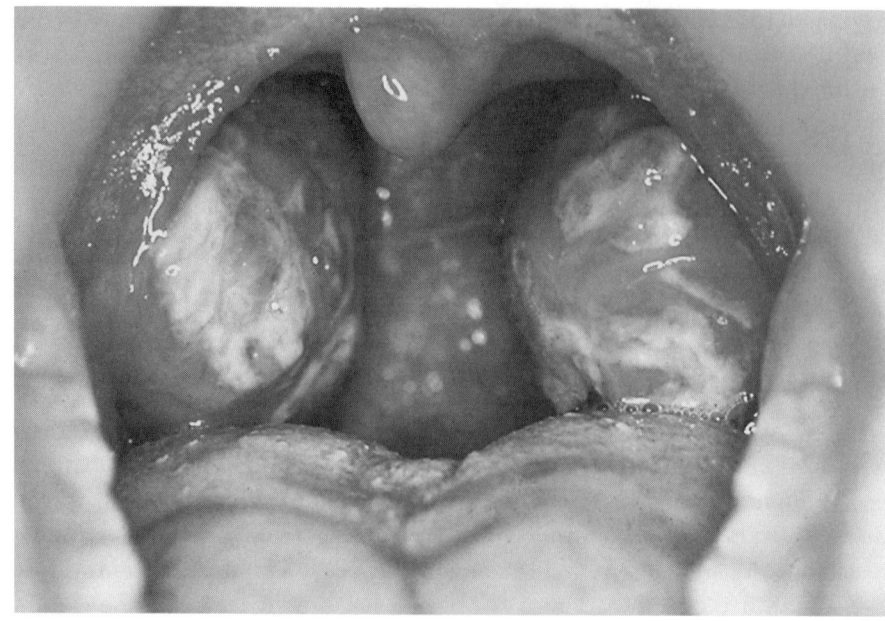

Glandular fever, or mononucleosis, is a viral infection that causes inflamed tonsils (shown here) and fever, and may cause an enlarged spleen. Symptoms most often appear in teens, but more than 80 percent of adults in the United States carry the virus and can transmit it. [Science Photo Library/Photo Researchers, Inc. Reproduced by permission.]

Internet Resources

Baby Center. "Baby Food Basics." Available from <http://www.babycenter.com>

Queens University. "A Guide to Infant Feeding—From Birth to 24 Months." Available from <http://www.queensu.ca/medicine>

Infection

microorganisms: bacteria and protists; single-celled organisms

bacteria: single-celled organisms without nuclei, some of which are infectious

respiratory system: the lungs, throat, and muscles of respiration, or breathing

gastrointestinal: related to the stomach and intestines

fatigue: tiredness

immune system: the set of organs and cells, including white blood cells, that protect the body from infection

antibiotic: substance that kills or prevents the growth of microorganisms

An infections is an illness caused by **microorganisms** or **bacteria** that invade the body. The body's defenses against infections begin with blocking the entry of microorganisms into the system. Hand washing is an effective strategy in preventing the entry of microorganisms into the body through the skin, the **respiratory system**, or the GI (**gastrointestinal**) tract.

Local infections may produce redness, tenderness, and swelling, but systemic infections produce more serious symptoms such as fever, chills, sweats, and **fatigue**. Many infections will go away on their own, however, as the body's **immune system** can successfully fight off many infections. Others, however, require treatment, such as the use of **antibiotic** medications. SEE ALSO IMMUNE SYSTEM.

Catherine Christie

Insulin

insulin: hormone released by the pancreas to regulate level of sugar in the blood

hormone: molecules produced by one set of cells that influence the function of another set of cells

glucose: a simple sugar; the most commonly used fuel in cells

diabetes: inability to regulate level of sugar in the blood

Insulin is a **hormone** produced by specialized cells in the pancreas. Secreted into the bloodstream at each meal, insulin helps the body use and store **glucose** (sugar) produced during the digestion of food. In people with **diabetes**, the pancreas either does not produce enough insulin or the body cannot use the insulin that is produced in an efficient manner.

Treatment for diabetes requires the delivery of insulin into the bloodstream by either an insulin pen, needle and syringe, or pump. An insulin pen is a device that looks like a pen but contains an insulin cartridge. Both the syringe and pen methods require injection of the insulin into the arm, thigh, or abdomen. Pump therapy, however, continuously administers insulin according to a programmed plan unique to the pump wearer. Several types of insulin exist, and they differ in when the insulin begins working after it is injected, when the insulin is working hardest, and how long the insulin lasts in the body.

Insulin release and glucose **absorption** depend on a number of factors, including the glycemic index of food and the co-ingestion of **fat** and **protein**. Consumption of high-glycemic foods causes **hyperglycemia** which results in the release of too much insulin. On the other hand, low-glycemic foods or the ingestion of fat and protein in a meal provide steady glucose absorption and release of insulin.

Exercise lowers blood glucose levels and increases the amount of insulin in the bloodstream, along with improving the body's use of insulin. A balance must exist between the sugar used for **energy**, the sugar available from food, and the insulin used in lowering blood sugar. Consequently, changes may have to be made to insulin, or food intake, or both, prior to and after exercise. SEE ALSO DIABETES MELLITUS; GLYCEMIC INDEX; HYPERGLYCEMIA; HYPOGLYCEMIA.

Julie Lager

absorption: uptake by the digestive tract

fat: type of food molecule rich in carbon and hydrogen, with high energy content

protein: complex molecule composed of amino acids that performs vital functions in the cell; necessary part of the diet

hyperglycemia: high level of sugar in the blood

energy: technically, the ability to perform work; the content of a substance that allows it to be useful as a fuel

Bibliography

Bode, Bruce W.; Sabbah, Hassan T.; Gross, Todd M.; Fredrickson, Linda P.; and Davidson, Paul C. (2002). "Diabetes Management in the New Millennium Using Insulin Pump Therapy." *Diabetes/Metabolism Research and Reviews* 18 (Suppl. 1):S14–S20.

DeWitt, Dawn E. and Hirsch, Irl B. (2003). "Outpatient Insulin Therapy in Type 1 and Type 2 Diabetes Mellitus: A Scientific Review." *Journal of the American Medical Association* 289(17):2254–2264.

Parmet, Sharon; Cassio, Lynm; and Glass, Richard M. (2003). "Insulin." *Journal of the American Medical Association* 289(17):2314.

Internet Resources

American Diabetes Association. "About Insulin." Available from <http://www.diabetes.org/>

National Library of Medicine. "Diabetes." Updated July 2, 2003. Available from <http://medlineplus.gov/>

Irradiation

Irradiation, or "electronic **pasteurization**," exposes food to a radiant source of energy, such as **gamma rays** or electron beams, for a brief period of time. Irradiation is a "cold" process that produces little heat, so food can remain packaged throughout the process—and until opened by the consumer. Irradiation decreases or eliminates harmful **bacteria**, insects, and **parasites**. It does not make a food radioactive, and it is allowed in nearly forty countries (including the United States, France, Israel, Russia, and China). It is also endorsed by many agencies, including the World Health Organization. Food Irradiation is not without controversy, however, and many consumer groups and organic farming organizations oppose it, believing that it can alter the cellular structure of foods and cause the production of **free radicals**. Other

pasteurization: heating to destroy bacteria and other microorganisms, after Louis Pasteur

gamma rays: very high energy radiation, more powerful than x rays

bacteria: single-celled organisms without nuclei, some of which are infectious

parasite: organism that feeds off of other organisms

free radical: highly reactive molecular fragment, which can damage cells

hazards cited by critics include the partial destruction of **vitamins** in irradiated foods, the destruction of beneficial bacteria as well as harmful bacteria, and the environmental hazard of nuclear irradiation facilities.

A logo called the "radura" is used internationally to indicate that the food has been irradiated, though some have suggested that this symbol is too benign to accurately represent the irradiation process, and that it is too similar to the symbol of the U.S. Environmental Protection Agency. SEE ALSO BIOTECHNOLOGY; FOOD SAFETY.

M. Elizabeth Kunkel
Barbara H. D. Luccia

Bibliography

Institute of Food Technologists' Expert Panel on Food Safety and Nutrition (1998). *Scientific Status Summary: Irradiation of Food.* Chicago, IL: Author.

Satin, Morton (1996). *Food Irradiation: A Guidebook,* 2nd edition. Lancaster, PA: Technomic Publishing.

Internet Resources

U.S. Department of Agriculture Food Safety and Inspection Service. Available from <http://www.fsis.usda.gov>

vitamin: necessary complex nutrient used to aid enzymes or other metabolic processes in the cell

isoflavones: estrogen-like compounds in plants

phytochemical: chemical produced by plants

biological: related to living organisms

physiological: related to the biochemical processes of the body

cancer: uncontrolled cell growth

heart disease: any disorder of the heart or its blood supply, including heart attack, atherosclerosis, and coronary artery disease

diabetes: inability to regulate level of sugar in the blood

estrogen: hormone that helps control female development and menstruation

cholesterol: multi-ringed molecule found in animal cell membranes; a type of lipid

tofu: soybean curd, similar in consistency to cottage cheese

protein: complex molecule composed of amino acids that performs vital functions in the cell; necessary part of the diet

Isoflavones

Isoflavones are **phytochemicals**, which are naturally occurring compounds found in plants that potentially have strong **biological** activity (and, therefore, a **physiological** effect) in the body. They may help lower the risk for various diseases, including **cancer**, **heart disease**, and **diabetes**. Similar in chemical structure to **estrogen**, isoflavones are, in fact, weak estrogens, and may have an effect similar to estrogens on the body. Nonestrogenic effects of isoflavones include reduction of **cholesterol** levels and inhibition of cancer-cell growth. Food sources include soy products such as soy milk, **tofu**, tempeh, and miso, but not soy sauce or soybean oil. Isoflavones may or may not be found in soy **protein**, depending on the processing method. SEE ALSO ANTIOXIDANTS; FUNCTIONAL FOODS; PHYTOCHEMICALS; SOY.

Susan Mitchel

Johnson, Howard
American businessman
1885–1972

Howard Deering Johnson had very humble beginnings in the food service business. Although he is mostly known for his motel, hotel, and restaurant chains, it was his branded ice cream that gave him a spectacular start in the business.

Howard Johnson was born in Boston, Massachusetts, in 1885. He quit school in the eighth grade to work in his father's cigar store and export business as a salesman. Johnson served in World War I as a part of the American Expeditionary Force. Soon after Johnson's return, his father died, leaving him the business and its heavy debt. He sold the business to pay off the

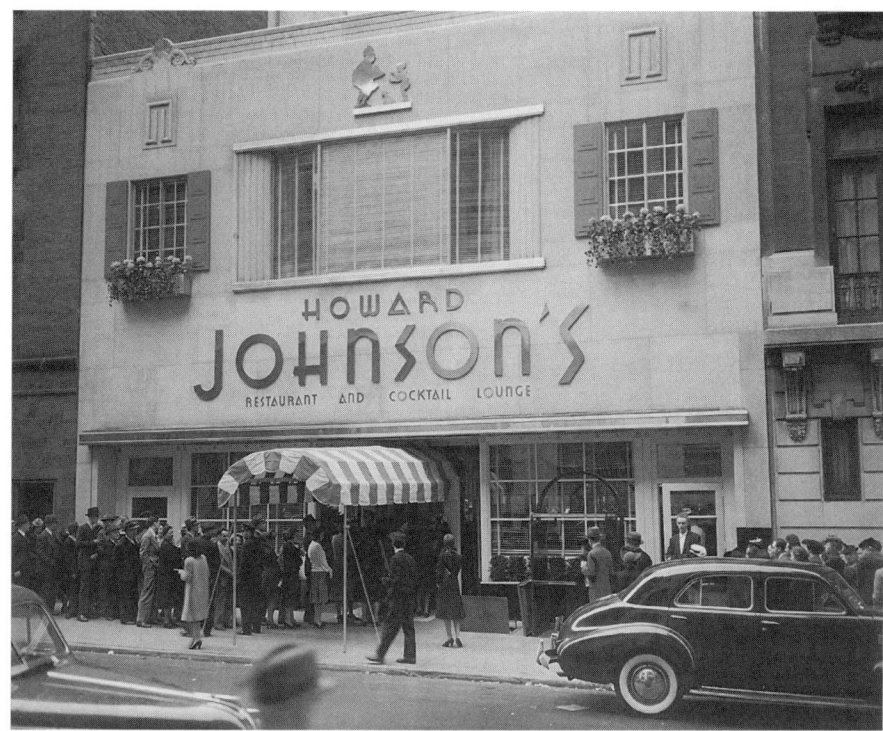

In the 1950s, Howard Johnson's restaurants dotted the American landscape, and travelers came to depend on the restaurants' consistency. This new way of doing business, called *franchising*, was perfected by the chain's founder, Howard Dearing Johnson.
[© Bettmann/Corbis. Reproduced by permission.]

debts in 1924. Johnson then borrowed $2,000 to buy a small corner drugstore and soda fountain in Wollaston, Massachusetts. He sold candy, newspapers, cigars, and medicine—and he was very successful.

The popularity of the soda fountain convinced him that having better-tasting ice cream would boost his business. At first, he used his mother's recipe. Not satisfied with this, he invested $300 in an ice cream recipe from an elderly German immigrant who was retiring. This premium ice cream recipe utilized natural flavors and twice the normal level of butterfat. Johnson began with three flavors, eventually increasing this to twenty-eight flavors. He also sold his ice cream at local beaches to boost business.

A local restaurant owner who purchased ice cream from the drug store asked to use the Howard Johnson name on his restaurant. Johnson agreed, which made him the exclusive source of supplies. The restaurant combined a lunch counter, **fast-food** takeout, an ice cream stand, and a sit-down restaurant—all in one location. Johnson soon began selling franchises of his restaurants. The white buildings trimmed with orange and sea blue became the Howard Johnson trademarks.

Johnson was very effective in maintaining quality control. At a Howard Johnson establishment, one could expect cleanliness and hospitality. The waitresses were hired for their courtesy, and high chairs were available for children at all restaurants, along with meal portions especially for children. By 1940, Johnson had about 135 restaurants.

During World War II, 90 percent of the restaurants closed due to gas rationing. The industrious Johnson contracted to manufacture candy and other goods for the armed forces. After the war, he began expanding his chains nationwide. More Americans were beginning to travel, and Johnson saw a need for better quality motels and hotels to meet the needs of these

fast food: food requiring minimal preparation before eating, or food delivered very quickly after ordering in a restaurant

travelers and their families. Johnson created motor hotels, offering good services and cleanliness. By 1965, the Howard Johnson name was to be found on 770 restaurants and 265 motor hotels.

Howard Johnson retired in 1959, leaving the company to his son. However, he continued to monitor his restaurants for cleanliness and proper food preparation, often performing unannounced inspections.

Howard Johnson's Restaurant's Smart Meals are based on the federal government's Dietary Guidelines for Americans. They rank lower in fat, **calories**, **cholesterol**, and sodium than traditional fast-food meals. The **nutrition** information is always clearly visible on the menu, so that diners are aware of what they are eating.

calorie: unit of food energy

cholesterol: multi-ringed molecule found in animal cell membranes; a type of lipid

nutrition: the maintenance of health through proper eating, or the study of same

As of 2002, only fifteen Howard Johnson restaurants and two ice cream shops remain in the United States and Puerto Rico, mainly due to increased competition from fast-food restaurants and their low prices. Menu items and the original-recipe ice cream can still be purchased in various supermarkets and in all Howard Johnson restaurants. There are nearly five hundred hotels in fourteen countries. In the 1980s, the restaurant chain separated from the franchised hotels when the Howard Johnson Corporation was sold to other corporations. In addition, the contract that had allowed Howard Johnson to be the "King of the Road" expired and was not renewed. This allowed fast-food chains to claim space on the nation's highways and turnpikes. Nevertheless, Howard Johnson made it possible for travelers and families on the go to eat nutritiously and enjoy a higher standard in all aspects of hospitality than was previously available. SEE ALSO DIETARY TRENDS, AMERICAN; FAST FOODS.

Slande Celeste

Bibliography

"Hitting the Road Healthfully." (1994). *Tufts University Diet and Nutrition Letter.* 12(5):7.

Lavine, S. A. (1965). *Famous Merchants.* New York: Dodd Mead.

Internet Resources

HoJo Land. "HoJo History." Available from <http://hojoland.homestead.com>

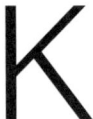

Kellogg, John Harvey
American physician
1852–1943

John Harvey Kellogg was an influential spokesman for vegetarianism, a leader in the invention of nut- and soy-based meat substitutes, a surgeon, and, for over fifty years, the director of the Battle Creek Sanitarium. In partnership with his brother Will, he made the Kellogg name famous. By studying food chemistry, Kellogg learned that an early step in **indigestion** is the conversion of starch to dextrin, or sugar. Cereal grains have a high starch content, and Kellogg discovered that prolonged baking almost completely dextrinized the starch in multigrain biscuits. He ground these up and served them to his patients, calling the creation "granola." In 1889, Kellogg invented the first flaked breakfast cereal, which was made from wheat. He later devised a method of producing corn flakes.

indigestion: reduced ability to digest food

Many **entrepreneurs**, including C. W. Post, the man most responsible for instigating Battle Creek's food "gold rush," came to make riches from breakfast cereal.

Born and raised near Battle Creek, the birthplace of the Seventh-day Adventist Church, Kellogg became intimately involved with the religious-medical-health doctrine of the Seventh-day Adventists. Yet, tragically, before his death he and his brother had split their business, he had given up the rights to use the Kellogg name, and he spent the final third of his life outside the Seventh-day Adventist Church, which expelled him in 1907 due to his divergent views on the Bible and his belief in pantheism, the belief that there is a divine presence in all living things.

Born to John Preston Kellogg and his second wife, Anne, on February 26, 1852, John Harvey Kellogg's family lived on a 160-acre farm in rural Tyrone Township in Livingston County, Michigan. When he was four years old, his family moved to Battle Creek. John Preston Kellogg invested money toward the building of the Battle Creek Sanitarium. However, it was the early church leaders, James and Ellen White, who encouraged Kellogg's ambition and steered him toward a career in medicine. He graduated in February 25, 1875, from Bellevue Hospital Medical School with an M.D. degree, after first spending twenty weeks in Florence Heights, New Jersey, at Dr. Russell Trall's Hygeio-Therapeutic College. Trall was a founding member and officer of the American Vegetarian Society and the author of *The Scientific Basis of Vegetarianism* (1860). He was also a leading figure in American hydropathy, an alternative system of medical practice that treated medical conditions with applications of water.

As a young man, Kellogg would often sit in on meetings concerning the Battle Creek Sanitarium during his visits home from school, and it soon became evident that he should work there. Four major Seventh-day Adventist leaders were situated in Battle Creek, James and Ellen White, Uriah Smith, and Professor Sidney Brownsberger, president of Battle Creek College. At the age of twenty-four, Kellogg agreed to be medical director of the Battle Creek Sanitarium for one year starting in 1876. At that time the institution had twenty patients.

By force of personality and hard work, Kellogg put Battle Creek Sanitarium on the map as the place for the wealthy to recuperate and rejuvenate. And he remained at the Battle Creek Sanitarium long after corn flakes had made Battle Creek the cereal center of the world. The sanitarium burned to the ground in 1902, and the boom in cereals helped to finance its rebuilding.

After initiating the production of granola in 1877, Dr. Kellogg organized the Sanitarium Food Company as a subsidiary of the Battle Creek Sanitarium in 1901. This company marketed a variety of oatmeal, graham and fruit crackers, and whole grain cereals and breads. In 1908 it became the Kellogg Food Company. After a long contentious dialogue, Kellogg and his brother parted ways, and in 1920 the rights to manufacture cereal went to Will along with the commercial use of the Kellogg name.

Unable to have children, Kellogg and his wife, Ella (née Eaton) were active in aiding children, many of whom were raised in their home. Together, they established the Haskell Home for Orphans in 1894, and at one time

entrepreneur: founders of new businesses

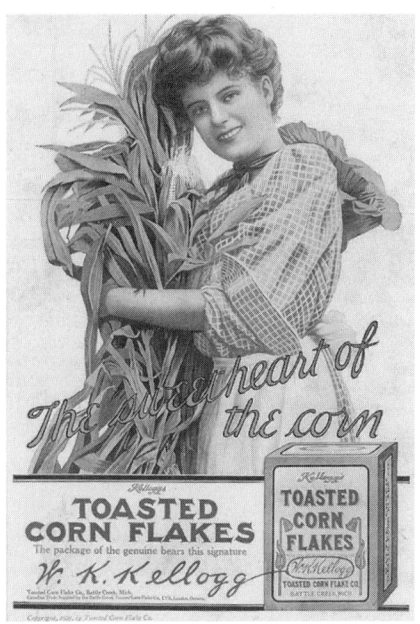

John Harvey Kellogg helped to invent Cornflakes cereal; but it was his brother, Will Keith Kellogg, who recognized the cereal's marketability. John Harvey preferred to focus on reforming the health of the nation, and to that end he promoted a vegetarian diet and abstinence from alcohol and tobacco.
[Courtesy of Mark LaFlaur. Reproduced by permission.]

they together helped as many as thirty individuals in one year. They assumed responsibility for forty-two children, legally adopting four or five of them. They hired private tutors for the children and provided them with jobs. Their efforts were not completely successful, however, as one of the children later became a drifter and blackmailed Kellogg with threats of embarrassment. At the age of seventy-eight, Kellogg moved to Florida and renovated the Country Club Hotel—which was donated by a previous patron, the pioneer aircraft manufacturer Glenn Curtiss—and opened the Miami–Battle Creek Sanitarium, a 100-bed establishment, which ran at capacity for his remaining thirteen years of life. SEE ALSO BATTLE CREEK SANITARIUM, EARLY HEALTH SPA; WHITE, ELLEN G.

Louise E. Schneider

Bibliography

Graybill, Ron (1992). "The Whites Come to Battle Creek: A Turning Point in Adventist History." Adventist Heritage. Loma Linda, CA: Department of Archives and Special Collections with the Department of History and the School of Religion.

Sabate, Joan (2001). *Vegetarian Nutrition.* Boca Raton, FL: CRC Press.

Schwartz, Richard W. (1970). *John Harvey Kellogg, M.D.* Nashville, TN: Southern Publishing Association.

Stoltz, Garth (1992). "A Taste of Cereal." Adventist Heritage. Loma Linda, CA: Department of Archives and Special Collections with the Department of History and the School of Religion.

Kroc, Ray
American businessman
1902–1984

Raymond Albert Kroc was born in Oak Park, Illinois, to Luis and Rose Kroc. He had two younger siblings, Robert and Lorraine. As a child, his mother called Ray "Danny Dreamer" because he would daydream all the time. Rose Kroc was a piano teacher, and she taught young Ray to play.

Kroc's first job was with his uncle, Earl Edmund Sweet, in a soda fountain the summer before he started high school. The next summer Ray dropped out of school, and he used the money he made the previous summer to rent a building with two friends. They sold sheet music and small instruments, but after a few months the business failed.

During World War I, Kroc lied about his age and became an ambulance driver for the Red Cross. He returned to Chicago after the war and held various jobs, including work as a jazz pianist and as a real-estate salesman. In the summer of 1919, Ray played in a band at Paw-Paw Lake, Michigan, where he met his future wife, Ethel Flemming. Ray and Ethel married in 1922, but only after he satisfied his father's requirement of getting a steady job—selling paper cups for the Lily Tulip Cup Company, where he worked for seventeen years.

In the early 1940s, Kroc became the exclusive distributor of a multi-mixer that could mix five milk shakes simultaneously. Two of his best customers were the McDonald brothers, Richard and Maurice (Mac), who bought eight of the mixers for their **fast-food** restaurants. The McDonalds had started with a group of hot-dog carts, and now had a chain of restau-

fast food: food requiring minimal preparation before eating, or food delivered very quickly after ordering in a restaurant

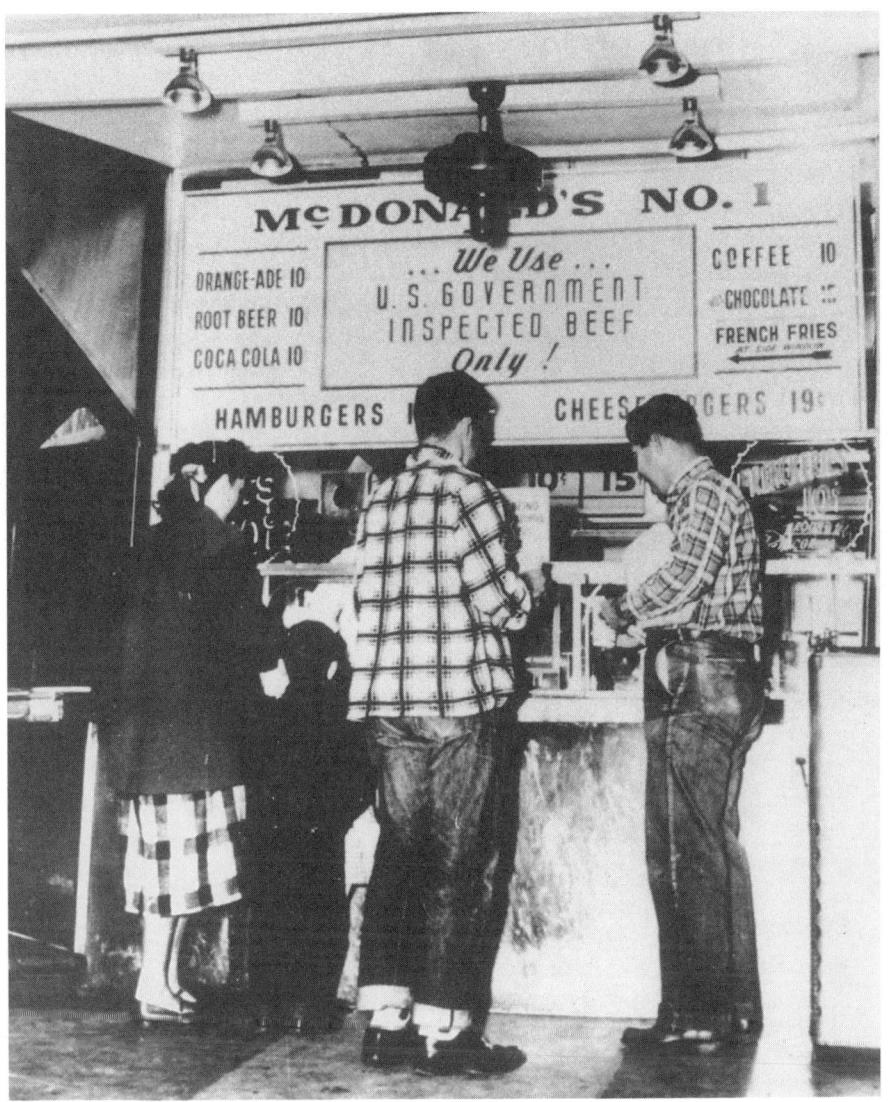

Customers line up at the very first McDonald's restaurant, which in 1954 inspired Ray A. Kroc to build a fast-food empire. Today there are more than 30,000 McDonald's restaurants worldwide. [AP/Wide World Photos. Reproduced by permission.]

rants—for which Richard McDonald designed the "golden arches" logo and the "number-of-hamburgers-sold" sign.

In 1954, Kroc went to San Bernardino, California, to see the McDonald brothers' restaurant, which used an assembly-line format to prepare foods. Kroc decided to set up a chain of drive-in restaurants based on the McDonalds' format and convinced the brothers to sell him the rights to franchise McDonald's restaurants nationwide. His first restaurant opened on April 15, 1955, in Des Plaines, Illinois. Kroc also began selling franchises on the condition that the owners managed their restaurants. Kroc was known for his obsessive cleanliness, and he wanted the restaurants kept very clean. In 1961, Kroc bought out the McDonald brothers for $2,700,000. At this time he had established 228 restaurants, and sales had reached $37,000,000. By 1963 more than 1 billion hamburgers had been sold.

Kroc served as the company's president from 1955 to 1968, as chairman of the board from 1968 to 1977, and as a senior chairman from 1977 until his death. He also was the owner of the San Diego Padres professional baseball team. Kroc died on January 14, 1984, in San Diego, California. He

McDonald's Worldwide

By 2004, McDonalds had become a $40 billion global enterprise with more than 30,000 restaurants in 120 countries and more than half its sales outside the United States. International outlets are adapted to local cultures. In Saudi Arabia, for example, single men are seated separately from women and children. Indian McDonald's restaurants serve no beef or pork, but feature instead such menu items as a Chicken Maharaja Mac, a Paneer Salsa Wrap, and a McAloo Tikki Burger. In Japan, where the "r" sound is difficult, Ronald McDonald goes by the name Donald McDonald. As the chain faces slowing sales in a mature domestic market, the pace of its international expansion has increased. In China, where there are already 500 McDonald's, the chain plans to open more than 100 new branches a year. The company has become a major employer worldwide, with more than 1 million employees. However, despite (or because of) its international success, McDonald's has frequently come under attack as a symbol of American cultural imperialism. In 2000, anti-globalization protesters in a French farm town smashed windows in a half-built McDonald's franchise, highlighting the struggle between small farmers and big business in the global agriculture market. And after the United States began bombing Afghanistan in 2001, McDonald's outlets in Pakistan and Indonesia were vandalized. Attacks on McDonald's have been recorded in more than 50 countries.

—*Paula Kepos*

---

is remembered as a pioneer in the fast-food industry, and was named as one of *Time* magazine's "Builders and Titans" of the twentieth century. SEE ALSO Dietary Trends, American; Fast Foods.

Delores C. S. James

Bibliography

Kroc, Raymond, A. (1977). *Grinding It Out*. Chicago, IL: Contemporary Books.

Schlosser, Eric (2001). *Fast Food Nation: The Dark Side of the All-American Meal*. New York: Houghton Mifflin.

Internet Resources

Britannica.com (2001). "Kroc, Ray." Available from <http://www.britannica.com>

Pepin, Jacques. (2000). "Ray Kroc." Available from <http://www.time.com/time>

Kwashiorkor

The term **kwashiorkor**, meaning "the disease of the displaced child" in the language of Ga, was first defined in the 1930s in Ghana. Kwashiorkor is one of the more severe forms of **protein malnutrition** and is caused by inadequate protein intake. It is, therefore, a **macronutrient** deficiency.

Kwashiorkor is largely a problem in the developing world, although it can be found in geriatric and hospitalized patients in Western nations. Generally, kwashiorkor occurs when drought, **famine**, or societal unrest leads to an inadequate food supply. Protein-depleted diets in such areas are mostly based on starches and vegetables, with little meat and animal products. A lack of maternal understanding regarding balanced diets further contributes to the problem. Finally, infections and other disease states negatively impact **nutrient** intake, digestion, and **absorption**.

---

kwashiorkor: severe malnutrition characterized by swollen belly, hair loss, and loss of skin pigment

protein: complex molecule composed of amino acids that performs vital functions in the cell; necessary part of the diet

malnutrition: chronic lack of sufficient nutrients to maintain health

macronutrient: nutrient needed in large quantities

famine: extended period of food shortage

nutrient: dietary substance necessary for health

absorption: uptake by the digestive tract

Children are most at risk due to their increased dietary needs. Inadequate caloric and protein intake manifests itself with certain physical characteristics. Symptoms may include any of the following: failure to gain weight, stunted linear growth, generalized **edema**, protuberant (swollen) abdomen, diarrhea, skin desquamation (peeling) and vitiligo (white spots on the skin), reddish pigmentation of hair, and decreased muscle mass. Mental changes include lethargy, apathy, and irritability. Physiologic changes include a fatty liver, **renal failure**, and **anemia**. During the final stages of kwashiorkor, patients can experience, **shock**, coma, and, finally, death.

Treatment of kwashiorkor begins with rehydration. Subsequent increase in food intake must proceed slowly, beginning with **carbohydrates** followed by protein supplementation. If treatment is initiated early, there can be a regression of symptoms, though full height and weight potential will likely never be reached. SEE ALSO MALNUTRITION; MARASMUS; NUTRITIONAL DEFICIENCY; PROTEIN.

Seema P. Kumar

edema: accumulation of fluid in the tissues

renal failure: inability of the kidneys to cleanse the blood

anemia: low level of red blood cells in the blood

shock: state of dangerously low blood pressure and loss of blood delivered to the tissues

carbohydrate: food molecule made of carbon, hydrogen, and oxygen, including sugars and starches

Bibliography

Latham, Michael (1997). *Human Nutrition in the Developing World*. Rome: Food and Agricultural Organization of the United Nations.

Trowell, H. C.; Davis, J. N. P.; and Dean, R. F. A. (1982). *Kwashiorkor*. New York: Academic Press.

Internet Resources

World Health Organization (1996). *WHO Global Database on Child Growth and Malnutrition*. Available from <http://www.who.int/nutgrowthdb>

Lactose Intolerance

Lactose intolerance is the inability to digest significant amounts of lactose, the primary sugar in milk. This inability results from a shortage of the **enzyme** lactase, which is normally produced by the cells that line the small intestine. Lactase breaks down lactose into simpler forms that can then be absorbed into the bloodstream during the digestive process. Common symptoms of lactose intolerance include **nausea**, cramps, bloating, gas, and diarrhea.

Structure and Functions of Lactose

Lactose is a **disaccharide carbohydrate**, composed of the two monosaccharides, **glucose** and galactose. When lactose reaches the digestive system, the lactase enzyme breaks down lactose into glucose and galactose. The liver then changes the galactose into glucose. If this process occurs normally, the glucose enters the bloodstream and raises the blood glucose level.

Prevalence

As many as 75 percent of all adults worldwide are lactose intolerant, and between 30 million and 50 million Americans are lactose intolerant. Certain racial or ethnic groups are more widely affected than others. As many as 75 percent of all African-American, Jewish, Native American, and Mexican-American adults, and 90 percent of Asian-American adults are lactose

lactose intolerance: inability to digest lactose, or milk sugar

enzyme: protein responsible for carrying out reactions in a cell

nausea: unpleasant sensation in the gut that precedes vomiting

disaccharide carbohydrate: molecule composed of two linked sugars

glucose: a simple sugar; the most commonly used fuel in cells

intolerant. The condition is least common among persons of northern European descent.

Types of Lactose Intolerance

There are three basic types of lactose intolerance: primary, secondary, and **congenital**. In primary lactose intolerance, the body begins to produce less lactase after about the age of two, depending on an individual's racial or ethnic background. This type is genetically determined and is a permanent condition.

Secondary lactose intolerance, on the other hand, is temporary and results from a disease or medications that damage the lining of the small intestine where lactase is normally active. Secondary lactose intolerance gradually disappears when the illness passes.

Congenital lactose intolerance is an extremely rare condition in which the lactase enzyme is completely absent at birth. Unlike other types of lactose intolerance, this type requires complete avoidance of lactose.

Clinical Diagnosis

The most common tests used to measure the **absorption** of lactose in the digestive system are the lactose tolerance test, the hydrogen breath test, and the stool **acidity** test.

The lactose tolerance test involves an individual drinking a liquid that contains lactose. The individual must fast before this test, in which several blood samples are taken over a two-hour period to measure the blood glucose level, which indicates how well the body is able to digest lactose. If lactose is incompletely absorbed, then the blood glucose level will not rise, confirming a diagnosis of lactose intolerance.

The hydrogen breath test measures the amount of hydrogen in the breath. Normally, no hydrogen is detectable in the breath. However, undigested lactose in the colon is fermented by **bacteria**, and various gases, including hydrogen, are produced. The hydrogen is absorbed from the **intestines**, carried through the bloodstream to the lungs, and exhaled. As with the previous test, a lactose-loaded beverage is consumed, and the individual then breathes into a machine that measures the amount of hydrogen in the breath.

The stool acidity test measures the amount of acid in a person's stool. Undigested lactose fermented by bacteria in the colon creates **lactic acid** and other short-chain **fatty acids** that can be detected in a stool sample. In addition, glucose may be present in the sample as a result of unabsorbed lactose in the colon.

Nutrition for People with Lactose Intolerance

There are degrees of intolerance for lactose. Studies have shown that many true lactose intolerants can consume moderate amounts of milk and dairy products without symptoms, particularly if milk is part of a meal.

Milk and other dairy products are a major source of **calcium**. Many people with lactose intolerance may be able to tolerate yogurt with active cultures, which is very high in calcium, even though it is fairly high in lactose. Evidence shows that the bacterial cultures used in making yogurt

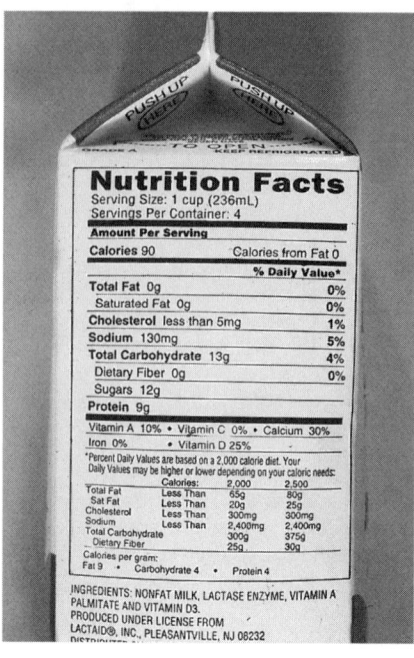

Between 30 and 50 million Americans are lactose intolerant, meaning they are deficient in the enzyme lactase. The majority of lactose-intolerant people can consume small amounts of lactose, or lactose in certain foods, but may experience symptoms of intestinal upset if they consume too much. *[Photograph by Leonard Lessin. Peter Arnold, Inc. Reproduced by permission.]*

congenital: present from birth

absorption: uptake by the digestive tract

acidity: measure of the tendency of a molecule to lose hydrogen ions, thus behaving as an acid

bacteria: single-celled organisms without nuclei, some of which are infectious

intestines: the two long tubes that carry out the bulk of the processes of digestion

lactic acid: breakdown product of sugar in the muscles in the absence of oxygen

fatty acids: molecules rich in carbon and hydrogen; a component of fats

calcium: mineral essential for bones and teeth

produce some of the lactase enzyme required for proper digestion. Lactose-intolerant individuals should also be able to tolerate cheese, as most of the lactose is removed, along with the whey, when the cheese is made.

However, people with lactose intolerance who do not drink milk or eat diary products can still get the calcium they need from dark-green, leafy vegetables such as broccoli, turnip or collard greens, and kale. Certain fish with soft, edible bones, such as herring, salmon, or sardines, are also good calcium sources.

Although milk and foods made from milk are the only natural sources, lactose is often added to **processed foods**, such as bread, cereal, and salad dressing. This is because dairy products can contribute to the required or desired flavor, color, and texture of many foods, in addition to increasing the nutritional value of processed foods. Some products that are labeled "nondairy," such as powdered coffee creamer and whipped toppings, may include ingredients that are derived from milk, and therefore contain lactose. It is important to carefully read food labels, looking not only for milk and lactose among the contents, but also for such terms as *whey, curds, milk by-products, dry milk solids,* and *nonfat dry milk powder,* all of which contain lactose. SEE ALSO AFRICAN AMERICANS, DIET OF; AFRICANS, DIETS OF; ASIANS, DIET OF; CARBOHYDRATES.

Gita C. Gidwani

processed food: food that has been cooked, milled, or otherwise manipulated to change its quality

Bibliography

National Digestive Diseases Information Clearinghouse (2002). "Lactose Intolerance." NIH Publication No. 02-2751. Available from <http://www.niddk.nih.gov>

Lay Health Advisor

One model utilized to counter public health budget cuts is the use of lay health advisors (LHAs). Potential LHAs are individuals in the community who have a reputation as a "natural helper" and are trusted by their friends, family, and neighbors. One of the primary objectives of an LHA is to bring together professionals and consumers to mobilize the resources of a community to foster support for preventive health actions. LHAs can facilitate behavior change, especially in underserved populations, by bringing notice to particular health issues that may be of detriment to that community.

Beth Hensleigh

Bibliography

Thomas, James; Eng, Eugenia; and Clark, Michele (1998). "Lay Health Advisors: Sexually Transmitted Disease Prevention through Community Involvement." *American Journal of Public Health* 88(8):1252.

Internet Resources

North Carolina Breast Cancer Screening Program. "NC-BCSP Lay Health Advisors." Available from <http://bcsp.med.unc.edu/pages/LHAs.htm>

Lead Poisoning

Lead is an indestructible **heavy metal** that can accumulate and linger in the body. Although the problem of lead exposure has been reduced in the United

heavy metal: lead, chromium, and other metals found in the middle section of the periodic table of the elements

States, minorities and disadvantaged individuals remain chronically exposed. In developing countries, occupational and environmental exposures still exist and are a serious public health problem.

Definition of Lead Poisoning

Lead poisoning, or plumbism, is defined as a toxic condition caused by the ingestion or inhalation of the metallic element lead, which is found in many places, including the air, soil, water, houses, ceramic cookware, and solder used in metal cans and pipes. Lead poisoning occurs when blood lead levels are equal to or greater than 10 µg/dl (micrograms per deciliter).

Symptoms of Lead Poisoning

Lead exposure results from either inhaling or ingesting lead. Low levels of exposure (up to 10 µg/dl) are associated with **anemia**, headaches, general weakness, **fatigue**, learning disabilities, impaired **development** of the **nervous system**, and delayed growth, while greater levels of exposure (70 µg/dl) include symptoms such as decreased appetite, vomiting, abdominal pain, **constipation**, and drowsiness. If blood lead levels exceed 70 µg/dl, coma, seizures, bizarre behavior, impaired muscular coordination, and even death can occur.

Populations at Risk

Lead poisoning is one of the greatest environmental threats to children. Lead **absorption** is five to eight times greater in children than in adults. Approximately 11 percent of ingested lead will reach the adult digestive tract, as compared to 30 to 70 percent in children. In addition, children absorb up to 50 percent of inhaled lead. Children that are at greatest risk are those living near highways and interstates, in urban and inner-city areas, or in low-income housing. While the United States government banned leaded gasoline in 1986, residual lead is still present in the soil around highways and interstates. Children that live in homes or play in playgrounds near those areas can ingest lead through dust on their hands. In developing countries where leaded gasoline is still used, children living near highways are exposed to lead through automobile and truck exhaust.

Children living in inner-city and urban areas are exposed to lead through leaded paint used in older homes (prior to 1978), as well as through the presence of pipes soldered with lead solder. Lead can leach into the water in the pipes, contributing to the blood lead levels of children (and adults) ingesting the water. The major sources of lead exposure today are household dust from paint and exterior soil. In addition, children of low **socioeconomic status** are at a nutritional disadvantage, for they often do not consume enough food to keep their stomachs full enough to slow absorption, and because they usually do not have enough **iron** and **calcium** in their diets.

In developing countries, both adults and children face a risk of lead poisoning due to exposure sources such as leaded gasoline, lead-based cosmetics, lead solder in food containers, ceramic cookware, folk remedies, and lead-based paint. Since adverse effects of lead poisoning are magnified in **malnourished** populations, it is critical that developing countries recognize the threat of unintentional lead exposure.

---

anemia: low level of red blood cells in the blood

fatigue: tiredness

development: the process of change by which an organism becomes more complex

nervous system: the brain, spinal cord, and nerves that extend throughout the body

constipation: difficulty passing feces

absorption: uptake by the digestive tract

socioeconomic status: level of income and social class

iron: nutrient needed for red blood cell formation

calcium: mineral essential for bones and teeth

malnourished: lack of adequate nutrients in the diet

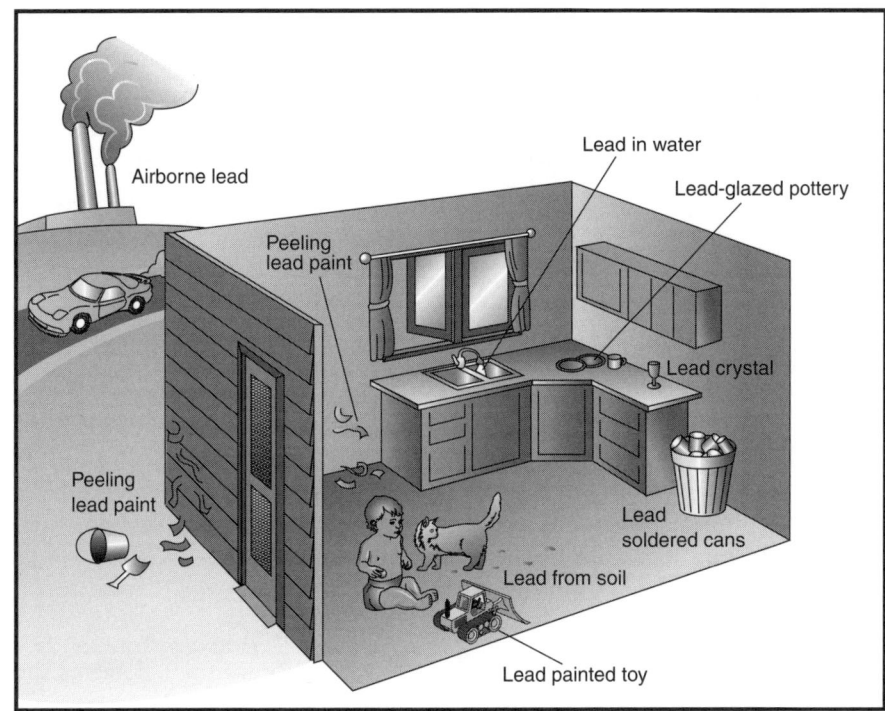

Lead is commonly found in and around the home, especially in older homes. Children are especially susceptible to lead poisoning, since they absorb lead more readily than adults. Even minor exposure to lead can severely affect a child's development. [Electronic Illustrators Group. Reproduced by permission.]

Sources of Lead

During the 1970s, Americans discontinued the use of leaded gasoline, and other sources of environmental lead exposure have gradually been reduced. While exposure to lead has diminished, residual amounts still remain in contaminated soil, dust, lakes, and streams.

A major source of environmental exposure for children is lead-based paint. While this type of paint is no longer manufactured in the United States, buildings constructed prior to 1978 may contain residual lead. Lead exposure occurs when lead-contaminated dust is inhaled or ingested. In addition, young children may eat contaminated paint chips or ingest contaminated paint dust while sucking their hands or fingers.

Other sources of lead exposure include ceramic cookware and lead solder. Lead contained in the glaze on ceramic cookware can leach out and enter food during the cooking process. In lead-soldered pipes, lead enters the water as it passes through or collects in the pipe. People living in older homes with lead-soldered pipes should drink bottled water or make certain that the water is allowed to run several minutes before it is ingested. Water that has sat in the pipes longer than six hours should not be consumed.

While lead solder is no longer used to seal cans in the United States, imported food remains a source of exposure. Once again, lead from the solder leaches into the food. Acidic foods and drinks, such as pickles or fruit juice, enhance the leaching process. Other exposure sources include a food coloring (*lozeena*) from Iraq that is sometimes used to color rice and meat, and to which lead is sometimes added; prune juice concentrate from France and raisins from Turkey (lead-containing preservatives and pesticides are used on foods such as prunes and raisins), and duck eggs from Taiwan (lead is used in the traditional method of preserving duck eggs). In addition, a

Prevalence of Lead Poisoning

As a result of public health initiatives, lead levels in children's blood have dropped steadily since the 1970s, but approximately 434,000 U.S. children between one and five years of age still have elevated lead levels. Lead poisoning remains a particular threat among certain racial and ethnic groups that are disproportionately affected. For example, 6 percent of white children living in older housing have elevated lead levels, while the numbers for African-American and Mexican-American children in similar housing are 22 percent and 13 percent, respectively. In developing countries, which commonly use unleaded gasoline, lead poisoning is the most significant environmental disease among children. According to the World Health Organization, fifteen to eighteen million children in the developing world have suffered permanent brain damage as a result of lead poisoning.

—Paula Kepos

nutritional deficiency: lack of adequate nutrients in the diet

mucosa: moist exchange surface within the body

fortified: altered by addition of vitamins or minerals

environment: surroundings

number of folk remedies from around the world, as well as imported leaded crystal, can be sources of lead exposure. Folk remedies of concern include: *koo sar* pills, used as a remedy for menstrual cramps in Asia; *azarcon*, an orange powder used for intestinal illness in Mexico; *ghasard*, an Indian folk remedy for babies; *kandu*, a red powder used to treat stomachache; *farouk*, a Middle Eastern teething remedy; and *hai gen fen*, a clamshell powder added to tea.

Nutritional Interventions

Nutritional deficiencies allow lead to accumulate in body tissues and organs. The absorption of lead is greatest when the stomach is empty; therefore, consuming regular meals is important. Unfortunately, the ability to afford three meals a day is sometimes a problem for populations at risk for lead poisoning.

In the body, calcium binds to lead and inhibits its absorption; therefore, dietary calcium interferes with the absorption of lead through the intestinal **mucosa**. Among high-risk populations, calcium supplements or the addition of milk and yogurt to meals and snacks is recommended.

Research has also demonstrated a link between iron deficiency and lead poisoning. Recognition of this link is important, since iron deficiency is the most common childhood nutritional problem worldwide. Iron supplementation, or consuming foods rich in iron, such as **fortified** cereals, prunes, beef, and calves liver, can interfere with lead accumulating in the body.

Educational Interventions

In many developed nations, information programs are available to advise homeowners of lead hazards in older homes. Programs offering proper methods of exposure reduction are important, since homeowners attempting to rid their homes of lead paint and pipes with lead solder can inadvertently increase their exposure through sanding and other activities. International groups, such as the World Health Organization, are working to increase international awareness of lead exposure issues and abatement programs. In 1998, the U.S. National Center for Environmental Health identified childhood lead poisoning as one of its five global priorities.

The most effective intervention for lead poisoning is removing all sources of lead from the **environment**. Since this is not possible for many high-risk populations, health care providers can provide parents and child-care workers with information on how to care for children's nails and on proper hand-washing techniques, as well as information on the dangers of consuming paint chips and/or paint dust.

Consumer-awareness campaigns relating to the potential hazards of imported cookware and dishes can also help adults and children avoid unintentional ingestion of lead. Individuals need to be aware of the potential presence of lead in products and food items from other countries, particularly those that lack environmental controls relating to lead, such as Mexico, Turkey, Pakistan, India, Indonesia, Nepal, Thailand, and many countries in the Middle East and Asia.

Medical Treatment

Typically, persons diagnosed with blood lead levels greater than 45 µg/dl will receive chelation therapy, which uses chemical agents that bind to lead in the body and cause it to be excreted in the urine or feces. High blood lead levels are considered a medical emergency requiring immediate attention, since the chances of serious complications rise as lead accumulates in the blood.

Virginia Jones Noland

Bibliography

Alters, S., and Schiff, W. (2001). *Essential Concepts for Healthy Living*, 2nd ed. Boston: Jones and Bartlett.

Binns, H.; Kim, D.; and Campbell, C. (2001). "Targeted Screening for Elevated Blood Lead Levels: Populations at High Risk." *Pediatrics* 108:1364–1366.

Chisolm, J. J. (2001). "The Road to Primary Prevention of Lead Toxicity in Children." *Pediatrics* 107:581–583.

Edlin, G.; Golanty, E.; and Brown, K. M. (1999). *Health and Wellness*, 6th ed. Boston: Jones and Bartlett.

Ellis, M., and Kane, K. (2000). "Lightening the Lead Load in Children." *American Family Physician* 62:545–565.

Lynch, R.; Boatright, D.; and Moss, S. (2000). "Lead-Contaminated Imported Tamarind Candy and Children's Blood Lead Levels." *Public Health Reports* 115:537–543.

Nadakavukaren, A. (1990). *Man and Environment: A Health Perspective*, 3rd ed. Prospect Heights, IL: Waveland Press.

Sargent, J. D. (1994). "The Role of Nutrition in the Prevention of Lead Poisoning in Children." *Pediatric Annals* 23:636–642.

Satcher, D. (2000). "The Surgeon General on the Continuing Tragedy of Childhood Lead Poisoning." *Public Health Reports* 115:579–580.

Simon, J., and Hudes, E. (1999). "Relationship of Ascorbic Acid to Blood Lead Levels." *Journal of the American Medical Association* 281:2289–2293.

Telljohann, S.; Symons, C.; and Miller, D. (2001). *Health Education: Elementary and Middle School Applications*, 3rd ed. Boston: McGraw Hill.

Tong, S.; Schirnding, Y; and Prapamontol, T. (2000). "Environmental Lead Exposure: A Public Health Problem of Global Dimensions." *Bulletin of the World Health Organization* 78:1068–1077.

Warren, C. (2000). *Brush with Death: A Social History of Lead Poisoning*. Baltimore, MD: Johns Hopkins University Press.

Whitney, E., and Nunnelley, E. (1987). *Understanding Nutrition*, 4th ed. New York: West Publishing.

Wright, R.; Shannon, M.; Wright, R.; and Hu, H. (1999). "Association between Iron Deficiency and Low-Level Lead Poisoning in an Urban Primary-Care Clinic." *American Journal of Public Health* 89(7):1049–1053.

Legumes

Legumes are the edible seeds of plants. They provide a good source of **protein**, thiamine, folic acid, vitamin E, and **fiber**. The **insoluble** fiber in legumes helps to lower blood **cholesterol**. Examples of legumes are: dried beans, peas, and seeds (including navy, broad, butter, northern, pinto, red, and black beans, as well as chick peas, soybeans, and peanuts).

Legumes are an important source of protein for vegetarians, especially **vegans**. The protein in legumes is considered incomplete, however, and needs to be eaten in combination with whole grains to make a complete (high-quality) protein (e.g., green beans, lentils, and rice; navy beans and barley; soybeans and sesame seeds; red beans and rice). Such combinations

legumes: beans, peas, and related plants

protein: complex molecule composed of amino acids that performs vital functions in the cell; necessary part of the diet

fiber: indigestible plant material which aids digestion by providing bulk

insoluble: not able to be dissolved in

cholesterol: multi-ringed molecule found in animal cell membranes; a type of lipid

vegan: person who consumes no animal products, including milk and honey

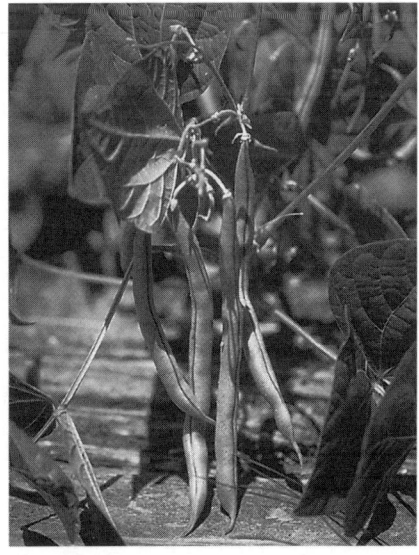

Legumes include many varieties of beans, including the popular green bean shown here. Legumes provide more fiber per serving than any other vegetable, and also provide plenty of protein. *[JLM Visuals. Reproduced with permission.]*

have been used for centuries in the diets of people practicing vegetarianism. SEE ALSO PLANT-BASED DIETS; SOY; VEGETARIANISM.

Simin B. Vaghefi

Life Expectancy

The term *life expectancy* is used to describe the average life span of an individual. Life expectancy can vary considerably in different areas of the world. Compared to other advanced countries, for example, people in the United States "die earlier and spend more time disabled" (WHO, 2000). Factors that affect life expectancy in the United States include: (1) the HIV epidemic, (2) cancers relating to tobacco, (3) high rates of **coronary heart disease**, (4) poor health among minority groups living in rural areas, and (5) high levels of violence.

coronary heart disease: disease of the coronary arteries, the blood vessels surrounding the heart

According to the World Health Organization (WHO) the Japanese have the longest healthy life expectancy (74.5) among 191 countries the organization examined in 2000. In contrast, the shortest life expectancy (26 years) exists among the people of Sierra Leone. These figures were based on a new method of calculating *healthy* life expectancy called Disability Adjusted Life Expectancy (DALE), which was developed by the WHO. DALE summarizes the expected number of years to be lived in adequate health, rather than just the expected number of years lived.

According to DALE the United States ranks twenty-fourth, with an average life expectancy of 70.0 years for babies born in 1999. (Examined by gender, U.S. female babies in 1999 could expect 72.6 years of life, while male babies could expect only 67.5 years.) Life expectancy based on DALE for other countries are: Australia, 73.2 years; France, 73.1; Sweden, 73.0; Spain, 72.8; Italy, 72.7; Greece, 72.5; Switzerland, 72.5; Monaco, 72.4; and Andorra, 72.3.

The world's average life expectancy at birth rose to 67 years in 1998 (from 61 years in 1980). Although individual countries vary in average life-span years, the average number of years has increased due to increases in intake of nutritious food, primary health care (including safe water, sanitation, and immunizations), and education. SEE ALSO INFANT MORTALITY RATE; MATERNAL MORTALITY RATE.

Daphne C. Watkins

Internet Resources

World Bank. "Life Expectancy." Available from <http://www.worldbank.org/depweb/english/modules>

World Health Organization (2000). "Japan Number One in New 'Healthy Life' System." Available from <http://www.int/inf-pr-2000/en/pr2000-life.html>

Lipid Profile

cardiovascular: related to the heart and circulatory system

atherosclerosis: build-up of deposits within the blood vessels

artery: blood vessel that carries blood away from the heart toward the body tissues

lipid: fats, waxes and steroids; important components of cell membranes

Cardiovascular disease (CVD) is a major cause of death in the world and is mainly due to **atherosclerosis** (hardening of the **arteries**). Abnormal blood **lipids** are risk factors for CVD.

OPTIMAL, BORDERLINE, AND HIGH LEVELS FOR EACH COMPONENT

Element	Optimal	Borderline	High risk
LDL Cholesterol	<100	130–159	160+
HDL Cholesterol	>60	35–45	<35
Triglycerides	<150	150–199	>200
Total Cholesterol	<200	200–239	>240
Cholesterol to HDL Ratio	<4	5	>6

SOURCE: National Heart, Lung, and Blood Institute.

Blood Lipids and Lipid Transport

Lipids are **insoluble** (does not dissolve) in water but are soluble (dissolves) in alcohol and other solvents. When dietary fats are digested and absorbed into the small intestine, they eventually re-form into **triglycerides**, which are then packaged into **lipoproteins**.

Dietary fats, including **cholesterol**, are absorbed from the small **intestines** and transported into the liver by lipoproteins called *chylomicrons*. Chylomicrons are large droplets of lipids with a thin shell of **phospholipids**, cholesterol, and **protein**. Once chylomicrons enter the bloodstream, an **enzyme** called *lipoprotein lipase* breaks down the triglycerides into fatty acid and **glycerol**. After a 12- to 14-hour fast, chylomicrons are absent from the bloodstream. Thus, individuals who are having a lipid profile done should fast overnight to ensure that chylomicrons have been cleared.

The liver removes the chylomicron fragments, and the cholesterol is repackaged for transport in the blood in *very low-density lipoproteins* (VLDLs), which eventually turn into *low-density lipoproteins* (LDL). LDL cholesterol (LDL-C)—the "bad cholesterol"—consists mainly of cholesterol. Most LDL particles are absorbed from the bloodstream by receptor cells in the liver. Cholesterol is then transported throughout the cells. Diets high in saturated fats and cholesterol decrease the uptake of LDL particles by the liver. LDL particles are also removed from the bloodstream by scavenger cells, or macrophages, which are **white blood cells** that bury themselves in blood vessels such as arteries. Scavenger cells prevent cholesterol from reentering the bloodstream, but they deposit the cholesterol in the inner walls of blood vessels, eventually leading to the **development** of plaque.

High-density lipoproteins (HDLs) are a separate group of lipoproteins that contain more protein and less cholesterol than LDL. **HDL** cholesterol (HDL-C) is also called "good cholesterol." HDL is produced primarily in the liver and intestine, and it travels in the bloodstream, picks up cholesterol, and gives the cholesterol to other lipoproteins for transport back to the liver.

Lipid Profile

A lipid profile measures total cholesterol, HDL cholesterol, LDL cholesterol, and triglycerides. A physician may order a lipid profile as part of an annual exam or if there is specific concern about CVD, especially coronary artery disease. The National Cholesterol Education Program recommends that individuals age twenty and over have a fasting lipoprotein profile every

---

insoluble: not able to be dissolved in

triglyceride: a type of fat

lipoprotein: blood protein that carry fats

cholesterol: multi-ringed molecule found in animal cell membranes; a type of lipid

intestines: the two long tubes that carry out the bulk of the processes of digestion

phospholipid: a type of fat used to build cell membranes

protein: complex molecule composed of amino acids that performs vital functions in the cell; necessary part of the diet

enzyme: protein responsible for carrying out reactions in a cell

glycerol: simple molecule that forms a portion of fats

white blood cell: immune system cell that fights infection

development: the process of change by which an organism becomes more complex

HDL: high density lipoprotein, a blood protein that carries cholesterol

HDL/LDL RATIO VALUES

Risk level	Men	Women
Very Low Risk	3.4	3.3
Low Risk	4.0	3.8
Average Risk	5.0	4.5
Moderate Risk	9.5	7.0
High Risk	>23	>11

SOURCE: National Heart, Lung, and Blood Institute.

five years. A lipid profile should be done after a nine- to twelve-hour fast without food, liquids, or medication. If fasting is not possible, the values for total cholesterol and HDL-C may still be useful. If total cholesterol is 200 milligrams per deciliter (mg/dl) or higher, or HDL-C is less than 40 mg/dl, the individual will need to have a follow-up lipoprotein profile done to determine LDL-C and triglyceride levels.

Depending on the physician's request, the lipid profile may include the ratio of cholesterol to HDL. This ratio is sometimes used in place of total blood cholesterol. The ratio is obtained by dividing the HDL cholesterol level by the total cholesterol. For example, if a person has total cholesterol of 200 mg/dl and an HDL cholesterol level of 50 mg/dl, the ratio is 4:1. The goal is to keep the ratio below 5:1, and optimally at 3.5:1. There are several **over-the-counter** cholesterol measuring devices on the market, but none has been endorsed by any medical organizations.

Treating Abnormal Blood Lipids

The National Cholesterol Education Program, the American College of Cardiology, and the American Heart Association recommend **diet** and lifestyle modification as the first line of defense against abnormal blood lipids. These recommendations include a diet low in total **fat, saturated fat,** and cholesterol; a diet high in **fiber**; weight loss or weight management; increased physical activity; smoking cessation; increased intake of plant **sterols** (e.g., margarines and salad dressings made with soybean sterols); and daily use of a low-dose aspirin. Drug therapy may be required for high-risk individuals. Cholesterol-lowering **drugs** works to lower LDL by reducing cholesterol synthesis and by binding **bile** acids in the small intestines. However, there are possible side effects to these drugs that patients should be aware of. SEE ALSO ARTERIOSCLEROSIS; ATHEROSCLEROSIS; CARDIOVASCULAR DISEASES; FATS.

Delores C. S. James

over-the-counter: available without a prescription

diet: the total daily food intake, or the types of foods eaten

fat: type of food molecule rich in carbon and hydrogen, with high energy content

saturated fat: a fat with the maximum possible number of hydrogens; more difficult to break down than unsaturated fats

fiber: indigestible plant material which aids digestion by providing bulk

sterol: building blocks of steroid hormones; a type of lipid

drugs: substances whose administration causes a significant change in the body's function

bile: substance produced in the liver which suspends fats for absorption

Bibliography

Birtcher, Kim K., et al. (February 2000). "Strategies for Implementing Lipid-Lowering Therapy: Pharmacy-Based Approach." *American Journal of Cardiology* 85(3):30–35.

National Cholesterol Education Program (2001). *Third Report of the National Cholesterol Education Program Expert Panel on Detection, Evaluation, and Treatment of High Blood Cholesterol in Adults (Adult Treatment Panel III), Executive Summary.* NIH Publication No. 01-3670. Washington, DC: National Institutes of Health.

Wardlaw, G.; Hampl, J.; and DiSilvestro, R. (2004). *Perspectives in Nutrition*, 6th edition. Boston, MA: McGraw-Hill.

Internet Resources

American Heart Association. "Cholesterol, Home Testing Devices." Available from <http:/www.americanheart.org>

Lab Tests OnLine. "Lipid Profile." Available from <http://www.labtestsonline.org>

National Heart Lung and Blood Institute. "Recommendations for Lipoprotein Measurement." Available from <http://www.nhlbi.nih.gov/prof/heart>

Low Birth Weight Infant

An infant born with a weight of less than five pounds (2,500 grams) at birth is classified as a low birth weight infant. Babies with low birth weight were either born prematurely or are small for their age because their growth was restricted in the womb. Poor maternal health and **nutrition** may cause low birth weight. Risk factors include inadequate prenatal nutrition, smoking during pregnancy, and infection during pregnancy. Low birth weight infants face a higher risk of death within the first year of life and have higher rates of disability and disease than other infants. Low birth weight is a leading cause of infant mortality throughout world.

Amy N. Marlow

nutrition: the maintenance of health through proper eating, or the study of same

Macrobiotic Diet

George Ohsawa (1893–1966) coined the term *macrobiotic* to describe a philosophy towards life, health, and healing. Macrobiotic means "way of long life." Macrobiotics is best described as a way of living according to the principles of yin and yang. Ohsawa, in his book, *Zen Macrobiotics*, describes twelve principles of yin and yang. On the simplest level, it means that individuals eat foods that keep them in balance with their **environment** (i.e., in a hot (yang) climate, more cooling (yin) foods are eaten, and vice versa). Oshawa outlined a ten-stage "Zen" macrobiotic **diet** in which each stage gets more restrictive. The diet is alleged to overcome all forms of illness. At the "highest level," the diet is nutritionally inadequate and has resulted in several deaths. Oshawa devoted much of his time trying to understand the "Order of the Universe," and eventually succumbed to the efforts of his experimentation.

More recently, macrobiotics has come to mean a dietary regimen used to prevent and treat many diseases. The macrobiotic diet is actually several diets ranging in restrictions from severe to moderate. The severe diet consists exclusively of whole cereal grains, while the moderate diet consists of whole cereal grains and certain types of vegetables, fruits, and soups. Today's leading proponent is Michio Kushi, who reformulated and popularized macrobiotics in the United States.

The standard macrobiotic diet avoids many foods including meat, poultry, animal fats, eggs, dairy products, refined sugar, and foods containing artificial sweeteners or other chemical additives. All recommended foods are preferably organically grown and minimally processed. Consumption of genetically modified, irradiated, processed, canned, and frozen foods is discouraged. The diet consists of five categories of foods (with a recommended weight percentage of total food consumed):

- Whole cereal grains (40%–60%).
- Vegetables, including smaller amounts of raw or pickled vegetables (20%–30%).

macrobiotic: related to a specific dietary regimen based on balancing of vital principles

environment: surroundings

diet: the total daily food intake, or the types of foods eaten

Macrobiotic Diet

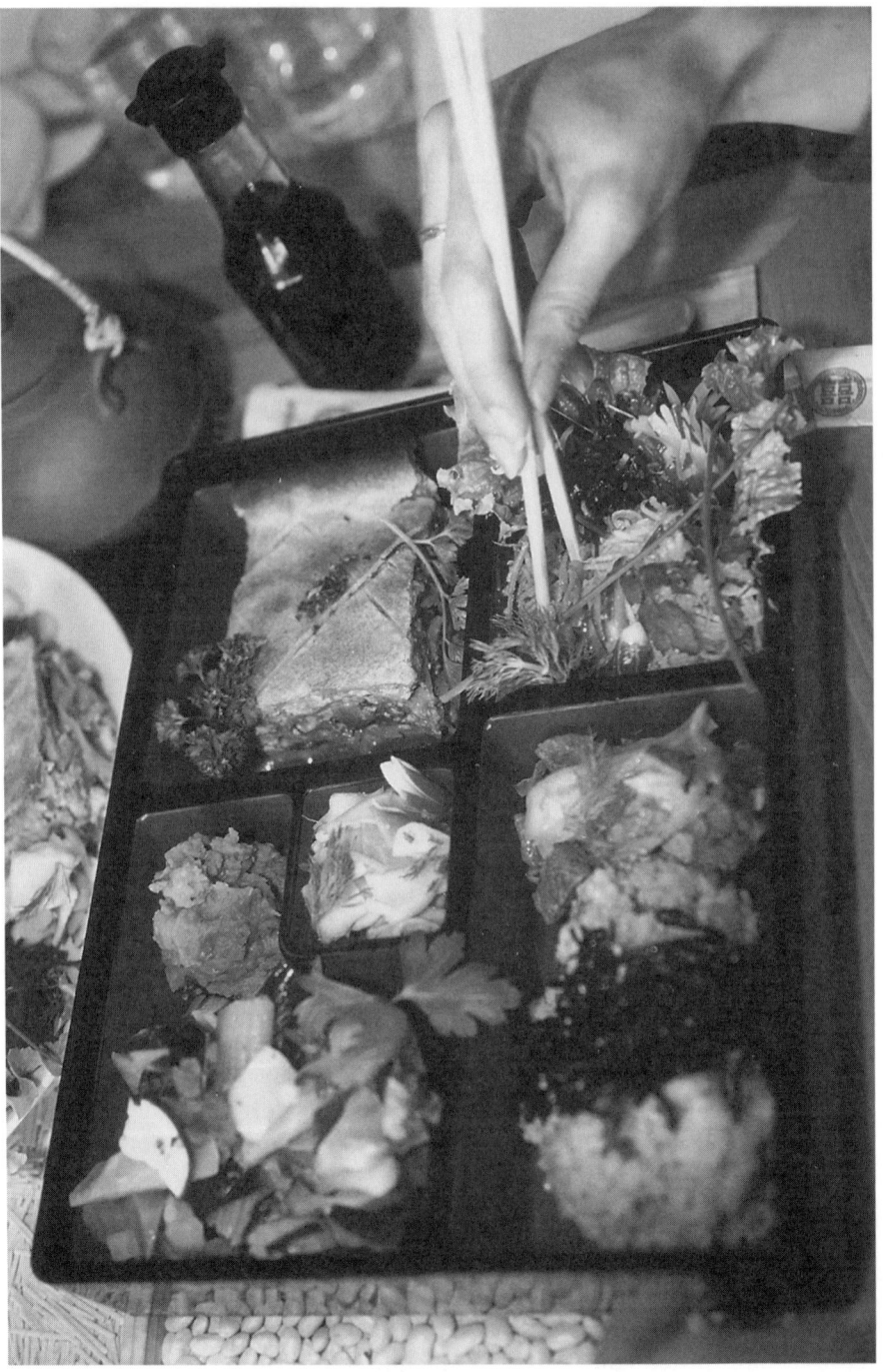

People who follow a macrobiotic diet limit their food intake to specific foods, especially whole grains, vegetables, and beans. Though certain aspects of the macrobiotic diet are nutritious, scientists dispute claims that it can cure cancer and other diseases. *[Thierry Orban/Corbis Sygma. Reproduced by permission.]*

- Beans and sea vegetables (5%–10%).
- Soups (which may be made with vegetables, sea vegetables, grains, or beans).
- Beverages including any traditional tea that does not have an aromatic fragrance or a stimulating effect and spring water or good-quality well water, without ice. Not recommended are tropical or semitropical fruits and fruit juices, soda, artificial drinks and beverages, coffee, and colored tea.
- Occasional foods include fruit, white fish, seeds, and nuts.

- Foods to eliminate from the diet include meat, animal **fat**, eggs, poultry, dairy products, refined sugars, chocolate, molasses, honey, vanilla, hot spices, artificial vinegar, and strong alcoholic beverages.

Although the range of intakes varies, macrobiotic diets are generally low in **energy**, **protein**, and fat. They are also likely to be inadequate in **vitamin D**, folic acid, vitamin B$_{12}$, riboflavin, **calcium**, and **iron**. **Clinical** cases of **malnutrition** and growth failure in children have been reported.

Proponents of the macrobiotic diet recommend it for **cancer** patients. It is alleged to slow progression of cancer by starving the rapidly reproducing cells responsible for the disease. Many patients with HIV/AIDS also turn to a macrobiotic diet to help combat the disease. However, these patients and others with immune-suppressed diseases are already losing alarming amounts of weight, and they also have other medical and nutritional complications. The macrobiotic diet may only exacerbate their problem and cause more **nutritional deficiencies**.

Delores C. S. James

Bibliography

Bowman, B. B.; Kushner, R. F.; Dawson, S. C.; Levin, B. (1984). "Macrobiotic Diets for Cancer Treatment and Prevention." *Journal of Clinical Oncology* 2(6):702–711.

Kushi M. (1987). *The Book of Macrobiotics: The Universal Way of Health and Happiness.* Tokyo: Japan Publications.

Internet Resources

Horowitz, J., and Tomita, M. (2002). "The Macrobiotic Diet as Treatment for Cancer: Review of the Evidence." *The Permanente Journal* 6(4). Available from <http://www.kaiserpermanente.org/medicine/permjournal>

Kushi Institute. "What is macrobiotics?" Available from <http://www.kushiinstitute.org/whatismacro.html>

fat: type of food molecule rich in carbon and hydrogen, with high energy content

energy: technically, the ability to perform work; the content of a substance that allows it to be useful as a fuel

protein: complex molecule composed of amino acids that performs vital functions in the cell; necessary part of the diet

vitamin D: nutrient needed for calcium uptake and therefore proper bone formation

calcium: mineral essential for bones and teeth

iron: nutrient needed for red blood cell formation

clinical: related to hospitals, clinics, and patient care

malnutrition: chronic lack of sufficient nutrients to maintain health

cancer: uncontrolled cell growth

nutritional deficiency: lack of adequate nutrients in the diet

Malnutrition

The **nutritional requirements** of the human body reflect the nutritional intake necessary to maintain optimal body function and to meet the body's daily **energy** needs. **Malnutrition** (literally, "bad **nutrition**") is defined as "inadequate nutrition," and while most people interpret this as **undernutrition**, falling short of daily nutritional requirements, it can also mean overnutrition, meaning intake in excess of what the body uses. However, undernutrition affects more than one-third of the world's children, and nearly 30 percent of people of all ages in the developing world, making this the most damaging form of malnutrition worldwide.

The **etiology** of malnutrition includes factors such as poor food availability and preparation, recurrent infections, and lack of nutritional education. Each of these factors is also impacted by political instability and war, lack of sanitation, poor food distribution, economic downturns, erratic health care provision, and by factors at the community/regional level.

People at Risk

Certain people are more susceptible to malnutrition than others. For example, individuals in rapid periods of growth, such as infants, adolescents,

nutritional requirements: the set of substances needed in the diet to maintain health

energy: technically, the ability to perform work; the content of a substance that allows it to be useful as a fuel

malnutrition: chronic lack of sufficient nutrients to maintain health

nutrition: the maintenance of health through proper eating, or the study of same

undernutrition: food intake too low to maintain adequate energy expenditure without weight loss

etiology: origin and development of a disease

In developing nations, more than half of all deaths among children under five years old are due to malnutrition. Malnourished children who survive may experience stunted growth, illness, and lifelong malnourishment. *[Photograph by Bruce Brander. National Audubon Society Collection/Photo Researchers, Inc. Reproduced by permission.]*

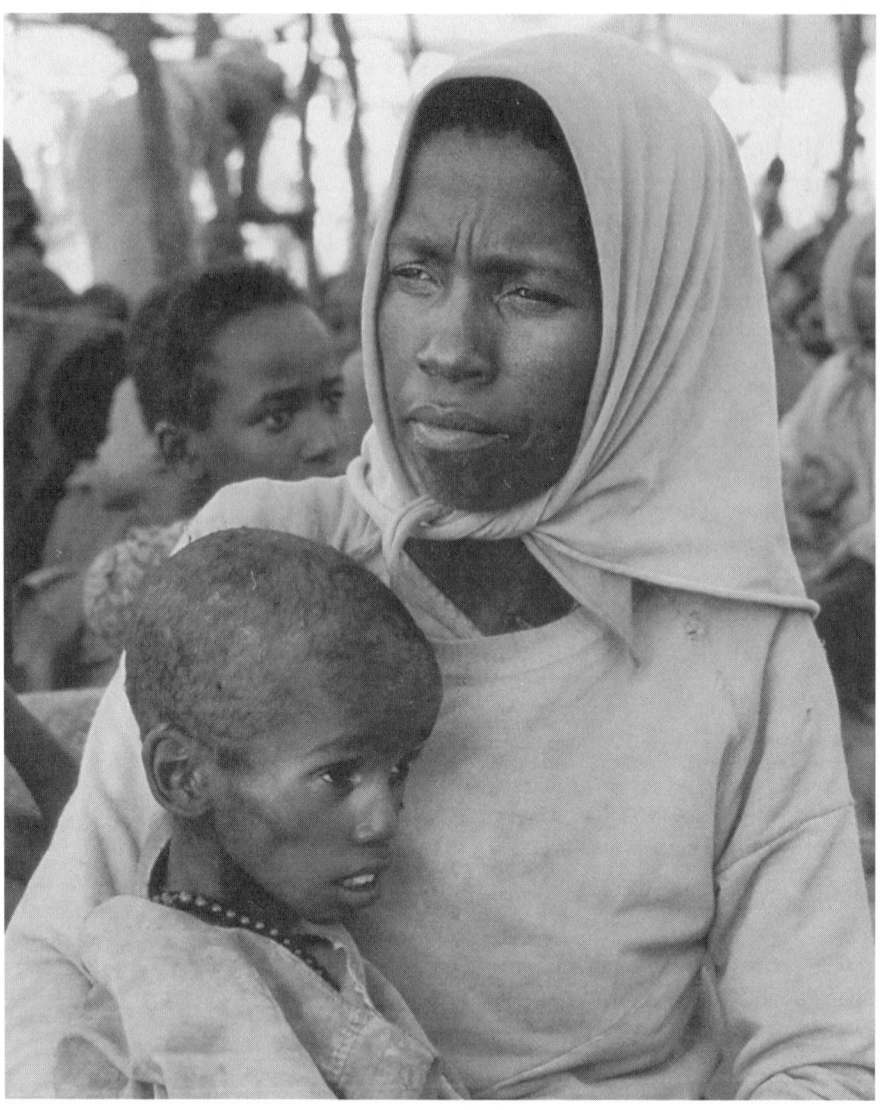

gastrointestinal: related to the stomach and intestines

chronic: over a long period

immune system: the set of organs and cells, including white blood cells, that protect the body from infection

absorption: uptake by the digestive tract

nutrient: dietary substance necessary for health

malnourished: lack of adequate nutrients in the diet

hookworm: parasitic nematode that attaches to the intestinal wall

malaria: disease caused by infection with Plasmodium, a single-celled protozoon, transmitted by mosquitoes

and pregnant women, have higher nutritional needs than others, and are therefore more susceptible to the effects of poor nutrition. Those living in deprived socioeconomic circumstances or that lack adequate sanitation, education, or the means to procure food are also at risk. Most importantly, individuals at risk for systemic infections (particularly **gastrointestinal**) and those who suffer with a **chronic** disease are at greatly increased risk because they require additional energy to support their **immune system** and often have decreased **absorption** of **nutrients**.

In fact, the relationship between malnutrition and infection is cyclical—infection predisposes one to malnutrition, and malnutrition, which impairs all immune defenses, predisposes one to infection. The World Health Organization (WHO) identifies malnutrition as "the single most important risk factor for disease" (WHO). Some research has identified **malnourished** children as being more likely to suffer episodes of infectious disease, as well as episodes of longer duration and greater severity, than other children. In particular, **hookworm**, **malaria**, and chronic diarrhea have been linked with malnutrition. These conditions are more prevalent in the developing world than in the industrialized world, though malnutrition exists worldwide, particularly in areas of poverty and among patients with chronic disease or who are hospitalized and on **enteric** feeding.

Necessary Nutrients

The WHO's Department of Nutrition for Health and Development is responsible for formulating dietary and nutritional guidelines for international use. Adequate total nutrition includes the following nutrients: **protein**, energy (**calories**), vitamin A and carotene, **vitamin D**, vitamin E, vitamin K, thiamine, riboflavin, **niacin**, vitamin B6, pantothenic acid, **biotin**, **folate**, vitamin C, **antioxidants**, **calcium**, **iron**, **zinc**, selenium, magnesium, and iodine. Most important are protein and the caloric/energy requirement needed to utilize protein. If these elements are inadequate, the result is a protein-energy malnutrition (PEM), or protein-calorie malnutrition (PCM), which affects one in every four children worldwide, with the highest concentration in Asia. Chronic deficiencies of protein and calories result in a condition called **marasmus**, while a **diet** high in **carbohydrates** but low in protein causes a condition called **kwashiorkor**.

Malnutrition and Growth

Malnutrition from any cause retards normal growth. Growth assessments are therefore the best way to monitor a person's nutritional status. While there are a variety of methods used to measure growth, the most common are known as **anthropometric** indices, which compare an individual's age, height, and weight, each of which is measured against the others. The values are expressed as percentages, or percentiles, of the normal distribution of these measurements. So, for example, a child with a given height and age might rank in the 90th percentile for height based on all children of that particular age, meaning that 90 percent of children that age are shorter than this particular child. Through anthropometric studies, researchers have found that particular measurements correlate with specific growth trends, based on how the body normally changes over time. Abnormal height-for-age (stunting) usually measures long-term growth faltering. Low weight-for-height (**wasting**) correlates with an **acute** growth disturbance.

Malnutrition can have severe long-term consequences. Children who suffer from malnutrition are more likely to have slowed growth, delayed development, difficulty in school, and high rates of illness, and they may remain malnourished into adulthood.

Limited growth patterns are distributed unevenly across the globe. Eighty percent of children affected by stunting or wasting live in Asia, with 15 percent in Africa and 5 percent in Latin America. Low weight-for-age (underweight) is usually used as an overall measurement of growth status. More than 35 percent of all preschool-age children in developing countries are underweight. There are differences, however, across regions. "The risk of being underweight is 1.5 times higher in Asia than in Africa, and 2.3 times higher in Africa than Latin America" (Onis, p. 10). In some ways, these indices also enable an indirect understanding of the societal factors in these regions that contribute to malnutrition as mentioned above.

The Universal Declaration of Human Rights, established by the United Nations (UN) in 1948, identifies nutrition as a fundamental human right.

enteric: pertaining to the intestine; delivered via a tube into the intestine

protein: complex molecule composed of amino acids that performs vital functions in the cell; necessary part of the diet

calorie: unit of food energy

vitamin D: nutrient needed for calcium uptake and therefore proper bone formation

niacin: one of the B vitamins, required for energy production in the cell

biotin: a portion of certain enzymes used in fat metabolism; essential for cell function

folate: one of the B vitamins, also called folic acid

antioxidant: substance that prevents oxidation, a damaging reaction with oxygen

calcium: mineral essential for bones and teeth

iron: nutrient needed for red blood cell formation

zinc: mineral necessary for many enzyme processes

marasmus: extreme malnutrition, characterized by loss of muscle and other tissue

diet: the total daily food intake, or the types of foods eaten

carbohydrate: food molecule made of carbon, hydrogen, and oxygen, including sugars and starches

kwashiorkor: severe malnutrition characterized by swollen belly, hair loss, and loss of skin pigment

anthropometric: related to measurement of characteristics of the human body

wasting: loss of body tissue often as a result of cancer or other disease

acute: rapid-onset and short-lived

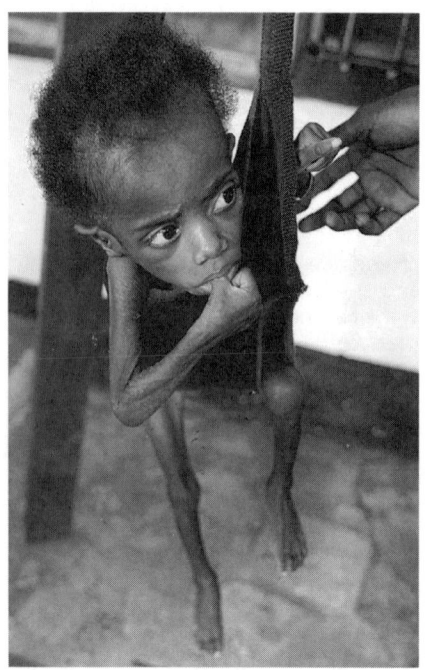

An acutely malnourished Liberian boy is weighed at a therapeutic feeding center. Such centers, operated by international relief organizations, provide intensive care and a specialized diet to rehabilitate severely malnourished children. [AP/Wide World Photos. Reproduced by permission.]

enrichment: addition of vitamins and minerals to improve the nutritional content of a food

hygiene: cleanliness

prevalence: describing the number of cases in a population at any one time

marasmus: extreme malnutrition, characterized by loss of muscle and other tissue

protein: complex molecule composed of amino acids that performs vital functions in the cell; necessary part of the diet

energy: technically, the ability to perform work; the content of a substance that allows it to be useful as a fuel

malnutrition: chronic lack of sufficient nutrients to maintain health

kwashiorkor: severe malnutrition characterized by swollen belly, hair loss, and loss of skin pigment

calorie: unit of food energy

wasting: loss of body tissue often as a result of cancer or other disease

acute: rapid-onset and short-lived

gastrointestinal: related to the stomach and intestines

Malnutrition remains one of the world's highest priority health issues, not only because its effects are so widespread and long lasting, but also because it can be eradicated. Given the multifactorial causes of malnutrition, interventions must be focused on both acute and broad goals. Current efforts are targeted at high-risk groups, particularly infants and pregnant women, for it is "in these populations and during these ages that nutritional interventions have the greatest potential for benefit" (Schroeder, p. 46). Even the simple supplementation of vitamin A or beta-carotene supplements during pregnancy can decrease maternal mortality by 40 percent. Interventions include direct food supplementation, food access, agricultural **enrichment**, nutritional education, and improved infrastructure related to **hygiene**, sanitation, and health care delivery. Each of these programs "must be tailored to the particular problems, cultural conditions, and resource constraints of the local context" (Schroeder, p. 417). Strategies for reducing the **prevalence** of malnutrition must effectively address its many causes. SEE ALSO KWASHIORKOR; MARASMUS; NUTRIENTS; NUTRITION.

Seema P. Kumar

Bibliography

Gillespie, Stuart, and Lawrence Haddad (2001). *Attacking the Double Burden of Malnutrition in Asia and the Pacific.* Washington, DC: International Food Policy Research Institute.

Onis, M.; Monteiro, C.; Akre, J.; and Clugston, G. (1993). "The Worldwide Magnitude of Protein-Energy Malnutrition." In *Bulletin of the World Health Organization* 71(6).

Schroeder, Dirk G. (2001). "Malnutrition." In *Nutrition and Health in Developing Countries*, ed. Richard Semba and Martin Bloem. Totowa, NJ: Humana Press.

Shannon, Joyce Brennflck (2001). *Worldwide Health Sourcebook.* Detroit, MI: Omnigraphics.

Marasmus

Marasmus is one component of **protein-energy malnutrition** (PEM), the other being **kwashiorkor**. It is a severe form of malnutrition caused by inadequate intake of protein and **calories**, and it usually occurs in the first year of life, resulting in **wasting** and growth retardation. Marasmus accounts for a large burden on global health. The World Health Organization (WHO) estimates that deaths attributable to marasmus approach 50 percent of the more than ten million deaths of children under age five with PEM.

The major factors that cause a deficit of caloric and protein intake include the following: the transition from breastfeeding to nutrition-poor foods in infancy, **acute** infections of the **gastrointestinal** tract, and **chronic** infections such as HIV or **tuberculosis**. The imbalance between decreased energy intake and increased energy demands result in a negative energy balance.

The physiologic response to a negative energy balance is to reduce energy consumption. Children who suffer from marasmus display decreased activity, lethargy, **behavioral** changes, slowed growth, and weight loss. The subsequent effects on the body are wasting and a loss of **subcutaneous fat** and muscle, resulting in growth retardation. The majority of children who suffer from marasmus never return to age-appropriate growth standards.

The cornerstone of therapy for marasmus is to supply the body with the necessary **nutritional requirements**. The nutritional needs of children in the rehabilitation stage require at least 150 kilocalories per kilogram per day. **Dehydration** must be addressed with oral rehydration therapy, while **micronutrient** deficiencies, such as vitamin A deficiency, require supplementation. Immunizations must be reviewed and given as necessary to reduce the burden of **infectious diseases** on children's bodies. Finally, family education must be ongoing to improve behavioral responses to such conditions. Some ready-to-use formulas and foods have also been developed. Such a broad approach must be taken to help reduce the **morbidity** and mortality caused by this condition. SEE ALSO CALORIE; INFANT MORTALITY RATE; KWASHIORKOR; MALNUTRITION; PROTEIN.

Seema Pania Kunar

chronic: over a long period

tuberculosis: bacterial infection, usually of the lungs, caused by Mycobacterium tuberculosis

behavioral: related to behavior, in contrast to medical or other types of interventions

subcutaneous: beneath the skin

fat: type of food molecule rich in carbon and hydrogen, with high energy content

nutritional requirements: the set of substances needed in the diet to maintain health

dehydration: loss of water

micronutrient: nutrient needed in very small quantities

infectious diseases: diseases caused by viruses, bacteria, fungi, or protozoa, which replicate inside the body

morbidity: illness or accident

Marketing Strategies

The American Marketing Association defines marketing as "the process of planning and executing the conception, pricing, promotion, and distribution of ideas, goods, and services to create exchanges that satisfy individual and organizational objectives." Marketers use an assortment of strategies to guide how, when, and where product information is presented to consumers. Their goal is to persuade consumers to buy a particular brand or product.

Successful marketing strategies create a desire for a product. A marketer, therefore, needs to understand consumer likes and dislikes. In addition, marketers must know what information will convince consumers to buy their product, and whom consumers perceive as a credible source of information. Some marketing strategies use fictional characters, celebrities, or experts (such as doctors) to sell products, while other strategies use specific statements or "health claims" that state the benefits of using a particular product or eating a particular food.

Impact and Influence

Marketing strategies directly impact food purchasing and eating habits. For example, in the late 1970s scientists announced a possible link between eating a high-fiber **diet** and a reduced risk of **cancer**. However, consumers did not immediately increase their consumption of high-fiber cereals. But in 1984 advertisements claiming a relationship between high-fiber diets and protection against cancer appeared, and by 1987 approximately 2 million households had begun eating high-fiber cereal. Since then, other health claims, supported by scientific studies, have influenced consumers to decrease consumption of foods high in **saturated fat** and to increase consumption of fruits, vegetables, skim milk, poultry, and fish.

Of course, not all marketing campaigns are based on scientific studies, and not all health claims are truthful. In July 2000 a panel of experts from the U.S. Department of Agriculture supported complaints made by the Physicians Committee for Responsible Medicine that the "Got Milk" advertisements contained untruthful health claims that suggested that milk consumption improved sports performance, since these claims lacked scientific

diet: the total daily food intake, or the types of foods eaten

cancer: uncontrolled cell growth

saturated fat: a fat with the maximum possible number of hydrogens; more difficult to break down than unsaturated fats

Companies often use characters to appeal to young consumers. Ronald McDonald first appeared on T.V. in 1963, portrayed by Willard Scott. The clown is known worldwide, and according to McDonald's, is the most recognizable figure next to Santa Claus. *[Photograph by Tim Clary. AP/Wide World Photos. Reproduced by permission.]*

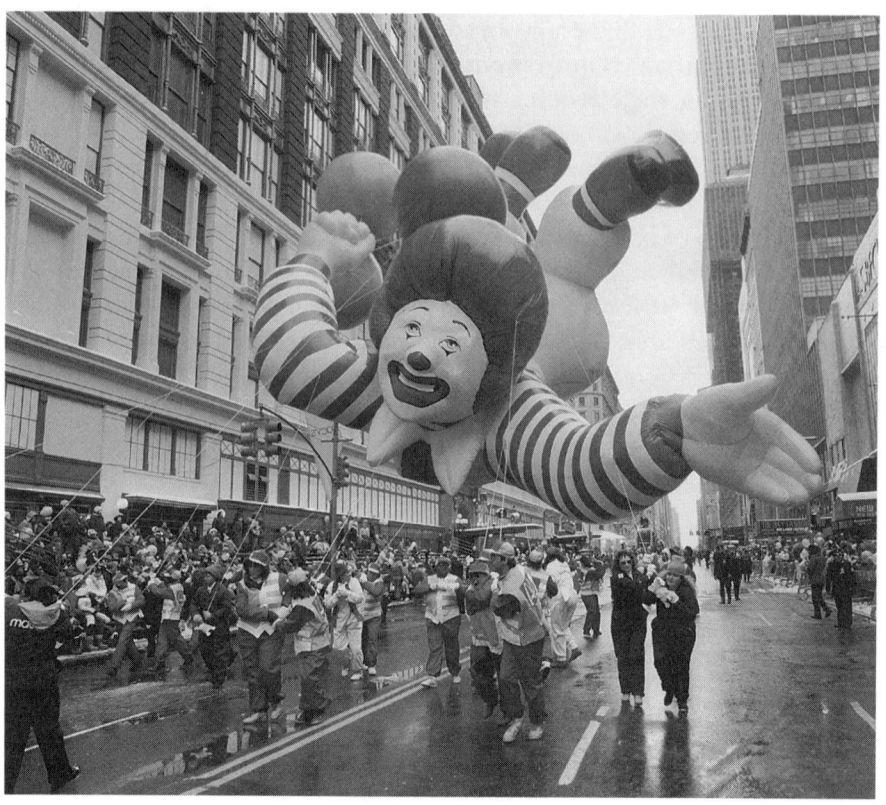

heart disease: any disorder of the heart or its blood supply, including heart attack, atherosclerosis, and coronary artery disease

prostate: male gland surrounding the urethra that contributes fluid to the semen

support. In addition, the panel agreed with the physicians' claim that whole milk consumption may actually increase the risk of **heart disease** and **prostate** cancer, and recommended that this information be included in advertisements.

The tremendous spending power and influence of children on parental purchases has attracted marketers, and, as a result, marketing strategies aimed at children and adolescents have increased. Currently, about one-fourth of all television commercials are related to food, and approximately one-half of these are selling snacks and other foods low in nutritional value. Many of the commercials aimed at children and adolescents use catchy music, jingles, humor, and well-known characters to promote products. The impact of these strategies is illustrated by studies showing that when a majority of television commercials that children view are for high-sugar foods, they are more likely to choose unhealthful foods over nutritious alternatives, and vice versa.

Inappropriate Advertisements

Attempts to sell large quantities of products sometimes cause advertisers to make claims that are not entirely factual. For instance, an advertisement for a particular brand of bread claimed the bread had fewer **calories** per slice than its competitors. What the advertisement did not say was that the bread was sliced much thinner than other brands.

calorie: unit of food energy

Deceptive advertising has also been employed to persuade women to change their infant feeding practices. Advertisers commonly urge mothers to use infant formula to supplement breast milk. Marketing strategies include

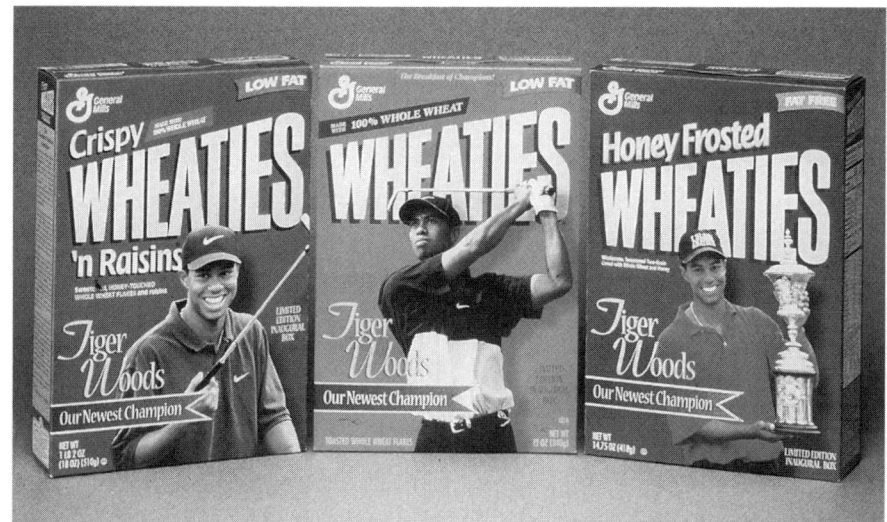

One strategy used by advertisers is to feature a celebrity in their advertisements or on their packaging. The implicit message is that the celebrity endorses the product, uses the product, and may even depend on the product for success. [AP/Wide World Photos. Reproduced by permission.]

giving women trial packs or coupons for several months of free formula. Often, women are not aware that supplementing breast milk with formula will reduce or stop their milk supply. When the samples and coupons are no longer available, women may try to "stretch" the formula by mixing it with water, unaware that diluting the formula places their infant at risk for **malnutrition**. Many groups have objected to the use of marketing strategies that include free formula and coupons, and infant-formula manufacturing companies have been forced to modify their marketing practices.

Other marketing strategies involve labeling foods as "light," meaning that one serving contains about 50 percent less **fat** than the original version (or one-third fewer calories). For example, a serving of light ice cream contains 50 percent less fat than a serving of regular ice cream. As a result, consumers mistakenly believe that eating light food means eating healthful food. However, they fail to realize that a serving of the light version of a food such as ice cream can still contain more fat and sugar than is desirable.

Food labels with conflicting information often confront consumers. For example, labels claiming "no fat" do not necessarily mean zero grams of fat. Food labeling standards define low-fat foods as those containing less than 0.5 gram of fat per serving. Therefore, consuming several servings may mean consuming one or two grams of fat, and people are often unaware of what amount of a food constitutes a "serving." In addition, foods low in fat may be high in sugar, adding additional calories to one's daily caloric intake. Too often, consumers mistakenly translate a claim of "no fat" into one of "no calories."

Other examples of conflicting claims include labels advertising foods as "high in fiber," without specifically indicating the presence of high levels of salt, sugar, or other **nutrients**. Also, labels advertising dairy products as high in **calcium**, and thus offering protection from **osteoporosis**, are often missing information relating to the high fat content and its possible contribution to the risk of heart disease.

Consumers are also misled by food comparisons. For example, one fruit drink may be advertised as containing more vitamin C than another, when in reality neither of the drinks are a good source of the vitamin. In addition,

malnutrition: chronic lack of sufficient nutrients to maintain health

fat: type of food molecule rich in carbon and hydrogen, with high energy content

nutrient: dietary substance necessary for health

calcium: mineral essential for bones and teeth

osteoporosis: weakening of the bone structure

labels on some fruit drinks claim that the product "contains real fruit juice" when, in reality, the fine print reveals that one serving contains "less than 10% fruit juice."

Recommendations for Responsible Food Marketing

Consumers rely on product advertisements and food labels for nutritional education. The American Association of Advertising Agencies states that responsible food marketing strategies should: (1) avoid vague, false, misleading, or exaggerated statements; (2) avoid incomplete or distorted interpretations of claims made by professional or scientific authorities; and (3) avoid unfair product comparisons. Advertisers must also consider the long-term consequences or potential for harm stemming from their claims. While these recommendations are important in developed countries, they become even more critical in international marketing campaigns.

It is also important for consumers to recognize their role in evaluating health claims and product comparisons. While advertisers are aware of the need for truth in advertising, sometimes their desire to sell products overshadows an accurate disclosure of product attributes. Advertisers should bear in mind that inaccurate or vague health claims have the potential to cause economic hardship, illness, and even death. Lastly, marketing strategies used in developing nations should be subjected to the highest standards of truth in advertising. SEE ALSO EATING HABITS; HEALTH CLAIMS.

Virginia Jones Noland

Bibliography

Belch, George E., and Belch, Michael A. (1995). *Introduction to Advertising and Promotion: An Integrated Marketing Communications Perspective*. Boston: Irwin.

Boyle, Marie A., and Morris, Diane H. (1994). *Community Nutrition in Action*. St. Paul, MN: West Publishing.

Chetley, Andrew (1986). *The Politics of Baby Foods: Successful Challenges to an International Marketing Strategy*. New York: St. Martin's.

Connor, John M., et al. (1985). *The Food Manufacturing Industries: Structure, Strategies, Performance, and Policies*. Lexington, KY: D.C. Heath.

Elder, John P. (2001). *Behavior Change and Public Health in the Developing World*. Thousand Oaks, CA: Sage.

EPM Communications (1998). "TV Is the Most-Often-Used Source of Health Information." *Research Alert* 16:7.

Goldberg, Jeanne P., and Hellwig, Jennifer P. (1997). "Nutrition Scientists in the Media: The Challenge Facing Scientists." *Journal of the American College of Nutrition* 16:544–550.

Jeffrey, D. B.; McLellarn, R. W.; and Fox, D. T. (1982). "The Development of Children's Eating Habits: The Role of Television Commercials." *Health Education Quarterly* 9:174–189.

Mathios, Alan D., and Ippolito, Pauline M. (1998). "Food Companies Spread Nutrition Information through Advertising and Labels." *Food Review* 21(2):38–44.

Nestle, Marion. (2000). "Soft Drink 'Pouring Rights': Marketing Empty Calories to Children." *Public Health Reports* 115:308–319.

Sutton, Sharon M.; Balch, George I.; and Lefebvre, Craig (1995). "Strategic Questions for Consumer-Based Health Communications." *Public Health Reports* 110:725–733.

Taras, H. L., et al. (1998). "Television's Influence on Children's Diet and Physical Activity." *Journal of Developmental and Behavioral Pediatrics* 10:176–180.

Taylor, Anna (1998). "Violations of the International Code of Marketing Breast Milk Substitutes: Prevalence in Four Countries." *British Medical Journal* 316:1117–1122.

Internet Resources

Baker, Linda (2000). "Breast-Feeding vs. Formula Feeding: Message in a Bottle." Available from <http://www.zipmall.com/bab-bott.html>

Center for a New American Dream. "Just the Facts About Advertising and Marketing to Children." Available from <http://www.newdream.org/campaign/kids/facts.html>

Infant Feeding Action Coalition (INFACT) Canada (2002). "Infant Foods and Health Claims." Available from <http://www.infactcanada.ca/claimsfall1998.htm>

Medical College of Wisconsin. "Health Claims on Food Labels: What Do They Really Mean?" Available from <http://healthlink.mcw.edu/article/974663611.html>

Optimal Wellness Center (2002). "USDA Confirms Milk Ads Make False Health Claims." Available from <http://www.mercola.com/2001/oct/3/milk_ads.htm>

Mastitis

Mastitis is a common infection among breastfeeding women. The infection causes the breast to become tender, red, and hot. The woman also experiences flu-like symptoms, such as fever, tiredness, and sometimes **nausea** and vomiting. Breast infections can occur when the milk ducts become plugged or when the nipples become cracked. In rare cases, the connective tissues of the breast may become infected.

Mastitis usually affects only one breast, and is treatable with **antibiotics**. Women with mastitis are encouraged to continue to breastfeed, or to pump the milk from both breasts, to prevent the breasts from becoming abscessed. Mastitis is not dangerous to the infant, since the milk is not infected. SEE ALSO BREASTFEEDING.

Delores C. S. James

nausea: unpleasant sensation in the gut that precedes vomiting

antibiotic: substance that kills or prevents the growth of microorganisms

Bibliography

Worthington-Roberts, Bonnie, S., and Rodwell Williams, Sue (1993). *Nutrition in Pregnancy and Lactation*, 6th edition. Madison, WI: Brown & Benchmark.

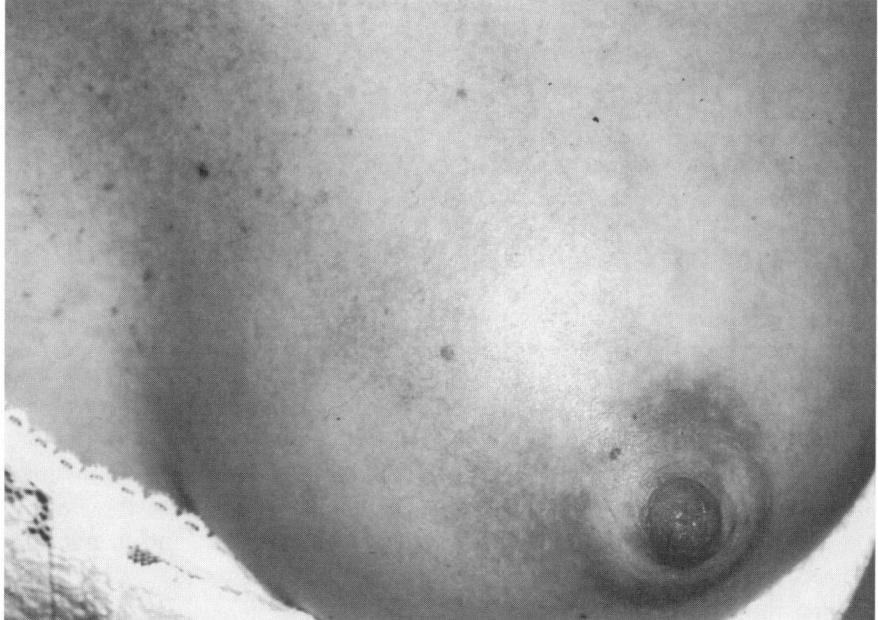

An inflamed, painfully tender breast combined with flu-like symptoms may indicate that a nursing mother has mastitis. Frequent feeding or pumping from the affected breast can help, as can rest and drinking lots of fluids. *[Photograph by Dr. P. Marazzi. Photo Researchers, Inc. Reproduced by permission.]*

Internet Resources

Tilson, Bonnie. "Mastitis." Available from <http://www.lalecheleague.org>

Maternal Mortality Rate

The maternal mortality rate reflects the number of maternal deaths in a population due to both direct obstetric causes and to conditions aggravated by pregnancy or childbirth. The maternal mortality rate in the United States is approximately 7.7 deaths per 100,000 pregnancies.

Research indicates that 88 to 98 percent of all maternal deaths can be prevented. Socioeconomic factors such as poverty, education level, and **malnutrition** have proven to be the underlying causes of most maternal deaths. Maternal mortality rates are substantially less in developed countries (1 in 1,800) than in developing countries (1 in 48), illustrating the impact of **socioeconomic status**. To keep the rates as low as possible, health officials in all nations must advocate for quality health services for all women during pregnancy and childbirth. SEE ALSO INFANT MORTALITY RATE.

Beth Hensleigh

malnutrition: chronic lack of sufficient nutrients to maintain health

socioeconomic status: level of income and social class

Internet Resources

Centers for Disease Control and Prevention. "Maternal Mortality: United States, 1982–1996." Available from <http://www.cdc.gov/epo/mmwr>

World Health Organization. "Reduction of Maternal Mortality. A Joint WHO/UNFPA/UNICEF/World Bank Statement." Available from <http://www.who.int/reproductive-health/publications>

Meals On Wheels

Meals On Wheels is a federal food assistance program aimed at improving the diets and nutritional status of homebound older adults. It is funded under Title III-C of the Older Americans Act (OAA) of 1965. The program provides one hot meal at noon five days a week. Each meal must supply approximately one-third of the recommended **nutrient** intakes. The meal pattern includes three ounces of meat or a meat alternate, two one-half cup portions of fruits and vegetables, one serving of bread, one teaspoon of butter or margarine, eight ounces of milk or a **calcium** equivalent, and one serving of dessert. SEE ALSO AGING AND NUTRITION; NUTRITION PROGRAMS IN THE COMMUNITY.

Beth Fontenot

nutrient: dietary substance necessary for health

calcium: mineral essential for bones and teeth

Meat Analogs

A meat analog is a manufactured food product that looks and tastes like meat. Vegetarians and other health-conscious individuals eat meat analogs because they are relatively high in **protein**. They are also very versatile and can be broiled, baked, or roasted. Soy, wheat **gluten**, beans, and/or nuts are used as the main protein source, with other ingredients used to provide texture and a meat-like taste. Meat analogs can be purchased to replace

protein: complex molecule composed of amino acids that performs vital functions in the cell; necessary part of the diet

gluten: a protein found in wheat

hamburger, steak, chicken, hot dogs, sausage, and many other meat products. SEE ALSO PROTEIN; SOY; VEGETARIANISM.

Lenore S. Hodges
Cheryl Flynt

Internet Resources

American Dietetic Association, Vegetarian Nutrition Practice Group. "Making the Change to a Vegetarian Diet." Available from <http://www.vegetariannutrition.net/articles.htm>

Seventh-day Adventist Dietetic Association. "Meatless Meats." Available from <http://www.sdada.org/meatlessmeats.htm>

Medical Nutrition Therapy

Medical **nutrition** therapy (MNT) is the development and provision of a nutritional treatment or therapy based on a detailed assessment of a person's medical history, psychosocial history, physical examination, and dietary history. It is used to treat an illness or condition, or as a means to prevent or delay disease or complications from diseases such as **diabetes**. The purpose of the assessment is to:

1. Determine the persons' need for therapy
2. Set parameters to plan a therapy
3. Develop a therapy plan
4. Determine the best method to initiate the therapy
5. Evaluate the effectiveness of the therapy

Assessment Components

A medical history includes the assessment of **acute** or **chronic** diseases or conditions, as well as any surgeries a person may have had. Medication and drug or alcohol use should also be determined. The evaluation of interactions between food and medications is included because medications may interfere with **nutrient absorption** or increase the excretion of nutrients. Vitamin, mineral, and **herbal** supplementation can affect nutritional balance, and interactions with medications are also possible. Knowing the types and amounts of any supplements being taken is important both to determine if the supplementation is needed and to determine if too much of a particular nutrient is being used, which might result in an overdose.

A physical examination includes an assessment of sex, age, and **anthropometric** data (measurement of height, weight, **body mass index**, and arm or wrist circumference). The physical appearance of the hair, skin, and nails can assist in identifying **nutritional deficiencies**. For example, spoon-shaped, pale, and brittle fingernails may indicate an **iron** deficiency. **Paralysis** or amputation can affect a persons' ability to eat and increase their risk of certain complications, such as bed sores, which require good nutrition to heal. A person's weight history, such as recent weight changes or rapid weight loss, can be an indicator of a nutritional problem. Knowing if any weight changes were voluntary can affect the direction of a medical nutrition therapy plan.

nutrition: the maintenance of health through proper eating, or the study of same

diabetes: inability to regulate level of sugar in the blood

acute: rapid-onset and short-lived

chronic: over a long period

nutrient: dietary substance necessary for health

absorption: uptake by the digestive tract

herbal: related to plants

anthropometric: related to measurement of characteristics of the human body

body mass index: weight in kilograms divided by square of the height in meters; a measure of body fat

nutritional deficiency: lack of adequate nutrients in the diet

iron: nutrient needed for red blood cell formation

paralysis: inability to move

A psychosocial assessment includes reviewing a person's economic status, ethnic and cultural background, living situation, education level, occupation, mental status, and access to adequate food sources to maintain good health. Each of these components plays a role in determining a person's ability to follow through on specific therapy plans. Handicaps such as mental retardation or blindness may affect a person's ability to prepare meals. The number of people in a household may limit food access or selection if they are on a limited income. In some situations, a recommendation for a change in the person's living situation may be made in order to improve their nutritional health. For example, an elderly person living alone may only eat one meal a day due to limited mobility and low income. Such a person would be a candidate for an **assisted-living** facility, where meals would be provided.

assisted-living: facility that provides aid in meal preparation, cleaning, and other activities to help maintain independent living

diet: the total daily food intake, or the types of foods eaten

fat: type of food molecule rich in carbon and hydrogen, with high energy content

A **diet** history includes an assessment of a person's usual dietary intake. This can be done by using any of the following methods: (1) a food frequency questionnaire, (2) a twenty-four-hour recall of food eaten, or (3) a three- to five-day food diary. Reviewing food preparation methods is helpful in determining the amount of sodium and **fat** in the diet. The frequency of meals eaten out is an important indicator of whether a person enjoys cooking, has access to cooking, or just prefers to eat out instead of cooking. These factors play a role in determining the details of a therapy plan. Other information that is obtained in a diet history includes:

1. Is the appetite level good or poor, and has it changed recently?
2. Have there been any taste alterations? If so, why?
3. Are there any chewing or swallowing difficulties?
4. What are the person's bowel habits and have they changed recently?
5. Are there any religious restrictions on the diet?
6. Are there any food **allergies** or intolerances?

allergy: immune system reaction against substances that are otherwise harmless

Therapy Provision

Medical nutrition therapy is provided by registered dietitians (RDs), who are the only health care professionals with nutrition-specific training. Education includes a bachelor's, master's, or doctoral degree from an accredited university. Required course work is approved by the Commission on Accreditation for Dietetics Education of the American Dietetic Association. After obtaining a degree focused on nutrition and dietetics and completion of a dietetic **internship**, a national credentialing exam is required. The Commission on Dietetic Registration administers the national examination. Registered dietitians must complete continuing education requirements to maintain their registration status. Advanced certifications can also be obtained through additional training and/or experience. The American Dietetic Association, the American Association of Diabetes Educators, and other nutrition-related organizations recognized within the dietetics profession award these certifications. Dietitians are also commonly referred to as nutritionists. Qualified nutritionists should also have the registered dietitian credentials, and many states require registered dietitians and nutritionist to be licensed.

internship: training program

Registered dietitians are employed in many settings, including: hospitals, health clinics, extended-care facilities, physician offices, home-care compa-

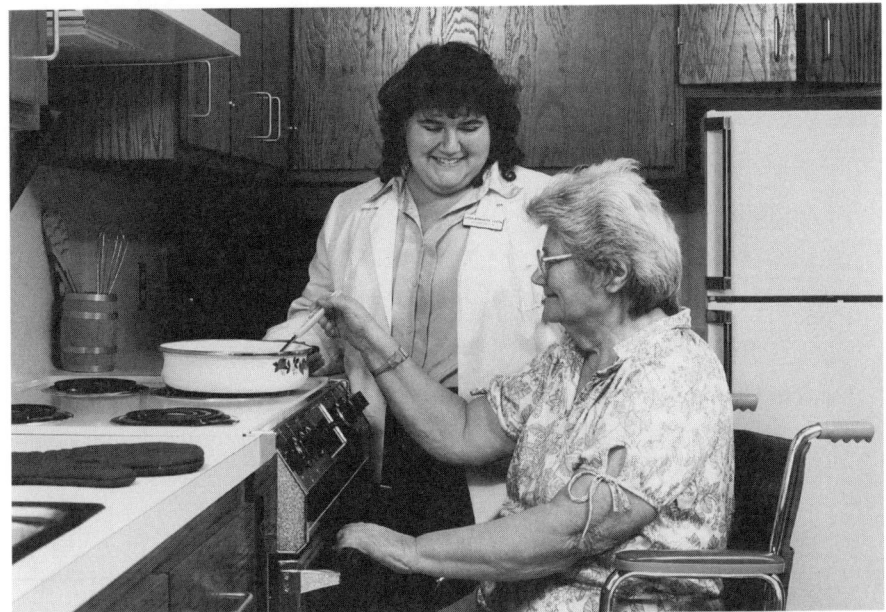

Registered dietitians who apply their expertise to treat illness practice medical nutrition therapy. The therapy may be designed to cure disease or to ensure that a patient's diet does not complicate recovery. In this picture, an RD helps a wheelchair-bound patient prepare a meal. [Royalty-Free/Corbis. Reproduced by permission.]

nies, private practice, community and public health programs, colleges and universities, school food service, state and federal health and nutrition programs, research organizations, and food or pharmaceutical organizations.

Insurance Coverage

Insurance coverage for the cost of MNT is inconsistent across the United States. Some private insurance companies have policies that pay the cost for a person to receive medical nutrition therapy based on protocols developed by the American Dietetic Association. Other companies leave the coverage to the discretion of a case manager or physician, while some refuse to provide reimbursement for any nutrition therapy.

Some U.S. states have laws that mandate that insurance companies provide coverage for MNT. Some of these states limit coverage to diabetes, while others include a wider range of diseases. In January 2002, the Medicare program began providing MNT coverage for persons with diabetes and **pre-renal** disease. (Medicare is a federal health insurance program for those over the age of sixty-five, those under sixty-five with certain disabilities, and for people with permanent kidney failure.) Congress is considering inclusion of other diagnoses, such as **cardiovascular** disease. This would expand the provision of MNT to those persons with coronary **artery** disease, congestive heart failure, and **hypertension**. Diabetes self-management training is a Medicare-covered benefit that includes MNT and education on issues such as blood **glucose** monitoring, disease complications, and prevention. Internationally, the cost of nutrition therapy is sometimes covered by a national health care system, or by a private system similar to that in the United States.

Medical Nutrition Therapy is physician directed. This means a person's primary care physician makes a referral to a registered dietitian for therapy. Many insurance carriers and state licensure laws require this referral to document the medical necessity of the therapy.

The expansion of insurance coverage for MNT by Medicare and private providers is vital to improving access to this type of care. Rising health

pre-renal: kidney disease caused by change in the blood supply to the kidney

cardiovascular: related to the heart and circulatory system

artery: blood vessel that carry blood away from the heart toward the body tissues

hypertension: high blood pressure

glucose: a simple sugar; the most commonly used fuel in cells

care costs and limited incomes often force choices between food and health care. Medical nutrition therapy has been shown to reduce health care cost for individuals, employers, hospitals, and insurance carriers. SEE ALSO DIETITIAN; NUTRITIONAL ASSESSMENT.

Mindy Benedict

Bibliography

American Dietetic Association (2000). *Manual of Clinical Dietetics*, 6th ed. Chicago, IL: Author.

Florida Dietetic Association (2002). *The Florida Dietetic Association Handbook of Medical Nutrition Therapy: The Florida Diet Manual*. Tallahassee, FL: Author.

Internet Resources

American Dietetic Association. "Medicare MNT Benefit Provider Information." Available from <http://www.eatright.org>

Mellanby, Edward
British physician
1884–1955

The British physician and pharmacologist Sir Edward Mellanby was born in West Hartlepool, England, the youngest son of John Mellanby, a shipyard owner, and his wife Mary Isabella Lawson. Mellanby attended Barnard Castle School and Emmanuel College in Cambridge, England, where he studied **physiology**. After working as a research student from 1905 to 1907, Mellanby studied medicine at St. Thomas's Hospital in London, and he held a fellowship for medical research from 1910 through 1912. He was married in 1914 to May Tweedy, of London, who was also a researcher in physiology. The following year Mellanby became a medical doctor.

From 1913 to 1920, Mellanby served as a lecturer at King's College for Women in London, where he later became a professor in physiology. In 1914, the Medical Research Committee of the college asked Mellanby to investigate the cause of **rickets**, a bone disease characterized by bone pain, skeletal deformity, impaired growth, and weakness.

Searching for a dietary deficiency that caused rickets, Mellanby decided to test porridge, the staple food of Scotland, by feeding a group of dogs a **diet** consisting exclusively of oats. Inadvertently, the dogs were kept indoors, without exposure to sunlight, during the experiment. In 1919, Mellanby reported that he produced rickets in the dogs through the restrictive diet. He then cured the dogs of rickets by adding cod-liver oil to their diet. Mellanby concluded that a component of cod-liver oil that the oats did not contain was essential in preventing rickets.

As a result, Mellanby proposed that rickets was caused by the absence of a dietary factor.

Scientists would later discover that rickets is prevented by **vitamin D**, which can either be consumed as a dietary factor or produced naturally by the body when exposed to sunlight. Mellanby's work laid the foundation for this conclusion, since the cod-liver oil fed to the dogs was a good source of vitamin D and the dogs were raised without exposure to sunlight.

---

physiology: the group of biochemical and physical processes that combine to make a functioning organism, or the study of same

rickets: disorder caused by vitamin D deficiency, marked by soft and misshapen bones and organ swelling

diet: the total daily food intake, or the types of foods eaten

vitamin D: nutrient needed for calcium uptake and therefore proper bone formation

In 1920, Mellanby was appointed chair of the pharmacology department at the University of Sheffield in England, and as an honorary physician to the Royal Infirmary. He held these positions until 1933, when he became secretary of the Medical Research Council, which had been established by the British government in 1913. He was closely involved with the planning of the new Institute of Medical Research, which opened in 1950 in London.

During World War II, Mellanby was involved with programs to create a wartime diet as well as programs to promote the welfare of both military and civilian personnel. After retiring from the Medical Research Council in 1949, he traveled to India, Australia, and New Zealand to serve as an advisor. After his return to England, he gave several public lectures. Mellanby died on January 30, 1955, while working in his London laboratory. SEE ALSO RICKETS.

Karen Bryla

Bibliography
Oxbury, Harold (1985). *Great Britons: Twentieth-Century Lives.* Oxford, England: Oxford University Press.

Internet Resources
National Academy of Sciences. "Unraveling the Enigma of Vitamin D: Closing in on Rickets." Available from <http://beyonddiscovery.org>

University of California, Riverside. "History of Vitamin D." Available from <http://vitamind.ucr.edu/history.html>

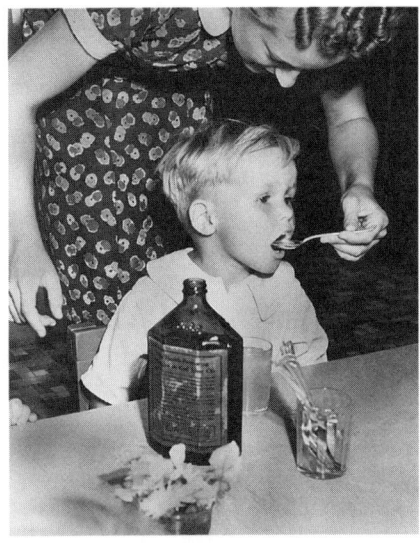

Research conducted by Sir Edward Mellanby led to the discovery that rickets is a disease of malnutrition, curable with regular doses of cod-liver oil. Scientists later determined that the condition is a result of vitamin D deficiency.
[Bettmann/Corbis. Reproduced by permission.]

Menopause

Young girls start menstruating between the ages of eleven and thirteen, when their reproductive systems reach maturity. Women have regular **menstrual cycles** every twenty-eight days until about the age of fifty, at which time menstruation becomes irregular. This irregularity signals the start of **menopause**. The natural cessation of menstruation occurs due to reduced production of the female **hormones estrogen** and progesterone, which generally occurs between the ages of forty and fifty-five. The age at which a woman enters menopause is affected by **genetics**, race, and environmental factors. Women can also go into premature menopause, either naturally or due to oophorectomy (the surgical removal of the ovaries).

Stages of Menopause

Women go through different phases of menopause, including perimenopausal, **menopausal**, and postmenopausal periods. During the perimenopausal period, the regular cyclical occurrence of menstruation is disrupted and menstruation becomes irregular. This phase may last anywhere from six months to a year. During the perimenopausal period, production of estrogen is reduced, and eventually stops. Menopause is defined as the cessation of the menstrual period. Women are described as postmenopausal when they have gone one year without a menstrual period.

Physiological Changes

The lack of estrogen and progesterone causes many changes in women's **physiology** that affect their health and well-being. These changes include:

menstrual cycles: the build-up and sloughing off of the lining of the uterus in women commencing at puberty and proceeding until menopause

menopause: phase in a woman's life during which ovulation and menstruation end

hormone: molecules produced by one set of cells that influence the function of another set of cells

estrogen: hormone that helps control female development and menstruation

genetics: inheritance through genes

menopausal: related to menopause, the period during which women cease to ovulate and menstruate

physiology: the group of biochemical and physical processes that combine to make a functioning organism, or the study of same

cholesterol: multi-ringed molecule found in animal cell membranes; a type of lipid

coronary heart disease: disease of the coronary arteries, the blood vessels surrounding the heart

calcium: mineral essential for bones and teeth

osteoporosis: weakening of the bone structure

basal metabolism: level of body energy consumption and chemical processes in the absence of exertion

cardiovascular: related to the heart and circulatory system

fatigue: tiredness

anxiety: nervousness

cancer: uncontrolled cell growth

aerobic: designed to maintain adequate oxygen in the bloodstream

phytoestrogen: plant-derived estrogen compound

legumes: beans, peas, and related plants

- Elevated levels of total **cholesterol** and LDL-cholesterol, which increases the risk of **coronary heart disease** (CHD) in women. During the reproductive years, estrogen prevents increased levels of blood cholesterol and maintains the activity of estrogen receptors in women, thus preventing the risk of CHD.

- **Calcium** loss from the bones is increased in the first five years after the onset of menopause, resulting in a loss of bone density. This bone loss then tapers off until about the age of seventy-five, when calcium loss accelerates again. This predisposes women to the risk of **osteoporosis** and bone fractures.

- The body composition of menopausal women also changes, with the percentage of body fat increasing and muscle mass decreasing. The increase in body-fat percentage is believed to be partly due to decreased physical activity.

- Decreased muscle mass reduces the rate of **basal metabolism**, which may be responsible for weight gain at this period of a woman's life.

- The abdominal-fat storage that occurs in women at this stage increases the risk for **cardiovascular** disease.

- The tissues in the urinary tract and reproductive organs atrophy.

Some other transient but unpleasant symptoms of menopause include hot flashes, **fatigue**, **anxiety**, sleep disturbance, and memory loss.

Treatments and Remedies: Benefits and Disadvantages of Each

Menopausal women are faced with many choices in terms of treatment or remedies for these problems. Some of the treatment choices are experimentally proven to be effective and relatively harmless, while other options such as herbs, teas, and dietary supplements have not been subjected to scientific experimentation and have not been proven to be without harm.

Estrogen replacement therapy (ERT) is the often-used medically prescribed treatment for menopausal and postmenopausal women. Although some studies have indicated a decreased risk of CHD and osteoporosis with ERT use, others have indicated it may increase the risk of breast **cancer**. The Women's Health Initiative, which was designed to study the effects of ERT on the health of elderly women, stopped the ERT part of the research in July 2002. The preliminary result of that study showed the risk of CHD was, in fact, increased in women on ERT.

Scientific investigations have shown that physical activity, including **aerobic** and muscular strengthening exercises, not only prevent bone mineral loss, they also help alleviate many menopausal symptoms, including the increased percentage of body fat, abdominal-fat storage, hot flashes, fatigue, and sleep disturbances.

Phytoestrogens, which are present in foods such as soy, red clover, flaxseed, and other beans and **legumes**, are natural plant estrogen-type chemicals that can help replace human estrogen without some of the risk factors of ERT. Epidemiological observations indicate that in some cultures where soy is a staple food, women do not suffer from hot flashes during and

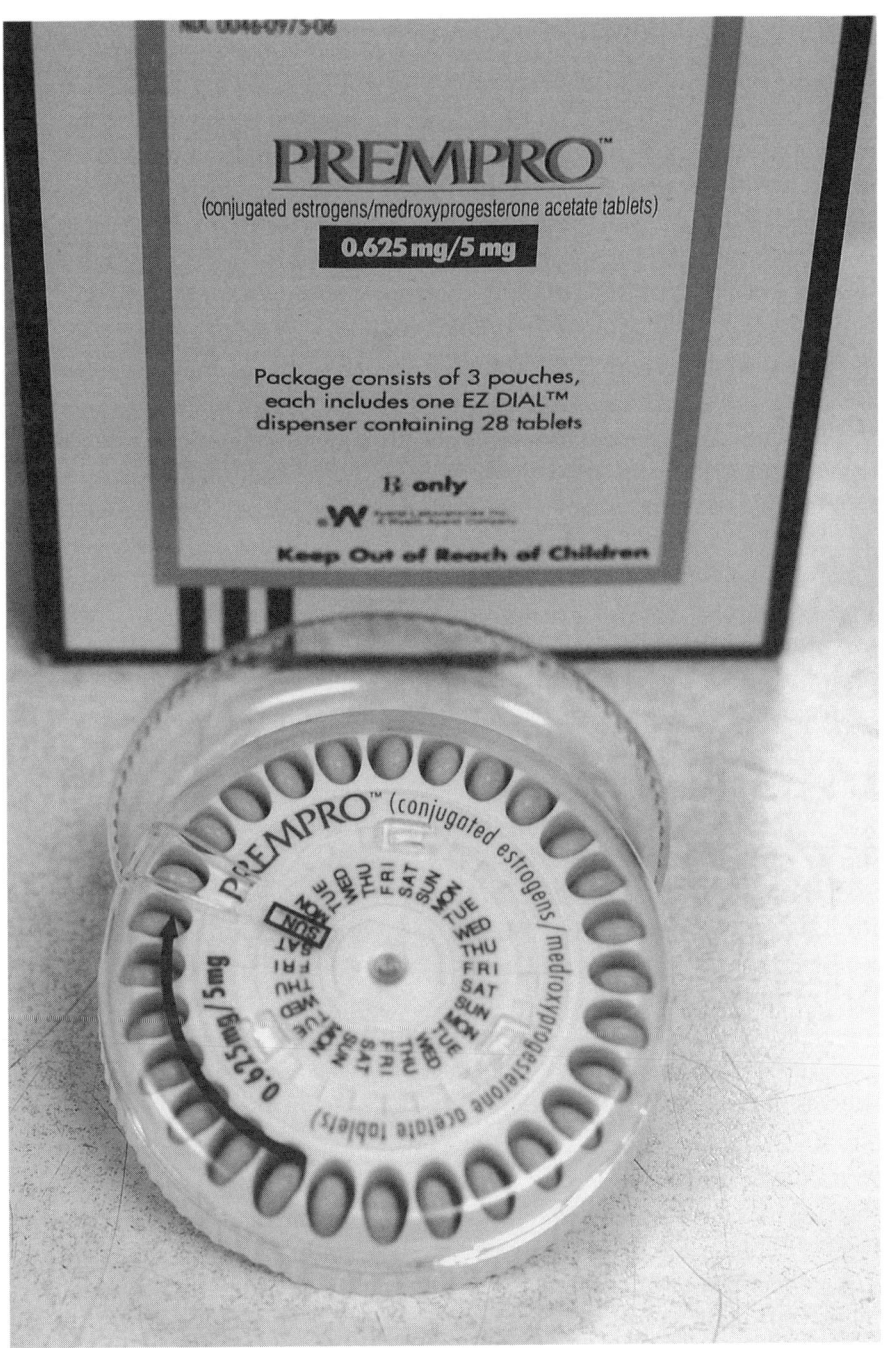

Hormone replacement pills are used by some women to reduce the symptoms of menopause. According to the Women's Health Initiative, women who use a combination of estrogen and the synthetic hormone progestin increase their risk of developing breast cancer and heart disease. [Stephen Chernin/Getty Images. Reproduced by permission.]

after menopause. The results of human experiments designed to study the effect of soy products on alleviating symptoms during menopause are new and inconsistent, but promising. In addition, the **isoflavones** in soy products are strong **antioxidants** and may be effective in reducing the risk of CHD in women of menopausal age.

Herbal supplements promoted by the supplement industry to prevent hot flashes, anxiety, sleep disturbances, and other symptoms of menopause have not been scientifically studied, and since the chemical composition of these supplements is not always known, they may contain harmful substances. Thus, these kinds of supplements are not generally recommended for menopausal women.

isoflavones: estrogen-like compounds in plants

antioxidant: substance that prevents oxidation, a damaging reaction with oxygen

herbal: related to plants

Dietary and Lifestyle Changes

Recommendations for dietary and lifestyle changes for women during menopause are a little different from that for women in general. Menopausal women need to eat less of foods that are high in **iron**. Because they are not menstruating, their requirement for iron is reduced, and is thus the same as for men, about 10 milligrams per day. This means that they need to cut down on red meat, organ meats such as liver and kidney, and other foods high in iron. If they are taking multivitamin and mineral supplements, ones with a low iron content are recommended.

Water intake is emphasized in older women and men, since the thirst sensation becomes dulled as people age. Six to eight glasses of fluid per day are recommended for this age group. Water, fruit juices, other nonalcoholic beverages, and fresh fruits can help provide variety in fluid intake. In addition, an increased consumption of legumes (e.g., dried chick peas, varieties of beans, lentils, soy and soy products) is recommended to provide phytoestrogens and isoflavones. There are other alternatives that are used by people around the world to reduce hot flashes and other symptoms of menopause, including herbs such as ginseng, black cohash, kava, and wild yam. However, there has been little scientific data to determine the effectiveness and safety of these supplements.

Menopausal women need to decrease their intake of total fat, **saturated fat**, and total **calories** to balance their **energy** expenditure and prevent weight gain, which is sometimes associated with this period in a women's life. It is believed that, on average, women gain about 1.2 pounds a year, with most of the weight gain in the form of abdominal fat. A study done in the 1990s found that a modest weight reduction program in premenopausal women, including **diet** and exercise, produced modest weight loss and favorable blood lipid changes that lasted five years through the women's menopausal period. This study (Simkin-Silverman et al.) proved that weight gain during menopause is not only related to hormonal changes, but also to decreased level of physical activity.

A woman's intake of dietary **fiber** must be increased during menopause to prevent **constipation**. This objective can be accomplished by following the Dietary Guidelines for Americans, which recommend consuming six servings of whole grains and cereals, three to five servings of vegetables, and two to four servings of fruit per day. Exercise is also very important for all older individuals. Thirty minutes of moderate daily exercise, such as speed walking, is recommended. Other exercises, such as flexibility and strength training to maintain lean muscle mass and bone density, can be very helpful if done two to three times a week. SEE ALSO WOMEN'S NUTRITIONAL ISSUES.

Simin Vaghefi

iron: nutrient needed for red blood cell formation

saturated fat: a fat with the maximum possible number of hydrogens; more difficult to break down than unsaturated fats

calorie: unit of food energy

energy: technically, the ability to perform work; the content of a substance that allows it to be useful as a fuel

diet: the total daily food intake, or the types of foods eaten

fiber: indigestible plant material which aids digestion by providing bulk

constipation: difficulty passing feces

Bibliography

Nelson, M. E.; Fiatrone, M. A.; Morganti, C. N. M.; et al. (1994). "Effects of High-Intensity Strength Training on Multiple Risk Factors for Osteoporotic Fractures." *Journal of the American Medical Association* 272:1909–1914.

Simkin-Silverman, L.; Wing, R. R.; Hansen, D. H.; et al. (1995). "Prevention of Cardiovascular Risk Factor Elevations in Healthy Premenopausal Women." *Preventive Medicine* 24:509–517.

Internet Resources

Women's Health Initiative. "Findings from the Women's Health Initiative." Available from <http://www.nhlbi.nih.gov/whi>

Men's Nutritional Issues

While many diseases and health care issues affect both men and women, certain diseases and conditions exhibited in men may require distinct approaches regarding diagnosis and management. Some of the major issues associated with men's health are related to **cancer**, **diabetes**, **heart disease**, **hypertension**, impotence, and **prostate** health. This entry highlights definitions, **etiology**, treatment, and **lifestyle** factors of men's health, as well as nutritional implications.

Cancer

Cancer is characterized as aberrant and uncontrolled cell growth. Cells divide more rapidly than normal, and these growths may metastasize (spread to other organs). It affects people of all ages and can attack any organ or tissue of the body. Some cancers are more responsive to treatment and lend themselves to a cure, while others seem to appear suddenly and resist treatment.

Much of what we know from nutritional epidemiology supports the role of **diet** as a means of staving off cancer. Particularly, a mostly plant-based diet—one high in fruits, vegetables, and whole grains—is the key. Men should aim for five to nine servings of fruits and vegetables daily and eat breads, cereals, and grains that are high in **fiber**, such as whole wheat bread, bran flakes, brown rice, and quinoa.

Apart from diet, the most important thing a man can do to reduce his cancer risk is stop smoking and cease using all tobacco products. Smoking is the number one preventable cause of death in the United States, claiming 400,000 lives per year, and it increases the risk for developing cancer. **Genetics** and environmental sources (e.g., ultraviolet light) are also linked with cancer.

Diabetes Mellitus

Carbohydrate intolerance—the inability to properly **metabolize** sugars—is known as diabetes mellitus, often just shortened to diabetes. The pancreas makes **insulin**, a **hormone** responsible for a cell's uptake of **glucose** (sugar) from blood for **energy**. People who have diabetes do not make enough insulin, or else the body cannot use what is made. Treatment includes achieving a healthy weight, engaging in exercise, and prescription medication. Sometimes people are able to cure their diabetes with diet and weight loss.

A proper diet for people with diabetes is comparable to what the average healthy person should already be eating. Basic tenets include: eat three meals daily, incorporate healthful snacks, focus on foods high in fiber, combine **protein** and carbohydrates with moderate amounts of unsaturated fat, and avoid sugar-sweetened beverages to reduce overall caloric intake.

Heart Disease

Heart disease, or coronary **artery** disease, is a result of improper function of the heart and blood vessels. There are many forms of heart disease. **Atherosclerosis** (hardening of the arteries) and hypertension (**high blood pressure**) are two of the most common. Fat deposits disrupt the flow of blood to the heart muscle, increasing the risk of myocardial infarction (**heart attack**).

---

cancer: uncontrolled cell growth

diabetes: inability to regulate level of sugar in the blood

heart disease: any disorder of the heart or its blood supply, including heart attack, atherosclerosis, and coronary artery disease

hypertension: high blood pressure

prostate: male gland surrounding the urethra that contributes fluid to the semen

etiology: origin and development of a disease

lifestyle: set of choices about diet, exercise, job type, leisure activities, and other aspects of life

diet: the total daily food intake, or the types of foods eaten

fiber: indigestible plant material which aids digestion by providing bulk

genetics: inheritance through genes

carbohydrate: food molecule made of carbon, hydrogen, and oxygen, including sugars and starches

metabolize: processing of a nutrient

insulin: hormone released by the pancreas to regulate level of sugar in the blood

hormone: molecules produced by one set of cells that influence the function of another set of cells

glucose: a simple sugar; the most commonly used fuel in cells

energy: technically, the ability to perform work; the content of a substance that allows it to be useful as a fuel

protein: complex molecule composed of amino acids that performs vital functions in the cell; necessary part of the diet

artery: blood vessel that carries blood away from the heart toward the body tissues

atherosclerosis: build-up of deposits within the blood vessels

high blood pressure: elevation of the pressure in the bloodstream maintained by the heart

heart attack: loss of blood supply to part of the heart, resulting in death of heart muscle

According to the National Cancer Institute, men are approximately 1.5 times as likely as women to develop colorectal cancer or heart disease. Both diseases may be prevented by eating well. The convenience and economic appeal of fast foods, such as hot dogs, can lead to poor dietary habits. *[Royalty-Free/Corbis. Reproduced by permission.]*

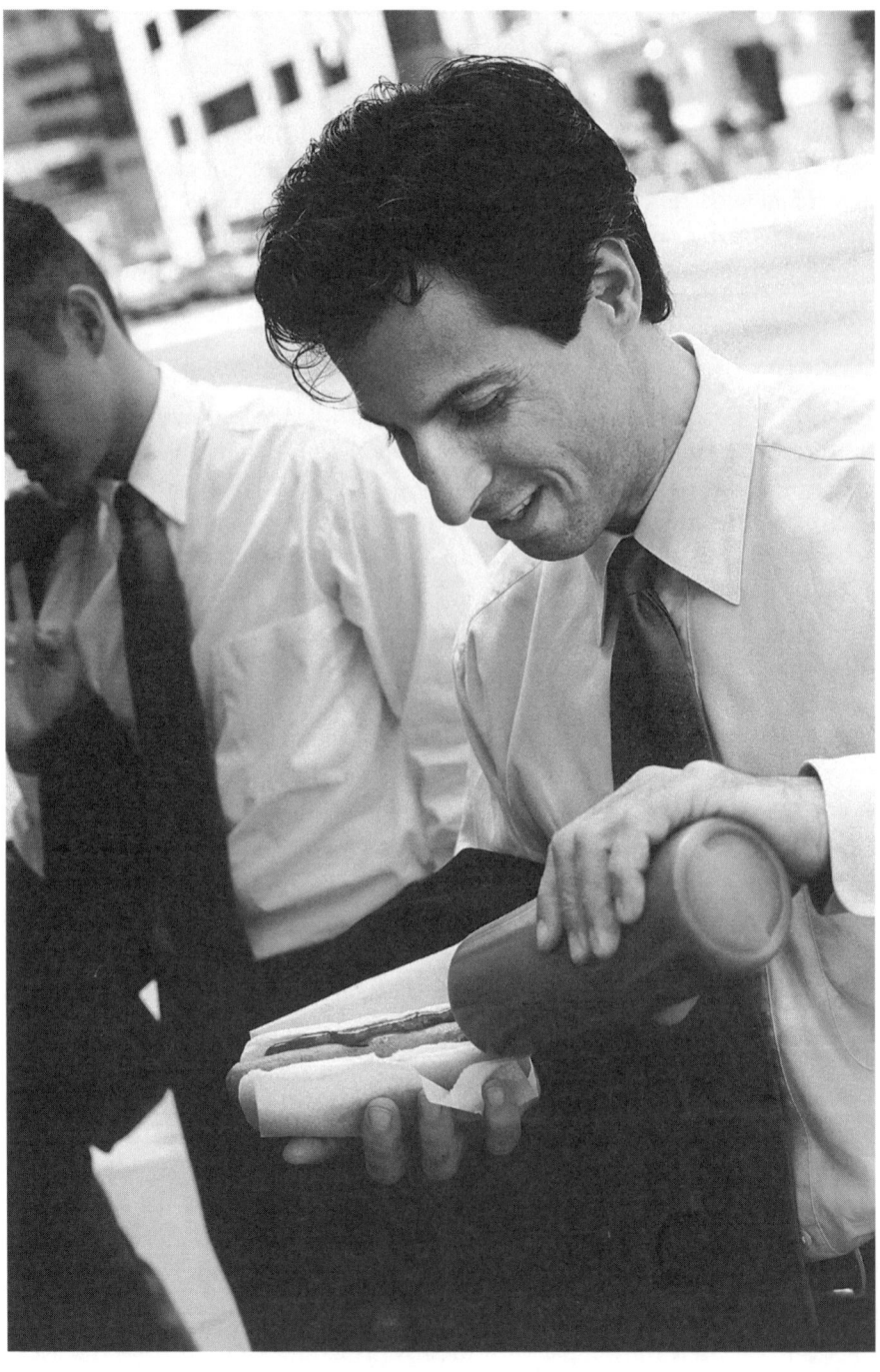

HDL: high density lipoprotein, a blood protein that carries cholesterol

cholesterol: multi-ringed molecule found in animal cell membranes; a type of lipid

Heart disease is the number one cause of death for men. According to the American Heart Association, 440,175 men died of heart disease in 2000. Apart from just being male, other risk factors are being forty-five years of age and older, low levels of high-density lipoprotein (**HDL**—the "good" **cholesterol**), high levels of low-density lipoprotein (LDL—the "bad" cholesterol), hypertension, smoking, excess body fat, diabetes, and a family history of heart disease.

The most important thing men should do to prevent heart disease is stop smoking and manage their weight. In terms of diet, dietitians recommend that men include more lean and healthier protein foods in their diets—such as white meat chicken and turkey, and sirloin instead of filet mignon. Additionally, eating fatty fish (e.g., salmon or mackerel) twice a week may have a cardioprotective effect. Baking and broiling are preferred over deep fat frying.

Hypertension

The Centers for Disease Control and Prevention (CDC) reports that 64 percent of men seventy-five and older have hypertension (high blood pressure), and African Americans are at a greater risk. Termed the "silent killer," hypertension often has no physical symptoms. Men often feel well enough to function normally in their day-to-days lives, and they do not view the risk as a serious one.

Being **obese** is associated with hypertension. Losing weight helps to control **blood pressure**, and sometimes men are able to decrease or discontinue their medication if their physicians determine it is no longer needed. Getting men to move away from large portions of fatty meat and potatoes and more toward three ounces of meat on a plate of overflowing vegetables is one sure method to help prevent **overweight** and manage hypertension. Additionally, some men are sensitive to dietary salt (sodium chloride). Eating too much salt can cause the body to retain water, resulting in increased blood pressure. **Processed foods** tend to be high in salt.

obese: above accepted standards of weight for sex, height, and age

blood pressure: measure of the pressure exerted by the blood against the walls of the blood vessels

overweight: weight above the accepted norm based on height, sex, and age

processed food: food that has been cooked, milled, or otherwise manipulated to change its quality

Impotence

Impotence, also known as erectile dysfunction, occurs when a man cannot maintain an erection to achieve orgasm in sexual intercourse. The National Institutes of Health report that 15 to 30 million American men have erectile dysfunction. Many things can prevent normal erection, including **psychological** interference, **neurological** problems, abnormal blood flow, and prescription medications. Certain health conditions, such as diabetes and heart disease, cause men to experience impotence as well. Treatment may consist of psychotherapy, prescription medication, and surgery.

psychological: related to thoughts, feelings, and personal experiences

neurological: related to the nervous system

Prostate Health

A small gland surrounding the urethra, the prostate supplies fluid that transports semen. The CDC reports that 31,078 men died of prostate cancer in 2000. Signs of prostate trouble are hesitant urination, weak urine flow and dribbling, and incontinence (inability to control urinary bladder). **Nutrition** may play a role in prostate health. Besides eating a varied diet focused on overall moderation, researchers have shown benefits from lycopene, a **phytochemical** (plant chemical) that gives plants a red color. Foods containing lycopene include processed tomato products, watermelon, and pink or red grapefruit.

nutrition: the maintenance of health through proper eating, or the study of same

phytochemical: chemical produced by plants

Conclusion

Nutrition impacts health. Eating a good diet promotes **wellness** and disease prevention for healthy men, and sound nutrition helps manage **chronic** diseases as well. Men often fall short of achieving a healthful diet due to busy work schedules, fear of or disinterest in cooking, and the stresses of daily living. Simple steps to improve time management and a willingness for experimentation in the kitchen are both reasonable suggestions to help men eat more healthful meals.

wellness: related to health promotion

chronic: over a long period

Apart from nutritious meals, men should visit their physicians regularly, both for checkups and to discuss the health implications of nutritional supplements (protein powder, vitamin E, etc.). Routine physical exams, including blood tests for cholesterol, blood pressure measurements, and cancer screenings, help identify problems early, which can dramatically improve outcomes. In addition, sixty minutes of exercise daily helps weight management. SEE ALSO ADULT NUTRITION; CANCER; DIABETES MELLITUS; HEART DISEASE; HYPERTENSION.

D. Milton Stokes

Bibliography

American Heart Association (2002). *Heart Disease and Stroke Statistics: 2003 Update.* Dallas, TX.: Author.

Perry, Angela, and Schacht, Marck, eds. (2001). *American Medical Association Complete Guide to Men's Health.* New York: Wiley.

Reichler, Gayle (1998). *Active Wellness.* New York: Time-Life Books.

Internet Resources

American Dietetic Association. <http://www.eatright.org>

Centers for Disease Control and Prevention, National Center for Health Statistics. "Fast Stats A to Z: Heart Disease." Available from <http://www.cdc.gov/nchs/fastats>

Centers for Disease Control and Prevention, National Center for Health Statistics. "Fast Stats A to Z: Prostate Disease." Available from <http://www.cdc.gov/nchs/fastats>

National Institute of Diabetes and Digestive and Kidney Diseases. "Erectile Dysfunction." Available from <http://www.niddk.nih.gov/health/>

Metabolism

metabolism: the sum total of reactions in a cell or an organism

catabolism: breakdown of complex molecules

carbohydrate: food molecule made of carbon, hydrogen, and oxygen, including sugars and starches

protein: complex molecule composed of amino acids that performs vital functions in the cell; necessary part of the diet

energy: technically, the ability to perform work; the content of a substance that allows it to be useful as a fuel

physiological: related to the biochemical processes of the body

metabolic: related to processing of nutrients and building of necessary molecules within the cell

oxygen: O_2, atmospheric gas required by all animals

atoms: fundamental particles of matter

glucose: a simple sugar; the most commonly used fuel in cells

mucosa: moist exchange surface within the body

glycogen: storage form of sugar

fat: type of food molecule rich in carbon and hydrogen, with high energy content

amino acid: building block of proteins, necessary dietary nutrient

biological: related to living organisms

diabetes: inability to regulate level of sugar in the blood

adipose tissue: tissue containing fat deposits

hormone: molecules produced by one set of cells that influence the function of another set of cells

insulin: hormone released by the pancreas to regulate level of sugar in the blood

Metabolism refers to the physical and chemical processes that occur inside the cells of the body and that maintain life. Metabolism consists of anabolism (the constructive phase) and **catabolism** (the destructive phase, in which complex materials are broken down). The transformation of the macronutrients **carbohydrates**, fats, and **proteins** in food to **energy**, and other **physiological** processes are parts of the **metabolic** process. ATP (adinosene triphosphate) is the major form of energy used for cellular metabolism.

Carbohydrate Metabolism

Carbohydrates made up of carbon, hydrogen, and **oxygen atoms** are classified as mono-, di-, and polysaccharides, depending on the number of sugar units they contain. The monosaccharides—**glucose**, galactose, and fructose—obtained from the digestion of food are transported from the intestinal **mucosa** via the portal vein to the liver. They may be utilized directly for energy by all tissues; temporarily stored as **glycogen** in the liver or in muscle; or converted to **fat**, **amino acids**, and other **biological** compounds.

Carbohydrate metabolism plays an important role in both types of **diabetes** mellitus. The entry of glucose into most tissues—including heart, muscle, and **adipose tissue**—is dependent upon the presence of the **hormone insulin**. Insulin controls the uptake and metabolism of glucose in these cells and plays a major role in regulating the blood glucose concentration. The reactions of carbohydrate metabolism cannot take place without the presence of the **B vitamins**, which function as coenzymes. Phosphorous, magnesium, **iron**, copper, manganese, **zinc** and chromium are also necessary as cofactors.

Carbohydrate metabolism begins with *glycolysis*, which releases energy from glucose or glycogen to form two **molecules** of pyruvate, which enter the **Krebs cycle** (or citric acid cycle), an oxygen-requiring process, through which they are completely oxidized. Before the Krebs cycle can begin, pyruvate loses a carbon dioxide group to form acetyl coenzyme A (acetyl-CoA). This reaction is irreversible and has important metabolic consequences. The conversion of pyruvate to acetyl-CoA requires the B vitamins.

The hydrogen in carbohydrate is carried to the electron transport chain, where the energy is conserved in ATP molecules. Metabolism of one molecule of glucose yields thirty-one molecules of ATP. The energy released from ATP through hydrolysis (a chemical reaction with water) can then be used for biological work.

Only a few cells, such as liver and kidney cells, can produce their own glucose from amino acids, and only liver and muscle cells store glucose in the form of glycogen. Other body cells must obtain glucose from the bloodstream.

Under **anaerobic** conditions, lactate is formed from pyruvate. This reaction is important in the muscle when energy demands exceed oxygen supply. Glycolysis occurs in the cytosol (fluid portion) of a cell and has a dual role. It degrades monosaccharides to generate energy, and it provides **glycerol** for **triglyceride** synthesis. The Krebs cycle and the electron transport chain occur in the **mitochondria**. Most of the energy derived from carbohydrate, protein, and fat is produced via the Krebs cycle and the electron transport system.

Glycogenesis is the conversion of excess glucose to glycogen. *Glycogenolysis* is the conversion of glycogen to glucose (which could occur several hours after a meal or overnight) in the liver or, in the absence of glucose-6-phosphate in the muscle, to lactate. *Gluconeogenesis* is the formation of glucose from noncarbohydrate sources, such as certain amino acids and the glycerol fraction of fats when carbohydrate intake is limited. Liver is the main site for gluconeogenesis, except during starvation, when the kidney becomes important in the process. Disorders of carbohydrate metabolism include diabetes mellitus, **lactose intolerance**, and **galactosemia**.

Protein Metabolism

Proteins contain carbon, hydrogen, oxygen, **nitrogen**, and sometimes other atoms. They form the cellular structural elements, are **biochemical** catalysts, and are important regulators of **gene expression**. Nitrogen is essential to the formation of twenty different amino acids, the building blocks of all body cells. Amino acids are characterized by the presence of a terminal carboxyl group and an amino group in the alpha position, and they are connected by peptide bonds.

Digestion breaks protein down to amino acids. If amino acids are in excess of the body's biological requirements, they are metabolized to glycogen or fat and subsequently used for energy metabolism. If amino acids are to be used for energy their carbon skeletons are converted to acetyl CoA,

B vitamins: a group of vitamins important in cell energy processes

iron: nutrient needed for red blood cell formation

zinc: mineral necessary for many enzyme processes

glycolysis: cellular reaction that begins the breakdown of sugars

molecule: combination of atoms that form stable particles

Krebs cycle: cellular reaction that breaks down numerous nutrients and provides building blocks for other molecules

anaerobic: without air, or oxygen

glycerol: simple molecule that forms a portion of fats

triglyceride: a type of fat

mitochondria: small bodies within a cell that harvest energy for use by the cell

lactose intolerance: inability to digest lactose, or milk sugar

galactosemia: inherited disorder preventing digestion of milk sugar, galactose

nitrogen: essential element for plant growth

biochemical: related to chemical processes within cells

gene expression: use of a gene to make the protein it encodes

which enters the Krebs cycle for oxidation, producing ATP. The final products of protein catabolism include carbon dioxide, water, ATP, urea, and ammonia.

Vitamin B_6 is involved in the metabolism (especially catabolism) of amino acids, as a cofactor in transamination reactions that transfer the nitrogen from one keto acid (an acid containing a keto group [-CO-] in addition to the acid group) to another. This is the last step in the synthesis of nonessential amino acids and the first step in amino acid catabolism. Transamination converts amino acids to L-glutamate, which undergoes **oxidative deamination** to form ammonia, used for the synthesis of urea. Urea is transferred through the blood to the kidneys and excreted in the urine.

The glucose-alanine cycle is the main pathway by which amino groups from muscle amino acids are transported to the liver for conversion to glucose. The liver is the main site of catabolism for all essential amino acids, except the branched-chain amino acids, which are catabolized mainly by muscle and the kidneys. **Plasma** amino-acid levels are affected by dietary carbohydrate through the action of insulin, which lowers plasma amino-acid levels (particularly the branched-chain amino acids) by promoting their entry into the muscle.

Body proteins are broken down when dietary supply of energy is inadequate during illness or prolonged starvation. The proteins in the liver are utilized in preference to those of other tissues such as the brain. The gluconeogenesis pathway is present only in liver cells and in certain kidney cells.

Disorders of amino acid metabolism include **phenylketonuria**, albinism, alkaptonuria, type 1 tyrosinaemia, nonketotic hyperglycinaemia, histidinaemia, homocystinuria, and maple syrup urine disease.

Fat (Lipid) Metabolism

Fats contain mostly carbon and hydrogen, some oxygen, and sometimes other atoms. The three main forms of fat found in food are glycerides (principally triacylglycerol [triglyceride], the form in which fat is stored for fuel), the **phospholipids**, and the **sterols** (principally **cholesterol**). Fats provide 9 kilocalories per gram (kcal/g), compared with 4 kcal/g for carbohydrate and protein. Triacylglycerol, whether in the form of chylomicrons (microscopic lipid particles) or other **lipoproteins**, is not taken up directly by any tissue, but must be hydrolyzed outside the cell to **fatty acids** and glycerol, which can then enter the cell.

Fatty acids come from the **diet**, adipocytes (fat cells), carbohydrate, and some amino acids. After digestion, most of the fats are carried in the blood as chylomicrons. The main pathways of lipid metabolism are lipolysis, beta-oxidation, **ketosis**, and lipogenesis.

Lipolysis (fat breakdown) and beta-oxidation occurs in the mitochondria. It is a cyclical process in which two carbons are removed from the fatty acid per cycle in the form of acetyl CoA, which proceeds through the Krebs cycle to produce ATP, CO_2, and water.

Ketosis occurs when the rate of formation of **ketones** by the liver is greater than the ability of tissues to oxidize them. It occurs during prolonged starvation and when large amounts of fat are eaten in the absence of carbohydrate.

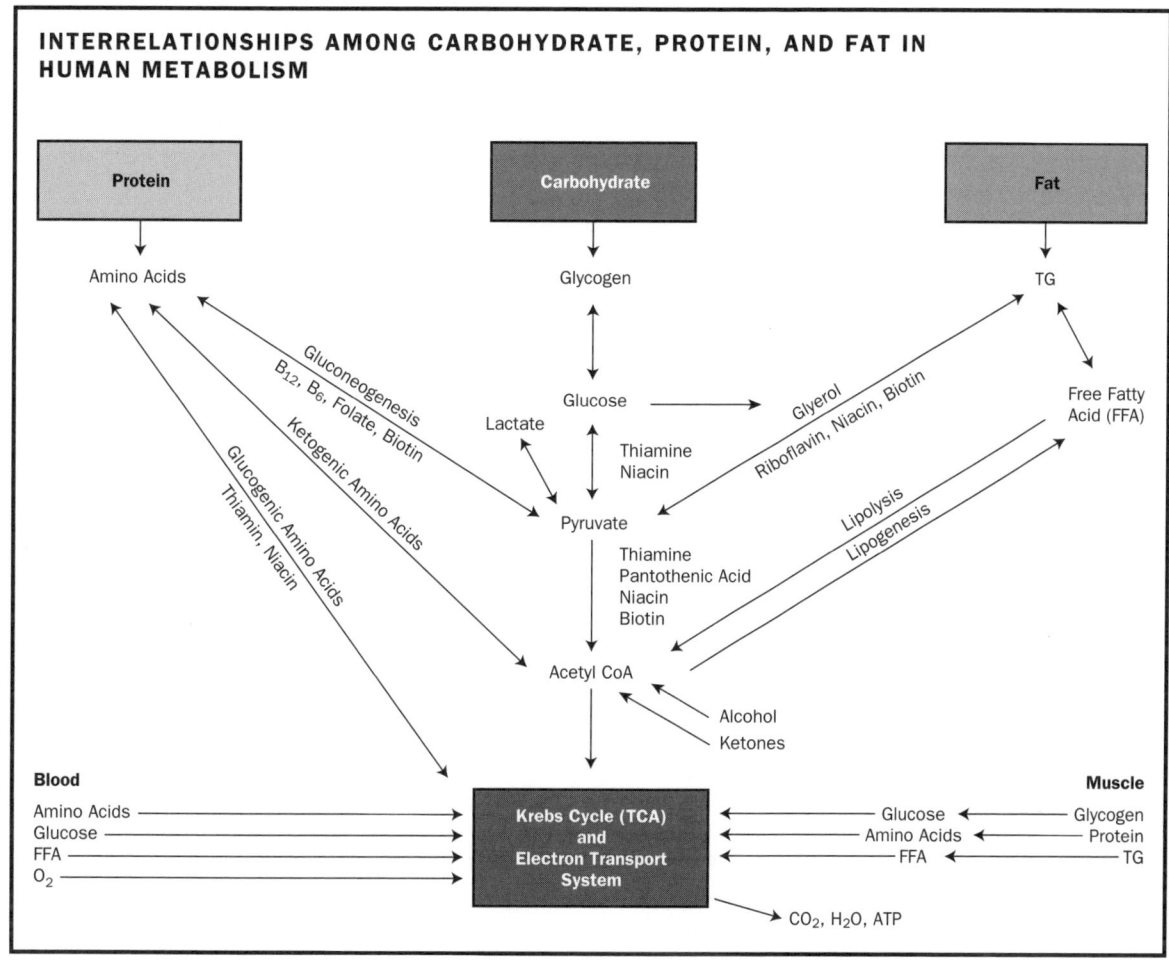

Lipogenesis occurs in the cytosol. The main sites of triglyceride synthesis are the liver, adipose tissue, and intestinal mucosa. The fatty acids are derived from the hydrolysis of fats, as well as from the synthesis of acetyl CoA through the oxidation of fats, glucose, and some amino acids. Lipogenesis from acetyl CoA also occurs in steps of two carbon atoms. NADPH produced by the pentose-phosphate shunt is required for this process. Phospholipids form the interior and exterior cell membranes and are essential for cell regulatory signals.

Cholesterol Metabolism

Cholesterol is either obtained from the diet or synthesized in a variety of tissues, including the liver, adrenal cortex, skin, intestine, testes, and aorta. High dietary cholesterol suppresses synthesis in the liver but not in other tissues.

Carbohydrate is converted to triglyceride utilizing glycerol phosphate and acetyl CoA obtained from glycolysis. Ketogenic amino acids, which are metabolized to acetyl CoA, may be used for synthesis of triglycerides. The fatty acids cannot fully prevent protein breakdown, because only the glycerol portion of the triglycerides can contribute to gluconeogenesis. Glycerol is only 5 percent of the triglyceride carbon.

Most of the major tissues (e.g., muscle, liver, kidney) are able to convert glucose, fatty acids, and amino acids to acetyl-CoA. However, brain and nervous tissue—in the fed state and in the early stages of starvation—depend almost exclusively on glucose. Not all tissues obtain the major part of their ATP requirements from the Krebs cycle. Red blood cells, tissues of the eye, and the kidney medulla gain most of their energy from the anaerobic conversion of glucose to lactate. SEE ALSO CARBOHYDRATES; FATS; NUTRIENTS; PROTEIN.

Gita Patel

Bibliography

Bland, Jeffrey S.; Costarella, L.; Levin, B.; Liska, DeAnn; Lukaczer, D.; Schiltz, B.; and Schmidt, M. A. (1999). *Clinical Nutrition: A Functional Approach.* Gig Harbor, WA: Institute of Functional Medicine.

Linder, Maria (1991). *Nutritional Biochemistry and Metabolism, with Clinical Applications,* 2nd edition. New York: Elsevier.

Newsholme E. A., and Leech, A. R. (1994). *Biochemistry for the Medical Sciences.* New York: Wiley.

Salway, J. G. 1999. *Metabolism at a Glance,* 2nd edition. Malden, MA: Blackwell Science.

Shils, M. E.; Olson, J. A.; Shike, M.; and Ross C. A.; eds. (1999). *Modern Nutrition in Health and Disease,* 9th edition. Baltimore, MD: Wilkins & Wilkins.

Wardlaw, Gordon M., and Kessel Margaret (2002). *Perspectives in Nutrition,* 5th edition. Boston: McGraw-Hill.

Williams, M. H. (1999). *Nutrition for Health, Fitness, and Sport,* 6th edition. Boston: McGraw-Hill.

Yeung, D. L., ed. (1995). *Heinz Handbook of Nutrition,* 8th edition. Pittsburgh, PA: Heinz Corporate Research Center.

Ziegler, Ekhard E., and Filer, L. J. (1996). *Present Knowledge in Nutrition,* 7th edition. Washington, DC: International Life Sciences Institute Press.

Zubay, Geoffrey L.; Parson, William W.; and Vance, Dennis E. (1995). *Principles of Biochemistry.* Dubuque, IA: William C. Brown.

Minerals

mineral: an inorganic (non-carbon-containing) element, ion, or compound

nutrient: dietary substance necessary for health

diet: the total daily food intake, or the types of foods eaten

metabolic: related to processing of nutrients and building of necessary molecules within the cell

energy: technically, the ability to perform work; the content of a substance that allows it to be useful as a fuel

protein: complex molecule composed of amino acids that performs vital functions in the cell; necessary part of the diet

trace: very small amount

calcium: mineral essential for bones and teeth

phosphorus: element essential in forming the mineral portion of bone

Minerals are inorganic elements that originate in the earth and cannot be made in the body. They play important roles in various bodily functions and are necessary to sustain life and maintain optimal health, and thus are essential **nutrients**. Most of the minerals in the human **diet** come directly from plants and water, or indirectly from animal foods. However, the mineral content of water and plant foods varies geographically because of variations in the mineral content of soil from region to region.

The amount of minerals present in the body, and their **metabolic** roles, varies considerably. Minerals provide structure to bones and teeth and participate in **energy** production, the building of **protein**, blood formation, and several other metabolic processes. Minerals are categorized into major and **trace** minerals, depending on the amount needed per day. Major minerals are those that are required in the amounts of 100 mg (milligrams) or more, while trace minerals are required in amounts less than 100 mg per day. The terms *major* and *trace,* however, do not reflect the importance of a mineral in maintaining health, as a deficiency of either can be harmful.

Some body processes require several minerals to work together. For example, **calcium**, magnesium, and **phosphorus** are all important for the formation and maintenance of healthy bones. Some minerals compete with each other for **absorption**, and they interact with other nutrients as well, which can affect their **bioavailability**.

Mineral Bioavailability

The degree to which the amount of an ingested nutrient is absorbed and available to the body is called bioavailability. Mineral bioavailability depends on several factors. Higher absorption occurs among individuals who are deficient in a mineral, while some elements in the diet (e.g., oxalic acid or oxalate in spinach) can decrease mineral availability by chemically binding to the mineral. In addition, excess intake of one mineral can influence the absorption and **metabolism** of other minerals. For example, the presence of a large amount of **zinc** in the diet decreases the absorption of **iron** and copper. On the other hand, the presence of **vitamins** in a meal enhances the absorption of minerals in the meal. For example, vitamin C improves iron absorption, and **vitamin D** aids in the absorption of calcium, phosphorous, and magnesium.

In general, minerals from animal sources are absorbed better than those from plant sources as minerals are present in forms that are readily absorbed and binders that inhibit absorption, such as **phytates**, are absent. **Vegans** (those who restrict their diets to plant foods) need to be aware of the factors affecting mineral bioavailability. Careful meal planning is necessary to include foods rich in minerals and absorption-enhancing factors.

Supplementation

It is generally recommended that people eat a well-balanced diet to meet their mineral requirements, while avoiding deficiencies and chemical excesses or imbalances. However, supplements may be useful to meet dietary requirements for some minerals when dietary patterns fall short of **Recommended Dietary Allowances** (RDAs) or **Adequate Intakes** (AIs) for normal healthy people.

The Food and Nutrition Board currently recommends that supplements or **fortified** foods be used to obtain desirable amounts of some nutrients, such as calcium and iron. The recommendations for calcium are higher than the average intake in the United States. Women, who generally consume lower energy diets than men, and individuals who do not consume dairy products can particularly benefit from calcium supplements. Because of the increased need for iron in women of childbearing age, as well as the many negative consequences of iron-deficiency **anemia**, iron supplementation is recommended for vulnerable groups in the United States, as well as in developing countries.

Mineral supplementation may also be appropriate for people with prolonged illnesses or extensive injuries, for those undergoing surgery, or for those being treated for alcoholism. However, extra caution must be taken to avoid intakes greater than the RDA or AI for specific nutrients because of problems related to nutrient excesses, imbalances, or adverse interactions with medical treatments. Although toxic symptoms or adverse effects from excess supplementation have been reported for various minerals (e.g., calcium, magnesium, iron, zinc, copper, and selenium) and tolerable upper limits set, the amounts of nutrients in supplements are not regulated by the

---

absorption: uptake by the digestive tract

bioavailability: availability to living organisms, based on chemical form

metabolism: the sum total of reactions in a cell or an organism

zinc: mineral necessary for many enzyme processes

iron: nutrient needed for red blood cell formation

vitamin: necessary complex nutrient used to aid enzymes or other metabolic processes in the cell

vitamin D: nutrient needed for calcium uptake and therefore proper bone formation

phytate: plant compound that binds minerals, reducing their ability to be absorbed

vegan: person who consume no animal products, including milk and honey

Recommended Dietary Allowances: nutrient intake recommended to promote health

adequate intake: nutrient intake that appears to maintain the state of health

fortified: altered by addition of vitamins or minerals

anemia: low level of red blood cells in the blood

Excesses of certain minerals can prevent the absorption of others, which is one reason that eating a balanced diet is superior to depending on mineral supplements. With the possible exception of iron and calcium, mineral deficiencies are rare among healthy people in developed nations. [AP/Wide World Photos. Reproduced by permission.]

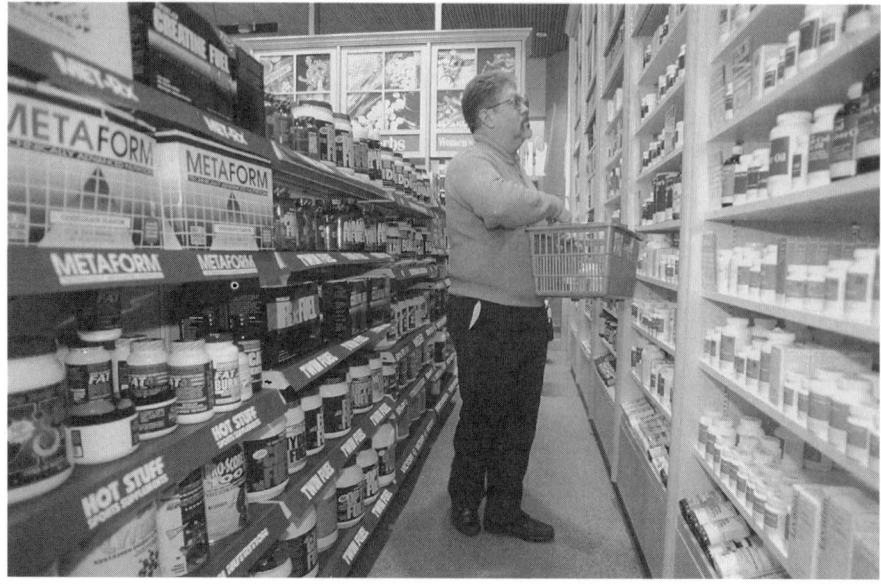

electrolyte: salt dissolved in fluid

blood pressure: measure of the pressure exerted by the blood against the walls of the blood vessels

glucose: a simple sugar; the most commonly used fuel in cells

amino acid: building block of proteins, necessary dietary nutrient

gastric: related to the stomach

enzyme: protein responsible for carrying out reactions in a cell

hormone: molecules produced by one set of cells that influence the function of another set of cells

fat: type of food molecule rich in carbon and hydrogen, with high energy content

blood clotting: the process by which blood forms a solid mass to prevent uncontrolled bleeding

high blood pressure: elevation of the pressure in the bloodstream maintained by the heart

hypertension: high blood pressure

cardiovascular: related to the heart and circulatory system

stroke: loss of blood supply to part of the brain, due to a blocked or burst artery in the brain

Food and Drug Administration (FDA). Therefore, supplement users must be aware of the potential adverse effects and choose supplements with moderate amounts of nutrients.

Major Minerals

The major minerals present in the body include sodium, potassium, chloride, calcium, magnesium, phosphorus, and sulfur.

Functions. The fluid balance in the body, vital for all life processes, is maintained largely by sodium, potassium, and chloride. Fluid balance is regulated by charged sodium and chloride ions in the extracellular fluid (outside the cell) and potassium in the intracellular fluid (inside the cell), and by some other **electrolytes** across cell membranes. Tight control is critical for normal muscle contraction, nerve impulse transmission, heart function, and **blood pressure**. Sodium plays an important role in the absorption of other nutrients, such as **glucose**, **amino acids**, and water. Chloride is a component of hydrochloric acid, an important part of **gastric** juice (an acidic liquid secreted by glands in the stomach lining) and aids in food digestion. Potassium and sodium act as cofactors for certain **enzymes**.

Calcium, magnesium, and phosphorus are known for their structural roles, as they are essential for the development and maintenance of bones and teeth. They are also needed for maintaining cell membranes and connective tissue. Several enzymes, **hormones**, and proteins that regulate energy and **fat** metabolism require calcium, magnesium and/or phosphorus to become active. Calcium also aids in **blood clotting**. Sulfur is a key component of various proteins and vitamins and participates in drug-detoxifying pathways in the body.

Disease prevention and treatment. Sodium, chloride, and potassium are linked to **high blood pressure** (**hypertension**) due to their role in the body's fluid balance. High salt or sodium chloride intake has been linked to **cardiovascular** disease as well. High potassium intakes, on the other hand, have been associated with a lower risk of **stroke**, particularly in people with hypertension. Research also suggests a preventive role for magnesium in hypertension and cardiovascular disease, as well as a beneficial effect in the treatment of **diabetes**, **osteoporosis**, and migraine headaches.

Osteoporosis is a bone disorder in which bone strength is compromised, leading to an increased risk of fracture. Along with other lifestyle factors, intake of calcium and vitamin D plays an important role in the maintenance of bone health and the prevention and treatment of osteoporosis. Good calcium nutrition, along with low salt and high potassium intake, has been linked to prevention of hypertension and **kidney stones**.

Deficiency. Dietary deficiency is unlikely for most major minerals, except in starving people or those with protein-energy **malnutrition** in developing countries, or people on poor diets for an extended period, such as those suffering from alcoholism, **anorexia nervosa**, or **bulimia**. Most people in the world consume a lot of salt, and it is recommended that they moderate their intake to prevent **chronic** diseases (high salt intake has been associated with an increased risk of death from stroke and cardiovascular disease). However, certain conditions, such as severe or prolonged vomiting or diarrhea, the use of **diuretics**, and some forms of kidney disease, lead to an increased loss of minerals, particularly sodium, chloride, potassium, and magnesium. Calcium intakes tend to be lower in women and vegans who do not consume dairy products. Elderly people with suboptimal diets are also at risk of mineral deficiencies because of decreased absorption and increased excretion of minerals in the urine.

Toxicity. Toxicity from excessive dietary intake of major minerals rarely occurs in healthy individuals. Kidneys that are functioning normally can regulate mineral concentrations in the body by excreting the excess amounts in urine. Toxicity symptoms from excess intakes are more likely to appear with **acute** or chronic kidney failure.

Sodium and chloride toxicity can develop due to low intake or excess loss of water. Accumulation of excess potassium in **plasma** may result from the use of potassium-sparing diuretics (medications used to treat high blood pressure, which increase urine production, excreting sodium but not potassium), insufficient aldosterone secretion (a hormone that acts on the kidney to decrease sodium secretion and increase potassium secretion), or tissue damage (e.g., from severe burns). Magnesium intake from foods has no adverse effects, but a high intake from supplements when kidney function is limited increases the risk of toxicity. The most serious complication of potassium or magnesium toxicity is cardiac arrest. Adverse effects from excess calcium have been reported only with consumption of large quantities of supplements. Phosphate toxicity can occur due to absorption from phosphate salts taken by mouth or in **enemas**.

Trace Minerals

Trace minerals are present (and required) in very small amounts in the body. An understanding of the important roles and requirements of trace minerals in the human body is fairly recent, and research is still ongoing. The most important trace minerals are iron, zinc, copper, chromium, fluoride, iodine, selenium, manganese, and molybdenum. Some others, such as arsenic, boron, cobalt, nickel, silicon, and vanadium, are recognized as essential for

diabetes: inability to regulate level of sugar in the blood

osteoporosis: weakening of the bone structure

kidney stones: deposits of solid material in kidney

malnutrition: chronic lack of sufficient nutrients to maintain health

anorexia nervosa: refusal to maintain body weight at or above what is considered normal for height and age

bulimia: uncontrolled episodes of eating (bingeing) usually followed by self-induced vomiting (purging)

chronic: over a long period

diuretic: substance that depletes the body of water

acute: rapid-onset and short-lived

plasma: the fluid portion of the blood, distinct from the cellular portion

enema: substance delivered via the rectum

some animals, while others, such as barium, bromine, cadmium, gold, silver, and aluminum, are found in the body, though little is known about their role in health.

biological: related to living organisms

oxygen: O₂, atmospheric gas required by all animals

hemoglobin: the iron-containing molecule in red blood cells that carries oxygen

myoglobin: oxygen storage protein in muscle

neurotransmitter: molecule released by one nerve cell to stimulate or inhibit another

genetic: inherited or related to the genes

insulin: hormone released by the pancreas to regulate level of sugar in the blood

oxidative: related to chemical reaction with oxygen or oxygen-containing compounds

Functions. Trace minerals have specific **biological** functions. They are essential in the absorption and utilization of many nutrients and aid enzymes and hormones in activities that are vital to life. Iron plays a major role in **oxygen** transport and storage and is a component of **hemoglobin** in red blood cells and **myoglobin** in muscle cells. Cellular energy production requires many trace minerals, including iron, copper, and zinc, which act as enzyme cofactors in the synthesis of many proteins, hormones, **neurotransmitters**, and **genetic** material.

Iron and zinc support immune function, while chromium and zinc aid **insulin** action. Zinc is also essential for many other bodily functions, such as growth, development of sexual organs, and reproduction. Zinc, copper and selenium prevent **oxidative** damage to cells. Fluoride stabilizes bone mineral and hardens tooth enamel, thus increasing resistance to tooth decay. Iodine is essential for normal thyroid function, which is critical for many aspects of growth and development, particularly brain development. Thus, trace minerals contribute to physical growth and mental development.

Role in disease prevention and treatment. In addition to clinical deficiency diseases such as anemia and goiter, research indicates that trace minerals play a role in the development, prevention, and treatment of chronic diseases. A marginal status of several trace minerals has been found to be associated with **infectious diseases**, disorders of the stomach, intestine, bone, heart, and liver, and **cancer**, although further research is necessary in many cases to understand the effect of supplementation. Iron, zinc, copper, and selenium have been associated with immune response conditions. Copper, chromium and selenium have been linked to the prevention of cardiovascular disease. Excess iron in the body, on the other hand, can increase the risk of cardiovascular disease, liver and colorectal cancer, and neurodegenerative diseases such as Alzheimer's disease. Chromium supplementation has been found to be beneficial in many studies of impaired glucose tolerance, a metabolic state between normal glucose regulation and diabetes. Fluoride has been known to prevent dental **caries** and osteoporosis, while potassium iodide supplements taken immediately before or after exposure to radiation can decrease the risk of radiation-induced thyroid cancer.

infectious diseases: diseases caused by viruses, bacteria, fungi, or protozoa, which replicate inside the body

cancer: uncontrolled cell growth

caries: cavities in the teeth

intravenous: into the veins

Deficiency. With the exception of iron, dietary deficiencies are rare in the United States and other developed nations. However, malnutrition in developing countries increases the risk for trace-mineral deficiencies among children and other vulnerable groups. In overzealous supplement users, interactions among nutrients can inhibit absorption of some minerals leading to deficiencies. Patients on **intravenous** feedings without mineral supplements are at risk of developing deficiencies as well.

Although severe deficiencies of better-understood trace minerals are easy to recognize, diagnosis is difficult for less-understood minerals and for mild deficiencies. Even mild deficiencies of trace minerals however, can result in poor growth and development in children.

Iron deficiency is the most common nutrient deficiency worldwide, including in the United States. Iron-deficiency anemia affects hundreds of millions of people, with highest **prevalence** in developing countries. Infants, young children, adolescents, and pregnant and lactating women are especially vulnerable due to their high demand for iron. Menstruating women are also vulnerable due to blood loss. Vegetarians are another vulnerable group, as iron from plant foods is less bioavailable than that from animal sources.

Zinc deficiency, marked by severe growth retardation and arrested sexual development, was first reported in children and adolescent boys in Egypt, Iran, and Turkey. Diets in Middle Eastern countries are typically high in **fiber** and phytates, which inhibit zinc absorption. Mild zinc deficiency has been found in vulnerable groups in the United States. Copper deficiency is rare, but can be caused by excess zinc from supplementation.

Deficiencies of fluoride, iodine, and selenium mainly occur due to a low mineral content in either the water or soil in some areas of the world. Fluoride deficiency is marked by a high prevalence of dental caries and is common in geographic regions with low water-fluoride concentration, which has led to the fluoridation of water in the United States and many other parts of the world. Goiter and **cretinism** (a condition in which body growth and mental development are stunted) have been eliminated by iodization of salt in the United States, but still occur in parts of the world where salt manufacture and distribution are not regulated. Selenium deficiency due to low levels of the mineral in soil is found in northeast China, and it has been associated with Keshan disease, a heart disorder prevalent among people of that area.

Toxicity. Trace minerals can be toxic at higher intakes, especially for those minerals whose absorption is not regulated in the body (e.g., selenium and iodine). Thus, it is important not to habitually exceed the recommended intake levels. Although toxicity from dietary sources is unlikely, certain genetic disorders can make people vulnerable to overloads from food or supplements. One such disorder, hereditary hemochromatosis, is characterized by iron deposition in the liver and other tissues due to increased intestinal iron absorption over many years.

Chronic exposure to trace minerals through cooking or storage containers can result in overloads of iron, zinc, and copper. Fluorosis, a discoloration of the teeth, has been reported in regions where the natural content of fluoride in drinking water is high. Inhalation of manganese dust over long periods of time has been found to cause brain damage among miners and steelworkers in many parts of the world.

In summary, minerals, both major and trace, play vital roles in human health, and care must be taken to obtain adequate intakes from a wide variety of whole foods. The most common result of deficiencies is poor growth and development in children. Minerals interact with each other and with other nutrients, and caution is required when using supplements, as excess intake of one mineral can lead to the deficiency of another nutrient. SEE ALSO ANEMIA; BIOAVAILABILITY; CALCIUM; DIETARY SUPPLEMENTS; OSTEOPOROSIS; VITAMINS, FAT-SOLUBLE; VITAMINS, WATER-SOLUBLE.

Sunitha Jasti

prevalence: describing the number of cases in a population at any one time

fiber: indigestible plant material which aids digestion by providing bulk

cretinism: arrested mental and physical development

Bibliography

Wardlaw, Gordon M. (1999). *Perspectives in Nutrition*, 4th edition. Boston: WCB McGraw-Hill.

Whitney, Eleanor N., and Rolfes, Sharon R. (1996). *Understanding Nutrition*, 7th edition. New York: West Publishing.

Internet Resources

The American Dietetic Association (2002). "Position of The American Dietetic Association: Food Fortification and Dietary Supplements." Available from <http://www.eatright.com>

The Linus Pauling Institute. "Minerals." Available from <http://osu.orst.edu/dept/lpi>

United States Department of Agriculture (2002). "Dietary Reference Intakes (DRI) and Recommended Dietary Allowances (RDA)." Available from <http://www.nal.usda.gov/fnic/>

Mood-Food Relationships

Research on the connection between a person's mood and the food he or she eats has reveled what many people have long believed, that eating a certain food can influence a person's mood—at least temporarily. Research by Judith Wurtman, a professor at the Massachusetts Institute of Technology (MIT), has focused on how certain foods alter one's mood by influencing the level of certain brain chemicals called **neurotransmitters**. While many other factors influence the level of these chemicals, such as **hormones**, heredity, **drugs**, and alcohol, three neurotransmitters—dopamine, norepinephrine, and **serotonin**—have been studied in relation to food, and this research has shown that neurotransmitters are produced in the brain from components of certain foods.

Effects of Neurotransmitters

Wurtman has reported that people are more alert when their brains are producing the neurotransmitters dopamine and norepinephrine, while serotonin production in the brain has been associated with a more calming, **anxiety**-reducing effect (and even drowsiness in some people). A stable brain serotonin level is associated with a positive mood state. It appears that women have a greater sensitivity than men to changes in this brain chemical. Mood swings during the menstrual cycle and **menopause** are thought to be caused by hormonal changes that influence the production of serotonin.

How does **diet** play a role? The foods that increase the production of serotonin in the brain are high in **carbohydrates**. Many kinds of foods carbohydrates, such as candy, cereal, and pasta, can produce a temporary increase in brain serotonin—and a subsequent calming or anxiety-reducing effect. This explains why people may feel drowsy in the afternoon after eating a large meal of pasta, since a rise in serotonin in the brain can also lead to drowsiness. Carbohydrates affect brain serotonin because they increase the amount of tryptophan in the brain. Tryptophan is the amino-acid precursor of serotonin.

The two other important brain chemicals that appear to be influenced by foods, dopamine and norepinephrine, produce a feeling of alertness, an increased ability to concentrate, and faster reaction times. There are two possible mechanisms for how this happens: (1) serotonin production is blocked by the consumption of protein-rich foods, resulting in increased alertness or concentration, or (2) levels of dopamine and norepinephrine are increased by the consumption of protein-rich foods.

---

neurotransmitter: molecule released by one nerve cell to stimulate or inhibit another

hormone: molecules produced by one set of cells that influence the function of another set of cells

drugs: substances whose administration causes a significant change in the body's function

serotonin: chemical used by nerve cells to communicate with one another

anxiety: nervousness

menopause: phase in a woman's life during which ovulation and menstruation end

diet: the total daily food intake, or the types of foods eaten

carbohydrate: food molecule made of carbon, hydrogen, and oxygen, including sugars and starches

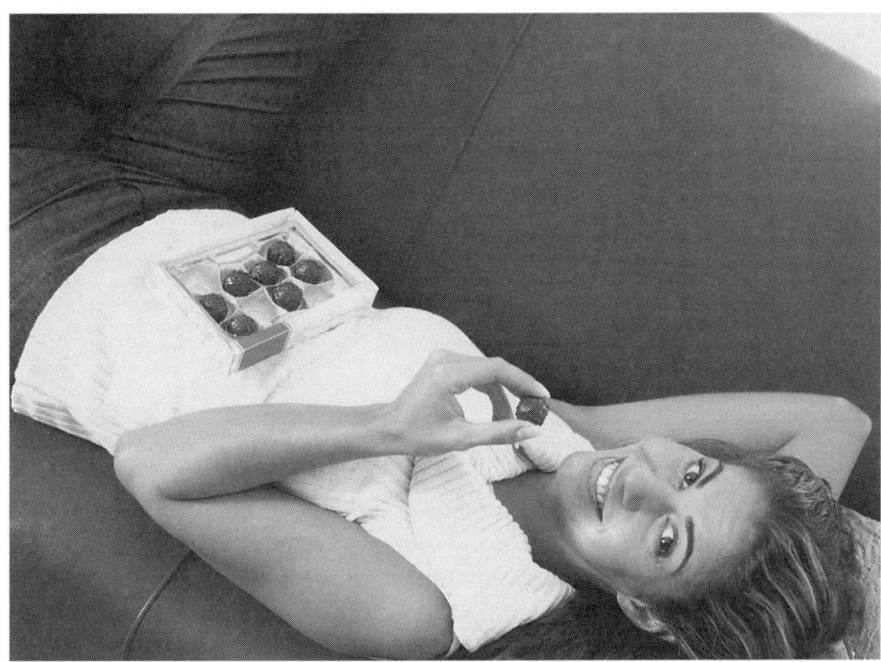

Chocolate consumption stimulates the release of serotonin and endorphin into the body, which combine to produce a relaxed or euphoric feeling. This may explain why some people crave chocolate when they're feeling depressed. [Royalty-Free/Corbis. Reproduced by permission.]

The food-mood response is short term. Eating tuna at lunch may increase alertness and concentration for two to three hours after eating, just as having pasta with tomato sauce will produce a calming response for two to three hours. Someday, there may be menus that offer foods for their intended mood effects. Such a menu might have selections such as "Smart Soup," "Happy Hamburger," "Serene Salad," or "Sleepy Spaghetti."

Size of Meal

Another factor that influences alertness and performance is the size of a meal. Large lunches containing 1,000 **calories** have been associated with decreased performance in the afternoon. Such high-calorie lunches tend to be high in **fat**. A lunch consisting of a double hamburger, french fries, and a shake would fit into this category. The size of a meal makes a difference because fat slows down **absorption**, and because blood flow to the stomach is increased for a longer period of time, resulting in less blood flow to the brain. The result is to feel sleepy and sluggish.

calorie: unit of food energy

fat: type of food molecule rich in carbon and hydrogen, with high energy content

absorption: uptake by the digestive tract

Circadian Rhythms

Circadian rhythms also affect eating and performance. These rhythms influence when individuals are more active, and when they are more likely to be sleepy. Research indicates there are different eating patterns for individuals with different rhythms. These eating patterns can enhance **energy** levels and performance. For example, "morning people" are usually at their best and most focused during the early hours of the day. Although breakfast is important, what foods these people eat becomes more important at lunch and throughout the afternoon. The energy level of a morning person begins to drop during the afternoon, and evening is their least alert and productive time. Thus, what they choose to eat at lunch and for snacks can make a difference in how they feel later in the day.

energy: technically, the ability to perform work; the content of a substance that allows it to be useful as a fuel

DIET-MOOD CONNECTION

Nutrient	Food sources	Neurotransmitter/mechanism	Proposed effect
Protein	Meat, Milk, Eggs, Cheese, Fish, Beans	Dopamine, Norepinephrine	Increased alertness, concentration
Carbohydrate (CHO)	Grains, Fruits, Sugars	Serotonin	Increased calmness, relaxation
Calories	All Foods	Reduced blood flow to the brain	Excess calories in a meal is associated with decreased alertness and concentration after the meal

amino acid: building block of proteins, necessary dietary nutrient

chronic: over a long period

acupuncture: insertion of needles into the skin at special points to treat disease

depression: mood disorder characterized by apathy, restlessness, and negative thoughts

---

Are You a Night Owl or an Early Bird?

Early Bird Traits

- Wakes up before the alarm goes off
- More energetic and productive during the morning
- Often up before daylight working on projects
- Energetic and alert during evening hours
- Typical bedtime around would be 9:00 to 10:00 p.m.

Night Owl Traits

- Only wakes up in the morning if the alarm is going off
- Ideal workday would begin at noon
- It takes several cups of coffee to function in the morning
- Most productive and alert in the afternoon and evening
- Typical bedtime would be after the late night news

Morning people need their protein-rich foods during the afternoon and evening, particularly if they need to be focused later in the day for a meeting or some other work requiring attention to detail. Instead of a lunch of pasta with marinara sauce, for example, morning people would be more alert in the afternoon if they added some grilled chicken, seafood, or other protein source to their pasta dish, thus increasing their levels of dopamine and norepinephrine.

Many people who are "evening persons," or "night owls," must nevertheless be at work at 9 a.m. For these people it is important not only to have breakfast, but to make sure that protein-rich food is part of the breakfast. Protein provides the brain with tyrosine, an **amino acid** that is a precursor of the chemicals that promote alertness. A mid-morning snack is another good time to include a protein-rich food, such as cheese or yogurt.

Positive Moods and Stress Reduction

Another group of chemicals that can influence mood and appetite are the endorphins. These are the body's natural opiate-like chemicals that produce a positive mood state, decreased pain sensitivity, and reduced stress. Endorphins are released when a person is in pain, during starvation, and during exercise—resulting in what is known as a "runner's high." Researchers are now looking at ways to utilize this response to alleviate **chronic** pain. Studies have shown that **acupuncture** may relieve pain by stimulating the release of endorphins.

A food substance related to endorphins is phenylethylamine, which is found in chocolate. Chocolate has always been a highly valued commodity in many cultures, and there is some evidence that chocolate may improve mood temporarily due to its high levels of sugar and fat, phenylethylamine, and caffeine. The sugar in chocolate is associated with a release of the neurotransmitter serotonin, and the fat and phenylethylamine are associated with an endorphin release. This combination produces an effect that has been called "optimal brain happiness." The caffeine in chocolate adds a temporary stimulant effect.

If changing one's diet does not produce a desired improvement in mood, or if feelings of sadness or disinterest occur much of the time, it is important to be evaluated for **depression**. In people who are depressed, brain serotonin levels are significantly lowered, and treatment usually involves a medication that can elevate serotonin levels to the normal range. Although food can provide a temporary lift, it does not provide enough serotonin to alleviate depression or changes in neurotransmitters associated with eating disorders.

Research on the food-mood connection has been aimed at understanding the effects of eating particular foods during particular mood states, as well as how foods can help to achieve a particular mood state. Future research will focus on the application of this research, such as to what degree food choices can influence worker productivity or affect circadian rhythm in cases of jet lag or lack of sleep. SEE ALSO ADDICTION, FOOD; CRAVINGS; EATING HABITS.

Catherine Christie

Bibliography

Mitchell, Susan, and Christie, Catherine (1998). *I'd Kill for a Cookie.* New York: Dutton.

Wurtman, J. (1989) "Carbohydrate Craving, Mood Changes, and Obesity." *Journal of Clinical Psychiatry* 49 (Suppl.) 37–39.

Wurtman, R. J., et. al. (1986) "Carbohydrate Cravings, Obesity and Brain Serotonin." *Appetite* 7 (Suppl.): 99–103.

Wurtman, R. J., and J. J. Wurtman (1989) "Carbohydrates and Depression." *Scientific American* (January): 68–75.

National Academy of Sciences (NAS)

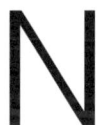

The National Academy of Sciences is a private agency that advises the federal government on scientific and technical matters. It is part of the National Academy, which also includes the National Academy of Engineering, the Institute of Medicine, and the National Research Council.

The NAS updates and publishes the **Recommended Dietary Allowances** (RDAs), which "represent the **nutrient** intake that is sufficient to meet the needs of nearly all healthy people in an age and gender group" (Wardlaw). More specific recommendations are needed for special populations, such as pregnant women, the elderly population, and those with medical conditions.

Recommended Dietary Allowances: nutrient intake recommended to promote health

nutrient: dietary substance necessary for health

In addition, since all nutrients and food components do not have established RDAs, **Dietary Reference Intakes** (DRIs) were developed as a guide to adequate and safe standards for nutrients such as **fiber**, **antioxidants**, and **trace** elements, and for upper level intakes of **vitamins** and **minerals**. SEE ALSO DIETARY REFERENCE INTAKE; RECOMMENDED DIETARY ALLOWANCES.

Pauline A. Vickery

Dietary Reference Intakes: set of guidelines for nutrient intake

fiber: indigestible plant material which aids digestion by providing bulk

antioxidant: substance that prevents oxidation, a damaging reaction with oxygen

trace: very small amount

vitamin: necessary complex nutrient used to aid enzymes or other metabolic processes in the cell

mineral: an inorganic (non-carbon-containing) element, ion, or compound

Bibliography

Wardlaw, Gordon M. (2000). *Contemporary Nutrition: Issues and Insights*, 4th edition. Boston: McGraw-Hill.

Whitney, E.; Catlado, C.; DeBruyne, L.; and Rolfe, S. (1996). *Nutrition for Health and Health Care.* Minneapolis, MN: West Publishing.

Williams, Sue R. (1993). *Nutrition and Diet Therapy*, 7th edition. St. Louis, MO: Mosby.

National Health and Nutrition Examination Survey (NHANES)

overweight: weight above the accepted norm based on height, sex, and age

obese: above accepted standards of weight for sex, height, and age

prevalence: describing the number of cases in a population at any one time

obesity: the condition of being overweight, according to established norms based on sex, age, and height

osteoporosis: weakening of the bone structure

nutrition: the maintenance of health through proper eating, or the study of same

clinical: related to hospitals, clinics, and patient care

cardiovascular: related to the heart and circulatory system

diabetes: inability to regulate level of sugar in the blood

infectious diseases: diseases caused by viruses, bacteria, fungi, or protozoa, which replicate inside the body

In the year 1999, 64 percent of the U.S. population was **overweight** or **obese**, while the **prevalence** of **obesity** among children and adolescents more than doubled during the previous two decades. Fifty-six percent of women over the age of fifty had low bone density, and 16 percent were suffering from the debilitating disease of **osteoporosis**. And while smoking prevalence hit an all-time low among adults, it has continued to increase among America's youth.

Statistics like these sell newspapers, inspire public-policy initiatives, and provide topics for classroom discussions. But where do these statistics come from? How can scientists determine the percentage of the *entire* U.S. population that suffers from conditions such as obesity and osteoporosis or engage in unhealthy habits such as smoking?

Statistics such as those listed above, along with a whole host of other health and **nutrition** data, are derived from the National Health and Nutrition Examination Survey, or NHANES. NHANES is arguably the largest and longest-running national source of objectively measured health *and* nutrition data. Through physical examinations, **clinical** and laboratory tests, and personal interviews, NHANES provides a "snapshot" of the health and nutritional status of the U.S. population. Findings from NHANES provide health professionals and policymakers with the statistical data needed to determine rates of major diseases and health conditions (e.g., **cardiovascular** disease, **diabetes**, obesity, **infectious diseases**) as well as identify and monitor trends in medical conditions, risk factors, and emerging public health issues, so that the appropriate public health policies and prevention interventions can be developed.

History of NHANES

The current NHANES was born out of The National Health Survey Act of 1956. This particular piece of legislation provided for the establishment of a continuing National Health Survey to obtain information about the health status of individuals residing in the United States, including the services received for or because of health conditions. The responsibility for survey development and data collection was placed upon the National Center for Health Statistics (NCHS), a research-oriented statistical organization housed within the Health Services and Mental Health Administration (HSMHA) of the Department of Health, Education, and Welfare (now the Department of Health and Human Services). Since its inception in 1959, eight separate Health Examination Surveys have been conducted and over 130,000 people have served as survey participants.

The first three National Health Surveys—National Health Examination Survey (NHES) I, II, and III—were conducted between 1959 and 1970, each with an approximate sample size of 7,500 individuals. NHES I (1959–1962) focused on selected **chronic** diseases of adults between 18 and 79 years of age, while NHES II (1963–1965) and NHES III (1966–1970) focused on the growth and development of children (6–11 years of age) and adolescents (12–17 years of age), respectively.

chronic: over a long period

Between the passage of the 1956 Act and the completion of NHES III, numerous nutrition-related studies were conducted that indicated that **malnutrition** remained a significant problem within certain segments of the U.S. population. This data, along with increasing scientific evidence linking dietary habits and risk for disease, prompted the Department of Health, Education, and Welfare to establish a continuing National Nutrition Surveillance System in 1969 (under the authority of the 1956 act) for the purposes of measuring the nutritional status of the U.S. population and monitoring the changes over time. Rather than conduct two separate surveys, which would require two separate samples and numerous additional hours of work, it was decided that the National Nutrition Surveillance System would be combined with the National Health Examination Survey, thereby forming the National Health and Nutrition Examination Survey, or NHANES.

malnutrition: chronic lack of sufficient nutrients to maintain health

Five NHANES have been conducted since 1970. NHANES I, the first cycle of the NHANES studies, was conducted between 1971 and 1975 and included a national sample of approximately 30,000 individuals between one and seventy-four years of age. Extensive dietary intake and nutritional status were collected by interview, physical examination, and a battery of clinical tests and measurements. NHANES II (1976–1980) included just slightly over 25,000 participants and expanded the age of the first NHANES sample somewhat by including individuals as young as 6 months of age. In addition, children and adults living at or below the poverty level were sampled at higher rates than their proportions in the general population ("oversampled") because these individuals were thought to be at particular nutritional risk.

While NHANES I and II provided extensive data regarding the health and nutritional status of the general U.S. population, it was somewhat biased against other ethnic groups residing in the United States, particularly Hispanics, whose numbers had been steadily increasing since data collection began in the 1960s. Thus, a Health and Nutrition Surveillance Survey specifically targeting the three largest Hispanic subgroups in the United States—Mexican Americans, Cuban Americans, and Puerto Ricans—was conducted between 1982 and 1984. The Hispanic Health and Nutrition Examination Survey (HHANES) was similar in design (i.e., similar instrumentation and data collection procedures) to the first two cycles of NHANES and included 16,000 individuals residing in regions across the United States with large Hispanic populations.

NHANES III (1988–1994) included a total of 40,000 individuals and expanded the age range even further than previous NHANES by including infants as young as two months of age, with no upper age limit on adults. In addition, to ensure the representativeness of both ethnicity and age, African Americans, Mexican Americans, infants, children, and those over sixty years old were oversampled. NHANES III also placed a greater emphasis on the effects of **environment** on health than either of the two previous NHANES (I and II). For example, data were gathered examining the levels of pesticide exposure, and the presence of carbon monoxide and various "**trace**" elements in the blood.

environment: surroundings

trace: very small amount

Beginning in 1999, NHANES became a "continuous survey." That is, unlike the previous NHANES surveys, which were conducted over a period of approximately four years with a "break" of at least one year between survey periods, the 1999–2000 survey was (and all subsequent surveys will be)

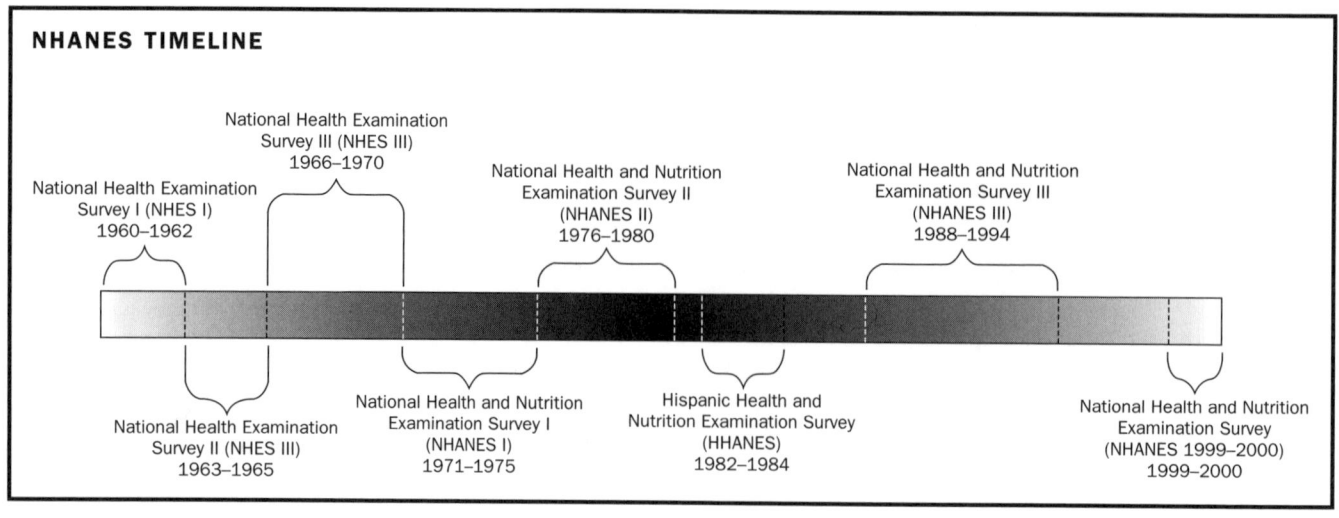

conducted without breaks, on a yearly basis. As the survey period is shorter in length, the subject sample will be smaller. The 1999–2000 survey included nutritional and medical data on approximately 8,837 individuals up to 74 years of age.

Procedures: How is NHANES Data Collected?

When NHES was originally conceived, it was determined that data would come from three primary sources:

1. Direct Interview: directly interviewing the survey participant and those within their household about their health.
2. Direct Examination: conducting clinical tests, **anthropometric**, **biochemical**, and radiological measurements, and physical examinations.
3. Physician Inquiry/Medical Records: reviewing participant's medical record.

In current practice, however, NHANES data are derived primarily from the first two sources; that is, via direct interview and direct clinical examination.

The NHANES data collection procedures have changed slightly over the years. These changes reflect not only the changing demographics of the United States over time, but also the changing nature of the survey (e.g., the inclusion of the nutrition component, the interest in the effects of environment upon health). Nonetheless, the basic tenets of data collection, particularly with regards to sampling, are similar.

Sampling. The goal of NHANES is to obtain a nationally "representative" yet manageable sample of noninstitutionalized persons residing in the United States. To achieve this goal, a nationwide probability sample of the population is selected via a complex series of statistical techniques. In very basic terms, the country is divided into geographic areas, also known as "primary sampling units" (PSUs). The PSUs are then combined to form strata, and each strata is then divided into a series of neighborhoods. Households are chosen at random from these neighborhoods, and inhabitants of those households are interviewed to determine if they are eligible for participation in the survey. Theoretically, each selected survey participant represents approximately 50,000 other U.S. residents.

---

anthropometric: related to measurement of characteristics of the human body

biochemical: related to chemical processes within cells

Data Collection Procedures. Once a household has been identified, a trained interviewer conducts an initial in-home interview with the potential survey participant to determine his or her study eligibility. Eligibility is determined by the collective responses to two in-depth questionnaires (the NHANES *Household Adult (or Youth) Questionnaire* and the *Family Questionnaire*) and from a series of **blood pressure** measurements. If the potential participant is deemed eligible for the study, an appointment is scheduled at a mobile examination center for the complete battery of medical and nutritional tests and measurements. The mobile examination centers (MEC) consist of four large trailers that contain all of the diagnostic equipment and personnel necessary to conduct a wide range of both simple and complex physical and biochemical evaluations. Four types of data collection methods are employed in the MEC:

1. A physical examination (including body measurements, a variety of X-rays, audiometry, electrocardiography, bone densitometry, allergy testing, and spirometry.
2. A dental examination.
3. Specimen collection (for hematological and urinary analysis).
4. Personal interview (to collect nutrition-related information; data on sensitive subjects such as tobacco use among youngsters, sexual experience, and **depression**; and tests of cognitive development and learning achievement).

The nutritional assessment component of NHANES was designed to include a variety of data sources, including:

- Dietary Intake Interviews: Quantitative and qualitative dietary information is collected using a 24-hour recall and food frequency questionnaire (FFQ).
- Nutrition-Related Interview: Information that is not sufficiently obtained via the dietary intake interview is included in this interview (e.g., water intake, vitamin and mineral supplementation, meal and snack patterns, infant feeding practices, alcohol intake, and food sufficiency).
- Anthropometric Data: Height, body weight, body composition, and various body circumferences are measured in order to determine body weight-fat distribution.
- Hematological and Nutritional Biochemistries: Blood lipid levels, blood **glucose** levels, vitamin and mineral status measures (e.g., **iron**, **calcium**, sodium, potassium, chloride, **folate**, **vitamins** such as B_{12}, A, and E), and **protein** status (total protein, albumin, and creatinine) are determined.
- Nutrition-Related Clinical Assessments: A combination of the above methodologies are used to assess risk for chronic diseases such as cardiovascular disease, diabetes, osteoporosis, and gallbladder disease.

Results: What Have We Learned from NHANES?

NHANES is probably best known for the prevalence data it provides on obesity. Indeed, as a result of data derived from NHANES, researchers, health professionals, and makers of public policy have been able to chart the

blood pressure: measure of the pressure exerted by the blood against the walls of the blood vessels

depression: mood disorder characterized by apathy, restlessness, and negative thoughts

glucose: a simple sugar; the most commonly used fuel in cells

iron: nutrient needed for red blood cell formation

calcium: mineral essential for bones and teeth

folate: one of the B vitamins, also called folic acid

vitamin: necessary complex nutrient used to aid enzymes or other metabolic processes in the cell

protein: complex molecule composed of amino acids that performs vital functions in the cell; necessary part of the diet

> ### NHANES in Action
>
> Data derived from NHES and NHANES surveys have been instrumental in the development and implementation of a number of health-related guidelines and reforms and public-policy initiatives. Examples include:
>
> - Growth Charts: Anthropometric data derived from NHES and NHANES has been instrumental in the development of growth charts used by pediatricians and health clinics across the United States and around the world.
>
> - Vitamin and Mineral Fortification of Food: Nutrient intake data derived from NHANES has aided in the determination of population groups at nutritional risk and spawned measures to address these nutritional inadequacies. For example, nutrient data from the first two NHANES indicated that certain segments of the U.S. population (women of childbearing age, young children and the elderly) were consuming inadequate amounts of iron. This information led to the fortification of grain and cereal products with iron. Similarly, NHANES data provided the additional proof of the connection between folate intake and neural tube defects needed to mandate the fortification of grain and cereal products with folate, a measure that has succeeded in significantly increasing blood folate levels in participants of the most recent (1999–2000) survey.
>
> - Lead Exposure: It was data derived from early NHANES that provided the first concrete evidence that blood levels of lead among Americans were becoming dangerously high. As a result, the Environmental Protection Agency called for a reduction in production and sales of consumer products containing relatively large amounts lead, most notably gasoline and household paints.

arthritis: inflammation of the joints

cancer: uncontrolled cell growth

fortification: addition of vitamins and minerals to improve the nutritional content of a food

increasing prevalence of obesity in the United States, as well as changes in obesity demographics (e.g., age, ethnicity, gender). Nonetheless, NHANES provides much more than just obesity prevalence data. NHANES issues vital data on the prevalence and correlates of chronic diseases such as **arthritis**, cardiovascular and respiratory diseases, diabetes, gallbladder and kidney diseases, osteoporosis, and **cancer**. In addition, NHANES supplies important information on the prevalence and trends of risk factors and other key health behaviors, including alcohol use, tobacco use and exposure, drug use, sexual experience, immunization histories, and physical activity. Data from NHANES has been instrumental in the development and implementation of a number of health-related guidelines and reforms and public-policy initiatives, including growth charts for children, folate **fortification** of grain products, and a reduction in the manufacturing and sales of lead-containing products.

Future Directions: Where Is NHANES Going from Here?

As previously mentioned, beginning in 1999, NHANES became a continuous, annual survey in order to provide more timely data on the health and nutritional status of the population. In addition, NHANES will eventually be linked with other related health and nutrition surveys of the U.S. population, including the National Health Interview Survey (NHIS) and the U.S. Department of Agriculture's Continuing Survey of Food Intakes by Individuals (CSFII). By combining and integrating the data from these extensive surveys, a more comprehensive evaluation of the current health and nutritional status of the U.S. population can be made.

Katherine A. Beals

Bibliography

McDowell, A.; Engel, A.; Massey, J. T.; Maurer, K. (1981). "Plan and Operation of the Second National Health and Nutrition Examination Survey, 1976–1980." *Vital and Health Statistics* 1(15):1–144.

National Center for Health Statistics (1965). "Cycle I of the Health and Examination Survey: Sample and Response. United States: 1960–1962." *Vital and Health Statistics* 1(4):1-43.

National Center for Health Statistics (1965). "Plan and Initial Program of the Health Examination Survey." *Vital and Health Statistics* 1(4):1–43.

National Center for Health Statistics (1978). "Plan and Operation of the Health and Nutritional Examination Survey, United States: 1971–1973. Programs and Collection Procedure." *Vital and Health Statistics* 10:1–46.

National Center for Health Statistics (1994). "Plan and Operation of the Third National Health and Nutritional Examination Survey, 1988–1994." *Vital and Health Statistics* 32:1–407.

Internet Resources

National Center for Health Statistics. "National Health and Nutrition Examination Survey." Available from <http://www.cdc.gov/nchs/nhanes> Updated April 3, 2003.

National Institutes of Health (NIH)

The U.S. National Institutes of Health (NIH) are charged with the vital mission of uncovering new knowledge that will lead to better health for everyone. To carry out this ambitious task, the NIH has become the largest agency for biomedical research in the world. It consists of twenty-seven separate institutes and centers and has a multibillion-dollar budget. However, it did not start out this way.

History of the National Institutes of Health

In 1887, the NIH began in Staten Island, New York, as a one-room federal laboratory within the Marine Hospital Service (MHS). At the time, it was called the Laboratory of **Hygiene**. The MHS was responsible for preventing the spread of **infectious disease** in the United States. For example, the staff at the MHS examined passengers on arriving ships for signs of communicable diseases such as **cholera** and yellow fever. By 1891, the federal government required the MHS to take on the additional responsibilities of developing and testing **vaccines**. That year, the service was relocated to Washington, D.C., and renamed the Hygienic Laboratory.

In 1902, Congress passed the Biologics Control Act to regulate vaccines sold in the U.S. This resulted in the Hygienic Laboratory adding divisions in chemistry, pharmacology, and zoology, all on a meager annual budget of $50,000. After ten years, this enterprise, now called the U.S. Public Health Service (PHS), was further authorized to study **chronic** diseases (e.g., **heart disease**, **diabetes**, and **cancer**) and infectious diseases (e.g., **tuberculosis**, influenza, and **malaria**). Despite working with limited funds, its investigators made several remarkable medical discoveries during this period. For example, in 1920, Joseph Goldberger discovered that *pellagra*, a skin disease widely considered to be infectious, was in fact the result of a vitamin deficiency that could be prevented by proper **nutrition**.

In 1930, the Hygienic Laboratory became the National Institutes of Health (NIH), and by 1938 the unit had moved to a privately donated estate

hygiene: cleanliness

infectious diseases: diseases caused by viruses, bacteria, fungi, or protozoa, which replicate inside the body

cholera: bacterial infection of the small intestine causing severe diarrhea, vomiting, and dehydration

vaccine: medicine that promotes immune system resistance by stimulating pre-existing cells to become active

chronic: over a long period

heart disease: any disorder of the heart or its blood supply, including heart attack, atherosclerosis, and coronary artery disease

diabetes: inability to regulate level of sugar in the blood

cancer: uncontrolled cell growth

tuberculosis: bacterial infection, usually of the lungs, caused by Mycobacterium tuberculosis

malaria: disease caused by infection with Plasmodium, a single-celled protozoon, transmitted by mosquitoes

nutrition: the maintenance of health through proper eating, or the study of same

in Bethesda, Maryland. Today, this is the primary home of the National Institutes of Health.

Pursuing the Mission of NIH

The activities of the NIH are overseen by the Public Health Service, which, in turn, is directed by the U.S. Department of Health and Human Services. However, the mission, goal, and activities of NIH distinguish it as a unique federation of biomedical research institutes. In pursuit of its broader mission, the specific goal of the NIH is to acquire biomedical knowledge that will enable researchers and practitioners to prevent, control, detect, and treat disease and disability. To achieve this goal, the NIH directs a number of programs and activities, including: (1) conducting research at the facility; (2) supporting scientific explorations of investigators in other settings (e.g., universities, medical schools, **clinical** centers) nationwide and internationally; (3) providing training for researchers; and (4) fostering the dissemination of medical information. The Office of the Director (OD) sets policy for planning, managing, and coordinating these programs and activities.

Within the OD is the Office of Legislative Policy and Analysis (OLPA). OLPA is responsible for making sure that the results of all of this research inform public policy and public health laws. To this end, the OLPA supervises legislative analysis and policy development, and also acts as a liaison between the NIH and Congress. As a result of the OLPA's participation in congressional hearings, for example, the Dietary Supplement Health and Education Act (DSHEA) was authorized in 1993. Consequently, the NIH established the Office of Dietary Supplements to conduct and coordinate research relating to dietary supplements and their impact on the health of the public.

The Institutes and Centers

To support its mission, the NIH has developed into a broad and complex federation consisting of a total of twenty institutes and seven centers. Each institute and center has its own medical or public health focus with well-defined priorities. For example, some institutes concentrate on a particular disease area (e.g., cancer, diabetes) whereas others support biomedical research (e.g., promoting diversity, providing medical resources).

One of the NIH's institutes is the famous U.S. National Library of Medicine (NLM), the world's largest medical library, holding nearly six million items, such as books, professional journals (e.g., *Science* and *Nature*), and photographs. A plethora of resources and search engines, including PubMed and MEDLINEplus, provide access to these materials through the World Wide Web.

In general, the institutes' research priorities are shaped by two things: (1) epidemiological assessments (i.e., studies of the distribution and determinants of diseases and injuries in populations), and (2) political pressure. In some cases, political concerns have affected plans for specific research directions regardless of the results of epidemiological assessments. For example, a wide variety of research supports the idea that stem cells (undifferentiated cells taken from human embryos) have great potential to reduce the burden of illness (stem cells can be used to create other body cells, such as blood

clinical: related to hospitals, clinics, and patient care

Accomplishments of the NIH

The NIH supports thousands of research projects every year. A small sample of the accomplishments from 2003 includes the following:

- The Human Genome Project—an ambitious international effort to identify the 30,000 genes in human DNA and determine the sequences of the three billion chemical base pairs that make up human DNA—was completed two years ahead of schedule. The data was made freely available to scientists around the world.

- New guidelines were published for the prevention, detection, and treatment of high blood pressure.

- A new Ebola vaccine proved successful in monkeys, with human trials to follow.

- The drug letrozol was shown to reduce recurrence of breast cancer.

- The serotonin transporter gene was discovered to influence the onset and severity of depression.

- Research showed that heart attack symptoms in women differ from those in men, which may help women and doctors identify the onset of an attack earlier.

- Scientists found that the levels of two proteins, beta-amyloid and tau, distinguish Alzheimer's patients from controls. This discovery may lead to the development of predictive and diagnostic tools.

- Combined estrogen and progestin therapy was found to increase the risk of dementia.

- Scientists discovered that a greater than usual number of copies of the a-synuclein gene may cause Parkinson's disease.

- A new West Nile Virus vaccine was shown to be effective in monkeys.

- An international research team found that using cloth to filter water in poor countries reduced the incidence of cholera by half.

—*Paula Kepos*

---

cells, or to regenerate tissue, bone, and muscle). However, despite the potential value of these applications, political concerns have threatened to end funding for this kind of research. On August, 9, 2001, President George W. Bush announced his decision to allow federal funds to support research on existing human embryonic stem cell lines under certain limited conditions.

Human Subjects: Protection and Ethics

Because much of the research supported by the NIH is conducted on human subjects, the NIH has several offices and programs in place to protect participants and address bioethical research issues. For example, to protect the rights and welfare of human subjects, the NIH has established at least fourteen separate Institutional Review Boards (IRBs). IRB committee members must review, and approve, all human-subject research activities prior to, and throughout, a study. Each principal investigator (the scientist in charge of directing a research project) must prove to the IRB that all of their human subjects provided **informed consent** before participating in study procedures. In addition, researchers must ensure the privacy of their participants is protected and their data are kept confidential.

informed consent: agreement to a procedure after understanding the risks

In addition to offices that protect research participants, the NIH contains a number of offices that address ethical concerns and appraise the potential social consequences of scientific pursuits. For example, the Office of Science Policy (OSP) advises the NIH director on policy issues that affect the

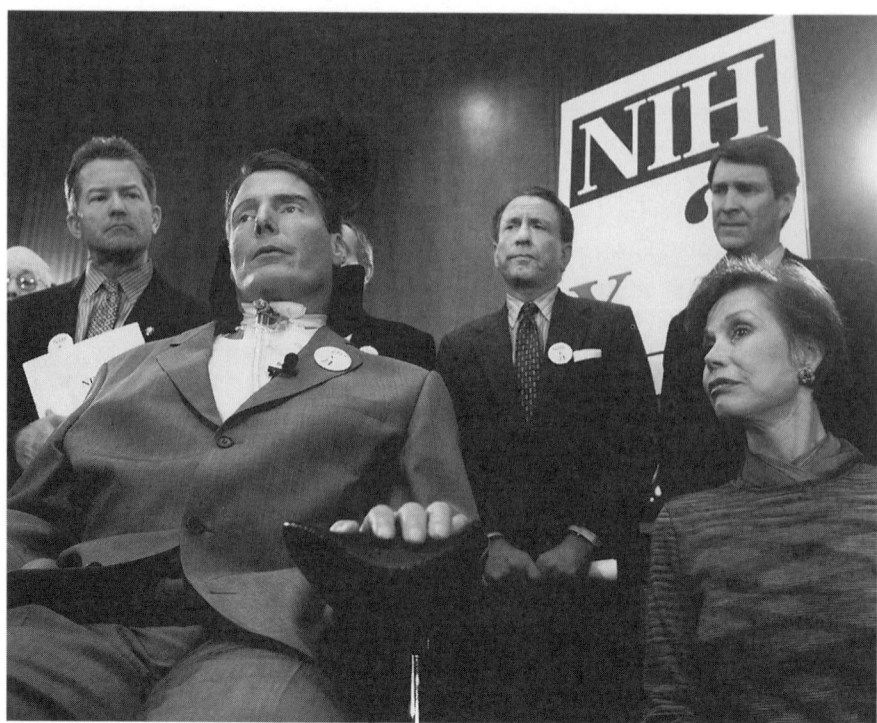

In 1998 the U.S. Congress committed to increase the budget of the National Institutes of Health to more than $27 billion. A press conference calling for the increase featured entertainers Christopher Reeve and Mary Tyler Moore. [AP/Wide World Photos. Reproduced by permission.]

research community. In addition, OSP coordinates the Trans-NIH Bioethics Committee (T-NBC), composed of scientists, ethicists, and IRB members. This group is explicitly responsible for developing policies and considering the ethical, legal, and social implications of NIH-funded research.

Funding Research Projects

The NIH's important role in health and medical research and training is reflected in a yearly budget of 23 billion dollars (as of fiscal year 2002), a sum generated almost entirely through taxes. Today, the NIH uses these funds to support over thirty thousand research projects conducted on the main campus (intramural) and away from campus (extramural) at universities, medical schools, and independent research institutions.

Although the intramural research conducted at the NIH is important, nearly 80 percent of the NIH's budget is spent on extramural grants to investigators and research institutions throughout the nation and the world. The grants program seeks to stimulate the discovery of biomedical knowledge by encouraging qualified scientists to participate in particular types of research. In addition, research grants and contracts guarantee that facilities, equipment, and human resources are available to conduct research.

Research and Biomedical Advances

Nationwide and internationally, over fifty thousand researchers have been awarded grants to conduct their studies away from NIH's main campus. Together, these researchers have made more scientific breakthroughs than could be listed in this book. Some noteworthy examples, however, include: (1) the discovery that antiretroviral **drugs** could prevent transmission of the HIV virus from mother to infant, (2) demonstrating that weight loss

drugs: substances whose administration causes a significant change in the body's function

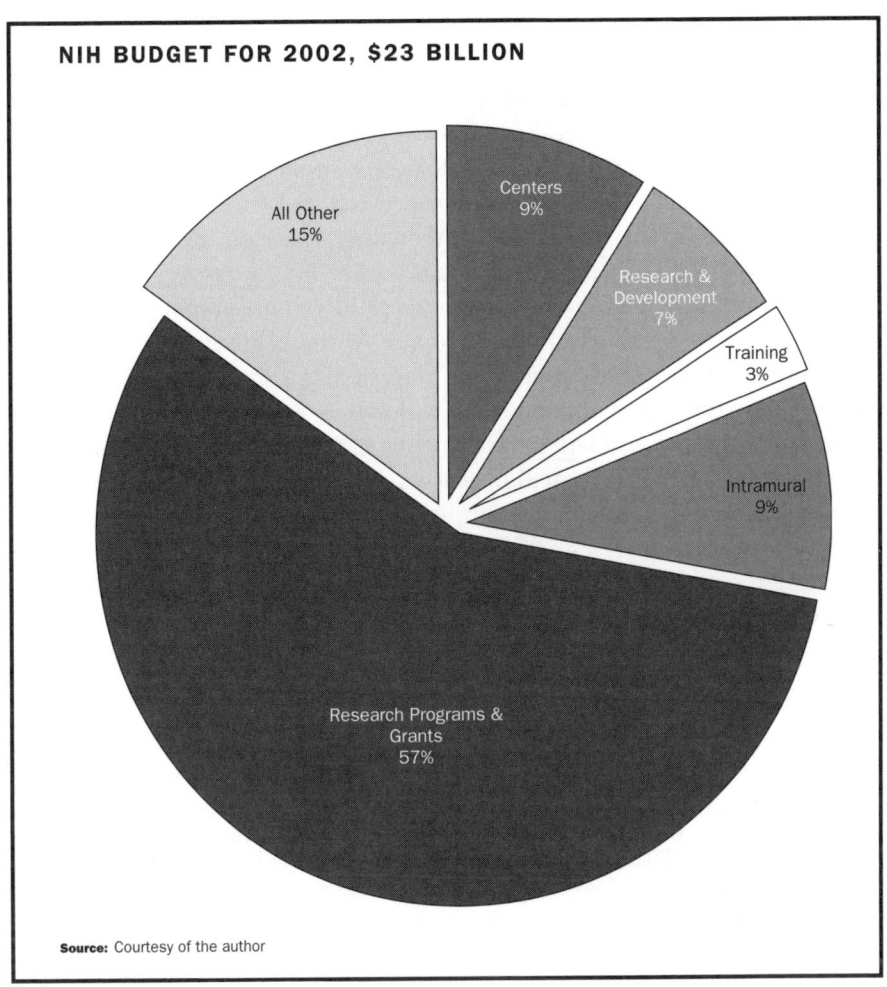

Source: Courtesy of the author

and restriction of dietary salt reduce the need for blood pressure-lowering drugs, (3) confirming that tight control of blood **glucose** (sugar) may help people living with diabetes prevent complications such as blindness, and (4) identifying leptin (a product of the "**obesity**" gene) and suggesting how it might be used to combat obesity in humans. A number of extramural investigators have also been honored with the Nobel Prize for their significant contributions to biomedical science. For example, the 1985 Nobel Prize in **Physiology** or Medicine was awarded jointly to Drs. Michael S. Brown and Joseph L. Goldstein for their discoveries concerning the regulation of **cholesterol metabolism** and its role in heart disease.

In addition to this work, research scientists, physicians, dentists, veterinarians, and nurses conduct more than two thousand intramural projects on the NIH campus. Several of these investigators have also received international attention for their discoveries. Currently, three Nobel laureates work at the NIH: Dr. Marshall W. Nirenberg (honored in 1968 for finding the key to cracking the **genetic** code), Dr. Julius Axelrod (honored in 1970 for discoveries concerning chemical transmitters in the **nervous system**), and Dr. D. Carleton Gajdusek (honored in 1976 for identifying the cause of kuru, a fatal infectious disease that affects the nervous system). Today, intramural researchers continue to work on projects that will, ultimately, improve the health of the public.

glucose: a simple sugar; the most commonly used fuel in cells

obesity: the condition of being overweight, according to established norms based on sex, age, and height

physiology: the group of biochemical and physical processes that combine to make a functioning organism, or the study of same

cholesterol: multi-ringed molecule found in animal cell membranes; a type of lipid

metabolism: the sum total of reactions in a cell or an organism

genetic: inherited or related to the genes

nervous system: the brain, spinal cord, and nerves that extend throughout the body

arthritis: inflammation of the joints

depression: mood disorder characterized by apathy, restlessness, and negative thoughts

biological: related to living organisms

diet: the total daily food intake, or the types of foods eaten

gene expression: use of a gene to make the protein it encodes

Since its humble beginning as a one-room laboratory of hygiene, the NIH has become the largest biomedical research enterprise in the world. This well-funded public program has enabled scientists to make tremendous strides in preventing, controlling, detecting, and treating disease. Still, there are enduring questions for researchers at each of the twenty-seven institutes and centers to tackle, such as ways to prevent and treat cancer, heart disease, blindness, **arthritis**, diabetes, Alzheimer's disease, **depression**, drug misuse, and AIDS. To pursue these and other issues, every year the NIH posts hundreds of requests for proposals (RFPs), encouraging scientists to submit grant proposals on different topics. At the beginning of the twenty-first century, the NIH is especially interested in supporting research that will improve the health of infants and children, women, older adults, and minorities. Future projects will help scientists, practitioners, and educators better understand how **biological** processes, behaviors, and lifestyle practices impact health and disease. For example, more will certainly be learned about nutrition-related illnesses and how **diet** influences **gene expression**. By directing research in these areas, the NIH is leading the way to better health for everyone. SEE ALSO GOLDBERGER, JOSEPH.

Jessica Schulman

Bibliography

Brown, Michael S., and Goldstein, Joseph L. (1984). "How LDL Receptors Influence Cholesterol and Atherosclerosis." *Scientific American* 251:52–60.

Pittenger, Mark F.; Mackay, Alastair, M.; Beck, Stephen C.; Jaiswal, Rama K.; Douglas, Robin; Mosca, Joseph D.; Moorman, Mark A.; Simonetti, Donald W.; Craig, Stewart; and Marshak, Daniel R. (1999). "Multilineage Potential of Adult Human Mesenchymal Stem Cells." *Science* 284:143–147.

Roe, Daphne A. (1973). *A Plague of Corn: A Social History of Pellagra*. New York: Cornell University Press.

Starr, Paul (1982). *The Social Transformation of American Medicine*. Washington, DC: Basic Books.

Internet Resources

National Institutes of Health (2001). "Press Release: FY 2002 President's Budget." Available from <http://www4.od.nih.gov/officeofbudget/press2002.pdf>

National Institutes of Health, Stetton Museum of Medical Research. "Historical Resources." Available from <http://history.nih.gov>

Native Americans, Diet of

When Christopher Columbus dropped anchor on the shores of San Salvador in the Caribbean Sea, he believed he reached India. Because he believed he was in India, Columbus named the inhabitants *Indians*, a term that was soon used to refer to all the native inhabitants of North America. Today, the term *Native American* is more commonly used.

The Hardships of Settlement

New settlers in North America had a difficult time learning how to grow food and harvest crops to sustain their colonies through the land's harsh winters. The Native Americans, on the other hand, were accustomed to the climate and the land's nuances, and were familiar with what types of food were available to them during the different times of the year. They did

RATES (%) OF OVERWEIGHT AND OBESITY IN MALE AND FEMALE NATIVE AMERICANS COMPARED TO ALL U.S. RACES

Age (in years)	Overweight: American Indians/ Alaska Natives (%)	Overweight: all races in U.S. (%)	Obese: American Indians/ Alaska Natives (%)	Obese: all races in U.S. (%)
Males				
Total (18+)	33.7	24.1	13.8	9.1
18–24	21.5	13.1	11.0	5.5
25–34	31.8	19.5	11.2	7.6
35–44	37.8	27.0	11.2	10.4
45–54	49.1	33.8	28.2	14.1
55–64	45.5	33.1	16.5	13.0
65+	25.2	23.0	11.1	5.4
Females				
Total (18+)	40.3	25.0	16.6	8.2
18–24	25.2	11.5	11.7	3.9
25–34	45.1	17.4	13.8	6.0
35–44	48.5	28.1	19.7	10.8
45–54	54.0	32.0	18.7	10.9
55–64	45.6	36.2	18.8	11.5
65+	45.6	30.1	20.7	7.7

SOURCE: Broussard, et al. (1991). "Prevalence of Obesity in American Indians and Alaska Natives." *American Journal of Clinical Nutrition.*

not go hungry as the settlers did. The Native Americans were skilled agriculturists, nomadic hunters, and food gatherers who lived in relatively egalitarian communities where both the women and men had equal responsibilities.

The portal that Columbus opened when he first stepped foot on the soil of the New World in 1492 triggered a steady influx of European settlers, indelibly affecting the lives of Native Americans. However, it was Thomas Jefferson's purchase of the Louisiana Territory from France in 1803 that fundamentally changed the course of Native Americans' future in North America. Hoping to expand the nation's size, Jefferson urged the Creek and Cherokee nations of Georgia to relocate to the newly acquired land. This began an era of devastating wars over land. The many years of struggle between Native American tribes and the U.S. government resulted in the near extinction of many Native American tribes.

General Diet before the Colonial Period

The Native American population, including American Indians and Alaska Natives, once totaled nearly 24 million, with over 500 tribes. The diets of Native Americans varied by geographic region and climate. They lived in territories marked by specific natural boundaries, such as mountains, oceans, rivers, and plains. Hunting, fishing, and farming supplied the major food resources. Native Americans survived largely on meat, fish, plants, berries, and nuts.

The most widely grown and consumed plant foods were maize (or corn) in the mild climate regions and wild rice in the Great Lakes region. A process called *nixtamalizacion* (soaking dry corn in lime water) was used to soften the corn into dough, called *nixtamal* or *masa*. This was prepared in a variety of ways to make porridges and breads. Many tribes grew beans and enjoyed them as *succotash*, a dish made of beans, corn, dog meat, and bear **fat**. Tubers

fat: type of food molecule rich in carbon and hydrogen, with high energy content

(roots), also widely eaten, were cooked slowly in underground pits until the hard tough root became a highly digestible gelatin-like soup. It is estimated that 60 percent of modern agricultural production in the United States involves crops domesticated by Native Americans.

Maple sugar comprised 12 percent of the Native American diet. The Native American name for maple sugar is *Sinzibuckwud* (drawn from the wood). Sugar was a basic seasoning for grains and breads, stews, teas, berries, vegetables. In the Southwest, the Native Americans chewed the sweet heart of the agave plant.

Many tribes preferred broth and herbed beverages to water. The Chippewa boiled water and added leaves or twigs before drinking it. Sassafras was a favorite ingredient in teas and medicinal drinks. Broth was flavored and thickened with corn silk and dried pumpkin blossoms. Native Americans in California added lemonade berries to water to make a pleasantly sour drink.

Sacred and Ceremonial Foods. Sacred foods included bear, organ meats, and *blood soup*. The Horns Society, a militant group of the Blackfoot Nation, used *pemmican*, made with berries, for its sacred communion meal. Boiled buffalo tongue was a delicacy and was served as the food of communion at the Sun Dance, a Lakota and Plains Indian courtship dance that also celebrated the renewal of spiritual life. Blood soup, made from a mixture of blood and corn flour cooked in broth, was used as a sacred meal during the nighttime Holy Smoke ceremony of the Sioux, a celebration of Mother Earth that involved the use of the "peace pipe." Wolves and coyotes were the only animals that were not hunted for food, because they were regarded as teachers or pathfinders and held as sacred by all tribes.

At marriage ceremonies, the bride and groom exchanged food instead of rings. The groom brought venison or some other meat to indicate his intention to provide for the household. The bride provided corn or bean bread to symbolize her willingness to care for and provide nourishment for her household.

Current Food Practices

Native American diets and food practices have possibly changed more than any other ethnic group in the United States. Although the current diet of Native Americans may vary by tribe, and by personal traits such as age (e.g., young versus old), it closely resembles that of the U.S. white population. Their diet, however, is poorer in quality than that of the general U.S. population. A recent study found that only 10 percent of Native Americans have a healthful diet, while 90 percent have a poor quality that needs improvement. The majority of Native Americans have diets that are too high in fat (62%). Only 21 percent eat the recommended amount of fruit on any given day, while 34 percent eat the recommended amount of vegetables, 24 percent eat the recommended amount of grains, and 27 percent consume the recommended amount of dairy products. Native Americans are also four times more likely to report not having enough to eat than other U.S. households.

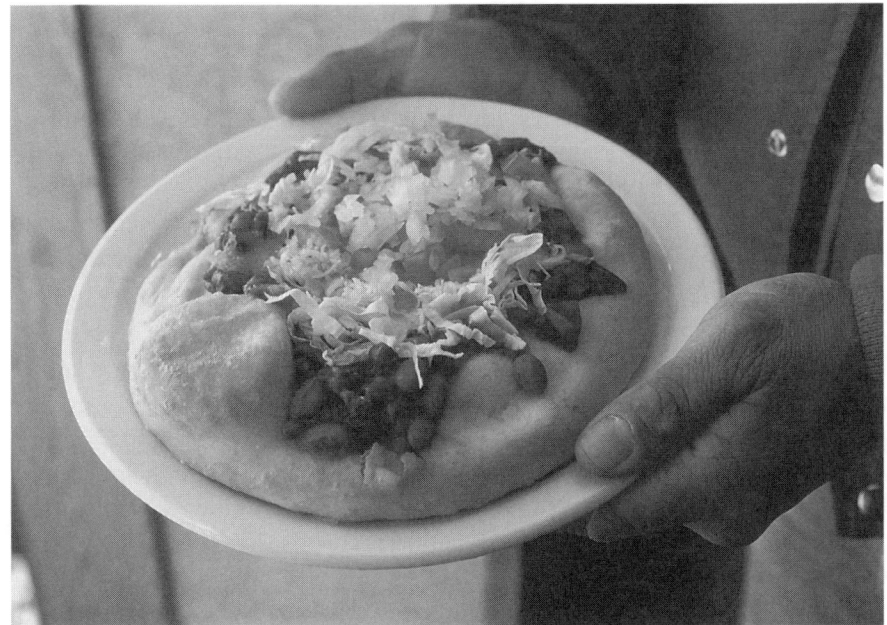

The frybread taco is a relatively recent addition to Native American fare. It requires white wheat flour, which came to the New World with Europeans.
[Photograph by Catherine Karnow. Corbis. Reproduced by permission.]

Diet-Related Health Issues

Heart disease is the leading cause of death among Native Americans. Risk factors, such as **high blood pressure**, cigarette smoking, high blood **cholesterol**, **obesity**, and **diabetes**, are health conditions that increase a person's chance for having heart disease. The more risk factors a person has, the greater chance a person may have for developing heart disease. Sixty-four percent of Native American men and 61 percent of women have one or more of these risk factors.

Diabetes. **Type II Diabetes** is one of the most serious health problems for Native Americans in the United States. It is estimated that 12.3 percent of Native Americans over nineteen years of age have type II diabetes, compared to about 6 percent of the general U.S. population—a statistic that has caused health experts to say diabetes has reached widespread proportions. On average, Native Americans are 2.8 times more likely to be diagnosed with diabetes than whites of a similar age. Diabetes is a major cause of health problems and deaths in most Native American populations. Diabetes rates for Native Americans vary by tribal group.

Obesity. Obesity is a major risk factor for both type II diabetes and heart disease. On average, 30 percent of all adult Native Americans are **obese**. Both males and females are consistently more **overweight** and obese than the total U.S. population. Among the Pima of Arizona and Mexico, for example, 95 percent of those with diabetes are also overweight. In addition to the increase in obesity among adults, obesity in children has also become a serious health problem. For both adults and children, the increasingly high rates of obesity have been associated with a high-fat diet and decreased levels of physical activity.

Conclusion

The history of the Native American people provides evidence of a culture strong enough to withstand the most difficult hardships. Though their lives

heart disease: any disorder of the heart or its blood supply, including heart attack, atherosclerosis, and coronary artery disease

high blood pressure: elevation of the pressure in the bloodstream maintained by the heart

cholesterol: multi-ringed molecule found in animal cell membranes; a type of lipid

obesity: the condition of being overweight, according to established norms based on sex, age, and height

diabetes: inability to regulate level of sugar in the blood

type II diabetes: inability to regulate the level of sugar in the blood due to a reduction in the number of insulin receptors on the body's cells

obese: above accepted standards of weight for sex, height, and age

overweight: weight above the accepted norm based on height, sex, and age

were changed in many ways over the centuries, their cooking and eating traditions have become mainstays of contemporary American cuisine. Many Native American recipes have been adopted by white populations in different regions in the United States, including succotash in the South, wild rice dishes in the northern Plains, pumpkin soup in New England, chili in the Southwest, broiled salmon in the Pacific Northwest, and corn on the cob in most areas of the country. Indeed, Native Americans have influenced American cuisine in ways the white population has yet to acknowledge.

Of greater importance, however, is the dire need to focus on the failing health of Native Americans. For complex reasons, Native Americans have not had the opportunity to access health care in ways that other Americans have. This has caused serious health problems. The limitations imposed on their living conditions, in concert with the socioeconomic obstacles that Native Americans face, challenge their livelihood. Though some programs have begun to target Native Americans' health problems, their future depends on receiving proper care for modern-day diseases. SEE ALSO CORN- OR MAIZE-BASED DIETS.

M. Cristina Flaminiano Garces
Lisa A. Sutherland

Bibliography

Brill, Steve, and Dean, Evelyn (1994). *Identifying and Harvesting Edible and Medicinal Plants.* New York: Hearst Books.

Centers for Disease Control and Prevention (2000). "Prevalence of Selected Cardiovascular Disease Risk Factors by Sociodemographic Characteristics among American Indians and Alaska Natives." *Morbidity and Mortality Weekly Report.*

Fiple, Kenneth F., and Coneè Ornelas, Krimhil, eds. (2000). *The Cambridge World History of Food*, Volumes 1 and 2. Cambridge, U.K.: Cambridge University Press.

Gohdes, D. (1995). "Diabetes in North American Indians and Alaska Natives." In *Diabetes in America.* Bethesda, MD: National Institute of Diabetes and Digestive and Kidney Diseases, National Institutes of Health.

Greaves, Tom, ed. (2002). *Endangered Peoples of North America: Struggles to Survive and Thrive.* Westport, CT: Greenwood Press.

Jennings, Francis (1975). *The Invasion of America: Indians, Colonialism, and the Cant of Conquest.* New York: W. W. Norton.

Jennings, Jesse D., ed. (1978). *Ancient Native Americans.* San Francisco, CA: W.H. Freeman.

Kavasch, Barrie (1977). *Native Harvests: Recipes and Botanicals of the American Indian.* New York: Vintage Books.

Lytle, L. A.; Dixon, L. B.; Cunningham-Sabo, L.; Evans, M.; Gittelsohn, J.; Hurley, J.; Snyder, P.; Stevens, J.; Weber, J.; Anliker, J.; Heller, K.; and Story, M. (2002). "Dietary Intakes of Native American Children: Findings from the Pathways Feasibility Study." *Journal of American Dietetic Association* 102(4):555–558.

National Institute of Diabetes and Digestive and Kidney Diseases (1995). *The Pima Indians: Pathfinders for Health.* Washington, DC: U.S. Government Printing Office.

Penner, Lucille Recht (1994). *A Native American Feast.* New York: Macmillan.

United States Department of Agriculture, Center for Nutrition Policy and Promotion (1999). "The Diet Quality of American Indians: Evidence from the Continuing Survey of Food Intakes by Individuals." *Nutrition Insights* 12.

Wolf, B. (1980). *The Ways of My Grandmothers.* New York: William Morrow.

Zinn, Howard (1980). *A People's History of the United States.* New York: Harper Collins.

Nongovernmental Organizations

The term *nongovernmental organization* (NGO) gained widespread use beginning in 1945, when it was used in the United Nations Charter to clearly distinguish between governmental and private organizations. To be considered an NGO, an organization must be free from government control, non-profit, not considered a political party, and not involved in criminal activity.

While NGOs are, by definition, independent from government, they often engage in political activities and work closely with governments. NGOs are involved in activities related to international development, including relief work, provision of health and human services, advocacy for human rights, and environmental protection. There are several types of NGOs, such as charity organizations, churches, research institutes, community-based organizations, and lobbying groups. Those whose primary focus is on the development and implementation of projects and programs are referred to as operational NGOs, and those whose primary focus is on defending or promoting a certain cause or influencing policies are called advocacy, or campaigning, NGOs. However, both operational and advocacy NGOs have to mobilize financial resources, needed materials, and volunteers in order to achieve their goals and purposes.

NGOs can be divided into three broad categories based on the scope of their work: community-based organizations (CBOs), national organizations, and international organizations. CBOs are usually established by members of a local community to serve their own needs. National organizations are formed to serve people within an entire country, and international organizations are usually headquartered in a developed country and provide services to more than one developing country. CBOs, national organizations, and international organizations may interact and work together. Since the mid-1970s the number of NGOs around the world has increased substantially—by the late twentieth century there were between 6,000 and 30,000 national NGOs and thousands of CBOs (the data on the number of NGOs is, unfortunately, very incomplete). SEE ALSO DISASTER RELIEF ORGANIZATIONS.

Laura Nelson

Bibliography

Basch, Paul F. (1999). *Textbook of International Health.* New York: Oxford University Press.

Internet Resources

Duke University Perkins Library. "Non-Governmental Organizations Research Guide." Available from <http://docs.lib.duke.edu/igo/guides/ngo>

Willetts, Peter (2002). "What is a Non-Governmental Organization?" Available from <http://www.staff.city.ac.uk/p.willetts>

World Bank. "NGO World Bank Collaboration." Available from <http://www.worldbank.org>

Northern Europeans, Diet of

The countries of northern Europe include the United Kingdom of Great Britain (England, Scotland, Wales, Northern Ireland), the Republic of Ireland (now a sovereign country), and France. (Although southern France is generally considered to be part of southern Europe, it will be included in this discussion.) These countries are all part of the European Union. England and France have a very diverse population due to the large number of immigrants from former colonies and current dependent territories. Catholicism and Protestantism are the dominant religions.

cardiovascular: related to the heart and circulatory system

coronary heart disease: disease of the coronary arteries, the blood vessels surrounding the heart

stroke: loss of blood supply to part of the brain, due to a blocked or burst artery in the brain

hypertension: high blood pressure

obesity: the condition of being overweight, according to established norms based on sex, age, and height

chronic: over a long period

heart disease: any disorder of the heart or its blood supply, including heart attack, atherosclerosis, and coronary artery disease

saturated fat: a fat with the maximum possible number of hydrogens; more difficult to break down than unsaturated fats

diet: the total daily food intake, or the types of foods eaten

protein: complex molecule composed of amino acids that performs vital functions in the cell; necessary part of the diet

Nutritional Status

Cardiovascular disease (e.g., **coronary heart disease**, **stroke**, **hypertension**) is the most common cause of death in these countries, and smoking rates are high. **Obesity** is the fastest growing **chronic** disease, especially among children. Alcoholism is high, especially among the Irish.

France's low rate of **heart disease** has been termed the "French Paradox." The theory is that France's low rate of heart disease is due to the regular consumption of wine, despite the high intake of saturated fats. However, recent evidence suggests that the rate of heart disease in France may have been underestimated and underreported, for while the rate of heart disease is lower in France than most countries, it is still the number one cause of death in France. In addition, the consumption of **saturated fat** has increased, which will eventually result in increased risk for coronary heart disease (CHD), regardless of wine intake.

Eating Habits and Meal Patterns

The northern European **diet** generally consists of a large serving of meat, poultry, or fish, accompanied by small side dishes of vegetables and starch. The traditional diet is high in **protein**, primarily from meat and dairy products. The diet tends to be low in whole grains, fruits, and vegetables. Immigrants from this region of the world brought this eating pattern to North America and it still influences the "meat and potatoes" American meal. The influence of each country's food habits on each other is also extensive.

England

English cuisine was primarily shaped during the Victorian era. The diet relies heavily on meats, dairy products, wheat, and root vegetables. The English are famous for their flower gardens, but they are also known for their kitchen gardens, which yield an abundance of herbs and vegetables. Breakfast is very hearty and generally consists of bacon, eggs, grilled tomato, and fried bread. Kippers (smoked herring) are also popular at breakfast. Many Britons still partake in afternoon tea, which consists of tiny sandwiches (no crust) filled with cucumber or watercress, scones or crumpets with jam or clotted cream, cakes or tarts, and a pot of hot tea. Tea shops abound in England, Wales, and Scotland, and Britons drink about four cups of tea a day. Coffee is also very popular with the younger generation.

The pub (short for "public house") is a central part of life and culture in the United Kingdom (Britain has over 61,000 pubs). British pubs are very cozy and homey, and they are famous for their beers, which are very strong. Pubs also serve food. The most common British pub meal is the "ploughman's lunch," named for traditional farmworkers. It consists of a large chunk of cheese, a hunk of homemade bread, pickled onion, and ale. Other popular menu items are shepherd's pie, Cornish pastry, Stargazy pie, and Lancashire hot pot. Britain's most famous dish is fish and chips, traditionally made with cod or pollack. There are some 8,500 fish-and-chip shops across the United Kingdom—they outnumber McDonald's eight to one.

Scotland

Scottish cuisine is centered on fresh raw ingredients such as seafood, beef, game, fruits, and vegetables. Porridge, or boiled oatmeal, is usually eaten

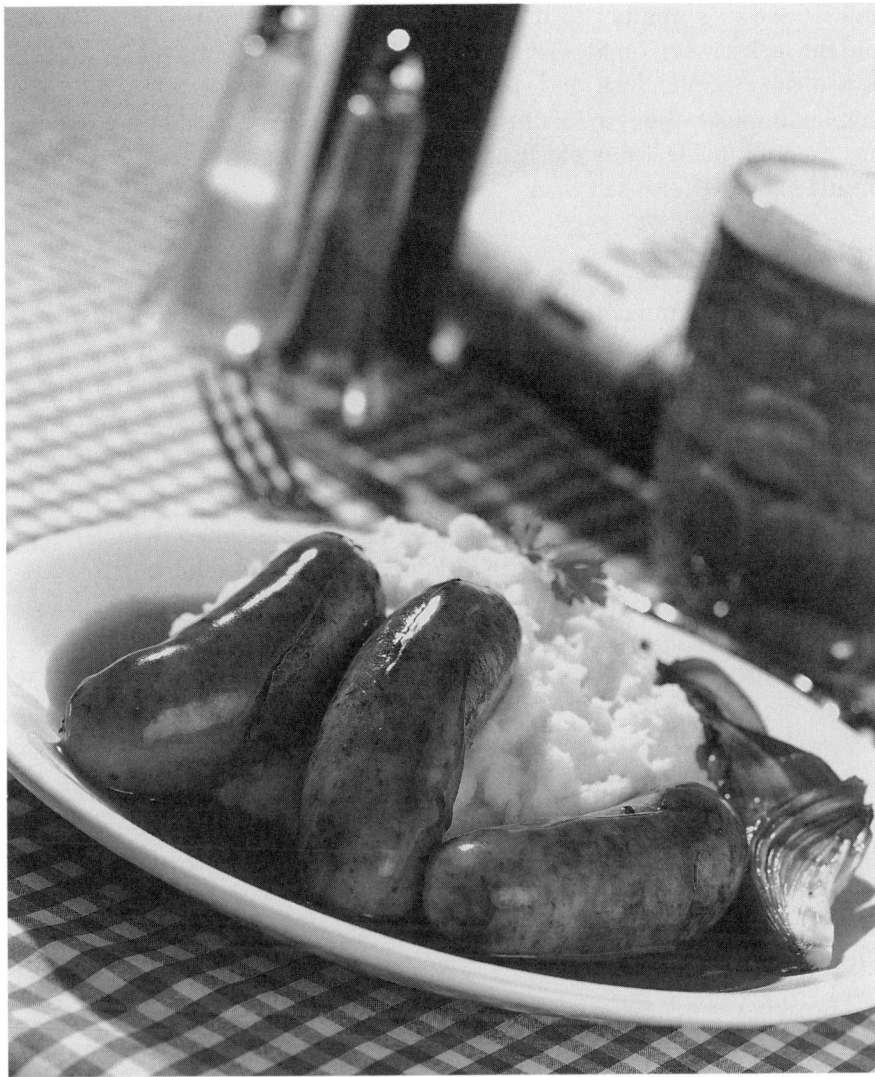

"Bangers and mash," a dish of sausage and mashed potatoes, is a favorite in English pubs. The Northern European diet is high in animal protein and fat, but it does not include many fruits or vegetables. [Royalty-Free/Corbis. Reproduced by permission.]

for breakfast. It is cooked with salt and milk—Scots do not usually eat their oatmeal with sugar or syrup.

The Aberdeen-Angus breed of beef cattle is widely reared across the world and is famous for rich and tasty steaks. Scottish lamb also has an excellent international reputation. Game such as rabbit, deer, woodcock, and grouse also plays an important role in the Scottish diet. Fish and seafood are abundant due to the numerous seas, rivers, and lochs (lakes). Scottish kippers and smoked salmon are international delicacies. As in other parts of the United Kingdom, there are numerous tea shops. Scotland is also known for its excellent whiskey and cheeses.

Scotland's national dish is haggis, which is made from sheep's offal. The windpipe, lungs, heart, and liver of the sheep are boiled and then minced. The mixture is then combined with beef suet and oatmeal. The mixture is placed inside the sheep's stomach, which is then sewn shut and boiled.

Wales

The food in Wales is pretty much the same as in Britain or Scotland, but there are a number of specialties. The leek (a vegetable) is a national emblem and is used in a number of dishes. St. David is the patron saint of Wales and the leek is worn on St. David's Day, March 1, a national holiday. Potato is a dietary staple. Fish and seafood are abundant, especially trout and salmon. Popular dishes in Wales include Welsh rarebit (or rabbit), poacher's pie, faggots (made from pig liver), Glamorgan sausage (which is actually meatless), and Welsh salt duck.

Ireland

The island of Ireland consists of Northern Ireland and the Republic of Ireland. The Republic of Ireland is a state that covers approximately five-sixths of the island, while the remaining sixth of the island is known as Northern Ireland and is part of the United Kingdom of Great Britain and Northern Ireland. Northern Ireland is predominantly Protestant and the Republic of Ireland is predominantly Catholic.

Milk, cheese, meat, cereals, and some vegetables formed the main part of the Irish diet before the potato was introduced to Ireland in the seventeenth century. The Irish were the first Europeans to use the potato as a staple food. The potato, more than anything else, contributed to the population growth on the island, which had less than 1 million inhabitants in the 1590s but had 8.2 million in 1840. However, the dependency on the potato eventually led to two major famines and a series of smaller famines.

The potato is still the staple food in Ireland, though other root vegetables, such as carrots, turnips, and onions, are eaten when in season. A traditional Irish dish is *colcannon*, made of mashed potatoes, onions, and cabbage. It came to the United States in the 1800s with the huge wave of Irish immigration, and is often served on St. Patrick's Day (March 17). Corned beef and cabbage are also eaten on St. Patrick's Day.

Breakfast is a large meal, usually consisting of oatmeal porridge, eggs, bacon, homemade bread, butter, and preserves. Strong black tea with milk and sugar is served with all meals. Lunch is the main meal of the day and is usually eaten at home with the whole family. Lunch is often a hearty soup, followed by meat, potatoes, vegetable, bread, and dessert. Afternoon tea is still common. A light supper is served later in the evening. Irish pubs are known throughout the world for their vibrant and friendly atmosphere. There are many different types of pubs, including dining pubs, music pubs, and pubs with accommodations (room and board). Irish whiskey and ale are also world-renowned.

France

One of modern France's greatest treasures is its rich cuisine. The French have an ongoing love affair with food. Families still gather together for the Sunday midday feast, which is eaten leisurely through a number of appetizers and main courses. Most French meals are accompanied by wine.

French cuisine is divided into classic French cuisine (*haute* cuisine) and provincial or regional cuisine. Classic French cuisine is elegant and formal and is mostly prepared in restaurants and catered at parties. More simple meals are usually prepared at home. Buttery, creamy sauces characterize classic French cuisine in the west, northwest, and north-central regions. The area surrounding Paris in the north-central region is the home of classic

French cuisine. The area produces great wine, cheese, beef, and veal. Fish and seafood are abundant in the northern region, and the famous Belon oysters are shipped throughout France. Apples are grown in this region and apple brandy and apple cider are widely exported. Normandy is known for its rich dairy products, and its butter and cheeses are among the best in the world. The Champagne district is located in the northernmost region, bordering Belgium and the English Channel, and is world-renowned for its sparkling wines. Only those produced in this region can be legally called "champagne" in France.

German cuisine has influenced French cuisine in the east and northeast parts of the country. Beer, sausage, sauerkraut, and goose are very popular, for example (goose fat is used for cooking). Famous dishes from these regions include *quiche Lorraine* and goose liver paté (*pâté de fois gras*). The south of France borders the Mediterranean Sea, and the cuisine in this region is similar to that of Spain and Italy. Olive oil, tomatoes, garlic, herbs, and fresh vegetables are all widely used. Famous dishes from this region are black truffeles, *ratatouille, salade Niçoise,* and *bouillabaisse.*

The French eat three meals a day and rarely eat snacks. They usually eat a light continental breakfast consisting of a baguette (French bread) or croissant with butter or jam. Strong coffee with hot milk accompanies breakfast (sometimes hot chocolate). Lunch is the largest meal of the day. Wine is drunk with lunch and dinner, and coffee is served after both meals. France is also known for its exquisite desserts such as *crème brûlée* and *chocolate mousse.* SEE ALSO CENTRAL EUROPEANS AND RUSSIA, DIETS OF; FRENCH PARADOX; SCANDINAVIANS, DIET OF.

Delores C. S. James

Bibliography

Kittler, P. G., and Sucher, K. P. (2001). *Food and Culture,* 3rd edition. Stamford, CT: Wadsworth.

Internet Resources

Frommer's. "Great Britain." Available from <http://www.frommers.com/destinations/greatbritain>

Diners Digest. "English Food." Available from <http://www.cuisinenet.com/glossary/england.html>

Linnane, John (2000). "A History of Irish Cuisine." Available from <http://www.ravensgard.org/prdunham/irishfood.html>

Nutrient Density

Nutrient density is a measure of the nutrients a food provides compared to the **calories** it provides. Foods low in calories and high in nutrients are *nutrient dense,* while foods high in calories and low in nutrients are *nutrient poor.* Nutrient-dense foods should be eaten often, whereas nutrient-poor foods should only be eaten occasionally. A healthful **diet** includes mostly nutrient-dense foods. People who restrict their calories should obtain as much **nutrition** as they can from the calories they consume by choosing nutrient-dense foods. Those who consistently choose nutrient-poor foods will not get the nutrients they need. SEE ALSO NUTRIENTS.

Beth Fontenot

nutrient: dietary substance necessary for health

calorie: unit of food energy

diet: the total daily food intake, or the types of foods eaten

nutrition: the maintenance of health through proper eating, or the study of same

Nutrient-Drug Interactions

Medications have become an integral part of life for many people. Medicine serves to help people when they are sick, allowing them to live longer and healthier lives. With rapidly growing research and technology, medications are more beneficial, and new ones continue to be discovered. **Drugs** do need to be taken with caution, however. All medications, whether prescribed by a doctor or bought **over-the-counter**, are capable of harmful side effects. The foods people eat contain **nutrients** that are used by the body to produce **energy**. Sometimes, certain medications may interact with both the food eaten and the nutrients the food gives to the body for proper functioning. When the body is unable to use a nutrient due to a drug that has been taken, a nutrient-drug interaction has occurred.

Function of a Drug

A drug is taken to prevent or treat sickness and disease. It is important to know what happens in the body when a drug is taken in order to better understand the interaction between nutrients and drugs. The action of a drug taken orally generally occurs in four steps: (1) the drug dissolves in the stomach, (2) the drug is absorbed into the blood and moves via the blood to the area of the body that needs it, (3) the body reacts to the medicine, and (4) the body gets rid of the drug by way of the kidney, liver, or both.

Adverse Effects of Nutrient-Drug Interactions

A nutrient-drug interaction may impact the body in several ways. Certain foods can affect the rate at which the body uses a medication. A drug will not work as well if a certain nutrient in a food speeds up or slows down the

drugs: substances whose administration causes a significant change in the body's function

over-the-counter: available without a prescription

nutrient: dietary substance necessary for health

energy: technically, the ability to perform work; the content of a substance that allows it to be useful as a fuel

NUTRIENT-DRUG INTERACTIONS

Drug	Indication	Possible Effects
Coumadin	Anticoagulant (blood thinner)	Vitamin K is a nutrient in the body that helps blood to clot. Vitamin K is present in foods such as green, leafy vegetables and fish. It will interfere with a blood thinner like coumadin.
Dilantin	Anticonvulsant (anti-seizure)	Vitamin D and folic acid levels in the body are decreased by the taking of these types of drugs.
Norvasc	Antihypertensive (for high blood pressure)	Consuming foods high in sodium (i.e., licorice, processed meats, canned foods) will decrease the effectiveness of the drug.
Aspirin	Anti-inflammatory/pain reliever	Taking large amounts of these drugs will cause a loss of Vitamin C in the body.
Birth control pills	Oral contraceptives	Women who take these drugs often have low levels of folic acid and Vitamin B_6 in the blood.
Dyazide/Thiazide	Diuretics (water-eliminating)	Taking diuretics often leads to a loss of potassium in the body.
Tetracycline	Antibiotic	Calcium may interact with the effectiveness of the antibiotic. Avoid dairy products for two to three hours before and after taking the medicine.
Lipitor/Zocor	Statins (cholesterol-lowering drugs)	Antioxidants (Vitamin A, C, E, B, folic acid) may interact with the drug by reversing its effect.
Prednisone	Corticosteroid	The drug may increase appetite thus increasing nutrient intake.
Lasix	Diuretic (water-eliminating)	The drug may decrease appetite thus decreasing nutrient intake.

SOURCE: Compiled from references in the bibliography.

drug's **absorption** into the body. Short- or long-term instances of nutrient-drug interactions may be life threatening. A nutrient-drug interaction may also impact the nutritional status of the body. Nutrient-drug interactions can occur with both prescription and over-the-counter medicine.

Impact of Food on Effectiveness of a Drug

A medication has ingredients, just as food does, that allow it to function correctly when taken in order to help the body in some way. A food may interfere with the effectiveness of a drug if the food interacts with the ingredients in the medication, preventing the drug from working properly. Nutrients in food may either delay absorption into the body or speed up elimination from the body, either or which can impact a drug's effectiveness. For example, the acidic ingredients in fruit juices are capable of decreasing the power of **antibiotics** such as penicillin. Tetracycline, another infection-fighting drug, is impacted by the consumption of dairy products. Many medications that are taken to fight **depression** can be dangerous if mixed with beverages or foods that consist of tyramine, which is found in items such as beer, red wine, and some cheeses.

Food can also impact the effectiveness of a drug due to the way it is consumed. Generally, medicine is to be taken at the same time food is eaten. This is because the medicine may upset the stomach if the stomach is empty. However, sometimes taking a drug at the same time that food is eaten can interfere with the way the medicine is absorbed by the body.

Impact on Nutritional Status

A drug has the capacity of interfering with a person's nutritional status. Appetite may be stimulated by a certain drug, resulting in an increase in nutrient intake due to more food being eaten. However, drugs may also cause a decrease in appetite, leading to a decrease in nutrient intake. In this case, a drug could possibly cause a nutritional deficiency. Nutritional status may also be impacted by a drug's effect on the three main nutrients: **carbohydrates**, **fat**, and **protein**. A drug may speed up or slow down the breakdown of these three nutrients, which are essential to the body's functioning. When a drug affects the absorption of nutrients from food into the body, less energy is available to be used by the body. The impact of the nutrient-drug interaction may vary according to the medicine taken, the dose of the medicine given, and the form taken (e.g., pill, liquid).

The Elderly and Nutrient-Drug Interactions

Elderly persons are at a significant risk for nutrient-drug interactions. This population often takes the highest amount of medications, and with the use of multiple drugs, certain problems may exist. A loss of appetite, a reduced sense of taste and smell, and swallowing problems all may result from medication use in elderly people.

Malnutrition is a common problem among older adults. Therefore, nutritional status may be already impacted by decreased nutrient intake. This may only worsen the effect of a possible nutrient-drug interaction. Elderly people who take many drugs on a routine basis for long periods of time are at greatest risk of nutrient depletion and **nutritional deficiencies**.

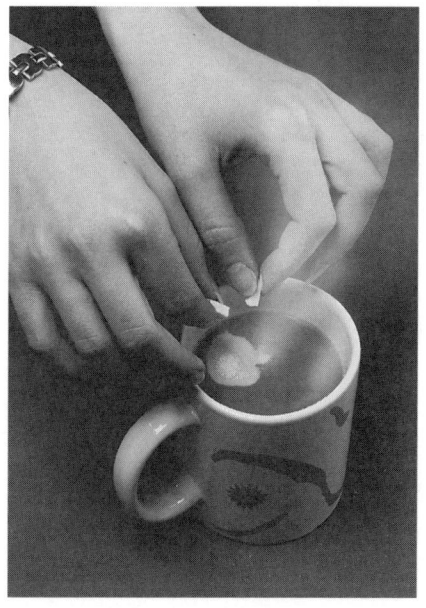

Some drugs may affect the absorption of nutrients, while some foods—for example, those containing caffeine—can amplify or modify the effects of certain drugs. Taking drugs with hot beverages could also make them less effective. *[Octane Photographic. Reproduced by permission.]*

absorption: uptake by the digestive tract

antibiotic: substance that kills or prevents the growth of microorganisms

depression: mood disorder characterized by apathy, restlessness, and negative thoughts

carbohydrate: food molecule made of carbon, hydrogen, and oxygen, including sugars and starches

fat: type of food molecule rich in carbon and hydrogen, with high energy content

protein: complex molecule composed of amino acids that performs vital functions in the cell; necessary part of the diet

malnutrition: chronic lack of sufficient nutrients to maintain health

nutritional deficiency: lack of adequate nutrients in the diet

Tips for Avoiding Interactions

There are ways to avoid placing the body at risk of an unwanted nutrient-drug interaction. The following are tips to remember about taking medications and will help avoid interactions:

- Be sure to read the label on a prescription medicine and ask a pharmacist or physician if something is not clear.
- Read all directions, warnings, and any possible side effects printed on all drug labels and information in the package.
- Always take medications with a full glass of water.
- A drug may not work correctly if a medicine is taken improperly; do not stir medication into food or take apart capsules (unless told to do so).
- Take vitamin and mineral supplements before or after medicine, as they may interact with certain drugs.
- Avoid stirring drugs into hot drinks such as coffee because the drug's effectiveness can be destroyed by the hot temperature.
- Do not drink alcohol when taking any medicine.
- Always tell a physician and pharmacist about all medicines being taken, including both prescription and over-the-counter drugs. SEE ALSO ADULT NUTRITION; ALTERNATIVE MEDICINES AND THERAPIES; NUTRIENTS; NUTRITIONAL DEFICIENCY.

D. Michelle Swords

Bibliography

Alonso-Aperte, E., and Varela-Moreiras, G. (2000). "Drugs-Nutrient Interactions: A Potential Problem during Adolescence." *European Journal of Clinical Nutrition* 54:S69–S74.

Heimburger, Douglas C., and Weinsier, Roland L. (1997). *Handbook of Clinical Nutrition*, 3rd edition. St. Louis, MO: Mosby.

Mahan, L. Kathleen, and Escott-Stump, Sylvia (1996). *Krause's Food, Nutrition, and Diet Therapy*, 9th edition. Philadelphia: W. B. Saunders Company.

Roe, Daphne A. (1994). "Medications and Nutrition in the Elderly." *Primary Care* 21:135–147.

Worthington-Roberts, Bonnie S., and Rodwell Williams, Sue (1996). *Nutrition throughout the Life Cycle*, 3rd edition. Boston: WCB/McGraw-Hill.

Internet Resources

College of Agricultural Sciences, Penn State Unviersity. "Facts about Food/Drug Interactions." Available from <http://www.penpages.psu.edu/>

University of Florida, Cooperative Extension Service, Institute of Food and Agricultural Sciences. "Food/Drug and Drug/Nutrient Interactions: What You Should Know about Your Medications." Available from <http://edis.ifas.ufl.edu/HE776>

Nutrients

An important aspect of **nutrition** is the daily intake of **nutrients**. Nutrients consist of various chemical substances in the food that makes up each person's **diet**. Many nutrients are essential for life, and an adequate amount of nutrients in the diet is necessary for providing **energy**, building and main-

---

nutrition: the maintenance of health through proper eating, or the study of same

nutrient: dietary substance necessary for health

diet: the total daily food intake, or the types of foods eaten

energy: technically, the ability to perform work; the content of a substance that allows it to be useful as a fuel

THE THREE FUNCTIONS OF NUTRIENTS		
Provide Energy	**Promote growth and development**	**Regulate body functions**
Carbohydrates	Proteins	Proteins
Proteins	Lipids	Lipids
Lipids (fats and oils)	Vitamins	Vitamins
	Minerals	Minerals
	Water	Water

taining body organs, and for various **metabolic** processes. People depend on nutrients in their diet because the human body is not able to produce many of these nutrients—or it cannot produce them in adequate amounts.

Nutrients are essential to the human diet if they meet two characteristics. First, omitting the nutrient from the diet leads to a nutritional deficiency and a decline in some aspect of health. Second, if the omitted nutrient is put back into the diet, the symptoms of nutritional deficiency will decline and the individual will return to normal, barring any permanent damage caused by its absence.

There are six major classes of nutrients found in food: **carbohydrates**, **proteins**, **lipids** (fats and oils), **vitamins** (both fat-soluble and **water-soluble**), **minerals**, and water. These six nutrients can be further categorized into three basic functional groups.

Carbohydrates

Carbohydrates are the major source of energy for the body. They are composed mostly of the elements carbon (C), hydrogen (H), and **oxygen** (O). Through the bonding of these elements, carbohydrates provide energy for the body in the form of kilocalories (kcal), with an average of 4 kcal per gram (kcal/g) of carbohydrates (a kcal is equivalent to a calorie on a nutritional label of a packaged food).

Carbohydrates come in a variety of sizes. The smallest carbohydrates are the simple sugars, also known as monosaccharides and disaccharides, meaning that they are made up of one or two sugar **molecules**. The best known simple sugar is table sugar, which is also known as **sucrose**, a disaccharide. Other simple sugars include the monosaccharides **glucose** and fructose, which are found in fruits, and the disaccharides, which include sucrose, lactose (found in milk), and maltose (in beer and malt liquors). The larger carbohydrates are made up of these smaller simple sugars and are known as polysaccharides (many sugar molecules) or complex carbohydrates. These are usually made up of many linked glucose molecules, though, unlike simple sugars, they do not have a sweet taste. Examples of foods high in complex carbohydrates include potatoes, beans, and vegetables. Another type of complex carbohydrate is dietary **fiber**. However, although fiber is a complex carbohydrate made up of linked sugar molecules, the body cannot break apart the sugar linkages and, unlike other complex carbohydrates, it passes through the body with minimal changes.

Although carbohydrates are not considered to be an essential nutrient, the body depends on them as its primary energy source. The body utilizes most carbohydrates to generate glucose, which serves as the basic functional

metabolic: related to processing of nutrients and building of necessary molecules within the cell

carbohydrate: food molecule made of carbon, hydrogen, and oxygen, including sugars and starches

protein: complex molecule composed of amino acids that performs vital functions in the cell; necessary part of the diet

lipid: fats, waxes and steroids; important components of cell membranes

vitamin: necessary complex nutrient used to aid enzymes or other metabolic processes in the cell

water-soluble: able to be dissolved in water

mineral: an inorganic (non-carbon-containing) element, ion or compound

oxygen: O_2, atmospheric gas required by all animals

molecule: combination of atoms that form stable particles

sucrose: table sugar

glucose: a simple sugar; the most commonly used fuel in cells

fiber: indigestible plant material which aids digestion by providing bulk

amino acid: building block of proteins, necessary dietary nutrient

molecule of energy within the cells of the human body (glucose is broken down to ultimately produce adenosine triphosphate, or ATP, the fundamental unit of energy). When the supply of carbohydrates is too low to adequately supply all the energy needs of the body, **amino acids** from proteins are converted to glucose. However, the typical American individual consumes more than adequate amounts of carbohydrates to prevent this utilization of protein.

Proteins

nitrogen: essential element for plant growth

biological: related to living organisms

enzyme: protein responsible for carrying out reactions in a cell

hormone: molecules produced by one set of cells that influence the function of another set of cells

Proteins are composed of the elements carbon (C), oxygen (O), hydrogen (H), and **nitrogen** (n). They have a variety of uses in the body, including serving as a source of energy, as substrates (starter materials) for tissue growth and maintenance, and for certain **biological** functions, such as making structural proteins, transfer proteins, **enzyme** molecules, and **hormone** receptors. Proteins are also the major component in bone, muscle, and other tissues and fluids. When used for energy, protein supplies an average of 4 kcal/g.

Proteins are formed by the linking of different combinations of the twenty common amino acids found in food. Of these, ten are essential for the human in the synthesis of body proteins (eight are essential throughout a human's life, whereas two become essential during periods of rapid growth, such as during infancy).

Protein may be found in a variety of food sources. Proteins from animal sources (meat, poultry, milk, fish) are considered to be of high biological value because they contain all of the essential amino acids. Proteins from plant sources (wheat, corn, rice, and beans) are considered to be of low biological value because an individual plant source does not contain all of the essential amino acids. Therefore, combinations of plant sources must be used to provide these nutrients.

kwashiorkor: severe malnutrition characterized by swollen belly, hair loss, and loss of skin pigment

marasmus: extreme malnutrition, characterized by loss of muscle and other tissue

Protein deficiency is not common in the American diet because most Americans consume 1.5 to 2 times more protein than is required for the body to maintain adequate health. This excess intake of protein is not considered to be harmful for the average healthy individual. However, when protein intake is inadequate, but total caloric intake is sufficient, a condition known as **kwashiorkor** may occur. Symptoms of kwashiorkor include an enlarged stomach, loss of hair and hair color, and an enlarged liver. Conversely, if protein and caloric intake are both inadequate, a condition known as **marasmus** occurs. Marasmus presents with a stoppage of growth, extreme muscle loss, and weakness.

Lipids

insoluble: not able to be dissolved in

glycerol: simple molecule that forms a portion of fats

triglyceride: a type of fat

Lipids, which consist of fats and oils, are high-energy yielding molecules composed mostly of carbon (C), hydrogen (H), and oxygen (O) (though lipids have a smaller number of oxygen molecules than carbohydrates have). This small number of oxygen molecules makes lipids **insoluble** in water, but soluble in certain organic solvents. The basic structure of lipids is a **glycerol** molecule consisting of three carbons, each attached to a fatty-acid chain. Collectively, this structure is known as a **triglyceride**, or sometimes it is called a triacylglycerol. Triglycerides are the major form of energy stor-

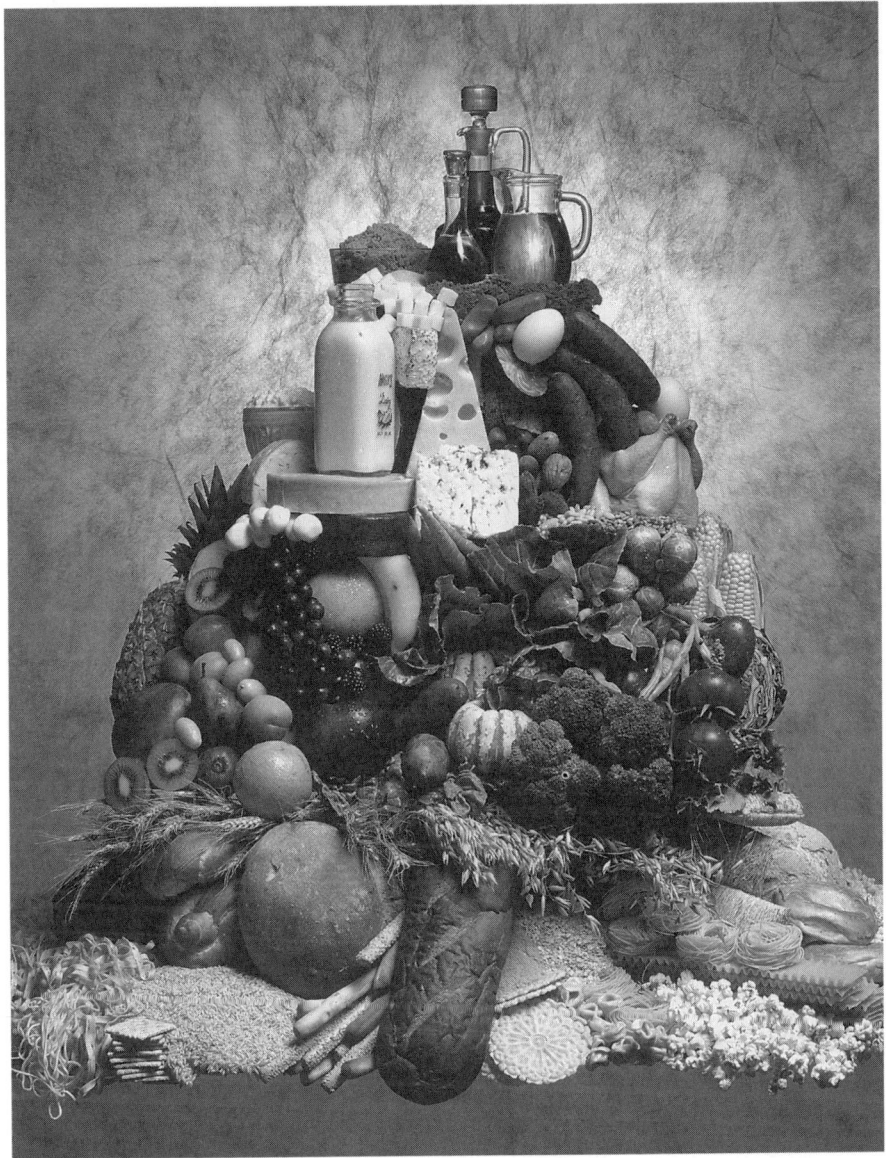

The Food Guide Pyramid groups foods together based on their nutrient content. In theory, a diet designed around the pyramid will include all the essential nutrients that the body needs to thrive. [Photograph by Gabe Palmer. Corbis. Reproduced by permission.]

age in the body (whereas carbohydrates are the body's major energy source), and are also the major form of fat in foods. The energy contained in a gram of lipids is more than twice the amount in carbohydrates and protein, with an average of 9 kcal/g.

Lipids can be broken down into two types, saturated and unsaturated, based on the chemical structure of their longest, and therefore dominant, fatty acid. Whether a lipid is solid or liquid at room temperature largely depends on its property of being saturated or unsaturated. Lipids from plant sources are largely unsaturated, and therefore liquid at room temperature. Lipids that are derived from animals contain a higher amount of saturated fats, and they are therefore solid at room temperature. An exception to this rule is fish, which, for the most part, contain unsaturated fat. The important difference between saturated and unsaturated **fatty acids** is that saturated fatty acids are the most important factor that can increase a person's **cholesterol** level. An increased cholesterol level may eventually result in the clogging of blood **arteries** and, ultimately, **heart disease**.

fatty acids: molecules rich in carbon and hydrogen; a component of fats

cholesterol: multi-ringed molecule found in animal cell membranes; a type of lipid

artery: blood vessel that carries blood away from the heart toward the body tissues

heart disease: any disorder of the heart or its blood supply, including heart attack, atherosclerosis, and coronary artery disease

essential fatty acids: particular molecules made of carbon, hydrogen, and oxygen that the human body must have but cannot make itself

blood pressure: measure of the pressure exerted by the blood against the walls of the blood vessels

absorption: uptake by the digestive tract

metabolism: the sum total of reactions in a cell or an organism

B vitamins: a group of vitamins important in cell energy processes

biotin: a portion of certain enzymes used in fat metabolism; essential for cell function

bacteria: single-celled organisms without nuclei, some of which are infectious

intestines: the two long tubes that carry out much of the processes of digestion

antibiotic: substance that kills or prevents the growth of microorganisms

physiological: related to the biochemical processes of the body

nervous system: the brain, spinal cord, and nerves that extend throughout the body

Not all fatty acids are considered harmful. In fact, certain unsaturated fatty acids are considered essential nutrients. Like the essential amino acids, these fatty acids are essential to a person's diet because the body cannot produce them. The **essential fatty acids** serve many important functions in the body, including regulating **blood pressure** and helping to synthesize and repair vital cell parts. It is estimated that the American diet contains about three times the amount of essential fatty acids needed daily. Lipids are also required for the **absorption** of fat-soluble vitamins, and they are generally thought to increase the taste and flavor of foods and to give an individual a feeling of fullness.

Vitamins

Vitamins are chemical compounds that are required for normal growth and **metabolism**. Some vitamins are essential for a number of metabolic reactions that result in the release of energy from carbohydrates, fats, and proteins. There are thirteen vitamins, which may be divided into two groups: the four fat-soluble vitamins (vitamins A, D, E, and K) and the nine water-soluble vitamins (the **B vitamins** and vitamin C). These two groups are dissimilar in many ways. First of all, cooking or heating destroys the water-soluble vitamins much more readily than the fat-soluble vitamins. On the other hand, fat-soluble vitamins are much less readily excreted from the body, compared to water-soluble vitamins, and can therefore accumulate to excessive, and possibly toxic, levels. This means, of course, that levels of water-soluble vitamins in the body can become depleted more quickly, leading to a vitamin deficiency if those nutrients are not replaced regularly. Deficiencies of vitamins may result from inadequate intake, as well as from factors unrelated to supply. For instance, vitamin K and **biotin** are both produced by **bacteria** that live within the **intestines**, and a person can become deficient if these bacteria are removed by **antibiotics**. Other factors that may result in a vitamin deficiency include disease, pregnancy, drug interactions, and newborn development (newborns lack the intestinal bacteria that create certain vitamins, such as biotin and vitamin K).

Minerals

Minerals are different from the other nutrients discussed thus far, in that they are inorganic compounds (carbohydrates, proteins, lipids, and vitamins are all organic compounds). The fundamental structure of minerals is usually nothing more than a molecule, or molecules, of an element. The functions of minerals do not include participation in the yielding of energy. But they do play vital roles in several **physiological** functions, including critical involvement in **nervous system** functioning, in cellular reactions, in water balance in the body, and in structural systems, such as the skeletal system.

Because minerals have a very simple structure of usually one or more molecules of an element, they are not readily destroyed in the heating or cooking process of food preparation. However, they can leak out of the food substance that contains them and seep into the water or liquid the food is being cooked in. This may result in a decreased level of minerals being consumed if the liquid is discarded.

There are many minerals found within the human body, but of the sixteen (or possibly more) essential minerals, the amount required on a daily basis varies enormously. This is why minerals are subdivided into two classes: macrominerals and microminerals. Macrominerals include those that are needed in high quantities, ranging from milligrams to grams. **Calcium**, phosphorous, and magnesium are macrominerals. Microminerals are those necessary in smaller quantities, generally between a microgram and a milligram. Examples of microminerals include copper, chromium, and selenium. Dietary requirements for some minerals have yet to be established.

calcium: mineral essential for bones and teeth

Water

Water makes up the last class of nutrients, though the fact that it is considered a nutrient is surprising to many people. Water, however, has many necessary functions in the human body. Some of its actions include its use as a solvent (a substance that other substances dissolve in), as a lubricant, as a conduction system for transportation of vital nutrients and unnecessary waste, and as a mode of temperature regulation.

There are many available sources of water other than tap water and bottled water. Some foods have a high water content, including many fruits and vegetables. In addition, the body can make small amounts of water from various metabolic prcesses that result in molecules of water as a by-product. This, however, is by no means sufficient for the body's needs of water. It is generally recommended that people drink eight cups (or nearly 2 liters) of water a day to maintain an adequate supply. SEE ALSO CARBOHYDRATES; FATS; KWASHIORKOR; MARASMUS; MINERALS; NUTRITIONAL DEFICIENCY; PROTEIN; VITAMINS, FAT-SOLUBLE; VITAMINS, WATER-SOLUBLE; WATER.

Susan S. Kim
Jeffrey Radecki

Bibliography

Harper, A. (1999). "Defining the Essentiality of Nutrients." In *Modern Nutrition in Health and Disease*, 9th edition, ed. M. E. Shills, et al. Baltimore, MD: Williams and Wilkins.

Morrison, Gail, and Hark, Lisa (1999). *Medical Nutrition and Disease*, 2nd edition. Cambridge, MA: Blackwell Science.

Subar, A. F., et al. (1998). "Dietary Sources of Nutrients in the U.S. Diet, 1989 to 1991." *Journal of the American Dietetic Association* 98:537.

Wardlaw, Gordon M., and Kessel, Margaret (2002). *Perspectives in Nutrition*, 5th edition. Boston: McGraw-Hill.

Nutrition

Nutrition is the science that studies the interactions between living organisms and food. Human nutrition includes the study of **nutrients** and other substances found in foods; how the human body uses nutrients for growth and maintenance; and the relationship between foods, food components, dietary patterns, and health. The study of nutrition encompasses all aspects of the ingestion, digestion, absorption, transport, **metabolism,** interaction, storage, and excretion of nutrients by the body. In a broader sense, the study of nutrition also includes the various psychological, sociological, cultural, technological, and economic factors that affect the foods and dietary patterns chosen by an individual.

nutrient: dietary substance necessary for health

metabolism: the sum total of reactions in a cell or an organism

Beth Fontenot

Nutrition Education

Nutrition education is a critical component of most major health promotion and disease prevention programs. Research indicates that **behavioral** change is directly related to the amount of nutrition education received. Nutrition Education involves the communication of nutrition-related information that will equip individuals, families, and communities to make healthful food choices. The media remain the primary source of nutrition information in the United States. Thus, nutrition education also focuses on discriminating between credible and noncredible sources of nutrition information. Nutrition messages and programs must be culturally relevant and specific to the target group. Registered dietitians are the professionals who are specifically trained to deliver information on food and nutrition.

Cindy Martin

nutrition: the maintenance of health through proper eating, or the study of same

behavioral: related to behavior, in contrast to medical or other types of interventions

Bibliography

American Dietetic Association (2003). "Nutrition Services: An Essential Component of Comprehensive School Health Programs." *Journal of the American Dietetic Association* 103:505–514.

Internet Resources

Ferme, Lori (2002). "Nutrition and You: Trends 2002." Available from <http://www.eatright.org>

Smith, Barbara (1995). "Past Experiences and Needs for Nutrition Education: Summary and Conclusions of Nine Case Studies." Available from <http://www.fao.org>

Nutrition Programs in the Community

In the United States, as in most developed countries, a number of services and programs exist to help those who are in need due to age, illness, poverty or adverse circumstances. This is often not the case in less-developed countries, where individuals and communities experience hardships due to a lack of social, health, and welfare services. In the United States, private charitable organizations, churches, and the government assist in providing what is often called a "safety net" of services, including **nutrition** or food services, to prevent or reduce deprivation for individuals and communities. The nutrition programs that have the greatest impact are those supported by the government, and in most cases the federal government provides resources to states through various funding methods.

nutrition: the maintenance of health through proper eating, or the study of same

FNS Programs

The Food and Nutrition Service (FNS) of the United States Department of Agriculture (USDA) was established in 1969. The purpose of this agency is to: (1) make food assistance available to the needy, (2) improve the eating habits of children, and (3) assist with the distribution of surplus foods, thereby stabilizing farm prices. A number of programs exist to achieve these goals.

National School Lunch Program.

The U.S. Congress established the National School Lunch Program (NSLP) in 1946 to safeguard the health and well-being of children and encourage the domestic consumption of nutritious agricultural commodities. Participating schools in all the states receive cash subsidies and free commodities from the USDA. Schools and residential child-care institutions are responsible for providing lunches that meet specific nutritional standards. Students are eligible to receive lunches free or at a reduced price depending on their family's income (some pay full price). Though based on the rationale that a child cannot learn if he or she is hungry, in recent years there have been more concerns with the possible overconsumption of some **nutrients**, particularly **fat**. Some evaluations have suggested that school lunches may not be as healthy as they could be.

nutrient: dietary substance necessary for health

fat: type of food molecule rich in carbon and hydrogen, with high energy content

School Breakfast Program. This program was established as a permanent program for public and nonprofit private schools in 1975. The School Breakfast Program (SBP) helps states to provide a free or reduced-price nutritious breakfast to students in participating schools. Breakfasts may be hot or cold, but they must meet exact standards, provide specific foods, and meet one-fourth of the RDAs (**Recommended Dietary Allowances**) over time. Eligibility requirements are similar to the NSLP.

Recommended Dietary Allowances: nutrient intake recommended to promote health

Summer Food Service Program for Children. During school vacations, eligible children are able to receive meals and snacks under this program. Community agencies, nonprofit organizations, governmental units, recreational facilities, and summer camps are allowed to sponsor this program in communities where 50 percent or more of the children are from households that are at or below 185 percent of the poverty level. This nutrition program was established in 1975.

Special Milk Program. Since 1966 this program has been available to provide cash reimbursement for each half-pint of milk provided to students in schools not participating in the National School Lunch Program. The purpose is to encourage the consumption of milk. Children are eligible to participate regardless of income.

The Women, Infants, and Children Program (WIC). This program provides, at no cost, assistance to purchase supplemental nutritious foods, nutrition education, and referrals to other agencies. Pregnant and postpartum women, infants, and children under five years of age who meet specific health risk and income requirements are eligible to participate. The WIC Farmers Market, where available, allows participants to acquire fresh produce. WIC was authorized in 1972 and has proven to be cost-effective in reducing and preventing problems such as **anemia** and poor birth outcomes in the populations served.

anemia: low level of red blood cells in the blood

Food Stamp Program. The purpose of the Food Stamp Program, established in 1977, is to improve the diets of people with low incomes. Assistance is provided, through food stamps, for purchasing foods. Recently, more efforts have been made to also provide some nutrition education.

Commodity Supplemental Food Program. Since 1973 this program has provided direct food distribution to persons over sixty years old, and to lower income people, in some states. Specific foods are provided to meet participants' nutritional needs. Persons participating in WIC are not eligible for this program.

Nutrition Programs in the Community

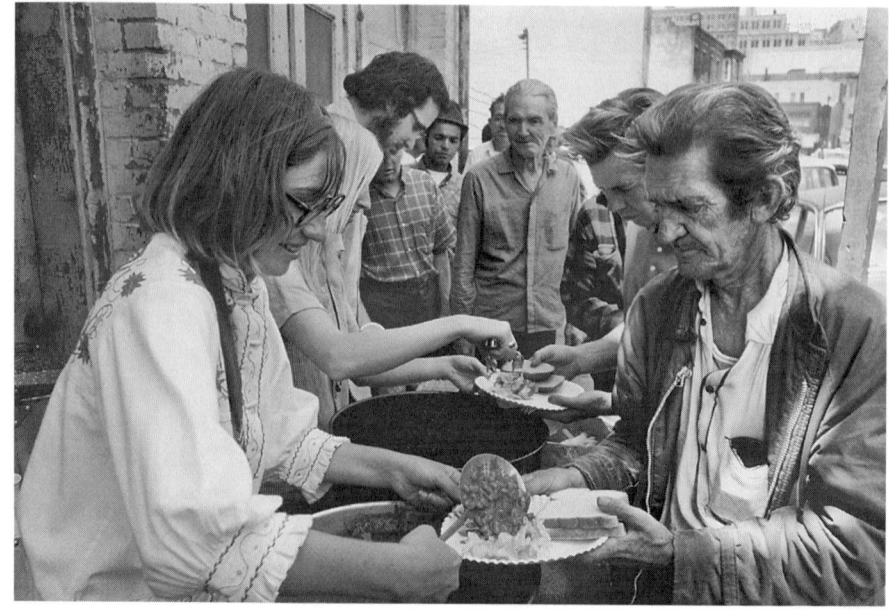

A variety of community nutrition programs receive aid from the federal government. For example, the U.S. Department of Agriculture distributes food surpluses to charitable institutions, which then provide the food to people in need. [Photograph by Vince Streano. Corbis. Reproduced by permission.]

Separate USDA programs also exist for providing commodities and surplus foods to charitable institutions, child- and adult-care programs, Indian reservations, and for temporary emergency food assistance. Other USDA programs, such as the Expanded Food and Nutrition Program and the Nutrition and Education Training Program, exist to increase nutrition knowledge and skills.

DHHS Programs

Another agency that plays a major role in meeting community nutrition needs is the U.S. Department of Health and Human Services (DHHS), which oversees a number of nutrition programs.

Nutrition Program for Older Americans.
Funds are given to state agencies on aging to coordinate a variety of services for the elderly, including congregate and home-delivered meals. A nutritious lunch, nutrition education, opportunities for social interaction, referral, and transportation assistance are provided. Meals are free, but participants may make a voluntary contribution. All persons over sixty years old, and their spouses (of any age), may participate, and income is not a factor for eligibility. This program was authorized in 1965.

Head Start Program.
Officially established in 1967, Head Start provides education, nutrition, and social and health services to participants. Specifically, nutritious meals, snacks, nutrition assessment, and nutrition education are provided to children and parents. To be eligible, children must be three to five years old and from a lower-income family.

DHHS also provides funding for the Title V Maternal Child Health Program, which does provide some nutrition assessment and nutrition education to children, adolescents, and women of childbearing age. This program provides a variety of other health-related services and specific programs for special-needs children and for those at risk for physical or developmental disabilities. States determine how these federal funds will be used, so the program does vary depending on the state.

While many programs are available, nutrition-related diseases and hunger still exist as real problems for some Americans. There are many who fail to gain the available benefits due to a variety of barriers. For example, homeless people often lack transportation and are unable to provide the required documentation to access some services.

Government agencies provide the majority of nutrition programs, but many religious and charitable organizations also assist in meeting the huge needs. Catholic Charities, Meals on Wheels, and the American Heart Association are examples of nonprofit groups that put forth extensive efforts to feed those in need and educate the public on relevant food and nutrition-related issues. SEE ALSO MEALS ON WHEELS; SCHOOL FOOD SERVICE; SCHOOL-AGED CHILDREN, DIET.

Leslene Gordon

Bibliography

Boyle, Marie A., and Morris, Diane H. (1994). *Community Nutrition in Action: An Entrepreneurial Approach.* New York: West Publishing.

Endres, Jeannette B. (1999). *Community Nutrition: Challenges and Opportunities.* New Jersey: Prentice Hall.

Frankle, Reva T., and Owen, Anita L. (1993). *Nutrition in the Community: The Art of Delivering Services.* St. Louis, MO: Mosby.

Nutritional Assessment

A **nutrition** assessment is an in-depth evaluation of both objective and subjective data related to an individual's food and **nutrient** intake, lifestyle, and medical history.

Once the data on an individual is collected and organized, the practitioner can assess and evaluate the nutritional status of that person. The assessment leads to a plan of care, or intervention, designed to help the individual either maintain the assessed status or attain a healthier status.

Elements of the Assessment

The data for a nutritional assessment falls into four categories: **anthropometric**, **biochemical**, clinical, and dietary.

Anthropometrics. Anthropometrics are the objective measurements of body muscle and **fat**. They are used to compare individuals, to compare growth in the young, and to assess weight loss or gain in the mature individual. Weight and height are the most frequently used anthropometric measurements, and skinfold measurements of several areas of the body are also taken.

As early as 1836, tables had been developed to compare weight and height in order to provide a reference for an individual's health status. The Metropolitan Life Insurance Company revised height and weight tables in 1942, using data from policyholders, to relate weight to disease and mortality. There has been much discussion about the relevance (and appropriateness) of using the individuals who buy life insurance as a basis for "ideal" height and weight. There are also a number of problems with using a table to determine whether an individual is at the right weight—or even what the "ideal

nutrition: the maintenance of health through proper eating, or the study of same

nutrient: dietary substance necessary for health

anthropometric: related to measurement of characteristics of the human body

biochemical: related to chemical processes within cells

fat: type of food molecule rich in carbon and hydrogen, with high energy content

Nutritional Assessment

1983 METROPOLITAN HEIGHT AND WEIGHT TABLES
Women

Height Feet-inches		Small frame	Medium frame	Large frame
4	10	102–111	109–121	118–131
4	11	103–113	111–123	120–134
5	0	104–115	113–126	122–137
5	1	106–118	115–129	125–140
5	2	108–121	118–132	128–143
5	3	111–124	121–135	131–147
5	4	114–127	124–138	134–151
5	5	117–130	127–141	137–155
5	6	120–133	130–144	140–159
5	7	123–136	133–147	143–163
5	8	126–139	136–150	146–167
5	9	129–142	139–153	149–170
5	10	132–145	142–156	152–173
5	11	135–148	145–159	155–176
6	0	138–151	148–162	158–179

1983 METROPOLITAN HEIGHT AND WEIGHT TABLES
Men

Height Feet-inches		Small frame	Medium frame	Large frame
5	2	128–134	131–141	138–150
5	3	130–136	133–143	140–153
5	4	132–138	135–145	142–156
5	5	134–140	137–148	144–160
5	6	136–142	139–151	146–164
5	7	138–145	142–154	149–168
5	8	140–148	145–157	152–172
5	9	142–151	148–160	155–176
5	10	144–154	151–163	158–180
5	11	146–157	154–166	161–184
6	0	149–160	157–170	164–188
6	1	152–164	160–174	168–192
6	2	155–168	164–178	172–197
6	3	158–172	167–182	176–202
6	4	162–176	171–187	181–207

weight" means. Tables should therefore be used only as a guide, and other measurements should be included in the data collection and evaluation.

In 1959, research indicated that the lowest mortality rates were associated with below-average weight, and the phrase "desirable weight" replaced "ideal weight" in the title of the height and weight table.

To further characterize an individual's height and weight, tables also include body-frame size, which can be estimated in many ways. An easy way is to wrap the thumb and forefinger of the nondominant hand around the wrist of the dominant hand. If the thumb and forefinger meet, the frame is medium; if the fingers do not meet, the frame is large; and if they overlap, the frame is small.

Determining frame size is an attempt at attributing weight to specific body compartments. Frame size identifies an individual relative to the bone size, but does not differentiate muscle mass from body fat. Because it is the muscle mass that is metabolically active and the body fat that is associated with disease states, **Body Mass Index** (BMI) is used to estimate the body-fat mass. BMI is derived from an equation using weight and height.

body mass index: weight in kilograms divided by square of the height in meters; a measure of body fat

To estimate body fat, skinfold measurements can be made using skinfold calipers. Most frequently, tricep and subscapular (shoulder blade) skinfolds are measured. Measurements can then be compared to reference data—and to previous measurements of the individual, if available. Accurate measuring takes practice, and comparison measurements are most reliable if done by the same technician each time.

To estimate desirable body weight for amputees, and for paraplegics and quadriplegics, equations have been developed from cadaver studies, estimating desirable body weight, as well as **calorie** and **protein** needs. Calorie needs are determined by the height, weight, and age of an individual, which determine an estimate of daily needs.

The **Harris-Benedict equation** is frequently used, but there are quicker methods to estimate needs using just height and weight. Opinions and methods vary on how to estimate calorie needs for the **obese**. As previously mentioned, body fat is less metabolically active and requires fewer calories for support than muscle mass. If an individual's current body weight is more than 125 percent of the desirable weight for the individual's height and age, then using body weight to estimate calories needs usually leads to an overestimation of those needs.

Biochemical data. Laboratory tests based on blood and urine can be important indicators of nutritional status, but they are influenced by non-nutritional factors as well. Lab results can be altered by medications, **hydration** status, and disease states or other **metabolic** processes, such as **stress**. As with the other areas of nutrition assessment, biochemical data need to be viewed as a part of the whole.

Clinical data. Clinical data provides information about the individual's medical history, including **acute** and **chronic** illness and diagnostic procedures, therapies, or treatments that may increase nutrient needs or induce **malabsorption**. Current medications need to be documented, and both prescription **drugs** and **over-the-counter** drugs, such as laxatives or analgesics, must be included in the analysis. **Vitamins**, **minerals**, and **herbal** preparations also need to be reviewed. Physical signs of **malnutrition** can be documented during the nutrition interview and are an important part of the assessment process.

Dietary data. There are many ways to document dietary intake. The accuracy of the data is frequently challenged, however, since both questioning and observing can impact the actual intake. During a nutrition interview the practitioner may ask what the individual ate during the previous twenty-four hours, beginning with the last item eaten prior to the interview. Practitioners can train individuals on completing a food diary, and they can request that the record be kept for either three days or one week. Documentation should include portion sizes and how the food was prepared. Brand names or the restaurant where the food was eaten can assist in assessing the details of the intake. Estimating portion sizes is difficult, and requesting that every food be measured or weighed is time-consuming and can be impractical. Food models and photographs of foods are therefore used to assist in recalling the portion size of the food. In a metabolic study, where accuracy in the quantity of what was eaten is imperative, the researcher may ask the individual to prepare double portions of everything that is

---

calorie: unit of food energy

protein: complex molecule composed of amino acids that performs vital functions in the cell; necessary part of the diet

Harris-Benedict equation: a formula for calculating a person's minimum energy expenditure

obese: above accepted standards of weight for sex, height, and age

hydration: degree of water in the body

metabolic: related to processing of nutrients and building of necessary molecules within the cell

stress: heightened state of nervousness or unease

acute: rapid-onset and short-lived

chronic: over a long period

malabsorption: decreased ability to take up nutrients

drugs: substances whose administration causes a significant change in the body's function

over-the-counter: available without a prescription

vitamin: necessary complex nutrient used to aid enzymes or other metabolic processes in the cell

mineral: an inorganic (non-carbon-containing) element, ion or compound

herbal: related to plants

malnutrition: chronic lack of sufficient nutrients to maintain health

eaten—one portion to be eaten, one portion to be saved (under refrigeration, if needed) so the researcher can weigh or measure the quantity and document the method of preparation.

Food frequency questionnaires are used to gather information on how often a specific food, or category of food is eaten. The Food Guide Pyramid suggests portion sizes and the number of servings from each food group to be consumed on a daily basis, and can also be used as a reference to evaluate dietary intake.

During the nutrition interview, data collection will include questions about the individual's lifestyle—including the number of meals eaten daily, where they are eaten, and who prepared the meals. Information about **allergies**, food intolerances, and food avoidances, as well as caffeine and alcohol use, should be collected. Exercise frequency and occupation help to identify the need for increased calories. Asking about the economics of the individual or family, and about the use and type of kitchen equipment, can assist in the **development** of a plan of care. Dental and oral health also impact the nutritional assessment, as well as information about **gastrointestinal** health, such as problems with **constipation**, gas or diarrhea, vomiting, or frequent heartburn.

allergy: immune system reaction against substances that are otherwise harmless

development: the process of change by which an organism becomes more complex

gastrointestinal: related to the stomach and intestines

constipation: difficulty passing feces

Evaluation

After data are collected, the practitioner uses past experience as well as reference standards to assimilate the information into an assessment that provides an understanding of the individual's nutritional status. The practitioner uses the anthropometric data to assess ideal and desirable weight, as well as skinfold measurements to determine body fat. Height, weight, and age are plugged into the Harris-Benedict equation to determine calorie and protein needs. Using the clinical, biochemical, and dietary data, influences on the nutritional status can be determined. A nutritional intervention, which usually includes dietary guidance and exercise recommendations, is then formulated and discussed with the individual. SEE ALSO ADOLESCENT NUTRITION; ADULT NUTRITION; ANTHROPOMETRIC MEASUREMENTS; BODY MASS INDEX; DIETARY ASSESSMENT; EATING HABITS; FOOD GUIDE PYRAMID; NUTRITION; NUTRITION EDUCATION; OBESITY.

Carole S. Mackey

Bibliography

Christie, Catherine, and Mitchell, Susan, eds. (2000). *Handbook of Medical Nutrition Therapy: The Florida Diet Manual.* Lighthouse Point, FL: Florida Dietetic Association.

Grant, Anne, and DeHoog, Susan (1999). *Nutrition Assessment and Support,* 5th edition. Seattle, WA: Grant and DeHoog.

Williams, Sue Rodwell (1997). *Nutrition and Diet Therapy,* 8th edition. St. Louis, MO: Mosby.

Winkler, Marion Feitelson, and Lysen, Lucinda (1993). *Suggested Guidelines for Nutrition and Metabolic Management of Adult Patients Receiving Nutrition Support.* Chicago, IL: American Dietetic Association.

Nutritional Deficiency

nutritional deficiency: lack of adequate nutrients in the diet

nutrient: dietary substance necessary for health

Nutritional deficiencies occur when a person's **nutrient** intake consistently falls below the recommended requirement. Nutritional deficiencies can lead

Nutritional Deficiency

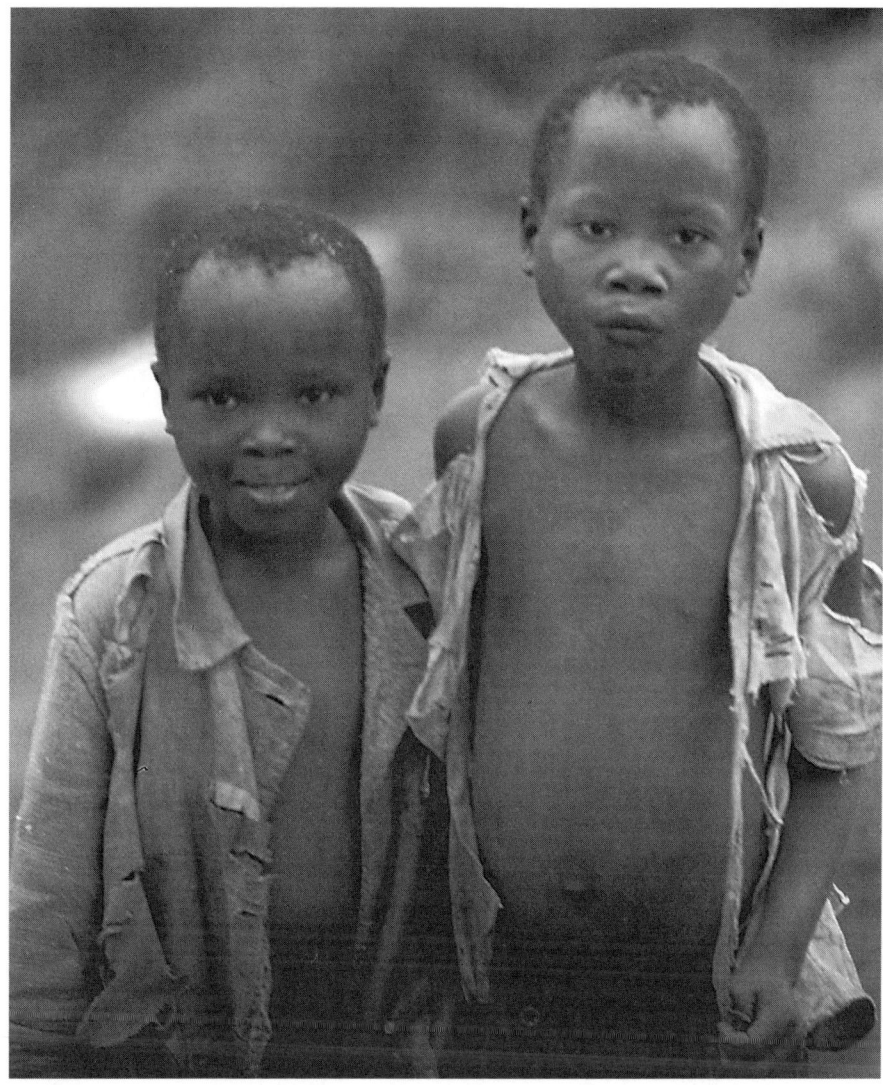

Children between 10–19 years of age face serious nutritional deficiencies worldwide, according to the World Health Organization. About 1,200 million, or 19 percent of adolescents suffer from poor nutrition that hurts their development and growth. *[Photograph by Jason Laure. Reproduced by permission.]*

to a variety of health problems, the most prevalent of which are **anemia**, beriberi, **osteoporosis**, pellagra, and **rickets**. Anemia occurs when the body does not have enough red blood cells to transport **oxygen** from the lungs to the body's cells. The most common symptom of anemia is a constant feeling of **fatigue**. Making sure that one's **diet** contains the proper amounts of **iron**, **folate**, and vitamin B_{12} can prevent anemia.

Prolonged thiamine deficiency can result in one of the more serious nutritional deficiencies, beriberi. Thiamine plays a major role in nerve processes, and a prolonged deficiency can result in nerve damage as well as heart and other muscle damage. Beriberi can be prevented by eating a diet containing foods rich in thiamine, such as meats, **legumes**, and whole-wheat breads.

Osteoporosis is an **asymptomatic** condition in which the loss of **minerals** can cause the body's bones to become porous and fragile. Making sure that one's diet contains the recommended amount of **calcium** and **vitamin D** can reduce the risk of developing osteoporosis.

The niacin-deficiency disease, pellagra, can produce symptoms such as dermatitis, **dementia**, diarrhea, and even death. Pellagra can be prevented through eating almost any protein-rich foods.

anemia: low level of red blood cells in the blood

osteoporosis: weakening of the bone structure

rickets: disorder caused by vitamin D deficiency, marked by soft and misshapen bones and organ swelling

oxygen: O_2, atmospheric gas required by all animals

fatigue: tiredness

diet: the total daily food intake, or the types of foods eaten

iron: nutrient needed for red blood cell formation

folate: one of the B vitamins, also called folic acid

legumes: beans, peas and related plants

asymptomatic: without symptoms

mineral: an inorganic (non-carbon-containing) element, ion or compound

calcium: mineral essential for bones and teeth

vitamin D: nutrient needed for calcium uptake and therefore proper bone formation

dementia: loss of cognitive abilities, including memory and decision-making

Rickets, or defective bone growth, is the result of an excessive vitamin D deficiency. It has been virtually wiped out in the United States due to the vitamin D **fortification** of milk. SEE ALSO ANEMIA; BERIBERI; OSTEOPOROSIS; PELLAGRA; RICKETS.

Beth Hensleigh

fortification: addition of vitamins and minerals to improve the nutritional content of a food

Internet Resources

Centers for Disease Control and Prevention. "CDC Identifies Nutritional Deficiencies Among Young Children." Available from <http://www.cdc.gov/nccdphp/dnpa/press/archive/nutritional_deficit.htm>

U.S. Food and Drug Administration. "Economic Characterization of the Dietary Supplement Industry Final Report." Available from <http://www.cfsan.fda.gov/∼comm/ds-econ4.html>

Nutritionist

Nutritionists are individuals who have studied the science of **nutrition**. Many nutritionists have a master's or doctoral degree in nutrition science and conduct research on food safety, eating habits, or the impact of food and nutrition on health. Some nutritionists are registered dietitians (RDs). An RD is a health professional who is trained to provide reliable nutrition advice and care in a variety of settings. In many states, nutritionists must be licensed or certified to practice in **clinical** and community settings. These licensed or certified nutritionists must meet the same requirements as an RD. Otherwise, many people with little or no education in nutrition science may be called nutritionists or nutrition counselors.

nutrition: the maintenance of health through proper eating, or the study of same

clinical: related to hospitals, clinics, and patient care

States regulate nutrition and dietetic professionals by one or more of the following methods:

- *Licensing*. Licensing statutes explicitly define the scope of practice, and it is illegal to practice without first obtaining a license from the state.

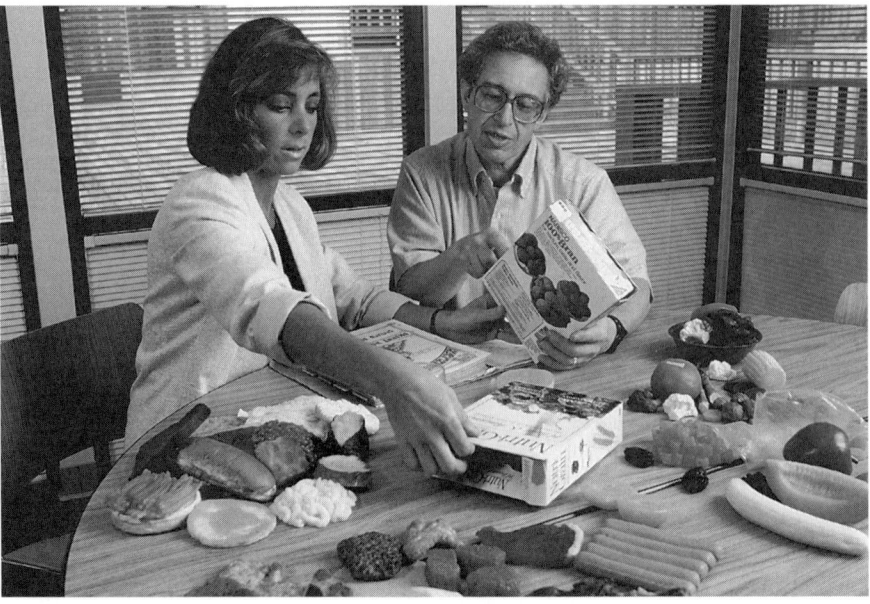

There is evidence that a healthy diet can improve longevity and prevent disease. Nutritionists research the diet's impact on overall health and advise patients, communities, hospitals, and companies about the science and methods of nutrition. *[Photograph by Nathan Benn. Corbis. Reproduced by permission.]*

- *Statutory certification.* Certification statutes limit the use of particular titles to persons meeting predetermined requirements. However, persons who are not certified may still practice the occupation or profession as long as they do not use the particular titles.

- *Registration.* This is the least restrictive form of state regulation. As with certification, unregistered persons may be permitted to practice the profession if they do not use the state-recognized title. Typically, exams are not given and enforcement of the registration requirement is minimal.

Many state licensure boards use the qualifications established by the American Dietetic Association (ADA) Commission on Dietetic Registration to establish who may practice in the discipline. These standards require that an individual:

1. Complete a bachelors degree and course work approved by the ADA Commission on Accreditation for Dietetics Education
2. Complete accredited and supervised practice components of at least 900 hours in clinical, community, and food-service settings
3. Pass a national exam administered by the Commission on Dietetic Registration
4. Complete continuing professional education requirements to maintain licensure or registration. SEE ALSO CAREERS IN DIETETICS; DIETITIAN.

Catherine Christie

Internet Resources

American Dietetic Association. "Becoming a Registered Dietitian." Available from <http://www.eatright.org/becomeanrd.html>

American Dietetic Association. "State Professional Regulation." Available from <http://www.eatright.org/gov/st042500.html>

Obesity

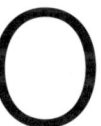

Obesity, defined as a **body mass index** of 30 or greater, is an epidemic in the United States and other industrialized nations, and it is rapidly becoming one in developing nations. As countries transition to westernized lifestyles, obesity tends to increase. Obesity rates vary from as little as 2 percent in some Asian countries to as much as 75 percent in some Pacific nations. There are more than 300 million **obese** persons in the world, and more than 750 million **overweight** persons. In the United States, 34 percent of adults are overweight and 30.5 percent are obese. Between 1980 and 2000, the percentage of overweight children ages six to eleven doubled, from 7 percent to 15 percent, and the percentage of overweight adolescents ages twelve to nineteen tripled, from 5 percent to 16 percent (Ogden, et al.). In Europe, the thinnest country is Sweden, with about 10 percent obesity, while the fattest is Lithuania, with about 79 percent obesity. The sad fact is the **prevalence** of obesity appears to be increasing in all countries.

An obese person has a 50 to 100 percent increased risk of premature death compared to someone of normal weight. In the United States, more than 300,000 deaths a year are attributable to obesity. Obesity is associated with type 2 **diabetes, coronary heart disease, stroke, hypertension,**

obesity: the condition of being overweight, according to established norms based on sex, age, and height

body mass index: weight in kilograms divided by square of the height in meters; a measure of body fat

obese: above accepted standards of weight for sex, height, and age

overweight: weight above the accepted norm based on height, sex, and age

prevalence: describing the number of cases in a population at any one time

diabetes: inability to regulate level of sugar in the blood

coronary heart disease: disease of the coronary arteries, the blood vessels surrounding the heart

stroke: loss of blood supply to part of the brain, due to a blocked or burst artery in the brain

hypertension: high blood pressure

cholesterol: multi-ringed molecule found in animal cell membranes; a type of lipid

cancer: uncontrolled cell growth

osteoarthritis: inflammation of the joints

gene: DNA sequence that codes for proteins, and thus controls inheritance

metabolism: the sum total of reactions in a cell or an organism

environment: surroundings

calorie: unit of food energy

fast food: food requiring minimal preparation before eating, or food delivered very quickly after ordering in a restaurant

sedentary: not active

blood pressure: measure of the pressure exerted by the blood against the walls of the blood vessels

glucose: a simple sugar; the most commonly used fuel in cells

diet: the total daily food intake, or the types of foods eaten

---

The Cost of Obesity

American spend more than $33 billion annually on weight loss, including low-calorie foods and fees at weight-loss clinics. A study estimated the health care cost of overweight and obesity to be $120 billion. This includes direct costs, such as doctor visits and medication, and indirect costs, such as wages lost by people too ill to work and the value of future earnings cut short by premature death. There are 63 million doctor visits per year related to obesity, and approximately 40 million workdays are lost.

—Paula Kepos

---

elevated blood **cholesterol**, some cancers (e.g., colon, endometrial, kidney, gallbladder, and postmenopausal breast **cancer**), **osteoarthritis**, gallbladder disease, and respiratory disease. In addition, obesity is often associated with discrimination and prejudice, causing some obese people to suffer poor self-esteem and reduced quality of life. The health care costs attributable to obesity exceed $100 billion a year in the United States, more than 6 percent of the total health care costs.

What Causes Obesity?

Obesity is caused by many factors. A person's weight is determined by a combination of **genes**, **metabolism**, behavior, culture, and **environment**. Genes and metabolism may help explain about 25 to 40 percent of body weight. However, a person's environment overwhelms the minor influences of biology. While genes may increase one's risk for obesity, they do not by themselves cause obesity. Genes certainly can't explain the rapidly increasing prevalence of obesity around the world.

For most people, obesity results from eating too much and not being active enough. The overwhelming factors responsible for obesity are environmental. Modern Western society encourages poor diets and lack of exercise. For example, portion sizes continue to increase. Americans were eating about 200 more **calories** per day in 2003 than they were in 1993. **Fast-food** restaurants encourage customers to "super size" and purchase "value" meals. Many target children, using well-known movie stars and cartoon characters in their advertising. Further, people eat out more often than in the past and many restaurants offer huge portion sizes. Americans seem determined to get as much food as they can for their money.

Television contributes to obesity through commercials urging people to buy food of low nutritional value, and by encouraging **sedentary** behavior. Many people tend to snack while watching television. Americans simply don't get enough physical activity. Less than one-third of American adults report that they do at least thirty minutes of brisk walking or other moderate activity on most days of the week, and almost half do no leisure-time activity at all. Almost half of U.S. high school students watch television more than two hours every day. This lack of physical activity is contributing to the increases in obesity and to other health-related conditions.

Treatment of Obesity

Weight loss in obese persons improves health. Weight losses of ten to twenty pounds have been shown to lower **blood pressure**, blood cholesterol, and blood **glucose** (in persons with type 2 diabetes), and to improve other health problems. An obese person does not have to lose fifty or a hundred pounds to realize health benefits, however, for even modest losses of weight can lead to major health benefits.

Diets

Reducing calories is one requirement for weight loss. Cutting only 100 extra calories a day from one's **diet** will lead to a weight loss of 10 pounds in a year, while cutting 500 calories a day will lead to a loss of 50 pounds in a year. Most health organizations recommend a specific distribution of calo-

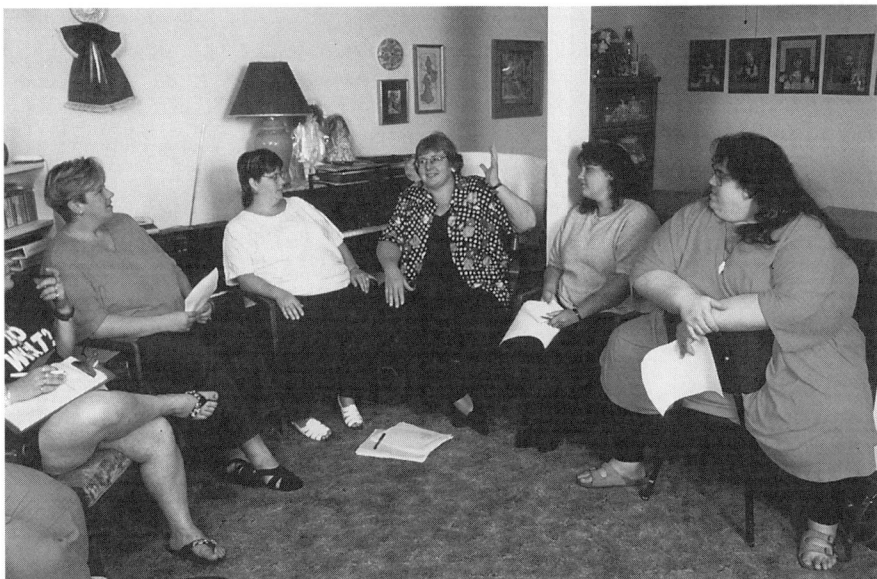

Joining a support group may help an obese person to lose weight. Losing weight can prevent a wide array of health problems that result from obesity and that generally lower the life expectancy of an obese person.
[Photograph by Carolyn A. McKeone. Photo Researchers, Inc. Reproduced by permission.]

ries. For example, about 25 to 30 percent of total calories should be from **fat** (mainly unsaturated fat, such as olive oil, corn oil, and safflower oil), 15 percent from **protein**, and 50 to 60 percent from **carbohydrates** (mainly complex carbohydrates, such as fruits and vegetables). Recommended total calories should be based on height, weight, age, and activity level. A plant-based diet, consisting of an abundance of fresh vegetables and fruit and limited in calories, seems to be a healthful one for most people.

fat: type of food molecule rich in carbon and hydrogen, with high energy content

protein: complex molecule composed of amino acids that performs vital functions in the cell; necessary part of the diet

carbohydrate: food molecule made of carbon, hydrogen, and oxygen, including sugars and starches

Physical Activity

Burning only an extra 100 calories a day by walking briskly for about 20 minutes will lead to a weight loss of about 10 pounds a year, while burning an extra 300 calories by walking briskly for about 60 minutes a day will lead to a weight loss of about 30 pounds. Physical activity contributes to weight loss, decreases abdominal fat, increases cardiorespiratory fitness, and helps with maintenance of lost weight. Any **aerobic** exercise, such as swimming, bicycling, jogging, skiing, or dancing, leads to these benefits, but for most obese people brisk walking seems to be the easiest activity to do. Other forms of exercise, such as resistance training or lifting weights, can also be helpful in a weight loss program. Finding ways to be more active every day, such as walking up a flight of stairs rather than taking the elevator, or walking somewhere rather than driving, can help a person burn calories without much effort.

aerobic: designed to maintain adequate oxygen in the bloodstream

Combined Diet and Exercise

The combination of a reduced-calorie diet and increased physical activity will lead to better weight loss than either one done separately. Small changes in diet and physical activity done each day is the key to long-term, successful weight loss for most obese people. SEE ALSO BODY IMAGE; BODY MASS INDEX; CHILDHOOD OBESITY; FAD DIETS; FAST FOODS; OVERWEIGHT; WEIGHT LOSS DIETS; WEIGHT MANAGEMENT.

John P. Foreyt

Bibliography

Flegal, Katherine M.; Carroll, Margaret D.; Ogden, Cynthia L.; and Johnson, Clifford L. (2002). "Prevalence and Trends in Obesity among U.S. Adults, 1999–2000." *Journal of the American Medical Association* 288(14):1723–1727.

Foreyt, John P.; McInnis, Kyle J.; Poston, Walker S. C.; and Rippe, James M.; eds. (2003). *Lifestyle Obesity Management*. Malden, MA: Blackwell.

Ogden, Cynthia L.; Flegal, Katherine M.; Carroll, Margaret D.; and Johnson, Clifford L. (2002). "Prevalence and Trends in Overweight among U.S. Children and Adolescents, 1999–2000." *Journal of the American Medical Association* 288(14):1728–1732.

Poston, Walker S. C., and Foreyt, John P. (1999). "Obesity Is an Environmental Issue." *Atherosclerosis* 146:201–209.

Omega-3 and Omega-6 Fatty Acids

Fatty acids are organic compounds composed of carbon chains of varying lengths, with an acid group on one end and hydrogen bound to all the carbons of the chain. **Essential fatty acids** (EFAs) are those that are necessary for health, but cannot be synthesized by the body. Therefore, it is important to supply the body with EFAs through one's daily dietary intake. EFAs are also called *vitamin F* or *polyunsaturates*. They are important ingredients for the growth and maintenance of cells. The body utilizes essential fatty acids for **hormone** production, specifically for the production of **prostaglandins**, which aid in reducing **hypertension**, migraine headaches, and **arthritis**.

Essential fatty acids offer many positive effects for the body, including the nourishment of skin and hair; reduction of **blood pressure**, **cholesterol**, and **triglyceride** levels; prevention of arthritis and inflammation; and the reduction of the risk of **blood clotting**. Furthermore, essential fatty acids help protect the body from **cardiovascular** disease, **candidiasis**, **eczema**, and **psoriasis**, and they play a critical role in brain development and in the transmission of nerve impulses.

Types of EFAs

There are basically two types of essential fatty acids, *omega-3* fatty acids, also known as linolenic acids, and *omega-6* fatty acids, which are also called linoleic acids. The two types are distinguished by their chemical structures. Omega-3 EFAs are found in deepwater fish, fish oil, and some vegetable oils, such as canola, flaxseed, and walnut oil. Nuts are also a good source of *omega-3* fatty acids, particularly hazelnuts, almonds, pecans, cashews, walnuts, and macadamia nuts. The best fish oil sources are salmon, mackerel, anchovies, sardines, and herring, which have a high **fat** content and provide more omega-3 than other fish. Flaxseeds are also a good source, and they are low in saturated fats and **calories** and have no cholesterol. Omega-6 fatty acids are found in raw nuts, seeds, **legumes**, and in unsaturated vegetable oils, such as borage oil, grape seed oil, primrose oil, sesame oil, and soybean oil.

Benefits of EFAs

There are many health benefits attributable to essential fatty acids. Research has shown that diets rich in monounsaturated fatty acids, which contain the *omega-3* variety, reduce total mortality by 70 percent in patients who have

---

fatty acids: molecules rich in carbon and hydrogen; a component of fats

essential fatty acids: particular molecules made of carbon, hydrogen, and oxygen that the human body must have but cannot make itself

hormone: molecules produced by one set of cells that influence the function of another set of cells

prostaglandin: hormone that helps regulate inflammation and other tissue processes

hypertension: high blood pressure

arthritis: inflammation of the joints

blood pressure: measure of the pressure exerted by the blood against the walls of the blood vessels

cholesterol: multi-ringed molecule found in animal cell membranes; a type of lipid

triglyceride: a type of fat

blood clotting: the process by which blood forms a solid mass to prevent uncontrolled bleeding

cardiovascular: related to the heart and circulatory system

candidiasis: a yeast infection

eczema: skin disease causing itching and flaking

psoriasis: skin disorder characterized by red, dry, scaly skin

fat: type of food molecule rich in carbon and hydrogen, with high energy content

calorie: unit of food energy

legumes: beans, peas, and related plants

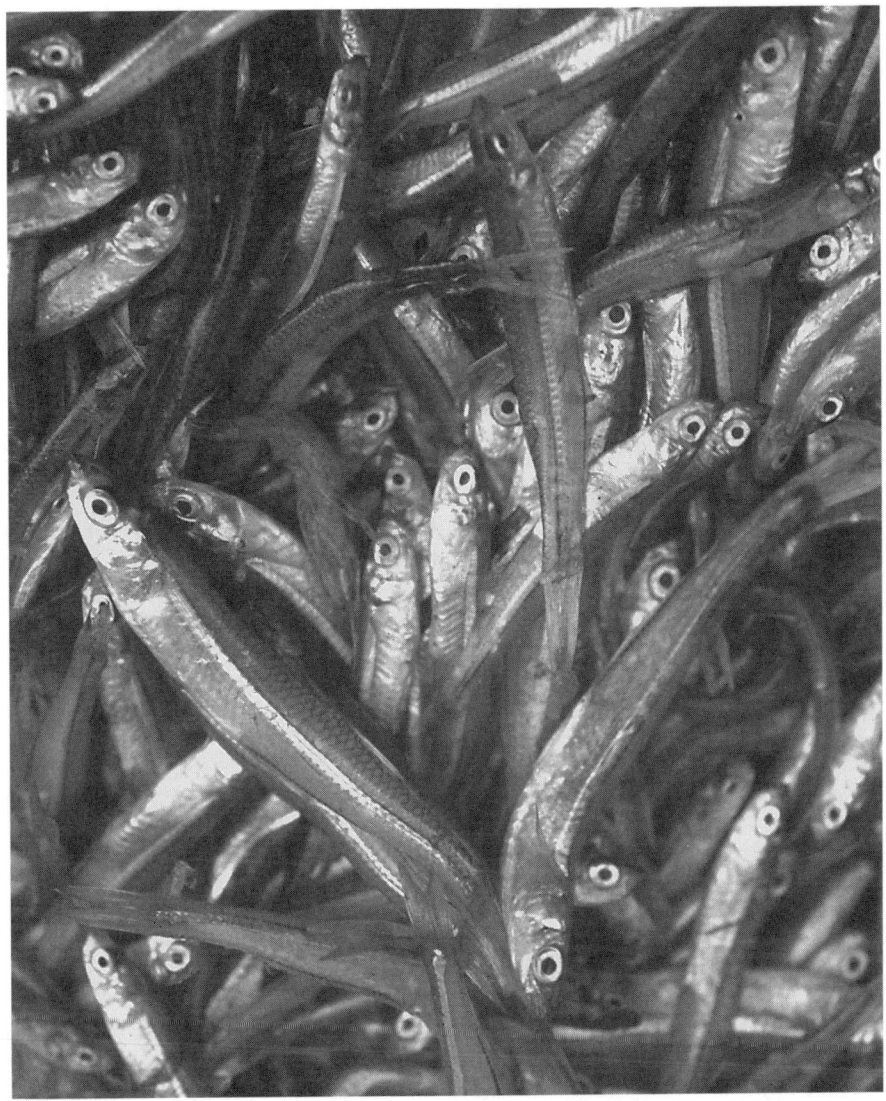

Omega-3 fatty acids have a balancing effect on omega-6 fatty acids. Both are essential nutrients, but they should be consumed in equal proportions. For Americans, that means substituting fish or nuts for fried foods once or more weekly. [National Audubon Society Collection/Photo Researchers, Inc. Reproduced by permission.]

already experienced a **heart attack**. This has led to a general recommendation to consume at least one meal a week of fish rich in *omega-3* fatty acids. It is generally accepted that *omega-3* fatty acids help to reduce the levels of triglycerides in the body, thus decreasing the risk of **heart disease**.

Omega-6 fatty acids have been shown to be beneficial in the reduction of cholesterol levels when they are substituted for saturated fats in a person's **diet**. The benefit in consuming *omega-6* fatty acids therefore lies in the fact that they reduce the **incidence** of coronary **artery** disease, which is a condition where excess cholesterol builds up on the arteries of the heart, eventually blocking the flow of blood and causing a heart attack. SEE ALSO FATS; HEART DISEASE; LIPID PROFILE.

Susan S. Kim
Jeffrey Radecki

heart attack: loss of blood supply to part of the heart, resulting in death of heart muscle

heart disease: any disorder of the heart or its blood supply, including heart attack, atherosclerosis, and coronary artery disease

diet: the total daily food intake, or the types of foods eaten

incidence: number of new cases reported each year

artery: blood vessel that carries blood away from the heart toward the body tissues

Bibliography

Masley, Steven C. (1998). "Dietary Therapy for Preventing and Treating Coronary Artery Disease." *American Family Physician* 57:1299–1305. Also available from <http://www.aafp.org>

Sizer, Frances, and Whitney, Eleanor (2000). *Nutrition: Concepts and Controversies*, 8th edition. Stamford CT: Wadsworth/Thomson Learning.

Oral Health

Oral tissues, such as the gingiva (gums), teeth, and muscles of mastication (chewing muscles), are living tissues, and they have the same **nutritional requirements** as any other living tissue in the body. When adequate, nutritious food is not available, oral health may be compromised by nutrient-deficiency diseases, such as **scurvy**. In contrast, when food is freely available, as in many industrialized societies, oral health may be compromised by both the continual exposure of the oral **environment** to food and the presence of **chronic** diseases, such as **diabetes**. The **diet** not only affects the number and kinds of carious lesions (cavities), but also is an important factor in the development of periodontal disease (gum disease).

According to the U.S. Surgeon General's report, *Healthy People 2010*, dental **caries** have significantly declined in the United States since the early 1970s. However, it remains an important concern, especially in specific subgroups in the U.S. population. For example, 80 percent of dental caries in children's permanent teeth are concentrated in 25 percent of the child and adolescent population, particularly in individuals from low socioeconomic backgrounds.

Factors Affecting Nutrition and Oral Health

Sugar, particularly the frequent ingestion of sweets (cakes, cookies, candy), is related to both dental caries and periodontal disease. For example, populations with a frequent exposure to sugar, such as agricultural workers in sugar-cane fields (who may chew on sugar cane while they work), have a greater number of decayed, missing, and restored teeth. Sugar (**sucrose**), has a unique relationship to oral health. Sucrose can supply both the substrate (building blocks) and the **energy** required for the creation of dental **plaque** (the mesh-like scaffold of **molecules** that harbor **bacteria** on tooth surfaces). Sucrose also releases **glucose** during digestion, and oral bacteria can **metabolize** the glucose to produce organic acids. However, oral bacteria can also produce organic acids from foods other than sugar.

Oral health may be related to many nutritional factors other than sugar, including the number of times a day a person eats or drinks, the frequent ingestion of drinks with low **acidity** (such as fruit juices and both regular and diet soft drinks), whether a person is exposed to fluoride (through fluoridated water, fluoridated toothpaste, or fluoride supplements), and whether an **eating disorder** is present. Not only can the diet affect oral health, but also oral health can affect eating patterns. This is particularly true in individuals with very poor oral health, who may not be able to chew without pain or discomfort. Older, *edentulous* (having no teeth) patients who have had a **stroke** with the accompanying chewing and swallowing problems may be at significant nutritional risk, particularly if they are living alone and on a limited income. Finally, **malnutrition** (both **undernutrition** and overnutrition) have specific effects on oral health.

---

nutritional requirements: the set of substances needed in the diet to maintain health

scurvy: a syndrome characterized by weakness, anemia, and spongy gums, due to vitamin C deficiency

environment: surroundings

chronic: over a long period

diabetes: inability to regulate level of sugar in the blood

diet: the total daily food intake, or the types of foods eaten

caries: cavities in the teeth

sucrose: table sugar

energy: technically, the ability to perform work; the content of a substance that allows it to be useful as a fuel

plaque: material forming deposits on the surface of the teeth, which may promote bacterial growth and decay

molecule: combination of atoms that form stable particles

bacteria: single-celled organisms without nuclei, some of which are infectious

glucose: a simple sugar; the most commonly used fuel in cells

metabolize: processing of a nutrient

acidity: measure of the tendency of a molecule to lose hydrogen ions, thus behaving as an acid

eating disorder: behavioral disorder involving excess consumption, avoidance of consumption, self-induced vomiting, or other food-related aberrant behavior

stroke: loss of blood supply to part of the brain, due to a blocked or burst artery in the brain

malnutrition: chronic lack of sufficient nutrients to maintain health

undernutrition: food intake too low to maintain adequate energy expenditure without weight loss

Undernutrition and Oral Health

Although oral diseases associated with vitamin deficiencies are rare in the United States and other industrialized countries, they may be common in emerging "third-world" nations. In these countries, the limited supply of nutrient-dense foods or the lack of specific nutrients in the diet (vitamin C, **niacin**, etc.) may produce characteristic oral manifestations. In addition, unusual food practices, such as chewing sugar cane throughout the day or other regional or cultural nutritional practices, may decrease the oral health of specific populations.

Vitamin-deficiency diseases may produce characteristic signs and symptoms in the oral cavity (mouth). For example, in a typical B-vitamin deficiency, a person may complain that the tongue is red and swollen and "burns" (*glossitis*), that changes in taste have occurred, and that cracks have appeared on the lips and at the corners of the mouth (angular cheilosis). In a vitamin C deficiency, petechiae (small, hemorrhaging red spots) may appear in the oral cavity, as well as on other parts of the body, especially after pressure has been exerted on the tissue. In addition, the gums may bleed upon probing with a dental instrument.

In humans, **calcium** deficiency rarely, if ever, causes the production of hypoplastic enamel (poorly mineralized enamel) similar to the **osteoporosis** produced in bone. Teeth appear to have a **biological** priority over bone when calcium is limited in the diet.

Oral health problems associated with **nutritional deficiencies** occur not only in populations with a limited food supply. Individuals whose chewing and swallowing abilities have been compromised by oral **cancer**, radiation treatment, or AIDS may also exhibit signs and symptoms of nutritional deficiencies.

Overnutrition and Oral Health

The proliferation of foods high in **calories**, **fat**, sugar, and salt, and low in nutritional content—such as that found in **fast-food** restaurants and vending machines—has created a "toxic" food environment in many industrialized countries, and this has had an important impact on oral health. Oral bacteria have the ability to synthesize the acids that dissolve tooth enamel from many different types of foods, not just sugar. Frequency of eating is a major factor related to poor oral health in infants, as well as children and adults. *Baby bottle tooth decay*, also called *nursing bottle caries*, is a term that refers to the caries formed when an infant is routinely put to sleep with a bottle. *Breastfeeding caries* is a condition associated with the constant exposure of an infant's oral environment to breast milk, while *pacifier caries* occurs when a pacifier is dipped in honey prior to inserting the pacifier into an infant's mouth.

Both childhood and adult **obesity** are on the rise, and they have reached epidemic proportions in some countries. Obesity is traditionally associated with increased rates of non-insulin-dependent diabetes; elevations in **blood pressure**; and elevated **serum** glucose, blood **cholesterol**, and **triglycerides** (blood fat)—but it is also associated with decreased oral health status. For example, the number of servings of fruit juice and soft drinks ingested each

---

niacin: one of the B vitamins, required for energy production in the cell

calcium: mineral essential for bones and teeth

osteoporosis: weakening of the bone structure

biological: related to living organisms

nutritional deficiency: lack of adequate nutrients in the diet

cancer: uncontrolled cell growth

calorie: unit of food energy

fat: type of food molecule rich in carbon and hydrogen, with high energy content

fast food: food requiring minimal preparation before eating, or food delivered very quickly after ordering in a restaurant

obesity: the condition of being overweight, according to established norms based on sex, age, and height

blood pressure: measure of the pressure exerted by the blood against the walls of the blood vessels

serum: non-cellular portion of the blood

cholesterol: multi-ringed molecule found in animal cell membranes; a type of lipid

triglyceride: a type of fat

Oral diseases like gingivitis (left) and periodontitis (right) may result from overnutrition. When food consumption is excessive, or when the foods consumed are frequently sugary or acidic, the enamel on teeth can dissolve and gums can be infected. [The Gale Group.]

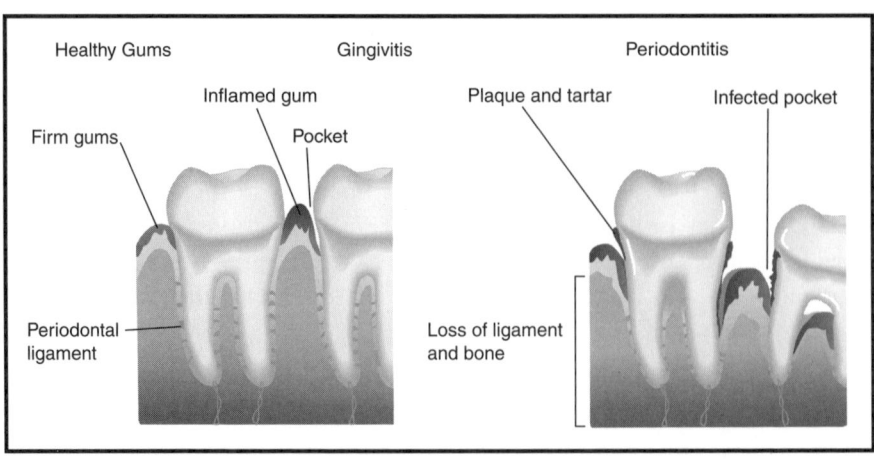

anorexia nervosa: refusal to maintain body weight at or above what is considered normal for height and age

micronutrient: nutrient needed in very small quantities

metabolism: the sum total of reactions in a cell or an organism

day is correlated not only with obesity in children, but also with increased caries. The American Academy of Pediatrics has warned parents on the overuse of fruit juices in children's diets.

Although diet soft drinks do not contain sugar, they do contain both carbonic and phosphoric acids and can directly destroy tooth enamel, particularly if the teeth are periodically exposed to a diet drink throughout the day. The direct demineralization of tooth enamel by regular and diet soft drinks has similarities to the demineralization of tooth enamel common in **anorexia** nervosa, in which forced regurgitation of food exposes lingual tooth surfaces (the side of the tooth facing the tongue) to stomach acids. In the case of enamel erosion produced by soft drinks and juices, effects are usually seen on all the tooth surfaces.

Fluoride and Oral Health

No discussion of nutrition and oral health would be complete without mentioning the role of the **micronutrient** fluoride. The addition of fluoride to the public drinking water supply is rated as one of the most effective preventive public health measures ever undertaken. Fluoride reduces dental caries by several different mechanisms. The fluoride ion may be integrated into enamel, making it more resistant to decay. In addition, fluoride may inhibit oral microbial **metabolism**, lowering the production of organic acids.

The relationship of nutrition to oral health includes much more than a simple focus on sugar's relationship to caries. It includes factors such as an individual's overall dietary patterns, exposure to fluoride, and a person's systemic health. SEE ALSO BABY BOTTLE TOOTH DECAY; BREASTFEEDING; FAST FOODS; OBESITY.

Warren B. Karp

Internet Resources

American Dental Association. "Oral Health Topics." Available from <http://www.ada.org>

American Dietetic Association. "Position of the American Dietetic Assoication: Oral Health and Nutrition." Available from <http://www.eatright.com>

U.S. Department of Health and Human Services. "Healthy People 2010." Available from <http://www.health.gov/healthypeople>

Oral Rehydration Therapy

Oral rehydration therapy (ORT) involves the replacement of fluids and **electrolytes** lost during an episode of diarrheal illness. Diarrheal illnesses are pervasive worldwide, and they have a particularly large impact in the developing world. Children under the age of five are the major victims and account for over 3 million deaths a year due to **dehydration** associated with diarrheal illness. The World Health Organization (WHO) estimates that over one million deaths are prevented annually by ORT. An oral rehydration solution (ORS) is the cornerstone of this treatment. Between 90 and 95 percent of cases of **acute**, watery diarrhea can be successfully treated with ORT.

Ancient civilizations in India and China made use of sugar and starch solutions to treat dehydration. Oral rehydration solutions make use of the ability of **glucose** to increase the resorption of fluids and salts into the intestinal wall. The current understanding of ORT was developed in 1968 by researchers responding to a **cholera** epidemic that began in 1958 in Bangladesh. **Intravenous** rehydration was inaccessible to much of the population that diarrhea affected, and it was found that oral rehydration solutions could replace such treatment cheaply and effectively. Most importantly, it was easily accessible in the form of prepackaged or homemade solutions.

WHO and UNICEF are the principal sponsors of global rehydration projects. These projects involve the development and distribution of prepackaged solutions, combined with education efforts for instruction in home preparation and delivery. There is some variation among packaged solutions, but the principle ingredients are glucose, sodium, and potassium. The UNICEF recipe for a simple homemade solution contains five cupfuls of boiled water, eight teaspoons of sugar, and one teaspoon of salt, resulting in one liter of solution. Double-sided measuring spoons have also been distributed to standardize measurement. In addition, fruit juices, coconut water, and other indigenous solutions can adequately approximate ORS.

Oral rehydration therapy has increased in use since its development, and it has potential for even greater use. However, severe cases of dehydration continue to need supervised medical care. SEE ALSO DEHYDRATION; DIARRHEA; MALNUTRITION; UNITED NATIONS CHILDREN'S FUND (UNICEF).

Seema Pania Kumar

electrolyte: salt dissolved in fluid

dehydration: loss of water

acute: rapid-onset and short-lived

glucose: a simple sugar; the most commonly used fuel in cells

cholera: bacterial infection of the small intestine causing severe diarrhea, vomiting, and dehydration

intravenous: into the veins

Bibliography

Agency for International Development (1988). *Oral Rehydration Therapy: A Revolution in Child Survival.* Weston, MA: Oegeschlager, Gunn & Hain.

Semba, Richard, and Bloem, Martin (2001). *Nutrition and Health in Developing Countries.* Totowa, NJ: Humana Press.

Internet Sources

Rehydration Project. Available from <http://rehydrate.org>

Organic Foods

In response to a need to standardize the use of such terms as *organic* and *natural*, the U.S. Congress passed the Organic Foods Production Act of

1990, which established the U.S. National Organic Standards Board (NOSB). In 1995, the NOSB defined *organic agriculture* as "an **ecological** production management system that promotes and enhances **biodiversity**, **biological** cycles and soil biological activity. It is based on minimal use of off-farm inputs and on management practices that restore, maintain and enhance ecological harmony." Organic production uses "materials and practices that enhance the ecological balance of natural systems and that integrate the parts of the farming system into an ecological whole," though such practices "cannot ensure that products are completely free of residues" of pesticides, herbicides, and other additives or contaminants. However, "methods are used to minimize pollution from air, soil, and water. Organic food handlers, processors, and retailers adhere to standards that maintain the integrity of organic agricultural products. The primary goal of organic agriculture is to optimize the health and productivity of interdependent communities of soil life, plants, animals and people" (NOSB).

Certification and Labeling of Organic Foods

According to regulations set forth by the United States Department of Agriculture (USDA), organic foods must come from farms or ranches certified by a state or private agency that has been accredited by the USDA. Foods labeled "100 percent organic" must contain only organically produced ingredients, excluding water and salt. Foods labeled "organic" must contain, by weight, at least 95 percent organically produced ingredients. Products meeting these requirements must display these terms on their principal display panel and may use the USDA seal and the seal or mark of certifying agents on packages and in advertisements. Foods labeled "made with organic ingredients" must contain, by weight, at least 70 percent organic ingredients. Up to three separate organic ingredients may be listed on the principal display label, and a certifying agent's seal or mark may be used on the package. The use of a USDA seal is prohibited, however. Livestock can be certified "organic" if they have been raised on organic foodstuffs for over one year.

Other labeling provisions include:

- Packaging of any product labeled "organic" must state the actual percentage of organic ingredients and use the word "organic" to modify each organically produced ingredient.
- The name and address of the certifying agent must be displayed on the label's information panel.
- There are no restrictions on the use of truthful labeling claims, such as "pesticide free," "no **drugs** or growth **hormones** used," or "sustainably harvested."
- Products made with less than 50 percent organic ingredients may make no claim other than designating specific organic ingredients with the ingredient information.

Over ninety private organizations and state agencies (certifying agents) currently accredit farms that produce organic food, but standards for growing and labeling organic food may differ. For example, different agencies may permit or prohibit the use of specific natural pesticides or fertilizers in growing organic food. In addition, some of the language contained on seals, labels, and logos approved by organic certifiers may differ.

Advantages of Organically Grown Foods

- Less artificial or synthetic pesticides, herbicides, fertilizer, and hormone residue.
- May contain higher concentration of nutrients and phytochemicals.
- May taste better.
- Environmental advantages, such as enhanced soil fertility, higher biodiversity, and increased water conservation.
- Decreased energy input for production.
- May have higher animal welfare standards.

Disadvantages of Organic Foods

- More expensive.
- May be fertilized with manure or sewage containing potentially harmful organisms.
- May have undesirable appearance.
- May be cross-contaminated with chemicals from other farms (also a risk with conventionally grown foods).
- Lower crop yield.
- Uncertainty over long-term sustainability of crop.

---

ecological: related to the environment and human interactions with it

biodiversity: richness of species within an area

biological: related to living organisms

drugs: substances whose administration causes a significant change in the body's function

hormone: molecules produced by one set of cells that influence the function of another set of cells

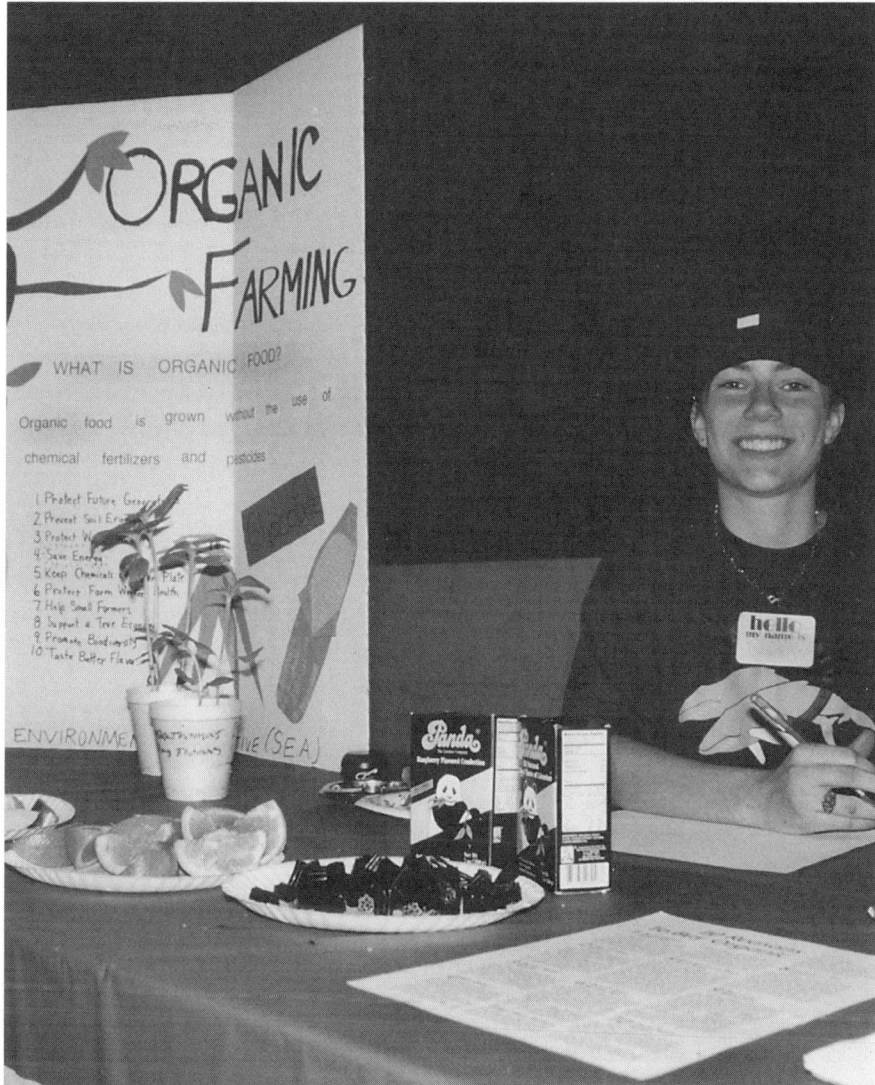

Science has not proven any nutritional difference between organically grown foods and conventionally grown foods. However, the methods employed by organic farmers may be more sustainable in the long term than conventional farming. *[Photograph by Robert J. Huffman. Field Mark Publications. Reproduced by permission.]*

The Market for Organic Foods

The global market for organic foods is expected to expand from $26 billion in 2001 to $80 billion in 2008. The greatest market growth has been in the European Union, where market revenues were forecast to expand by a third in 2001 to reach $12 billion, largely due to growth in Germany, Italy, France, and the United Kingdom. In all these countries, except the United Kingdom, growth has resulted from organic foods moving into mainstream marketing channels and from increased consumer interest. Japan is the third largest market for organic foods and accounts for the bulk of Asian organic market revenues. High growth is also occurring in Singapore, Hong Kong, and Taiwan, though these markets remain much smaller than the Japanese market.

The U.S. organic foods marketplace reached $6.95 billion in sales in 2001, up 19 percent from 2000. Sales are expected to increase in the United States, reaching $20 billion by 2008. The largest market for organic products worldwide is in fresh produce. Other popular organic foods include soy foods, meat, poultry, eggs, and meat and dairy alternatives.

Safety and Nutritional Value of Organic Foods

The **nutrient** content of plants is determined primarily by heredity, and organic foods generally contain no less **fat** or sodium, or more **vitamins**, **minerals**, or **fiber**, than the same food grown using conventional methods.

However, organic farming methods can enhance soil fertility, resulting in an increased concentration of some minerals and phtyochemicals in organic food. Organic food cannot be guaranteed pesticide-free, though organic farmers use only naturally occurring pesticides such as sulfur, copper, nicotine, and *Bacillus thuringiensis* (a naturally occurring bacterial disease of insects). Organic foods may contain pesticide residues that have drifted from farm to farm, or residual pesticides found in soil or water, though the amounts of such residues are certainly greater in conventionally produced foods, where pesticides are directly applied to the crops.

Furthermore, there is no evidence of consistent differences in appearance, flavor, or texture between organic foods and conventionally produced foods. Organic foods may be more susceptible to microbiological contamination. Several food-borne illness outbreaks resulting from *Salmonella enteriditis*, *Listeria monocytogenes*, and *E. coli* O157:H7 have been associated with consumption of organically grown produce.

Organic foods can be more costly than conventionally grown foods. The USDA Economic Research Service, in *USDA/ERS Food Cost Review 1950–97*, reports that in 1995 an average American household with two parents and two children spent $6,992 on food. Purchasing only organic foods would increase total food costs by $4,000 to $10,977 per year. However, as the organic market grows, the cost is likely to continue to drop.

Organic agriculture is generally seen to be environmentally friendly. Organic agriculture decreases the amount of nitrogen-containing chemicals that seep into groundwater supplies, decreases soil deterioration via crop rotation, and minimizes exposure of farm workers and livestock to potentially harmful compounds. However, use of animal manures may increase the risk of food-borne illness, and a dependence on nitrogen-fixing, green-manure crops uses large amounts of land. On the other hand, these methods can make nutrients more available to subsequent crops, increase crop productivity, and conserve water resources.

Many kinds of pesticides, including insecticides and herbicides, are commonly used in producing and marketing the food supply. High doses of some of these chemicals have been shown to cause **cancer** in laboratory animals, though the low concentrations found in some foods are generally well within established limits. Environmental pollution by slowly degrading pesticides can lead to food-chain bioaccumulation and persistent residues in body fat. These residues may increase the risk for certain cancers. Studies have shown that concentrations in tissues are low, and the evidence has not been conclusive. Continued research regarding pesticide use is therefore essential to insure food safety, improved food production, and reduced environmental pollution.

Sensible food practices can significantly reduce pesticide residue on foods. Such practices include washing and scrubbing fresh produce under running water, peeling and trimming produce when possible, removing the outer leaves of leafy vegetables, and trimming fat from meat and skin from

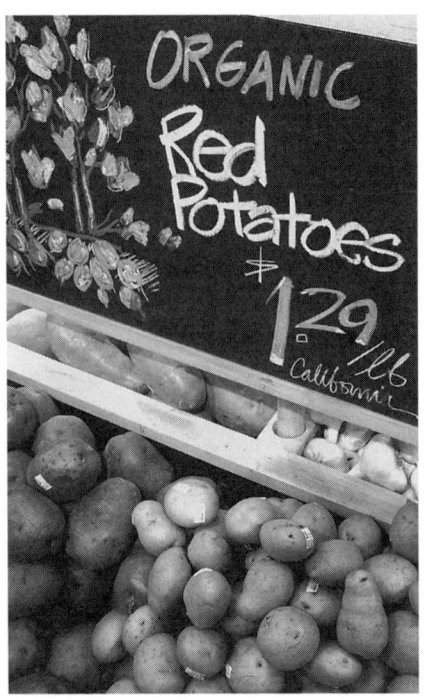

Fresh produce is the top-selling organic food, but organic dairy products are rapidly gaining popularity. Organic foods can be significantly more expensive than their conventionally grown counterparts, and research has not proven that health reasons alone justify their cost. [AP/Wide World Photos. Reproduced by permission.]

nutrient: dietary substance necessary for health

fat: type of food molecule rich in carbon and hydrogen, with high energy content

vitamin: necessary complex nutrient used to aid enzymes or other metabolic processes in the cell

mineral: an inorganic (non-carbon-containing) element, ion or compound

fiber: indigestible plant material which aids digestion by providing bulk

cancer: uncontrolled cell growth

poultry and fish. Eating a variety of foods from a variety of sources will reduce the likelihood of exposure to a single pesticide.

Organic foods are produced with ecologically based practices, such as biological pest management and composting. To be labeled "organic," foods must have been produced on certified organic farms and conform to established labeling requirements. From a scientific viewpoint, organic foods are no safer or nutritious than conventionally produced foods. Most major health organizations maintain that the health benefits of consuming a **diet** rich in fruits, vegetables, and whole grains significantly outweigh any health risk from residual pesticide, herbicide, or fertilizer consumption. According to the American Institute for Cancer Research, there is no convincing evidence that eating foods containing **trace** amounts of chemicals such as fertilizers, pesticides, herbicides, and drugs used on farm animals increases the risk for cancer. Organic agriculture provides consumers with an additional choice when purchasing food, however, and also provides some assurance of where a food was produced and how it was produced. SEE ALSO Food Labels; Food Safety; Vegetarianism.

diet: the total daily food intake, or the types of foods eaten

trace: very small amount

M. Elizabeth Kunkel
Barbara H. D. Luccia

Bibliography

Berlau, John (1999). "The Risky Nature of Organics: Growing Produce in Manure Raises Concerns." *Investor's Business Daily*, March 3.

Bourn, D., and Prescott, J. (2002). "A Comparison of the Nutritional Value, Sensory Qualities, and Food Safety of Organically and Conventionally Grown Produced Foods." *Critical Reviews in Food Science and Nutrition* 42(1):1–34.

Hartman Group (2000). *Organic Lifestyle Shopper Study: Mapping the Journey of Organic Consumers*. Bellevue, WA: Author.

Williams, P. R., and Hammitt, J. K. (2001). "Perceived Risks of Conventional and Organic Produce: Pesticides, Pathogens, and Natural Toxins." *Risk Analysis* 21(2):319–330.

Internet Resources

Elitzak, Howard (1999). "USDA/ERS Food Cost Review 1950–97." Available from <http://www.ers.usda.gov/publications/aer780/>

National Organic Standards Board. "National Organic Program." Available from <http://www.ams.usda.gov/nosb>

Nutrition Business Journal (2001). "Organic Foods Report 2001." Available from <http://www.nutritionbusiness.com>

Organisms, Food-Borne

Food-borne organisms are **bacteria, viruses,** and **parasites** that can cause illnesses which are either infectious or toxic in nature. They enter the body through the ingestion of contaminated food or water. Every person is at risk of food-borne illness, although infants, the elderly, the **immunocompromised**, and the **malnourished** are particularly at risk. Food-borne illness may be mild, seriously debilitating, or even fatal. Illness is typically characterized by diarrhea, vomiting, or both, but it can also involve other parts of the body, such as the central **nervous system**. Food-borne illness outbreaks most often result from inadequate cooking, inadequate holding temperatures, cross-contamination, unsafe food sources, and poor personal **hygiene**.

bacteria: single-celled organisms without nuclei, some of which are infectious

virus: noncellular infectious agent that requires a host cell to reproduce

parasite: organism that feeds off other organisms

immunocompromised: having a weakened immune system

malnourished: lack of adequate nutrients in the diet

nervous system: the brain, spinal cord, and nerves that extend throughout the body

hygiene: cleanliness

> **Mad Cow and Creutzfeldt-Jakob**
>
> New variant Creutzfeldt-Jakob disease (vCJD) is a rare, fatal brain disorder that is contracted by eating meat from cows infected with bovine spongiform encephalopathy (BSE, or "mad cow disease"). The disease has an incubation period lasting years or decades and has no known cure. As of December 2003, 153 cases of vCJD had been reported worldwide, the vast majority of which were in people who had lived in the United Kingdom during a BSE epidemic that lasted from 1980 to 1996. In 2003 a cow with BSE was discovered in the United States for the first time.
>
> —Paula Kepos

incidence: number of new cases reported each year

malnutrition: chronic lack of sufficient nutrients to maintain health

pathogen: organism that causes disease

cholera: bacterial infection of the small intestine causing severe diarrhea, vomiting, and dehydration

globalization: development of worldwide economic system

microorganisms: bacteria and protists; single-celled organisms

hepatitis: liver inflammation

salmonellosis: food poisoning due to Salmonella bacteria

Escherichia coli: common bacterium found in human large intestine

listeriosis: infectious disease caused by Listeria bacteria

Magnitude of Food-Borne Illness

Most of the available food-borne illness data is from industrialized nations, but the situation in poorer nations is probably worse. Developing countries may not have the resources needed to identify and document food-borne illness outbreaks, or outbreaks may go unreported in an effort to prevent negative publicity, which could affect a nation's tourism and trade industries.

Food-borne illnesses are a widespread and growing public health problem, both in developed and developing countries. The global **incidence** of food-borne illness is difficult to estimate, but it has been reported that, in 1998 alone, 2.2 million people, including 1.8 million children, died from diarrheal diseases, with a great proportion of these cases attributed to contaminated food and drinking water. Furthermore, diarrhea is a major cause of **malnutrition** in infants and young children.

In industrialized countries, the percentage of people suffering from food-borne illness each year has been reported to be as high as 30 percent. In the United States, for example, around 76 million cases of food-borne illness, resulting in 325,000 hospitalizations and 5,000 deaths, are estimated to occur each year. According to the U.S. Department of Agriculture, just seven food-borne organisms cause between 3.3 million and 12.3 million cases, and between 3,000 and 9,000 deaths, each year. While less well documented, developing countries bear the brunt of the problem due to the presence of a wide range of food-borne illness, including those caused by parasites and underlying food-safety problems.

Food contamination creates an enormous social and economic burden on communities and their health systems. In the United States, illness caused by the major **pathogens** alone are estimated to cost up to $37.1 billion annually in medical costs and lost productivity. The cost of food-borne illness in Australia is estimated at about $487 million to $1.9 billion per year. The re-emergence of **cholera** in Peru in 1991 resulted in the loss of $700 million in fish and fishery-product exports.

Historical Outbreaks

Food-borne illnesses emerge as a result of several factors. These include the **globalization** of the food supply, the inadvertent introduction of pathogens into new geographic areas, individual or group exposure to unfamiliar food-borne hazards while abroad, evolution of **microorganisms**, increases in the immunocompromised human population (those who are aging, HIV positive, or malnourished), and increases in the numbers of people eating away from home.

Food-borne illness outbreaks can take on massive proportions. In 1988, for example, an outbreak of **hepatitis** A resulting from the consumption of contaminated clams affected some 300,000 individuals in China. In 1994 an outbreak of **salmonellosis** due to contaminated ice cream occurred in the United States, affecting an estimated 224,000 persons. In 1996 an outbreak of **Escherichia coli** O157:H7 in Japan affected over 6,300 school children and resulted in two deaths. Outbreaks of **listeriosis** have been reported in many countries, including Australia, Switzerland, France, and the United States (outbreaks in France in 2000 and in the United States in 1999 were caused by contaminated pork tongue and hot dogs, respectively). As of

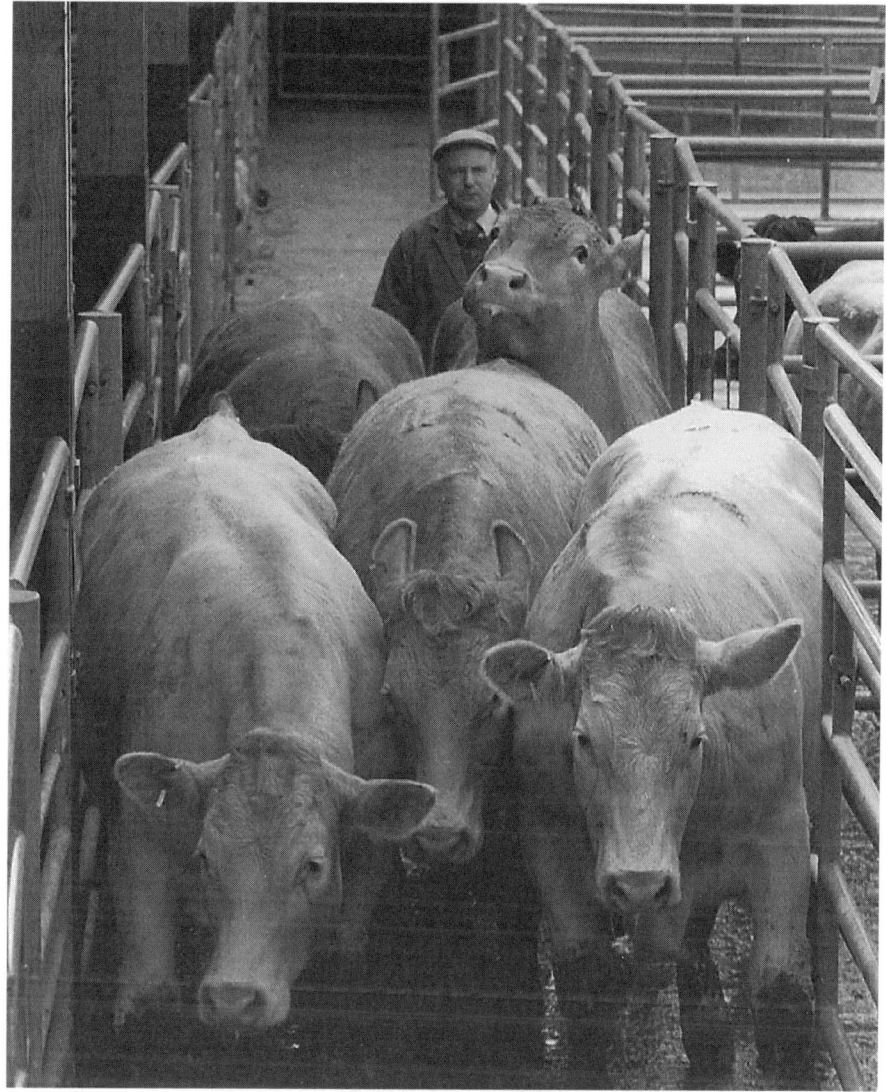

In December 2003, the USDA announced a recall of 10,410 pounds of beef that may have been exposed to the tissues of an animal that suffered from bovine spongiform encephalopathy, or so-called "mad cow disease." The recall generated a sensational response, even though other food-borne illnesses present a far greater danger to U.S. consumers. [AP/Wide World Photos. Reproduced by permission.]

January 2002, 119 people had developed variant Creutzfeldt-Jakob disease (the human variant of mad cow disease) secondary to exposure to infected animal products. Most of those cases were in Great Britain, but five cases were reported in France.

Types of Food-Borne Pathogens

Bacteria causing food-borne illness include *Escherichia coli* O157:H7, *Campylobacter jejuni*, *Salmonella*, *Staphylococcus aureus*, *Listeria monocytogenes*, *Clostridium perfringens*, *Vibrio parahaemolyticus*, *Vibrio vulnificus*, and *Shigella*. Bacteria are responsible for more cases of food-borne illness than any other organisms. Food can be contaminated with vegetative bacteria as well as spores. Vegetative bacteria can be reduced in food by proper sanitation and cooking techniques. When conditions become ideal for growth, bacterial spores germinate and reproduce rapidly and produce **toxins**, which result in illness.

toxins: poisons

Viruses, such as hepatitis A virus and Norwalk virus, can also cause food-borne illness. Viruses require a living host (human or animal) to grow and reproduce; they do not multiply in foods. However, a susceptible individual

MICROORGANISMS RESPONSIBLE FOR COMMON FOOD-BORNE ILLNESS

Microorganism	Food-borne illness	Symptoms	Common food sources	Incubation
Bacillus cereus	Intoxication	Watery diarrhea and cramps, or nausea and vomiting	Cooked product that is left uncovered—milk, meats, vegetables, fish, rice, and starchy foods	0.5–15 hours 2–5 days
Campylobacter jejuni	Infection	Diarrhea, perhaps accompanied by fever, abdominal pain, nausea, headache, and muscle pain	Raw chicken, other foods contaminated by raw chicken, unpasteurized milk, untreated water	
Clostridium botulinum	Intoxication	Lethargy, weakness, dizziness, double vision, difficulty speaking, swallowing, and/or breathing; paralysis; possible death	Inadequately processed, home-canned foods; sausages; seafood products; chopped bottled garlic; kapchunka; molona; honey	18–36 hours
Clostridium perfringens	Infection	Intense abdominal cramps, diarrhea	Meats, meat products, gravy, Tex-Mex type foods, other protein-rich foods	8–24 hours
Escherichia coli group	Infection	Watery diarrhea, abdominal cramps, low-grade fever, nausea, malaise	Contaminated water, undercooked ground beef, unpasteurized apple juice and cider, raw milk, alfalfa sprouts, cut melons	12–72 hours
Listeria Monocytogenes	Infection	Nausea, vomiting, diarrhea; may progress to headache, confusion, loss of balance and convulsions; may cause spontaneous abortion	Ready-to-eat foods contaminated with bacteria, including raw milk, cheeses, ice cream, raw vegetables, fermented raw sausages, raw and cooked poultry, raw meats, and raw and smoked fish	Unknown; may range from a few days to 3 weeks
Salmonella species	Infection	Abdominal cramps, diarrhea, fever, headache	Foods of animal origin; other foods contaminated through contact with feces, raw animal products, or infected food handlers. Poultry, eggs, raw milk, meats are frequently contaminated.	12–72 hours
Shigella	Infection	Fever, abdominal pain and cramps, diarrhea	Fecally contaminated foods	12–48 hours
Staphylococcus aureus	Intoxication	Nausea, vomiting, abdominal cramping	Foods contaminated by improper handling and holding temperatures—meats and meat products, poultry and egg products, protein-based salads, sandwich fillings, cream-based bakery products	1–12 hours
Hepatitis A	Infection	Jaundice, fatigue, abdominal pain, anorexia, intermittent nausea, diarrhea	Raw or undercooked molluscan shellfish or foods prepared by infected handlers	15–50 days
Norwalk-type viruses	Infection	Nausea, vomiting, diarrhea, abdominal cramps	Shellfish grown in fecally contaminated water; water and foods that have come into contact with contaminated water	12–48 hours
Giardia lamblia	Infection	Diarrhea, abdominal cramps, nausea	Water and foods that have come into contact with contaminated water	1–2 weeks
Trichinella spiralis	Infection	Nausea, diarrhea, vomiting, fatigue, fever, abdominal cramps	Raw and undercooked pork and wild game products	1–2 days

only needs to ingest a few viral particles to become ill. Frequent and proper handwashing is the most effective way to control the spread of food-borne viruses.

Parasites such as *Giardia lamblia, Cyclospora cayetanensis,* and *Cryptosporidium parvum* are another origin of food-borne illness. Parasites are small or microscopic creatures that, like viruses, require a living host to survive. **Parasitic** infection is far less common than bacterial or viral food-borne illness.

parasitic: feeding off another organism

biotoxin: poison made by living organisms

Other food-borne organisms include naturally occurring toxins such as mycotoxins, marine **biotoxins**, cyanogenic glycosides (compounds that can form cyanide when ingested), and toxins occurring in poisonous mushrooms. These can all cause severe illnesses. Mycotoxins, such as aflatoxin and ochratoxin A, are found at measurable levels in many staple foods, and the health implications of long-term exposure to such toxins are poorly understood. Although not considered food-borne organisms, cleaning solutions, some **food additives**, pesticides, herbicides, and heavy metals may also cause illness associated with ingestion of contaminated food.

food additive: substance added to foods to improve nutrition, taste, appearance or shelf-life

Prevention of Food-Borne Illness at Home and in Institutions

The World Health Organization has issued ten guidelines for developing culture-specific food-safety education:

1. Choose foods processed for safety, such as pasteurized dairy products and juices, or meat and poultry treated with ionizing radiation.

2. Cook food thoroughly—cook roasts to 145°F, ground beef to 160°F, and poultry to 180°F. Cook eggs until yolks and whites are firm. Use a meat thermometer.

3. Eat cooked foods immediately—food-borne organisms reproduce rapidly as food cools to room temperature.

4. Store cooked foods carefully—cooked foods should be held below 40°F or above 140°F.

5. Reheat cooked foods thoroughly—reheat all cooked foods to 165°F.

6. Avoid contact between raw foods and cooked foods—contact surfaces include cutting boards, utensils, and hands.

7. Wash hands repeatedly. Washing hands with warm water and soap before handing foods, after every interruption, and between handling raw and cooked foods is the most effective way to prevent food-borne illness.

8. Keep all kitchen surfaces meticulously clean—every food scrap, crumb, or dirty spot is a potential reservoir for organisms.

9. Protect foods from pests. Insects, rodents, and other animals frequently carry organisms that can cause food-borne illness.

10. Use safe water. If there is any doubt of the safety of the water supply, boil water before drinking it, using it in food preparation, or making ice.

The Hazard Analysis Critical Control Point (HACCP) system is used by institutions to anticipate and prevent food safety violations before they occur. HACCP flowcharts allow food managers to identify the critical control points, which are operations (practice, preparation step, or procedure) in the production of a food, and to make corrections as needed to prevent or eliminate hazards, or reduce them to acceptable levels. HACCP recipes provide detailed guidelines to food-service workers, and records assist health department personnel as they perform routine inspections of a facility. SEE ALSO ADDITIVES AND PRESERVATIVES; FOOD SAFETY; ILLNESSES, FOOD-BORNE; PESTICIDES.

M. Elizabeth Kunkel
Barbara H. D. Luccia

Bibliography

Cody, Mildred, and Kunkel, M. Elizabeth (2002). *Food Safety for Professionals*, 2nd edition. Chicago: American Dietetic Association.

Marriott, Norma G. (1999). *Principles of Food Sanitation*, 4th edition. Gaithersburg, MD: Aspen.

McSwane, David; Rue, Nancy; and Linton, Richard (1998). *Essentials of Food Safety and Sanitation.* Upper Saddle River, NJ: Prentice Hall.

Scott, Elizabeth, and Sockett, Paul (1998). *How to Prevent Food Poisoning: A Practical Guide to Safe Cooking, Eating, and Food Handling.* New York: John Wiley.

World Health Organization (2002). *Emerging Foodborne Diseases.* Geneva: Author.

Osteomalacia

osteomalacia: softening of the bones

vitamin D: nutrient needed for calcium uptake and therefore proper bone formation

calcium: mineral essential for bones and teeth

phosphorus: element essential in forming the mineral portion of bone

metabolism: the sum total of reactions in a cell or an organism

absorption: uptake by the digestive tract

bowel: intestines and rectum

lactose intolerance: inability to digest lactose, or milk sugar

malaise: illness or lack of energy

osteoporosis: weakening of the bone structure

incidence: number of new cases reported each year

Osteomalacia is a disease in which insufficient mineralization leads to a softening of the bones. Usually, this is caused by a deficiency of **vitamin D**, which reduces bone formation by altering **calcium** and **phosphorus metabolism**. Osteomalacia can occur because of reduced exposure to sunlight (which, after touching the skin, causes the body to make vitamin D), insufficient intake of vitamin D–enriched foods (like vitamin D–fortified milk), or improper digestion and **absorption** of food with vitamin D (as in **bowel** disorders such as **lactose intolerance** or celiac disease).

This disease causes the bending and misshaping of bones, such as bow-legging of the lower limbs, and is called rickets when it occurs in children. Affected children are usually listless and irritable. Symptoms in adults are often delayed until the disorder has advanced. These include easy fatigability, **malaise**, diffuse bone pain, and spasms. Muscular weakness occurs in severe cases. Osteomalacia should not be confused with **osteoporosis**, which is a disease of normal mineralization but decreased amounts of bone.

Osteomalacia can be diagnosed by blood and urine tests and confirmed by bone biopsy and X-rays. Treatment consists of oral doses of vitamin D, calcium, and phosphorus as well as increased exposure to ultraviolet light.

The easy availability of vitamin D–fortified milk has reduced the **incidence** of osteomalacia in developed countries to 0.1 percent. In areas with high levels of vegetarianism, such as in Asia, the incidence has been reported to be nearly 15 percent. Vitamin D, a fat-soluble vitamin, while not readily found in vegetables, is available in cheese, butter, cream, fish, oysters, fortified milk, and fortified cereals. SEE ALSO CALCIUM; OSTEOPOROSIS; RICKETS; VITAMINS, FAT-SOLUBLE.

Chandak Ghosh

Internet Resources

WebMD Health. "Osteomalacia." Available from <http://www.my.webmd.com>

University of Washington, Department of Medicine. "Osteoporosis and Bone Physiology: Osteomalacia." Available from <http://courses.washington.edu/bonephys/>

Osteopenia

osteoporosis: weakening of the bone structure

Osteopenia is defined as the stage of low bone density that precedes **osteoporosis**. At this stage, bone density is below average but not as low as occurs with osteoporosis. The World Health Organization formed a committee in 1994 to define osteoporosis, and four categories were defined: normal, osteopenia, osteoporosis, and established osteoporosis. All of these categories are measured by bone density and the prevalence of fractures. In osteopenia, bone density falls between one standard deviation and 2.5 standard deviations below average. Risk factors include age, race, and ethnicity, and the use of **hormones**. Although treatment for osteopenia is largely affected by age and the presence of fractures, women between the ages of fifty and seventy can prevent it by taking **estrogen** with **calcium** and exercising regularly.

According to the National Osteoporosis Foundation, approximately 10 million women and 2 million men in the United States have osteoporosis. Men have bones that are much larger and stronger than women's bones, which is why women suffer from the condition more often than men. However, both men and women share similar risk factors for osteoporosis (e.g., prolonged exposure to certain medications, **chronic** diseases that affect vital organs, undiagnosed low levels of **testosterone**, lifestyle habits, age, heredity, race), so methods of intervention are similar. SEE ALSO CALCIUM; OSTEOMALACIA; OSTEOPOROSIS; RICKETS; VITAMINS, FAT-SOLUBLE.

Daphne C. Watkins

hormone: molecules produced by one set of cells that influence the function of another set of cells

estrogen: hormone that helps control female development and menstruation

calcium: mineral essential for bones and teeth

chronic: over a long period

testosterone: male sex hormone

Internet Resources

Simmons, Sandra. "Common Myths about Osteopenia." Available from <http://www.ctds.info/osteopenia-2.html>

National Osteoporosis Foundation. "Osteoporosis: What Is It?" Available from <http://www.nof.org>

Osteoporosis

Osteoporosis, which is characterized by a decrease in the mass of otherwise normal bone is the most common **metabolic** bone disease. Normal bone is made of a hard outer shell (the cortex) and an inner network of spicules (fibers), called trabeculae, that give bone its characteristic strength. Bone mass is maintained at a progressive and then constant level until around the age of thirty-five. This maintenance is accomplished through bone remodeling, a cycle of breaking down and building up of bone. This cycle is controlled by **osteoblast** cells, which make bone, and osteoclast cells, which destroy bone. Beginning around age forty, the rate at which bone breaks down can exceed that at which it is built, resulting in diminished mass and a diminished amount of **calcium** in the bone. For women, in addition to this normal age-related bone loss, **menopause** and its subsequent reduction in female **hormone** levels (specifically **estrogen**) cause a specific loss in cortical and trabecular bone. In those who develop osteoporosis, the reduction in cortical and trabecular bone can be up to 30-40 percent, resulting in fragile bones that are prone to fracture.

Several factors contribute to the development of osteoporosis. Smoking, alcohol, and a **sedentary** lifestyle have all been shown to increase the risk of developing the disorder. Age and gender are also contributory factors. Women who have low estrogen levels (e.g., after menopause) are more likely to develop osteoporosis than others. Also, men generally maintain a higher bone density than women, making them less susceptible to the condition. Race can also play a role. Africans and people of African descent, for example, have a naturally higher bone density than Europeans and people of European descent and are therefore less likely to develop osteoporosis. A family history of osteoporosis certainly predisposes an individual to the

osteoporosis: weakening of the bone structure

metabolic: related to processing of nutrients and building of necessary molecules within the cell

osteoblast: cell that forms bone

calcium: mineral essential for bones and teeth

menopause: phase in a woman's life during which ovulation and menstruation end

hormone: molecules produced by one set of cells that influence the function of another set of cells

estrogen: hormone that helps control female development and menstruation

sedentary: not active

condition, and research is currently underway to identify **genes** linked to it. Other risk factors include long-term **steroid** therapy, Cushing's disease, hyperparathyroidism, and hyperthyroidism.

Traditionally, low intake of calcium and **vitamin D**, both of which are essential to bone building and maintenance, have been associated with osteoporosis as well. However, the role of dietary calcium remains controversial. Countries in Europe and North America, where the dietary intake of calcium is adequate, still show very high rates of osteoporosis. Studies have shown that high-protein diets, like those found in Europe and North America, raise the body's calcium requirement, thereby creating a calcium deficit in some.

One of the difficulties in understanding and managing osteoporosis is that its signs and symptoms are not apparent until the late stages of the disease, and many people with the osteoporosis are not diagnosed or treated until a fracture occurs. Hip and wrist fractures are very common, and vertebral compression fractures can occur with as little **stress** as that from sneezing or bending. These compressions can cause **chronic** backaches or cause patients to seemingly "lose height" as the vertebrae progressively curve into what is known as the "dowager's hump." Fractures also occur in the ribs, pelvis, and humerus (upper arm bone). Hip fractures can be the most devastating, often leading to death or long-term disability.

The most commonly used method to diagnose osteoporosis is to measure bone mineral density using dual energy X-ray absorbitometry (DEXA scans). This test is performed routinely in people who have risk factors or a prior diagnosis of osteoporosis. Density is usually measured in the lower spine or the hip, and the procedure is noninvasive and well tolerated. Quantitative CT (computerized tomography) scans and densitometry are also used, though less commonly. Blood levels of calcium, **phosphorus**, and parathyroid hormone—three hormones directly involved in bone building and remodeling—are usually normal. A more recent test that measures calcium excretion in urine may prove to be a helpful way of identifying risks for osteoporosis.

Early intervention and treatment of osteoporosis can halt or slow its progress. In some cases treatment can even reverse changes in bone density due to osteoporosis at least to a certain degree. Research regarding primary prevention of osteoporosis is ongoing. Supplements of dietary calcium and vitamin D, as well as weight-bearing exercises for the upper body, have been shown to slow bone loss. The use of supplementary estrogen (hormone replacement therapy) is very controversial. While estrogen has been shown to decrease bone loss and reduce the risks of certain fractures, it may also increase the risk of certain cancers and **heart disease**. **Drugs** called *bisphosphonates* stop osteoclast activity, increase bone density, and decrease the risk of fracture. In addition, supplements of calcitonin, a protein naturally made by the thyroid, can inhibit bone resorption by osteoclasts. It is important to identify those who may be at risk as early as possible, so that a healthy lifestyle, including a **diet** high in calcium and vitamin D, as well as exercise and early screening can be instituted.

According to the National Osteoporosis Foundation, 10 million people in the United States suffer from osteoporosis, while 34 million have early signs of bone density loss that could lead to osteoporosis (as of 2003). But despite what is known about populations at risk and potential treatments

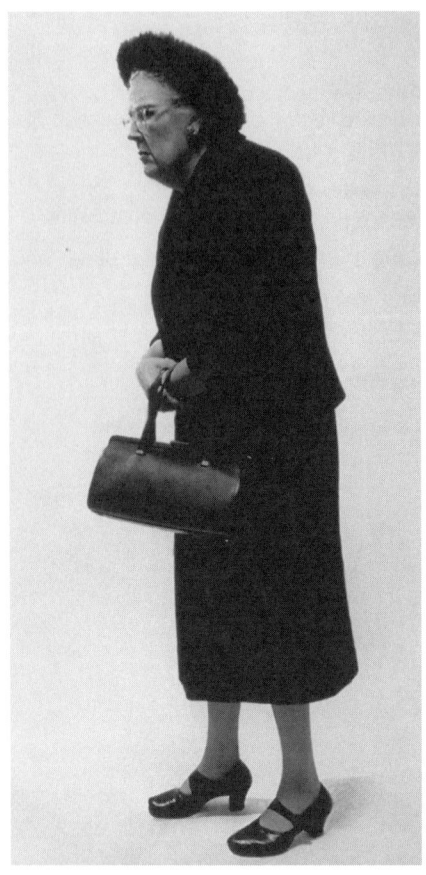

An elderly woman exhibits a dowager's hump, which is one symptom of osteoporosis. The hump is caused by repeated compression fractures of weakened vertebrae, which cause the upper spine to curve forward. [© Lester V. Bergman/Corbis. Reproduced by permission.]

gene: DNA sequence that codes for proteins, and thus controls inheritance

steroid: class of hormones composed of carbon rings, necessary for sexual development and mineral balance

vitamin D: nutrient needed for calcium uptake and therefore proper bone formation

stress: heightened state of nervousness or unease

chronic: over a long period

phosphorus: element essential in forming the mineral portion of bone

heart disease: any disorder of the heart or its blood supply, including heart attack, atherosclerosis, and coronary artery disease

for osteoporosis, some research reports that up to 40 percent of Caucasian women in the postmenopausal age group will sustain an osteoporotic fracture during the course of their lifetime (see Schnitzer). Approximately 20 percent of those women who sustain hip fractures will die within one year of the fracture, and those who survive will most likely require nursing-home care (see Andreoli). As populations around the world live longer, osteoporosis may continue to be an epidemic, and understanding how to identify, diagnose, and treat populations at risk will be of paramount importance. SEE ALSO AGING AND NUTRITION; CALCIUM; OSTEOMALACIA; OSTEOPENIA; RICKETS; VITAMINS, FAT-SOLUBLE; WOMEN'S NUTRITIONAL ISSUES.

Seema P. Kumar
Neela Pania

drugs: substances whose administration causes a significant change in the body's function

diet: the total daily food intake, or the types of foods eaten

Bibliography

Andreoli T. E., ed. (2001). "Osteoporosis." In Cecil *Essentials of Medicine*, 5th edition. Philadelphia: W. B. Saunders.

Looker A. C.; Orwell, E. S.; Johnston C. C., Jr.; et al. (1997). "Prevalence of Low Femoral Bone Density in Older U.S. Adults from NHANES III." *Journal of Bone Mineral Research* 12:1761–1768.

Internet Resources

National Osteoporosis Foundation. <http://www.nof.org>

Schnitzer, T. J. (2002). "Diagnosis and Treatment for Osteoporosis: Current Status and Expectations for the New Millennium." Available from http://www.medscape.com/viewprogram/605.

Overweight

The term *overweight* is used to describe an excess amount of total body weight including all tissues (fat, bone, muscle, etc.) and water. **Obesity**, in contrast, is an excess amount of body fat. An adult woman or man who has a body-fat percentage exceeding 35 percent (for women) or 25 percent (for men) is considered **obese**. A person can be overweight without being obese, as many professional football players and bodybuilders are, for such individuals have large amounts of muscle but not much fat. Likewise, a person can be obese without being overweight, such as some elderly individuals or lazy "couch potatoes," who may not weigh a lot but have too much body fat. However, almost all obese people are also overweight.

Because body fat is very difficult to measure accurately, height and weight are used to estimate overweight and obesity. **Body mass index** (BMI) is a formula that combines both height and weight. It is computed as weight in kilograms divided by height in meters squared, or as weight in pounds times 703 divided by height in inches squared. Normal weight for adults is represented by a BMI of 18.5 to 24.9; overweight by a BMI of 25 to 29.9; and obesity by a BMI of 30 or greater. SEE ALSO OBESITY; WEIGHT LOSS DIETS; WEIGHT MANAGEMENT.

John P. Foreyt

overweight: weight above the accepted norm based on height, sex, and age

obesity: the condition of being overweight, according to established norms based on sex, age, and height

obese: above accepted standards of weight for sex, height, and age

body mass index: weight in kilograms divided by square of the height in meters; a measure of body fat

Bibliography

Foreyt, John P., and St. Jeor, Sachiko T. (1997). "Definitions of Obesity and Healthy Weight." In *Obesity Assessment: Tools, Methods, Interpretation*, edited by Sachiko St. Jeor. New York: Chapman & Hall.

Poston, Walker S. C., and Foreyt, John P. (2002). "Body Mass Index: Uses and Limitations." *Strength and Conditioning Journal* 24(4):15–17.

U.S. Department of Health and Human Services (2001). *The Surgeon General's Call to Action to Prevent and Decrease Overweight and Obesity*. Rockville, MD: U.S. Department of Health and Human Services, Public Health Service, Office of the Surgeon General.

Internet Resources

National Heart, Lung, and Blood Institute. "Clinical Guidelines on Overweight and Obesity." Available from <http://www.nhlbi.nih.gov>

Pacific Islander Americans, Diet of

The Pacific Islands contain 789 habitable islands and are divided into the three geographic areas: Polynesia, Melanesia, and Micronesia. According to the 2000 U.S. Census, there are over a million Pacific Islanders in the United States, most of whom live in California, Hawaii, Washington, Utah, and Texas. Pacific Islander ethnicities in the United States include Carolinian, Fijian, Guamanian, Hawaiian, Kosraean, Melanesian, Micronesian, Northern Mariana Islander, Palauan, Papua New Guinean, Ponapean, Polynesian, Samoan, Solomon Islander, Tahitian, Tarawa Islander, Tongan, Trukese (Chuukese), and Yapese. Prior to 1980, Pacific Islander Americans (except Hawaiians) were classified with Asian Americans under the classification of "Asian and Pacific Islander American." Today, the U.S. Census Bureau includes Pacific Islander Americans under the classification of "Native Hawaiian and Other Pacific Islander." Pacific Islanders are a racially and culturally diverse population group, and they follow a wide variety of religions and have an array of languages.

Nutrition and Health Status

Accurate mortality and **morbidity** statistics for this population are limited, mainly because data on Pacific Islander Americans were classified with Asian Americans until a few years ago. Pacific Islander Americans have a high rate of **obesity**, and Native Hawaiians and Samoans are among the most **obese** people in the world. Dietary and lifestyle changes, as well as a likely **genetic** predisposition to store fat, are possible causes for this high rate. Lifestyles have changed from an active farming- and fishing-based subsistence economy to a more **sedentary** lifestyle. Pacific Islanders may be genetically predisposed to store fat for times of scarcity (the "thrifty gene" phenotype), and there is evidence that prenatal **undernutrition** modifies fetal development, predisposing individuals to adult obesity and **chronic** diseases.

Besides obesity, Pacific Islander Americans have high rate of **diabetes**, **hypertension**, **cardiovascular** disease, and **stroke**. Data collected from 1996 to 2000 suggest that Native Hawaiians are 2.5 times more likely to have diagnosed diabetes than white residents of Hawaii of similar age. Guam's death rate from diabetes is five times higher than that of the U.S. mainland, and diabetes is one of the leading causes of death in American Samoa. Overall, Pacific Islander Americans have much lower rates of **heart disease** than other minority groups in the United States, but it is still the leading cause of death within this population. Risk factors for and mortality from heart disease are high partly because of higher rates of obesity, diabetes, and **high**

---

morbidity: illness or accident

obesity: the condition of being overweight, according to established norms based on sex, age, and height

obese: above accepted standards of weight for sex, height, and age

genetic: inherited or related to the genes

sedentary: not active

undernutrition: food intake too low to maintain adequate energy expenditure without weight loss

chronic: over a long period

diabetes: inability to regulate level of sugar in the blood

hypertension: high blood pressure

cardiovascular: related to the heart and circulatory system

stroke: loss of blood supply to part of the brain, due to a blocked or burst artery in the brain

heart disease: any disorder of the heart or its blood supply, including heart attack, atherosclerosis, and coronary artery disease

NATIVE HAWAIIAN AND OTHER U.S. PACIFIC ISLANDER POPULATION, 2000		
National Origin	Population	Percent
Total	**874,414**	**100.0%**
Polynesian		
Native Hawaiian	401,162	45.9
Samoan	133,281	15.2
Tongan	36,840	4.2
Tahitian	3,313	0.4
Tokelauan	574	0.1
Polynesian, not specified	8,796	1.0
Micronesian		
Guamanian or Chamorro	92,611	10.6
Mariana Islander	141	*
Saipanese	475	0.1
Palauan	3,469	0.4
Carolinian	173	*
Kosraean	226	*
Pohnpeian	700	0.1%
Chuukese	654	0.1
Yapese	368	*
Marshallese	6,650	0.8
I-Kiribati	175	*
Micronesian, not specified	9,940	1.1
Melanesian		
Fijian	13,581	1.6
Papua New Guinean	224	*
Solomon Islander	25	*
Ni-Vanuatu	18	*
Melanesian, not specified	315	*
Other Pacific Islander	174,912	20.0

*Less than 0.1%.
SOURCE: U.S. Census Bureau, Census 2000.

The numbers by national origin do not add up to the total population figure because respondents may have put down more than one country. Respondents reporting several countries are counted several times. The total includes Native Hawaiian and other Pacific Islanders alone or in combination with other races or groups. Native Hawaiian and Pacific Islander population alone in 2000 was 398,835.

blood pressure. The poor health status of Pacific Islander Americans is also linked to socioeconomic indicators—Native Hawaiians have the worst socioeconomic indicators, the lowest health status, and the most diet-related maladies of all American minorities.

Eating Habits and Meal Patterns

The cuisine of Pacific Islander Americans varies slightly from culture to culture and is a blend of native foods and European, Japanese, American, and Asian influences. As with many cultures, food plays a central role in the culture. Pacific Islander Americans typically eat three meals a day. Breakfast is usually cereal and coffee; traditional meals are eaten for lunch or dinner; and fruits, fruit juices, vegetables, and nuts (e.g., peanuts and macadamia) are eaten in abundance. Milk and other dairy products are uncommon and there is a high **prevalence** of **lactose intolerance** among Pacific Islander Americans. Thus, **calcium** deficiency is prevalent.

Starchy foods are the foundation of the traditional diet. For example, the traditional Hawaiian diet is 75 to 80 percent starch, 7 to 12 percent fat, and 12 to 15 percent **protein**. Starch in the traditional diet comes primarily from root vegetables (e.g., taro, cassava, yam, green bananas, and breadfruit). In addition, the traditional diet is plentiful in fresh fruits, juices, nuts, and greens. Traditional meals include *poi* (boiled taro), breadfruit, green bananas, fish, or pork. Many dishes are cooked in coconut milk, and seaweed is often used as a vegetable or a condiment.

high blood pressure: elevation of the pressure in the bloodstream maintained by the heart

prevalence: describing the number of cases in a population at any one time

lactose intolerance: inability to digest lactose, or milk sugar

calcium: mineral essential for bones and teeth

protein: complex molecule composed of amino acids that performs vital functions in the cell; necessary part of the diet

Nutritional Transition

Many Pacific Islander Americans now eat an **Americanized** diet consisting of fast foods and highly processed foodstuffs such as white flour, white sugar, canned meat and fish, butter, margarine, mayonnaise, carbonated beverages, candies, cookies, and sweetened breakfast cereals. Rice is now a staple food, having taken over yam and taro in popularity in the 1980s and 1990s. This nutritional transition has resulted in an increase in cardiovascular disease (i.e., **coronary heart disease**, stroke, hypertension), obesity, and type 2 diabetes.

Nutrition education is needed to stimulate nutrition-related indigenous knowledge and the consumption of traditional nutrient-rich local foods as a more healthful alternative to fast foods and **processed foods**. There is also an urgent need for increased awareness of the health perils of obesity, especially among individuals with low **socioeconomic status**. Many health professionals are now emphasizing eating traditional "native" foods and encouraging residents to get back to a healthy lifestyle and to their cultural roots. Language is a major barrier to health education and medical interventions, however, and more health professionals need to be recruited from this population into health and medical fields in specific geographic areas. Professionals from the dominant (white) culture also need to become more culturally competent. SEE ALSO CARDIOVASCULAR DISEASE; DIETARY TRENDS, AMERICAN; OBESITY.

Ranjita Misra
Delores C. S. James

Americanized: having adopted more American habits or characteristics

coronary heart disease: disease of the coronary arteries, the blood vessels surrounding the heart

processed food: food that has been cooked, milled, or otherwise manipulated to change its quality

socioeconomic status: level of income and social class

Bibliography

Galanis D. J.; McGarvey, S. T.; Quested, C.; Sio, B.; and Afele-Fa'amuli, S. A. (1999). "Dietary Intake of Modernizing Samoans: Implications for Risk of Cardiovascular Disease." *Journal of the American Dietetic Association* 99(2):184–90.

Kittler, P. G., and Sucher, K. P. (2001). *Food and Culture*, 3rd edition. Stamford, CT: Wadsworth.

Wang, C. Y.; Abbot, L.; Goodbody, A. K.; and Hui, W. T. (2002). "Ideal Body Image and Health Status in Low-Income Pacific Islanders." *Journal of Cultural Diversity* 9(1):12–22.

Internet Resources

National Institute of Diabetes and Digestive and Kidney Diseases (NIDDK). "Diabetes in Asian and Pacific Islander Americans." Available from <http://diabetes.niddk.nih.gov/>

U.S. Geological Survey, Biological Resources Division. "The Status and Trends of the Nation's Biological Resources: Hawaii and the Pacific Islands." Available from <http://biology.usgs.gov/>

Pacific Islanders, Diet of

The Pacific Ocean—the world's largest ocean—extends about 20,000 kilometers from Singapore to Panama. There are 789 habitable islands within the "Pacific Islands," a geographic area in the western Pacific comprising Polynesia, Melanesia, and Micronesia. Polynesia includes 287 islands and is triangular, with Hawaii, New Zealand, and Easter Island at the apexes. Other major Polynesian islands include American (Eastern) Samoa, Western Samoa, Tonga, Tahiti, and the Society Islands. The Hawaiian Islands have been studied more than most other Pacific islands primarily because Hawaii is part of the United States of America. The Melanesian Islands (Melanesia) include the nations of Fiji, Papua New Guinea, Vanuatu, the Solomon Islands and New Caledonia (a French dependent). The 2,000 small islands of Micronesia include Guam (American), Kiribati, Nauru, the Marshall Islands, the Northern Mariana Islands, the Gilbert Islands, Palau, and the Federated States of Micronesia. Migration is very fluid between Polynesia, Melanesia, and Micronesia, and many Pacific Islanders also migrate to the United States and other countries. Pacific Islanders are a racially and culturally diverse population, and the people of the islands follow a wide variety of religions.

Nutritional Status

Mortality and **morbidity** statistics are limited, mainly because data on Pacific Islanders are often included with those on other Asians. A high percentage of Pacific Islanders live in poverty, though **nutritional deficiencies** are rare when there are adequate **calories**. Because Pacific Islander diets are based on whole foods found in nature and prepared without excess cooking, the recommended daily amounts of many **vitamins** and **minerals** can be met in only one meal. In addition, all of the fresh fruits consumed (mainly in the morning and during the afternoon) are abundant in **nutrients**.

Anemia, riboflavin deficiency, and **calcium** deficiency are common nutritional problems in the rural and urban areas of many islands, while **heart disease**, **hypertension**, type 2 **diabetes**, **obesity**, and other **chronic** diseases are on the rise. This is primarily due to a transition from traditional nutritious diets of fresh fruits, vegetables, poultry, and seafood to a **diet** with large amounts of imported and highly refined Western foods that are low in **fiber** and high in **fat** and sugars. Cigarette smoking, an increase in alcohol consumption, and a decreased level of physical activity are also contributing factors.

Obesity among Pacific Islanders is among the highest in the world, regardless of the island. Obesity may be due to a **genetic** predisposition and a cultural preference toward being heavy, but there is a high **prevalence** of physical inactivity among this population. Attitudes toward obesity are slowly changing, however, and it is gradually being viewed as unhealthy. Small studies that have placed **obese** and diabetic individuals on traditional diets have shown very good results, as individuals lost weight and diabetics were able to reduce or eliminate the need for **insulin**.

Eating Habits and Meal Patterns

While the islands are geographically close, the Pacific Island region is racially and culturally diverse. The cuisine varies slightly from island to island and is a blend of native foods with European, Japanese, and American influences. The cuisine is also influenced by the Asian Indians, Chinese, Korean, and Filipino agricultural workers who arrived in the eighteenth century. Food plays a central role in Pacific Islander culture; it represents prosperity, generosity, and community support. Hospitality is extended to visitors, who are usually asked to share a meal. Even if a visitor is not hungry, he or she will generally eat a small amount of food so that the host is not disappointed. Food is also often given as a gift, and a refusal of food is considered an insult to the host or giver.

morbidity: illness or accident

nutritional deficiency: lack of adequate nutrients in the diet

calorie: unit of food energy

vitamin: necessary complex nutrient used to aid enzymes or other metabolic processes in the cell

mineral: an inorganic (non-carbon-containing) element, ion or compound

nutrient: dietary substance necessary for health

anemia: low level of red blood cells in the blood

calcium: mineral essential for bones and teeth

heart disease: any disorder of the heart or its blood supply, including heart attack, atherosclerosis, and coronary artery disease

hypertension: high blood pressure

diabetes: inability to regulate level of sugar in the blood

obesity: the condition of being overweight, according to established norms based on sex, age, and height

chronic: over a long period

diet: the total daily food intake, or the types of foods eaten

fiber: indigestible plant material which aids digestion by providing bulk

fat: type of food molecule rich in carbon and hydrogen, with high energy content

genetic: inherited or related to the genes

prevalence: describing the number of cases in a population at any one time

obese: above accepted standards of weight for sex, height, and age

insulin: hormone released by the pancreas to regulate level of sugar in the blood

Pacific Islanders, Diet of

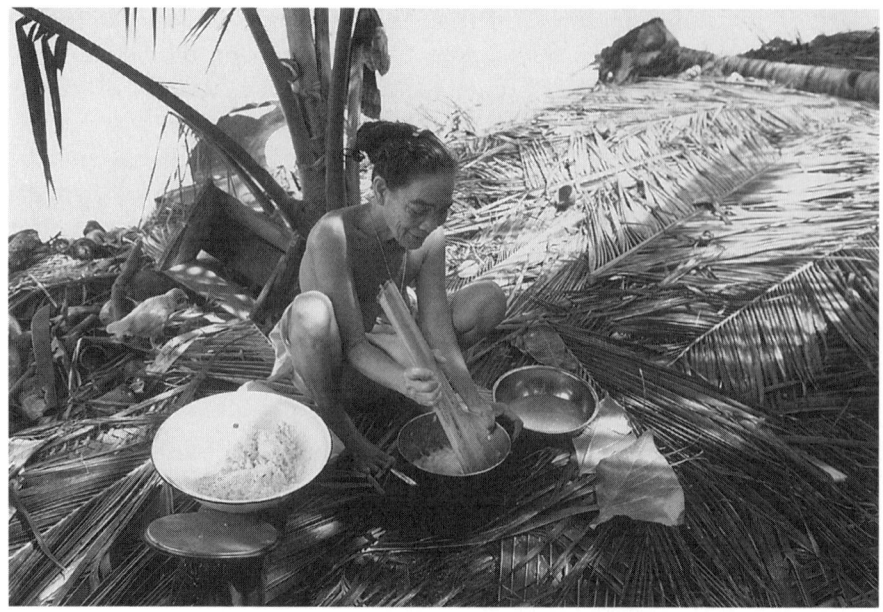

Breadfruit (being prepared here) is one of many starchy fruits traditionally eaten by Pacific Islanders. The diet also includes abundant fresh vegetables, fish, and nuts. [Photograph by Wolfgang Kaehler. Corbis. Reproduced by permission.]

lactose intolerance: inability to digest lactose, or milk sugar

Fruits, fruit juices, vegetables, and nuts (e.g., peanuts, macadamia, and litchi) are eaten in abundance, while milk and other dairy products are uncommon (there is a high prevalence of **lactose intolerance** among Pacific Islanders). Coconuts are plentiful, and both the milk and dried fruit are used to flavor meals. Pigs, chickens, and cows exist on the Pacific Islands, but in areas like Fiji they are expensive, so local villagers tend to purchase them only for large celebrations and feasts. Modern conveniences exist in many areas, but it is not uncommon for villagers to cook on outdoor fires or kerosene stoves. Many villagers still eat with their hands, and a bowl of water is provided for washing hands (a guest may request one before the meal if it is not offered).

Pacific Islanders typically eat three meals a day. Breakfast usually includes cereal and coffee, while traditional meals are eaten for lunch and dinner. However, in areas such as Hawaii, Samoa, and Guam, traditional foods now contribute only minimally to daily intake, most of which is made up of imported foods or fast food.

Traditional Cooking Methods and Food Habits

The traditional Pacific Islander diets are superior to Western diets in many ways. The weaknesses of the traditional Pacific Island diets are minimal and the strengths are immense. Traditional foods are nutrient-dense, meals are prepared in healthful ways, and oils are used sparingly. The high-fiber, low-fat nature of these diets reduces the risk for heart disease, hypertension, **stroke**, diabetes, obesity, and certain types of **cancer**.

stroke: loss of blood supply to part of the brain, due to a blocked or burst artery in the brain

cancer: uncontrolled cell growth

protein: complex molecule composed of amino acids that performs vital functions in the cell; necessary part of the diet

Starchy foods are the foundation of the traditional diet. For example, the traditional Hawaiian diet is 75 to 80 percent starch, 7 to 12 percent fat, and 12 to 15 percent **protein**. Starch in the diet comes primarily from root vegetables and starchy fruits, such as taro, cassava, yam, green bananas, and breadfruit. In addition, the traditional diet is plentiful in fresh fruits, juices, nuts, and the cooked greens of the starch vegetables (e.g., taro, yam). Traditional meals include *poi* (boiled taro), breadfruit, green bananas, fish, or pork. *Poi* is usually given to babies as an alternative to cereal. Many dishes are cooked in coconut milk, and more than forty varieties of seaweed are eaten, either as a vegetable or a condiment. Local markets with fresh foods are still abundant in most islands.

As expected, fish and other seafood are abundant in the Pacific Islands and are eaten almost every day in some islands. Most fish and seafood are stewed and roasted, but some are served marinated and uncooked. Pork is the most common meat, and it is used in many ceremonial feasts. Whole pigs are often cooked in pits layered with coals and hot rocks. Throughout the Pacific Islands, pit-roasted foods are used to commemorate special occasions and religious celebrations. The part of the pig one receives depends on one's social standing.

Samoans usually welcome visitors with a *kava* ceremony. Kava is made from the ground root of a pepper plant and is mixed with water. It is strained and usually served in a stone bowl or a half of a coconut shell. It looks like dirty water and tastes somewhat like dirty licorice. Guests are expected to drink it in one gulp. In Hawaii, *luaus* are common. A *luau* usually features pit-roasted pig, chicken, fish, and vegetables.

Traditional meals are highly seasoned with ginger, lime or lemon juice, garlic, onions, or scallions, depending on the dish. Lard and coconut oil (both saturated fats) are the most common fats used in cooking and give foods a distinctive flavor. Traditional beverages include fruit juices, coconut water, local alcoholic concoctions, and teas (primarily introduced by Asian immigrants).

Nutritional Transition

Many Pacific Islanders have moved to a more Western diet consisting of fast foods and **processed foods**, and as a result the **incidence** of both obesity and diabetes have soared. Pacific Islanders now rely on imported foods that are highly processed, such as white flour, white sugar, canned meat and fish, margarine, mayonnaise, carbonated beverages, candies, cookies, and breakfast cereals. Many locals sell their fruits and vegetables and then in turn purchase imported foods. On many islands, 80 to 90 percent of the foods are now imported. Imported rice is becoming the staple food in some areas, instead of locally grown provisions, and the ability to purchase imported foods is now a status symbol. Agricultural production also plays a role in the dietary transition. Local fruits and vegetables are increasingly less available due to population growth, urbanization, exporting of produce, and selling produce to hotels for the tourism industry. Traditional methods of hunting and gathering wild food, farming, processing, storing, and preserving traditional foods have all but disappeared in some areas.

Even though the health focus has been on the increase in obesity and diabetes, a different problem has occurred in Fiji. A dramatic increase in disordered eating among teenage girls has been observed in this nation, beginning with the introduction of television in 1995. In 1998 a researcher on Fiji reported that:

- 74 percent of girls reported feeling "too big or fat" at least sometimes.
- Of those who watched television at least three nights per week, 50 percent perceived themselves as too fat and 30 percent were more likely to diet.
- 62 percent reported dieting in the previous month, a comparable or higher proportion than reported in U.S. samples.

processed food: food that has been cooked, milled, or otherwise manipulated to change its quality

incidence: number of new cases reported each year

Many health professionals in the Pacific Islands, especially Hawaii, are now emphasizing eating traditional foods and encouraging residents to get back to a healthy lifestyle and to their cultural roots. Programs may now need to be developed to target eating disorders and disturbances.

The natural beauty of the Pacific Islands makes them popular destinations for ecotourists, and food-borne and water-borne diseases are the number one cause of illness among travelers. Visitors are therefore advised to wash their hands often and to drink only bottled or boiled water or carbonated drinks in cans or bottles. They also should avoid tap water, fountain drinks, and ice cubes. SEE ALSO ASIANS, DIET OF; DIABETES MELLITUS; DIETARY TRENDS, INTERNATIONAL; OBESITY; PACIFIC ISLANDER AMERICANS, DIET OF.

Delores C. S. James

Bibliography

Becker, A.; Burwell, R.; Navara, K.; and Gilman, S. (2003). "Binge Eating and Binge-Eating Disorder in a Small-Scale, Indigenous Society: The View From Fiji." *International Journal of Eating Disorders* 34(4):423–432.

Kittler, P. G., and Sucher, K. P. (2001). *Food and Culture*, 3rd edition. Stamford, CT: Wadsworth.

Internet Resources

Union College. "Fiji: A Digital Ethnography." Available from <http://fiji.union.edu>

U.S. Geological Survey, Biological Resources Division. "The Status and Trends of the Nation's Biological Resources: Hawaii and the Pacific Islands." Available from <http://biology.usgs.gov/>

Pasteur, Louis

French chemist and microbiologist
1822–1895

Louis Pasteur was born in Dole, France, on December 27, 1822. He was the only son of Jean Pasteur, a poorly educated leather tanner. Pasteur was not a very good student in elementary school and he preferred fishing and painting to studying. As he got older, however, he began to show an interest in scientific subjects, especially chemistry. Although he demonstrated a lot of talent as a painter, Pasteur's father encouraged him to study throughout high school and he was accepted to the best university in France, the École Normale in Paris.

While at the university, Pasteur began to pursue his interests in science and discovery. He became a professor and researcher after graduating from college and was most interested in applying his knowledge of science to help people live healthier lives. Throughout his lifetime, Pasteur made incredible contributions to the fields of medicine, chemistry, and biology by sharing his ideas and inventions with the world. He first discovered the dangers of germs that spread infections. He also discovered treatments for deadly diseases such as tetanus, **tuberculosis**, **diphtheria**, and rabies.

Pasteur was best known for inventing the process that became known as **pasteurization**. In 1864, the emperor of France, Napoleon III, asked Pasteur to investigate why wine and beer became sour shortly after they were made. The souring of wine and beer was a major economic problem in France, since many farmers relied on the sale of these beverages to earn a living.

tuberculosis: bacterial infection, usually of the lungs, caused by Mycobacterium tuberculosis

diphtheria: infectious disease caused by Cornybacterium diphtheriae, causing damage to the heart and other organs

pasteurization: heating to destroy bacteria and other microorganisms, after Louis Pasteur

Pasteur traveled to a vineyard to study this problem and was able to demonstrate that **bacteria** and other microscopic organisms were causing the wine to spoil. These were the same types of harmful bacteria that would cause food to spoil and make some people sick.

Pasteur discovered that the tiny organisms in the wine could be destroyed by heat, without damaging the wine. Later, Pasteur demonstrated that his technique could be applied to the preservation of other beverages such as milk and juice, as well as solid foods such as cheese and meat. Using the first form of pasteurization, a food product would have to be heated at 130 degrees Fahrenheit for thirty minutes. However, Pasteur later discovered an easier method in which beverages and foods could be pasteurized for a shorter time at a higher temperature.

When Pasteur died on September 28, 1895, he was named a national hero by the French government for his important contributions to science, health, and food safety. During Pasteur's lifetime, it was not easy for him to convince others of his ideas, which were sometimes seen as controversial in the 1800s. Today, the food industry around the world continues to use the process of pasteurization to ensure that harmful organisms are eliminated from foods. SEE ALSO Food Safety; Organisms, Food-Borne.

Melissa C. Morris

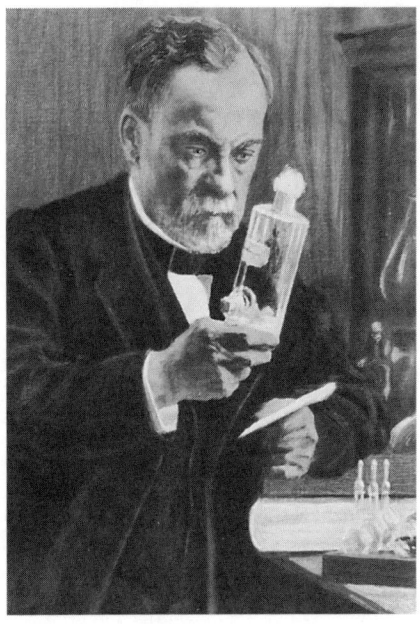

Hailed as the founder of microbiology, Louis Pasteur contributed immensely to the fields of medicine and food safety. He invented pasteurization, which prevents food spoilage, and he developed the technique of vaccination. *[Bettman/Corbis. Reproduced by permission.]*

bacteria: single-celled organisms without nuclei, some of which are infectious

Internet Resources

Bellis, Mary (2003). "Louis Pasteur." Available from <http://inventors.about.com>

Cohn, David V. (1996). "The Life and Times of Louis Pasteur." Available from <http://louisville.edu/library/>

Pasteur Institute (2003). "Louis Pasteur's Biography (1822–1895)." Available from <http://www.pasteur.fr/>

Pasteurization

Pasteurization, a process discovered by Louis Pasteur (while trying to inactivate spoilage organisms in beer and wine), occurs when a product is heated to a specific temperature for a specified length of time. This process is now applied to a wide array of food products, such as milk, fruit juice, cheese, and water. Milk is heated to 145°F (63°C) for thirty minutes (or to 160°F [71°C] for fifteen seconds) and then rapidly cooled to 50°F (10°C) for storage. In developing countries, heating water to 149°F (65°C) for six minutes will kill enough contaminates to make the water safe to drink. Pasteurization protects consumers from harmful **pathogens** such as Mycobacterium **tuberculosis** and Coxiella Burnetii in milk, and pasteurized products benefit from longer shelf life. SEE ALSO Food Safety.

Diane L. Golzynski

pasteurization: heating to destroy bacteria and other microorganisms, after Louis Pasteur

pathogen: organism that causes disease

tuberculosis: bacterial infection, usually of the lungs, caused by Mycobacterium tuberculosis

Pauling, Linus

American chemist
1901–1994

Linus Carl Pauling was born in Portland, Oregon, on February 28, 1901, to Herman and Lucy Pauling. Growing up in Oregon, Pauling and his family

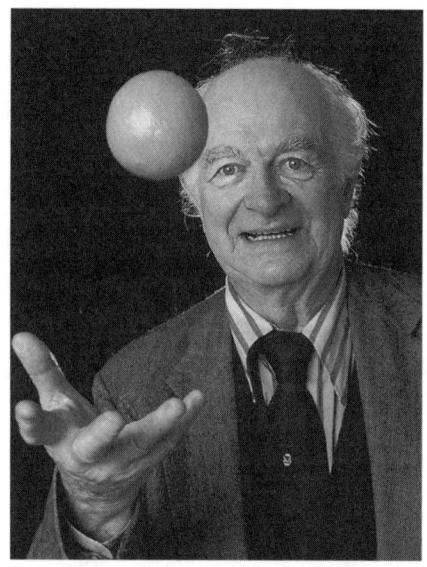

Two-time Nobel Prize winner Linus Pauling. Pauling's early work in chemistry earned him the world's respect, but his later work on nutrition was controversial. [© Roger Ressmeyer/Corbis. Reproduced by permission.]

molecule: combination of atoms that form stable particles

nutrition: the maintenance of health through proper eating, or the study of same

vitamin: necessary complex nutrient used to aid enzymes or other metabolic processes in the cell

mineral: an inorganic (non-carbon-containing) element, ion or compound

cancer: uncontrolled cell growth

heart disease: any disorder of the heart or its blood supply, including heart attack, atherosclerosis, and coronary artery disease

did not have much in the way of material wealth, especially after his father's death when he was only nine years old. However, Pauling was exceptionally bright and found many ingenious ways to make money, including delivering milk, running film projectors, and working at the local shipyard, to support his mother and two younger sisters.

Pauling was a gifted student and earned a scholarship to Oregon State University where he earned his Bachelor of Science degree and later went on to earn a Ph.D. in chemistry at the California Institute of Technology. As a young scientist, Pauling first became known to the world of chemistry with his use of X-rays to examine the molecular structure of crystals. Pauling later began to focus his research on the way **molecules** bond and his insight led to the creation of many of the medicines, dyes, plastics, and synthetic fibers people continue to use today. His work was so influential that he was recognized in 1954 with the prestigious Nobel Prize for Chemistry. In fact, Pauling is the only person to ever win two unshared Nobel Prizes—he was awarded the Nobel Peace Prize in 1962.

After being awarded his second Nobel Prize, Pauling began to study the role of **nutrition** in fighting disease. Pauling had spoken about the importance of **vitamins** and **minerals** to maintain health in the late 1930s, but he did not pursue research on the subject until almost thirty years later. Pauling proposed that large doses of vitamin C could protect a person from the common cold, and he wrote the book *Vitamin C and the Common Cold* in 1970. It quickly became a bestseller. He also believed in vitamin C's power to combat the flu, certain types of **cancer**, **heart disease**, infections, and even old age. In addition, Pauling suggested that other vitamins, such as vitamin E, and vitamin B also worked to fight disease and prolong life. In fact, Pauling believed that virtually all illnesses could be attributed to some form of vitamin deficiency.

Although Pauling was recognized all over the world for his theory on the power of nutritional medicine, medical doctors and nutrition scientists often criticized his beliefs. Many scientists did not agree with Pauling's ideas about vitamin therapy and the impact of vitamins and minerals on a person's health. They even tried to disprove Pauling's ideas by conducting research studies to show that vitamin C did not prevent colds or cancer. However, many of these studies were flawed, and Pauling was always able to respond with his own research data and logical reasoning to support his beliefs.

Pauling died of cancer at the age of 93 in August 19, 1994, at his ranch near Big Sur on the California coast. Before he died, he said that vitamin C had delayed the cancer's onset for twenty years. Pauling was awarded many prizes and received distinguished honors for his contributions to the fields of chemistry and humanity. He has been recognized as one of the most influential scientists of the twentieth century.

Melissa C. Morris

Internet Resources

Linus Pauling Institute (2003). "Linus Pauling—Scientist for the Ages." Available from <http://lpi.oregonstate.edu/lpbio/lpbio2.html>

Nobel e-Museum (2003). "Linus Pauling—Biography." Available from <http://www.nobel.se/chemistry/laureates/1954/pauling-bio.html>

Pellagra

Pellegra is a disease caused by a dietary deficiency of, or a failure to absorb, **niacin** (vitamin B$_3$) or the **amino acid** tryptophan, a precursor of niacin. First reported in 1735 by Don Gasper Casal, a Spanish physician, *pellagra* means "rough skin." Primary symptoms include the "3 Ds": **dementia** (mental symptoms), dermatitis (scaly skin sores), and diarrhea. A pellagra epidemic emerged during the 1900s in the United States, when corn (maize) began to replace other sources of dietary **protein** among the rural poor. Niacin in corn is tightly bound to protein, and thus poorly absorbed. Niacin **enrichment** of cereal grains and diets adequate in protein and **calories** eventually eradicated pellagra from the United States. Seasonal epidemics still occur in parts of Southeast Asia and Africa, however.

Kiran B. Misra

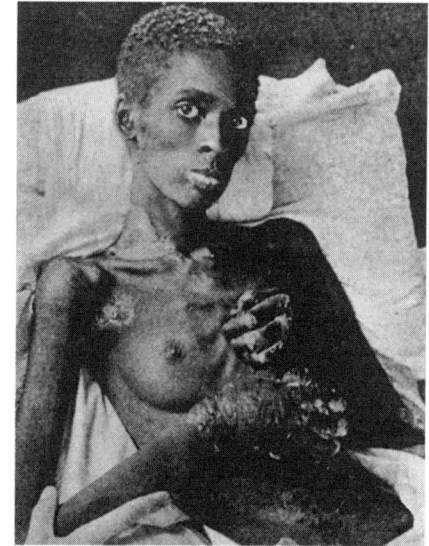

This woman's hands show scars from dermatitis, one of the primary symptoms of pellagra. The photo was taken in South Carolina, where thousands of rural poor succumbed to the illness at the start of the twentieth century.

niacin: one of the B vitamins, required for energy production in the cell

amino acid: building block of proteins, necessary dietary nutrient

dementia: loss of cognitive abilities, including memory and decision making

protein: complex molecule composed of amino acids that performs vital functions in the cell; necessary part of the diet

enrichment: addition of vitamins and minerals to improve the nutritional content of a food

calorie: unit of food energy

Pemberton, John S.

American pharmacist
1831–1888

John Stith Pemberton was born in Knoxville, Georgia, and spent his childhood in Rome, Georgia. He graduated from Southern Botanico Medical College of Georgia in 1850. Pemberton briefly practiced as a traditional Thomsonian "steam doctor," modeled after Samuel Thomson's *Complete System of Practice* as outlined in his book *New Guide to Health*. Steam doctors used steam baths, herbs, and other products to induce sweating, which they believed would restore the body to proper health. Pemberton later obtained a degree in pharmacy from a school in Philadelphia. In 1855, Pemberton moved to Columbus, Georgia, with his wife, Anna Eliza Clifford Lewis, and their only son, Charles Ney Pemberton. Here, he practiced primarily as a druggist for fourteen years, though he also performed other medical procedures. Pemberton was a member of the first licensing agency for pharmacists in Georgia.

In May 1862, Pemberton enlisted as a first lieutenant in the Confederate Army, and he organized Pemberton's Calvary to guard the town. In Pemberton's last battle he was shot and cut with a saber across the chest. He used morphine for his pain, and eventually became a morphine addict.

For five years after the war, Pemberton worked as a partner with Dr. Austin Walker, a local and wealthy physician. During this time, Pemberton invested all of his money in researching and developing a line of proprietary items, which included perfumes and **botanical** medicines. During this time, there was a large demand for home remedies and tonics in the United States, especially in large cities. In 1869, Pemberton moved to Atlanta, Georgia, to start a lucrative business—he developed, and successfully sold, a drink he called "French Wine Coca." Based on a similar European product called "Vin Mariana," Pemberton's tonic combined wine and the extract from coca leaves, the source of cocaine. Coca extract was commonly used at the time in medicines and "temperance drinks" to increase sexual drive, treat digestive problems, calm nerves, and extend longevity. It also was used to "cure"

botanical: related to plants

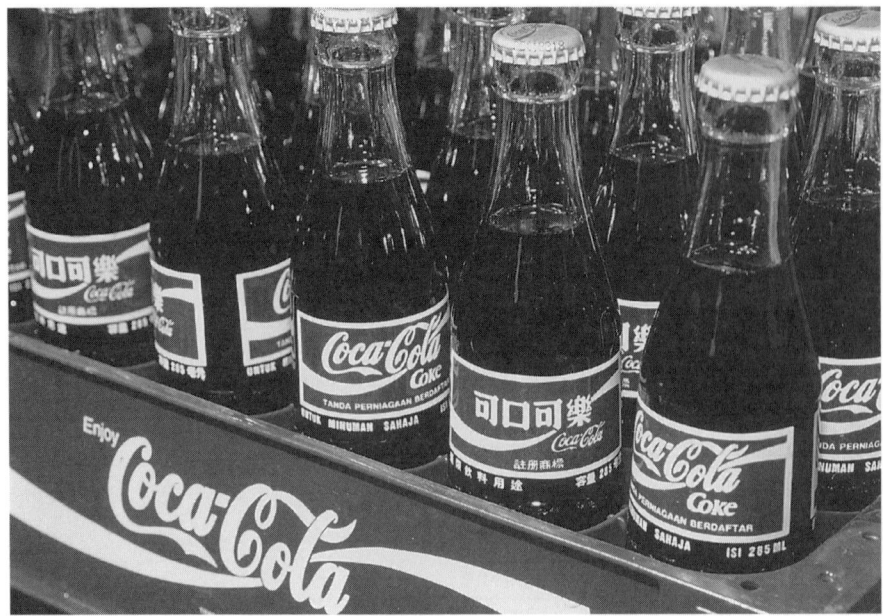

John S. Pemberton's 1886 Coca-Cola recipe contained a highly addictive stimulant extracted from coca leaves. That recipe was replaced in 1905 with one more similar to the modern beverage, which is distributed in 200 countries worldwide. [© Sergio Dorantes/Corbis. Reproduced by permission.]

addictions to morphine, nicotine, and alcohol. This was Pemberton's first well-known and widely sold drink. Pemberton himself endorsed his "wine" as a cure for morphine addiction.

In 1885, with talk of Prohibition, Pemberton developed a drink without alcohol. Pemberton added the extract from cola nuts, a strong stimulant containing caffeine, along with the coca, and he replaced the wine with sugar syrup. On May 18, 1886, Pemberton decided on a final formula for his new drink, and Frank Robinson, one of Pemberton's partners and a part owner of his company, came up with the name Coca-Cola and the trademark logo. On June 28, 1887, the Coca-Cola trademark patent was granted. Jacobs Pharmacy, in Atlanta, Georgia, was the first place to serve Coca-Cola from a soda fountain. The cocaine was eventually removed from the drink in 1905.

cancer: uncontrolled cell growth

Pemberton's financial troubles, along with his morphine addiction, led him to sell, trade, and give away portions of his company to various individuals. Coca-Cola eventually became one of the most prosperous businesses in the United States. Pemberton died on August 16, 1888, of stomach **cancer**, leaving behind many unfinished formulas. Pemberton also developed the first state-run laboratory to conduct tests on soil and crop chemicals. The facility is currently run by the Georgia Department of Agriculture.

Delores C. S. James

Bibliography

Pendergrast, Mark (2000). *For God, Country, and Coca-Cola.* New York: Basic Books.

Internet Resources

Britannica.com (2001). "The Coca-Cola Company." Available from <http://www.britannica.com>

Business Heroes Newsletter. "John Pemberton, Inventor of Coca Cola." Available from <http://www.businessheroes.com>

Hayes, Jack (1996). "Dr. John S. Pemberton (Inventor of Coca-Cola)." *Nation's Restaurant News* 30 (February):120–121. Available from <http://memory.loc.gov/ammem/ccmphtml/colainvnt.html>

Pesticides

Pesticide use is widespread in agriculture throughout the world, raising serious questions about the dangers theses substances pose to human health and the **environment**. Pesticides are substances intended to prevent, destroy, or repel injurious plants or animals. The term is frequently defined more broadly to include insecticides, herbicides (used to inhibit the growth and reproduction of certain plants), and fungicides (used to inhibit the growth of molds, mildews, and yeasts).

environment: surroundings

The main argument for pesticides use is an economic one. Pesticides can protect crops against sudden pest outbreaks and allow increased production, and they can ensure the production of more attractive fruits and vegetables. By delaying the rotting of produce, pesticides permit longer shipping times and extend the shelf life of fresh produce.

The dangers of pesticide use can be difficult to pinpoint, since exposure may be small but cumulative. Prolonged pesticide exposure in humans may negatively affect the nervous, reproductive, and immune systems and also raises the possibility of increased risk of some cancers. Their use also leads to the **development** of pesticide-resistant bugs, creating a need for newer and more powerful pesticides. SEE ALSO FOOD SAFETY; ORGANIC FOODS; REGULATORY AGENCIES.

development: the process of change by which an organism becomes more complex

Kim Schenck

Bibliography

Wardlaw, Gordon; Hampl, Jeffrey; and DiSilvestro, Robert (2004). *Perspectives in Nutrition*. New York: McGraw-Hill.

Internet Resources

United States Environmental Protection Agency. "Pesticides." Available from <http://www.epa.gov/pesticides/>

Phenylketonuria (PKU)

Phenylketonuria (fee-nyl-key-ton-uria), or PKU, is an inherited **metabolic** disease that results in severe developmental delay and **neurological** problems when treatment is not started very early and maintained throughout life. The disease is caused by the absence of the **enzyme** phenylalanine hydroxylase, which normally converts the **amino acid** phenylalanine to another amino acid, tyrosine. This results in a build-up of phenylalanine and a low level of tyrosine, which causes a variety of problems, including cognitive decline, learning disabilities, behavior or neurological problems, and skin disorders.

phenylketonuria: inherited disease marked by the inability to process the amino acid phenylalanine, causing mental retardation

metabolic: related to processing of nutrients and building of necessary molecules within the cell

neurological: related to the nervous system

PKU occurs in about 1 in 10,000 births. It is an autosomal recessive disorder, meaning the affected person inherits two copies of the defective gene, one from each parent. Newborn screening for PKU began in the mid-1960s and is now carried out in every state in the United States, as well as in many other countries.

enzyme: protein responsible for carrying out reactions in a cell

amino acid: building block of proteins, necessary dietary nutrient

The treatment for PKU consists of a special phenylalanine-restricted **diet** designed to maintain levels of phenylalanine in the blood between 2 and 6 mg/dl (milligrams per deciliter). All **proteins** are made up of amino acids; therefore, the diet for PKU consists of foods that contain only enough

diet: the total daily food intake, or the types of foods eaten

protein: complex molecule composed of amino acids that performs vital functions in the cell; necessary part of the diet

protein to provide the amount of phenylalanine necessary for growth and **development**. Foods allowed are primarily vegetables, fruits, and some cereals and grains. A synthetic formula containing all the amino acids except phenylalanine provides the remaining protein and **calories** for individuals with PKU. SEE ALSO AMINO ACIDS; ARTIFICIAL SWEETENERS; INBORN ERRORS OF METABOLISM.

Patricia D. Thomas

Internet Resources

National PKU News. Available from <http://www.pkunews.org>

development: the process of change by which an organism becomes more complex

calorie: unit of food energy

Phytochemicals

Phytochemicals are naturally occurring chemicals in plants that provide flavor, color, texture, and smell. Phytochemicals have potential health effects, as they may boost **enzyme** production or activity, which may, in turn, block **carcinogens**, suppress **malignant** cells, or interfere with processes that can cause **heart disease** and **stroke**. Phytochemical-rich foods include *cruciferous* vegetables (e.g., broccoli, Brussels sprouts, cauliflower, cabbage), *umbelliferous* vegetables (e.g., carrots, celery, parsley, parsnips), *allium* vegetables (e.g., garlic, onions, leek), berries, citrus fruits, whole grains, and **legumes** (e.g., soybeans, beans, lentils, peanuts). In the early twenty-first century, identification of the role of phytochemicals in health is an emerging area of science, and the global health community does not recommend supplementation with any specific phytochemicals. SEE ALSO ANTIOXIDANTS; FUNCTIONAL FOODS.

M. Elizabeth Kunkel
Barbara H. D. Luccia

phytochemical: chemical produced by plants

enzyme: protein responsible for carrying out reactions in a cell

carcinogen: cancer-causing substance

malignant: spreading to surrounding tissues; cancerous

heart disease: any disorder of the heart or its blood supply, including heart attack, atherosclerosis, and coronary artery disease

stroke: loss of blood supply to part of the brain, due to a blocked or burst artery in the brain

legumes: beans, peas and related plants

Bibliography

Meskin, M. S.; Bidlack, A. J.; and Davies, A. J. (2002). *Phtyochemicals in Nutrition and Health*. Boca Raton, FL: CRC Press.

Pica

Pica is defined as a compulsion to consume nonfood substances. Persons with pica crave items such as dirt, clay, paint chips, plaster, chalk, cornstarch, laundry starch, baking soda, coffee grounds, cigarette ashes, burnt match heads, cigarette butts, and rust. The cause of pica is poorly understood, but this strange behavior is often seen in those who are iron-deficient, particularly pregnant woman, even though none of the craved items contain significant amounts of iron. Pica can be dangerous during pregnancy, since consuming large amounts of some substances may cause **nutrient** deficiencies, intestinal problems, or lead to toxicity, placing both mother and baby at risk. SEE ALSO CRAVINGS; PREGNANCY.

Beth Fontenot

nutrient: dietary substance necessary for health

Plant-Based Diets

Plant-based diets are comprised of meals made predominately from a variety of vegetables, fruits, grains, beans, and nuts, with minimal amounts of

processed foods. Many professional organizations recommend a plant-based **diet** to help prevent **chronic** diseases such as **cancer, heart disease**, and **obesity**. This is because such a diet is usually high in **fiber** and low in **fat**.

Many times, modest amounts of meat are included in a plant-based diet, so it is not synonymous with a vegetarian diet. However, the bulk of the diet consists of fruits, vegetables, and whole grains. SEE ALSO MACROBIOTIC DIET; MEAT ANALOGS; VEGAN; VEGETARIANISM.

Lenore Hodges

Internet Resources

American Dietetic Association, Vegetarian Nutrition Practice Group. "Articles on Vegetarian Nutrition." Available from <http://www.vegetariannutrition.net/articles/html>

Seventh-day Adventist Dietetic Association. "Plant-Based Diets: Fact and Fiction." Available from <http:/www.sdada.org/facts&fiction/htm>

processed food: food that has been cooked, milled, or otherwise manipulated to change its quality

diet: the total daily food intake, or the types of foods eaten

chronic: over a long period

cancer: uncontrolled cell growth

heart disease: any disorder of the heart or its blood supply, including heart attack, atherosclerosis, and coronary artery disease

obesity: the condition of being overweight, according to established norms based on sex, age, and height

fiber: indigestible plant material which aids digestion by providing bulk

fat: type of food molecule rich in carbon and hydrogen, with high energy content

Popular Culture, Food and

Food is very much a part of popular culture, and the beliefs, practices, and trends in a culture affect its eating practices. Popular culture includes the ideas and objects generated by a society, including commercial, political, media, and other systems, as well as the impact of these ideas and objects on society.

Current Trends

There has been an increasing trend in the United States toward **consumerism**, a trend that is reflected in more people eating away from home; the use of dietary and **herbal** supplements; foods for specific groups (e.g., dieters, women, athletes, older adults); the use of convenience and **functional foods**; and ethnic diversity in diets. Mainstream populations in developed countries want low-calorie, low-fat foods, as well as simple, natural, and fresh ingredients.

Internationally, there has been an "Americanization" of diets through the growth and use of fast-food restaurants and **convenience foods**. In developing countries there is still a need for some basic foods, and governments and the food industry are working to develop products that can reduce international food shortages and **nutrient** deficiency problems.

Eating Away from Home

Internationally, the proportion of money spent on food eaten away from home, as well as the number of restaurants, has been steadily increasing since the second half of the twentieth century. People may dine at formal, sit-down restaurants, at **fast-food** eateries, at cafes, or they may purchase food from street vendors.

Fast-food restaurants have become very common, and are visited by all types of people. The growth and popularity of fast food has come to be known as the "McDonaldization" of America. In the United States, eating in these restaurants has decreased slightly among heavy users in the 18–34 age group, but has increased among other groups. Their popularity has also increased internationally.

consumerism: reliance on buying, rather than making, items necessary for living

herbal: related to plants

functional food: food whose health benefits are claimed to be higher than those traditionally assumed for similar types of foods

convenience food: food that requires very little preparation for eating

nutrient: dietary substance necessary for health

fast food: food requiring minimal preparation before eating, or food delivered very quickly after ordering in a restaurant

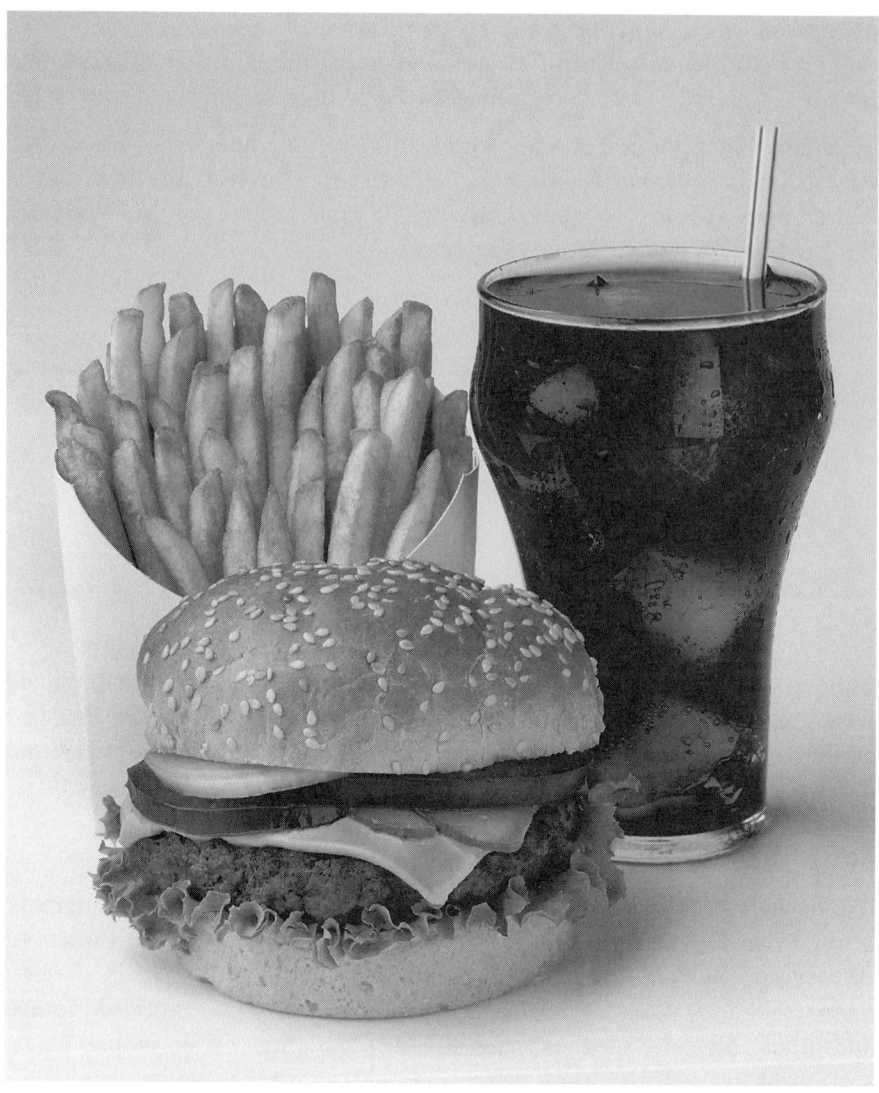

This simple meal demonstrates the complicated relationship between a culture and its food. In the twentieth century, Americans' preference for quick, portable meals popularized the fast-food burger. Over time the popularity of fast foods in America contributed to an epidemic of obesity. [Photograph by Lois Ellen Frank. Corbis/Lois Ellen Frank. Reproduced by permission.]

sedentary: not active

lifestyle: set of choices about diet, exercise, job type, leisure activities, and other aspects of life

obesity: the condition of being overweight, according to established norms based on sex, age, and height

body mass index: weight in kilograms divided by square of the height in meters; a measure of body fat

overweight: weight above the accepted norm based on height, sex, and age

obese: above accepted standards of weight for sex, height, and age

bulimia: uncontrolled episodes of eating (bingeing) usually followed by self-induced vomiting (purging)

binge: uncontrolled indulgence

anorexia nervosa: refusal to maintain body weight at or above what is considered normal for height and age

Many eateries now offer the option of larger serving (portion) sizes for a nominal additional fee (a "super size"). Eating away from home, and the shift to a more **sedentary lifestyle**, has been linked to the increasing rates of **obesity** in the United States.

Obesity and Malnutrition

Obesity, a form of malnutrition, is commonly defined as a **body mass index** over 30. Being **overweight** is defined as a body mass index of 25–30. There has been an increasing rate of obesity in the United States, especially among children. Obesity is now considered a national epidemic in many developed countries (such as the United States) but some persons feel that this concern has also caused a stigmatization of the **obese**.

Eating disorders can result in malnutrition. **Bulimia** is a condition marked by periods of **binge** eating followed by purging. This differs from compulsive overeating, or binge eating, which occurs when an individual eats compulsively but does not purge and becomes overweight. Starvation, either from the lack of available food or from self-imposed starvation, as in **anorexia** nervosa, will also cause malnutrition.

Despite a growing rate of obesity in developed countries, **undernutrition** remains the most common nutritional problem in developing nations. The combination of **protein** deficiency and **energy** deficiency is commonly known as *protein-energy malnutrition* (PEM). This form of malnutrition is most common in underveloped and developing countries, but also appears in geographic pockets of developed countries.

Dieting

About half of all Americans try to lose weight, or maintain their weight, every year. In an effort to lose weight people purchase weight loss pills; special herbal supplements; and formulated weight loss drinks, foods, and **diet** bars. People also join health clubs or spas, or buy special weight loss and exercise equipment, in an effort to lose weight and improve their health.

Among the common types of diets people follow are food-focused, celebrity, exchange, and supplement-based diets. Food-focused plans, such as the grapefruit diet, the banana diet, or a wine drinker's diet, emphasize consumption of only one, or a few, foods. Celebrity plans generally have the backing of a celebrity, and exchange plans lump together into food groups items with similar calories, **carbohydrates**, proteins, and fats. Some diets incorporate a commercial meal, snack bar, food, or beverage that must be purchased.

Supplements

Pills, liquids, or powders that contain nutrients and other ingredients are now readily available in stores. Supplements that contain herbs (or some herbal components) are growing in popularity. However, supplement production and use is not always well regulated, so consumers must be careful about what they purchase and consume.

Convenience Foods

To satisfy individuals who want to eat well at home but are short on time or do not want to prepare elaborate meals, many eateries also offer take-out meals or items. Fully or partially prepared "TOTE" (take-out-to-eat) foods, including home-delivered meals, are generally referred to as *convenience foods*. As more women (the traditional preparers of family meals) enter the labor force, people's desire to save time increases along with the use of convenience foods.

Functional Foods

The term *functional food* is often used in reference to foods that have nutrients (or non-nutrients) that might protect against disease. The term is used when referring to foods that have been **fortified**, have specific **phytochemicals** or active **microorganisms** added, or have been developed using **genetic** engineering techniques. However, all foods can support health in some way, and there is no legal definition of *functional food*. In addition, the actual benefit of these foods, if any, can vary and is open to interpretation. For example, both a candy bar and orange juice may have additional **calcium** added, and can therefore be called functional foods. The consumer must determine the benefit of such items.

---

undernutrition: food intake too low to maintain adequate energy expenditure without weight loss

protein: complex molecule composed of amino acids that performs vital functions in the cell; necessary part of the diet

energy: technically, the ability to perform work; the content of a substance that allows it to be useful as a fuel

diet: the total daily food intake, or the types of foods eaten

carbohydrate: food molecule made of carbon, hydrogen, and oxygen, including sugars and starches

fortified: altered by addition of vitamins or minerals

phytochemical: chemical produced by plants

microorganisms: bacteria and protists; single-celled organisms

genetic: inherited or related to the genes

calcium: mineral essential for bones and teeth

The TV Dinner

The "TV Dinner," a registered trademark of the Swanson company, first appeared in the early 1950s as women began leaving the kitchen for work outside the home, changing the way America ate. According to company lore, the product was invented by a sales representative who was left with 270 tons of unsold Thanksgiving turkey after the holiday. Inspired by a food tray with compartments he had seen on an airline, the representative proposed a frozen, prepared dinner for retail sale. The first frozen dinners—featuring turkey, stuffing, gravy, sweet potatoes, and peas—went into production in 1954. The following year, Swanson sold 25 million of them.

—Paula Kepos

Ethnic Foods

People now eat foods with origins in cultures other than their own, especially in the United States, where almost all dishes originated elsewhere but have been modified to suit the tastes and popularity of the mainstream population. Since the late twentieth century, however, there has been an increased incorporation of ethnic **cuisines** into the American diet, including foods from Asia, the Middle East, and Latin America. This trend is part of a larger movement toward diversity in all aspects of life.

Although all humans need food to survive, people's food habits (how they obtain, prepare, and consume food) are the result of **learned behaviors**. These collective behaviors, as well as the values and attitudes they reflect, come to represent a group's popular culture. SEE ALSO CONVENIENCE FOODS; DIETING; EATING HABITS; FAST FOODS; FUNCTIONAL FOODS; OBESITY.

Judith C. Rodriguez

cuisine: types of food and traditions of preparation

learned behaviors: actions that are acquired by training and observation, in contrast to innate behaviors

Bibliography

Carney, George O., ed. (1995). *Fast Foods, Stock Cars, and Rock 'n' Roll: Place and Space in American Pop Culture.* Lanham: Rowman & Littlefield.

Gabaccia, Donna R. (1998). *We Are What We Eat.* Cambridge, MA: Harvard University Press.

Gernmov, John, and Williams, Lauren (1999). *A Sociology of Food and Nutrition.* Oxford: Oxford University Press.

Maltby, Richard, ed. (1989). *Dreams for Sale: Popular Culture in the 20th Century.* London: Harrap.

Mukerji, Chandra, and Schudson, Michael (1991). *Rethinking Popular Culture.* Berkeley: University of California Press.

Scapp, Ron, and Seitz, Brian, eds. (1998). *Eating Culture.* Albany: State University of New York Press.

Schlosser, Eric (2001). *Fast Food Nation: The Darker Side of the All-American Meal.* New York: Houghton Mifflin.

Sizer, Frances, and Whitney, Eleanor (2002). *Nutrition Concepts and Controversies,* 9th edition. Belmont, CA: Wadsworth Thomson Learning.

Warde, Alan, and Martens, Lydia (2000). *Eating Out.* Cambridge, UK: Cambridge University Press.

Internet Resources

National Institutes of Health. "Weight Loss and Control." Available from <http://www.niddk.nih.gov/index.htm>

Pregnancy

Nutrition during the preconception period, as well as throughout a pregnancy, has a major impact on pregnancy outcome. Among prepregnancy considerations, the prepregnancy **Body Mass Index** (BMI), folic acid status, and **socioeconomic status** are the most important.

Prepregnancy BMI is an important factor in predicting pregnancy outcome, since both low prepregnancy and high prepregnancy BMI are associated with an increased risk for a negative pregnancy outcome.

Folic acid, a B vitamin, has been shown to prevent birth defects of the brain and spinal cord known as *neural tube defects* (NTDs). The most common NTDs are spina bifida and anencephaly. Folic acid is therefore needed

nutrition: the maintenance of health through proper eating, or the study of same

body mass index: weight in kilograms divided by square of the height in meters; a measure of body fat

socioeconomic status: level of income and social class

RECOMMENDED TOTAL WEIGHT-GAIN RANGES FOR PREGNANT WOMEN BY PREPREGNANCY BODY MASS INDEX (BMI)

Weight-for-height category	Recommended total weight gain	
	kg	lb
Low (BMI<19.8)	12.5–18	28–40
Normal (BMI of 19.8 to 26.0)	11.5–16	25–35
High (BMI >26.0 to 29.0)	7–11.5	15–25

Young adolescents and black women should strive for gains at the upper end of the recommended range. Short women (157 cm, or 62 inches) should strive for gains at the lower end of the range. The recommended target weight gain for obese women (BMI >29.0) is at least 6.8 kg (15 lb).

BMI is calculated using metric units.

SOURCE: Institute of Medicine.

---

both in preconception and early pregnancy. Since studies indicate that most women get less than half the recommended amount of folic acid, the March of Dimes recommends women consider a supplement of 400 micrograms of folic acid preconceptually to prevent the **incidence** of neural tube defects. In addition, it is suggested women capable of becoming pregnant consume a **diet** high in folic acid. Good sources of folic acid include oranges, green leafy vegetables, and **fortified** bread and cereals.

There is also a direct correlation between ethnicity, age, marital status, and educational status with increased negative pregnancy outcomes, such as low birth weight.

Pregnancy Weight Gain

Pregnancy is divided into three trimesters, with each trimester lasting three months, or approximately thirteen weeks (a normal pregnancy lasts 40 weeks). Recommendations for weight gain during pregnancy are based on the Institute of Medicine (IOM) definitions of prepregnancy BMI range. The BMI is defined as weight in pounds, divided by height in inches, divided by height in inches, multiplied by 703 (or weight in kilograms, divided by height in centimeters, divided by height in centimeters, multiplied by ten-thousand). The majority of weight gain should occur in the second and third trimesters. Weight gain can vary greatly in normal pregnancies with normal birth outcomes. Few studies have included women in their first trimester, so the importance of first-trimester weight gain on pregnancy outcome is unclear. However, a slow and steady rate of weight gain is considered ideal. The current recommended weight gain for the BMI ranges are outlined in the accompanying figure.

Poor weight gain during pregnancy is associated with prematurity, low birth weight, and small for gestational age. Among normal-weight women, weight gain above the recommended level corresponds to maternal fat stores and is not of benefit to fetal growth. In other words, fat gain during pregnancy parallels gestational weight gain, and women with greater weight gain also gain more fat. In addition, an inverse relationship exists between pre-pregnancy BMI and weight gain during pregnancy: women with a low pre-pregnancy BMI tend to gain more weight than women with a high pre-pregnancy BMI. On average, **overweight** women gain less weight than their thinner counterparts, though it is not unusual for **obese** women to achieve normal birth outcomes with less than the recommended weight gain.

incidence: number of new cases reported each year

diet: the total daily food intake, or the types of foods eaten

fortified: altered by addition of vitamins or minerals

overweight: weight above the accepted norm based on height, sex, and age

obese: above accepted standards of weight for sex, height, and age

DAILY NUMBER OF SERVINGS SUGGESTED FOR PREGNANCY

(Approximately 2200 calories)

Bread Group (one serving= 1 slice bread, ½ cup cereal, noodles, or rice)	9
Fruit Group (one serving = ½ cup fruit/fruit juice or one medium fruit)	3
Vegetables Group (One serving = ½ cup cooked or one cup raw)	4
Meat Group (one ounce chicken, beef, etc.)	6
Milk Group (one serving = 1 cup milk, 1 ounce cheese)	3
Total Fat (grams)*	73
Total added sugars (teaspoons)*	2

* Values for total fat and added sugars include fat and added sugars that are in food choices from the five major food groups, as well as fat and added sugars from foods in the fats, oils, and sweets group.

SOURCE: USDA Center for Nutrition Policy and Promotion.

---

obesity: the condition of being overweight, according to established norms based on sex, age, and height

calorie: unit of food energy

sedentary: not active

lifestyle: set of choices about diet, exercise, job type, leisure activities, and other aspects of life

nutrient: dietary substance necessary for health

glucose: a simple sugar; the most commonly used fuel in cells

diabetes: inability to regulate level of sugar in the blood

hypertension: high blood pressure

homeostasis: regulation of the proper internal state

In adolescent pregnancies, there are no established BMI recommendations regarding prepregnancy weight and weight gain. Excess weight gain, however, has been associated with postpartum **obesity** in adolescents.

Pregnancy Nutrition Requirements

Traditionally, caloric requirements during pregnancy have been estimated to be around an additional 300 **calories** per day. However, this must be adjusted for physical activity and prepregnancy weight (see accompanying figure) for the recommended number of servings of food groups. To meet weight-gain recommendations, a woman with a low prepregnancy BMI and a high activity level would require more calories than a woman with a high prepregnancy BMI and a **sedentary lifestyle**. A variety of foods from all food groups is important, since foods within the same food group do not contain exactly the same amount of **nutrients**. If increased weight gain is recommended, an emphasis should be placed on high-calorie food group items that contain a higher fat and sugar content. When less weight gain is recommended, women should choose from the lower-calorie food group choices.

Recommendations regarding sugar intake for pregnant women depend on weight gain and maternal blood **glucose** levels. A high sugar intake would not be advisable for women gaining more than the recommended weight or for those women who are having difficulty controlling normal blood glucose levels, while a high sugar intake would be beneficial for women requiring increased weight gain. A high sugar intake for women who are experiencing excessive weight gain or having difficulty maintaining normal glucose levels could result in increased maternal risk for complications associated with too much weight gain, such as **diabetes**, **hypertension**, premature delivery, and a large for gestational age fetus.

Adequate fluid intake is important to maintain hemodynamics (blood circulation) and **homeostasis** (fluid and tissue balance) and to reduce the risk of urinary tract infections. All pregnant women are encouraged to consume at least 64 ounces of fluid daily. Women at risk of gaining too much weight should be cautioned to limit their intake of sweetened fluids, including juice, and to consume more water. Exercise is considered healthful for most pregnant women, who should be encouraged to continue to exercise at prepregnancy levels. However, women should be cautious about

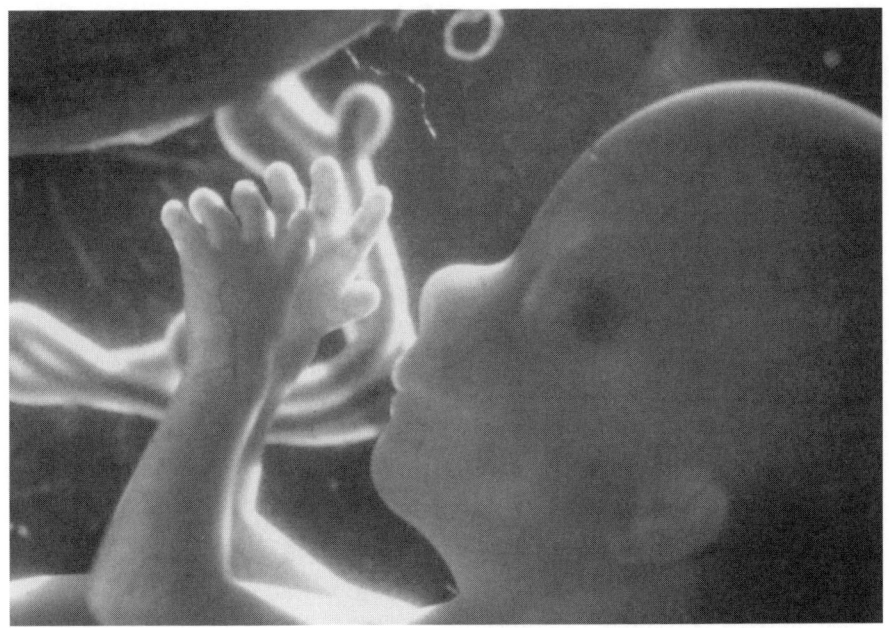

This human fetus is in the second trimester of development, a time when fetal weight gain begins to accelerate. Pregnant women should increase caloric intake by approximately 300 calories per day to account for rapid fetal growth. Calcium and iron supplements may also be necessary. [Photo Researchers, Inc. Reproduced by permission.]

beginning any new exercise program during pregnancy, and, if medically advised, should avoid certain activities. Health care providers may recommend bed rest and limiting physical activity (such as work) when preterm labor is present or when weight gain is poor. Increased physical activity will control excess weight gain, in addition to the normal beneficial physical and emotional effects.

Vitamin and Mineral Requirements

Iron is the only recommended nutrient for which requirements cannot be reasonably met by diet alone during pregnancy. Thirty milligrams of ferrous iron is recommended, and iron should be taken on an empty stomach. When more than 30 mg of iron is given to treat **anemia**, it is suggested to also take approximately 15 mg of **zinc** and 2 mg of copper, since iron interferes with **absorption** and utilization of these materials.

According to some studies, caffeine decreases the availability of certain nutrients, such as **calcium**, zinc, and iron. Current recommendations, therefore, include limiting the consumption of caffeinated containing products.

Calcium supplementation may be suggested if the average daily intake of calcium is less than 600 mg. Calcium intake is of particular concern among pregnant women under the age of twenty-five, since bone mineral density is still increasing in these women. Calcium supplements, if recommended, should be taken with meals. Additionally, **vitamin D** may be necessary if sunlight exposure is minimal. For vegetarians, the current recommendations also include a daily supplement of 2 mg of Vitamin B_{12}.

For women who don't ordinarily consume an adequate diet, or for those in high-risk categories (such as those carrying twins, heavy smokers, and drug abusers) a prenatal vitamin supplement is recommended, beginning in the second trimester. The supplement should contain the following: iron (30 mg); zinc (15 mg); copper (2 mg); calcium (250 mg); vitamin B_6 (62 mg); **folate** (300 mg); vitamin C (50 mg); vitamin D (5 mg).

iron: nutrient needed for red blood cell formation

anemia: low level of red blood cells in the blood

zinc: mineral necessary for many enzyme processes

absorption: uptake by the digestive tract

calcium: mineral essential for bones and teeth

vitamin D: nutrient needed for calcium uptake and therefore proper bone formation

folate: one of the B vitamins, also called folic acid

Special Nutrition Concerns

Food cravings during pregnancy are common and are not cause for concern, provided other nutrient needs are met and weight gain is in the target range. Pica—the ingestion of nonfood substances of nutritional value—is associated with anemia and can be a source of lead poisoning, bacterial infection, and dental problems. Pregnant women should be encouraged to avoid pica and discuss it with their medical provider.

Gestational diabetes is associated with high prepregnancy BMI and excess pregnancy weight gain. Infants of gestational-diabetic mothers are usually born large for gestational age (macrosomia) and are at higher risk for cesarean delivery and **hypoglycemia** postpartum.

Symptoms of toxemia of pregnancy, also known as preeclampsia, include swelling (**edema**) and proteinuria (excess **protein** in the urine). The cause of toxemia has not been determined, but the risk is associated with first pregnancies, advanced maternal age, African-American ethnicity, and women with a past history of diabetes, hypertension, or kidney disease. In severe cases, delivery is frequently induced.

Tips for common pregnancy discomforts include avoidance of offending foods (and their odor) when **nausea** and heartburn occur. Many pregnant women find that spicy, fatty foods can increase problems with nausea and heartburn. Frequent, small, and blander meals are often better tolerated. Some women find eating dry crackers before rising from bed in the morning helpful for nausea. However, since nausea and vomiting usually subside by the end of the first trimester, they do not have a significant impact on the final weight gain in most pregnancies. Hyperemesis gravidarum, or intractable vomiting during pregnancy, can rapidly result in **dehydration**, so medical intervention is required.

When **constipation** is a concern, increased consumption of whole grains, fruits, and vegetables is advisable, as well as increased fluid intake and physical activity.

Breastfeeding is the recommended method of infant nutrition, with a few exceptions. It benefits both mother and infant by providing protective **antibodies** to human disease, and breastfed babies are generally healthier and have higher I.Q. levels than bottle-fed babies. The development of jaw alignment problems and **allergies** are also far less likely in breastfed babies, while mothers who breastfeed have less postpartum complications and are considered to be at lower risk for breast **cancer**.

In the United States, women with HIV infection should not breastfeed. This is not a contraindication in developing countries, however, as the benefits may outweigh the possibility of infection. Untreated **tuberculosis** is also a contraindication for breastfeeding, while hepatitis C is currently not a contraindication for breastfeeding.

The Women, Infants, and Children (WIC) Program

The WIC program was established in the 1970s as a supplemental food and nutrition-education program. Eligibility requirements include a household income of up to 185 percent of the federal poverty level, as well as nutrition-risk criteria. The WIC program goals include improving pregnancy outcomes

---

hypoglycemia: low blood sugar level

edema: accumulation of fluid in the tissues

protein: complex molecule composed of amino acids that performs vital functions in the cell; necessary part of the diet

nausea: unpleasant sensation in the gut that precedes vomiting

dehydration: loss of water

constipation: difficulty passing feces

antibody: immune system protein that protects against infection

allergy: immune system reaction against substances that are otherwise harmless

cancer: uncontrolled cell growth

tuberculosis: bacterial infection, usually of the lungs, caused by Mycobacterium tuberculosis

by helping participants achieve recommended weight gain. Nutritional food choices and calorie levels based on recommended weight gain are emphasized. The program has been shown to significantly reduce a number of negative pregnancy outcomes, including low birth weight. SEE ALSO ADOLESCENT NUTRITION; BREASTFEEDING; LOW BIRTH WEIGHT INFANT; PICA; SMALL FOR GESTATIONAL AGE; WOMEN'S NUTRITIONAL ISSUES.

Mary Parke

Bibliography

Edwards, Cecile H. (1994) "African American Women and Their Pregnancies: Research Papers from the Program Project: Nutrition, Other Factors, and the Outcome of Pregnancy." *Journal of Nutrition* 124(6):917s–1027s.

Institute of Medicine, Committee on Nutritional Status during Pregnancy (1990). *Nutrition during Pregnancy*. Washington, DC: National Academy Press.

"Recent Developments in Maternal Nutrition and Their Implications for Practitioners." (1994). *American Journal of Clinical Nutrition* 59(2):437s–545S.

Stevens-Simon, Catherine, and McAarney, Elizabeth R. (1992). "Adolescent Pregnancy: Gestational Weight Gain and Maternal and Infant Outcomes." *American Journal of Diseases of Children* 146:1359–1364.

Suitor, Carol W. (1991). "Perspectives on Nutrition during Pregnancy." *Journal of the American Dietetic Association* 91:96–98.

Internet Resources

March of Dimes. "Folic Acid." Available from <http://www.marchofdimes.com/professionals/690.asp>

March of Dimes. "National Perinatal Statistics." Available from <http://www.marchofdimes.com/professionals/680_1239.asp>

MEDLINEplus Medical Encyclopedia. "Preeclampsia." Available from <http://www.nlm.nih.gov>

National Institute of Child Health and Human Development (2002). "Understanding Gestational Diabetes." Available from <http://www.nichd.nih.gov>

United States Department of Agriculture (USDA) Center for Nutrition Policy. Available from <http://www.usda.gov/cnpp>

Premenstrual Syndrome

Premenstrual syndrome (PMS) is characterized by emotional and physical symptoms that can be troubling and cause moderate discomfort for women the week or two before the onset of their menstrual cycle. PMS is estimated to affect up to 40 percent of reproductive-aged women. Approximately 5 to 10 percent of these women experience symptoms so severe that it totally impairs their everyday **lifestyle**. This severe form of PMS is known as premenstrual dysphoric disorder (PMDD). The precise **etiology** of PMS is still unknown; however, it is increasingly believed that the sensitive equilibrium between female sex **steroids** (the **hormones estrogen** and progesterone) and **neurotransmitters** in the brain is altered in women with PMS.

With a wide range of symptoms, both emotional and physical, the first step in successfully treating PMS is for a woman to recognize the changes in her body and mood. Keeping a close record of symptoms, their severity, and the dates they occur within the menstrual cycle is an important tool. Discussing this with a gynecologist can lead to a very successful treatment plan.

lifestyle: set of choices about diet, exercise, job type, leisure activities, and other aspects of life

etiology: origin and development of a disease

steroids: group of hormones that affect tissue build-up, sexual development, and a variety of metabolic processes

hormone: molecules produced by one set of cells that influence the function of another set of cells

estrogen: hormone that helps control female development and menstruation

neurotransmitter: molecule released by one nerve cell to stimulate or inhibit another

Symptoms

A woman is diagnosed with premenstrual syndrome if she has at least one emotional and one physical symptom during the five days before the onset of her period for three consecutive **menstrual cycles**. The specific symptom is not as important for diagnosis as is the cyclic fashion in which it appears. Emotional symptoms include minor **fatigue**, **depression**, angry outbursts, irritability, **anxiety**, confusion, social withdrawal, mood swings, and crying spells. Physical symptoms include headaches, bloating, acne, appetite changes and cravings, breast tenderness, and swelling of extremities.

Treatments

Diet. To help alleviate the symptoms of PMS, many treatments, both traditional and alternative, are being sought by thousands of women daily. According to some experts, the majority of PMS symptoms are a result of hormonal imbalances where there is too much estrogen in the body in comparison with the amount of progesterone. Studies have shown that a number of foods, such as, soy, vegetables and fruit, and nuts and seeds can actually help with hormonal balance. PMS sufferers are advised to increase their intake of fruits, vegetables, whole grains, low-fat dairy products and omega-3 **fatty acids** (mostly found in seafood and nuts). Eating small, frequent meals at the same time each day can help reduce bloating and fullness.

Several **clinical** trials have shown that supplementation of **calcium** and magnesium can play a crucial role in the prevention of PMS. Nine hundred to 1,200 milligrams of calcium per day was found to be effective in reducing food cravings and mood swings, and 200 to 500 milligrams of magnesium reduced bloating and breast tenderness. Studies of vitamin B_6 and vitamin E intake have had varied results. A daily multivitamin-mineral supplement is believed to be beneficial for all PMS sufferers.

Besides additions to the diet, it is suggested that women suffering from PMS should avoid caffeine, in the form of soft drinks, coffee, or chocolate; refined sugars; sodium; and saturated fats. Drinking plenty of water is a complement to cutting back on sodium. The effects of alcohol are usually magnified in premenstrual women, and therefore it is also advised that alcohol consumption be decreased or stopped totally.

Exercise. Scientific studies have shown that any type of physical exercise can help improve mood, decrease anxiety, and reduce **stress** reactions. As little as twenty to thirty minutes of **aerobic** type exercise three to five times a week, such as brisk walking, has shown to decrease some PMS symptoms. Some studies have also shown that doing nonaerobic exercises may also work, but to a smaller degree.

Complementary Medicine. Based on some preliminary scientific research, the herb chasteberry, also known as vitex agnus-castus, has been shown to relieve several PMS symptoms. According to a clinical trial, reported in January 2001 in a European scientific journal, more than half the women who received 20-milligram chasteberry tablets had a significant improvement in all their symptoms except bloating. Black cohosh and evening primrose oil are other herbs that are gaining popularity, though studies to date are inconclusive.

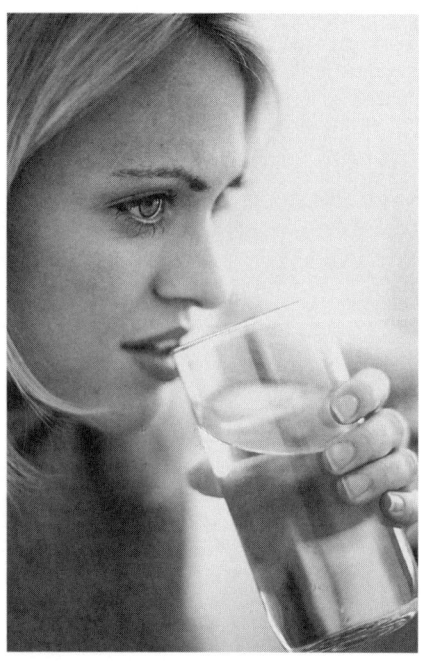

Up to 40 percent of reproductive-aged women experience symptoms of premenstrual syndrome (PMS). Eating certain foods and drinking plenty of water may help alleviate some of the discomfort of PMS. *[Photograph by Michael Keller. Corbis. Reproduced by permission.]*

menstrual cycles: the build-up and sloughing off of the lining of the uterus in women commencing at puberty and proceeding until menopause

fatigue: tiredness

depression: mood disorder characterized by apathy, restlessness, and negative thoughts

anxiety: nervousness

fatty acids: molecules rich in carbon and hydrogen; a component of fats

clinical: related to hospitals, clinics, and patient care

calcium: mineral essential for bones and teeth

stress: heightened state of nervousness or unease

aerobic: designed to maintain adequate oxygen in the bloodstream

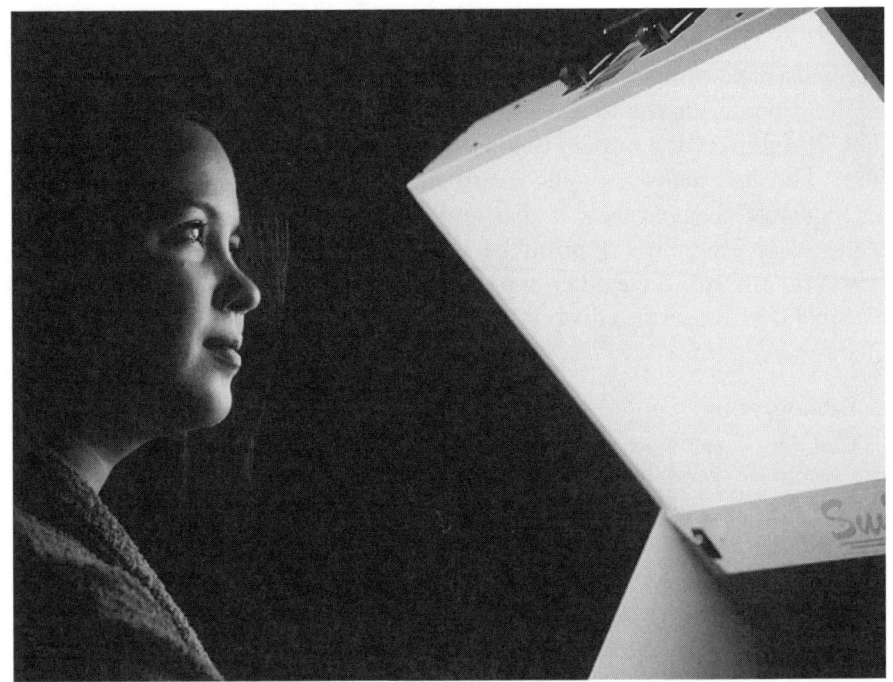

Light therapy can help alleviate the symptoms of PMS in some women. The results may be due to the relationship between melatonin, which is produced as a response to changes in visible light, and serotonin, which is a neural transmitter that contributes to a person's emotional outlook. [Najlah Feanny/Corbis. Reproduced by permission.]

Some studies have shown that women with PMS who are treated with bright-light therapy can have a substantial improvement in their mood. Bright-light therapy consists of sitting under a bright light of predetermined intensity for thirty minutes for one to two weeks before the onset of a menstrual cycle.

Many other alternative treatments are being explored for relieving PMS symptoms. To date, reflexology, massage therapy, and **acupuncture** are in the forefront of potential alternative treatments; however, future studies are needed to confirm their overall effectiveness.

acupuncture: insertion of needles into the skin at special points to treat disease

Pharmacologic. Since premenstrual symptoms are thought to be related to the changing levels of estrogen and progesterone, these hormones were among the first to be tested as a possible treatment. Although some early research reported positive findings, more recent studies have revealed that progesterone, whether natural of artificial, is not successful in the management of PMS.

A form of pharmacologic treatment that has shown positive results is the suppression of ovulation, which eliminates both the cyclic rhythm of hormone production and eliminating cyclic mood symptoms. The most common medications used for ovulation suppression are gonadotropin-releasing hormone (GnRH) agonists. Currently, the use of GnRH agonists is experimental; however, studies have shown that 75 percent of women treated with GnRH agonists have experienced reductions in tension, depression, mood swings, and breast tenderness.

Evidence from numerous controlled trials has clearly demonstrated that low-dose selective **serotonin** reuptake inhibitors (SSRIs) also have excellent **efficacy** with minimal side effects in treating women with severe PMS symptoms. SSRIs are a group of medications primarily used in treating depression and anxiety disorders. These medications have been shown to be best taken during the luteal phase of the menstrual cycle only.

serotonin: chemical used by nerve cells to communicate with one another

efficacy: effectiveness

Conclusion

Premenstrual syndrome, and its effect on millions of women, received a lot of attention during the 1990s, and many treatment modalities have emerged. The first step is for a woman to identify her symptoms and seek professional help. Through many available treatments, both traditional and alternative, and lifestyle changes such as diet and exercise, women no longer have to suffer so severely on a monthly basis. Research in this area is still needed, however, and more treatments need to be explored. SEE ALSO CRAVINGS; MOOD-FOOD RELATIONSHIPS; WOMEN'S NUTRITIONAL ISSUES.

Keri M. Gans

Bibliography

Dell, Diana, and Svec, Carol (2003). *The PMDD Phenomenon: Breakthrough Treatments for Premenstrual Dysphoric Disorder (PMDD) and Extreme Premenstrual Syndrome (PMS)*. New York: McGraw-Hill.

Northrup, Christiane (1998). *Women's Bodies, Women's Wisdom*. New York: Bantam.

Internet Resources

American College of Obstetricians and Gynecologists. "Dealing with PMS." *Spotlight on Women's Health*. Available from <http://www.acog.com>

Mayo Clinic. "Premenstrual Syndrome." Available from <http://www.mayclinic.com>

National Association for Premenstrual Syndrome. Available from <http://www.pms.org.uk/>

Nusbaum, Murray, and Schwarz, Richard. "Coping with PMS." American College of Obstetricians and Gynecologists. Available from <http://www.acog.com>

Lichten, Edward M. "Medical Treatment of Premenstrual Syndrome." Available from <http://www.usdoctor.com/pms.htm>

Preschoolers and Toddlers, Diet of

puberty: time of onset of sexual maturity

development: the process of change by which an organism becomes more complex

lifestyle: set of choices about diet, exercise, job type, leisure activities, and other aspects of life

growth spurts: periods of rapid growth

plateaus: periods during which growth is greatly reduced

anxiety: nervousness

nutritional requirements: the set of substances needed in the diet to maintain health

nutrient: dietary substance necessary for health

At approximately age one, children enter the latent period of growth. During this period, until the onset of **puberty**, growth and **development** are more gradual than during the first year. Physical growth steadies, and the body begins to look more proportioned as it prepares for an "upright" **lifestyle**.

The immediate stages following infancy are toddlerhood (ages one through three) and the preschool years (ages three through five). Characterized by temper tantrums, exploration, and endless questions, these periods can be trying for parents. Individual children experience **growth spurts** and **plateaus**—during which growth seems to stop completely. Food intake, and a liking of certain foods, may change constantly, causing a great deal of **anxiety** for parents.

Parents need to recognize that these changes are a normal part of development. Understanding the **nutritional requirements** of these age groups may help parents adapt to the new challenges. In addition, parents should be aware of the potential problems associated with feeding young children—and the ways to prevent them.

Nutritional Requirements

Compared to adults, small children need more **nutrients** in proportion to their body weight. As bones, muscles, teeth, and blood volume are develop-

Preschoolers and Toddlers, Diet of

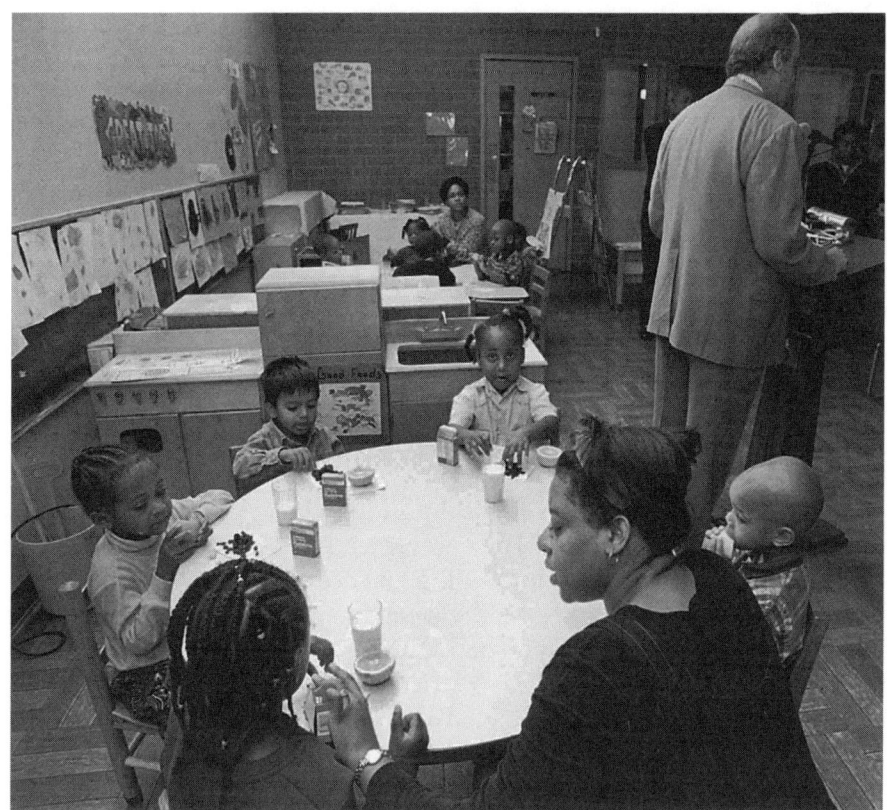

Former U.S. Secretary of Agriculture Dan Glickman promotes federal food programs at a daycare center while the children behind him enjoy lunch. *[Photograph by Mike Derer. AP/Wide World Photos. Reproduced by permission.]*

ing, nutrient intake needs to be adequate to support this process, and also to keep up with the growing child's increasing activity. A challenge also arises when growth spurts alternate with periods of no growth or slowed growth.

The **Dietary Reference Intakes** (DRIs), which include the **Recommended Dietary Allowances** (RDAs) and **Adequate Intakes** (AIs), should serve as a guide to prevent deficiencies in this age group. However, most of the levels set for preschoolers and toddlers are based on values established for infants and adults. In addition, the DRIs include a built-in margin of safety that exceeds the requirements for most children in the United States. Therefore, an intake that is less than that specified in the DRIs is not necessarily a reason for concern. For parents, a more practical approach to ensuring proper nutrient intake is to use the Food Guide Pyramid for Young Children, devised by the U.S. Department of Agriculture (USDA).0

Most people do not follow the requirements specified in these guides. Although severe nutrient deficiencies are rare in the United States, **calcium**, **iron**, **zinc**, vitamin B6, folic acid, and vitamin A are the nutrients most likely to be low in children as a result of poor dietary habits. Ensuring that children eat the recommended number of servings from each of the food groups in the pyramid is the best way to be certain that all nutritional requirements are met. A good rule of thumb for serving sizes is one tablespoon per year of age.

Energy and Protein Needs. **Basal metabolic rate**, growth, and physical activity all affect a child's daily energy. Regardless of the total intake, the composition should resemble the following: 50 to 60 percent of **calories** from **carbohydrates**, 25 to 35 percent of calories from fat, and 10 to

Dietary Reference Intakes: set of guidelines for nutrient intake

Recommended Dietary Allowances: nutrient intake recommended to promote health

adequate intake: nutrient intake that appears to maintain the state of health

calcium: mineral essential for bones and teeth

iron: nutrient needed for red blood cell formation

zinc: mineral necessary for many enzyme processes

basal metabolic rate: rate of energy consumption by the body during a period of no activity

calorie: unit of food energy

carbohydrate: food molecule made of carbon, hydrogen, and oxygen, including sugars and starches

fat: type of food molecule rich in carbon and hydrogen, with high energy content

RECOMMENDED DIETARY ALLOWANCES FOR ENERGY AND PROTEIN FOR CHILDREN.

Age (years)	Kilocalories			Grams of protein	
	daily	per kg	per cm	daily	per kg
1–3	1,300	102	14.4	16	1.2
4–6	1,800	80	16.0	24	1.1

SOURCE: Mahan L. Kathleen and Escott-Stump, Sylvia, eds. (2000). *Krause's Food, Nutrition & Diet Therapy*, 10th ed. Philadelphia, PA: W. B. Saunders Company.

15 percent of calories from protein (see accompanying table.) It should be remembered, however, that this is simply an estimate, and intake may need to be adjusted to suit each child.

Protein is a vital dietary component for preschoolers and toddlers, as it is needed for optimal growth. Enough protein should be consumed every day to allow for proper development. Protein deficiencies are rare in the United States, since most U.S. children consume plenty of protein each day. When protein **malnutrition** does occur, it is usually seen in those from low-income homes, those who follow a strict **vegan diet** excluding all animal sources, and those with multiple food **allergies**.

Vitamin and mineral needs. Iron is a vital component of **hemoglobin**, the carrier of **oxygen** in the blood. As a young child grows, blood volume increases, and so does the need for iron. Preschoolers and toddlers typically eat less iron-rich foods than they did in infancy. In addition, the iron that children get is usually non-heme iron (from plant sources), which has a lower availability than heme iron (from animal sources). As a result, children up to three years of age are at high risk for iron-deficiency **anemia**. The RDA for iron for both toddlers and preschoolers is ten milligrams (mg) per day.

Calcium is needed for bone and teeth mineralization and maintenance. The amount of calcium a child needs is determined in part by the consumption of other nutrients, such as protein, **phosphorus** and **vitamin D**, as well as the child's rate of growth. During this period of development, children need two to four times as much calcium per kilogram of body weight as adults do. The AI for toddlers is 500 mg/day, while for preschoolers it is 800 mg/day. Since dairy foods are the primary source of calcium, children who do not consume enough dairy or have an aversion to dairy products may be at risk for calcium deficiency.

The body can produce vitamin D in the skin in response to sun exposure. The amount of vitamin D needed daily thus depends mainly on how much time a child spends outside and on geographical location. The RDA for children living in tropical areas is between zero and 2.5 micrograms (μg) per day, depending on the amount of sun exposure. For those living in **temperate zones**, the RDA increases to 10 mc/day. Vitamin D–fortified milk is the best source.

Zinc is essential for proper development. It is needed for wound healing, proper sense of taste, proper growth, and normal appetite. Preschoolers and toddlers are sometimes at risk for marginal zinc deficiencies because the best sources are meats and seafoods, foods they may not eat regularly. The recommended intake of zinc is 10 mg/day.

---

malnutrition: chronic lack of sufficient nutrients to maintain health

vegan: person who consumes no animal products, including milk and honey

diet: the total daily food intake, or the types of foods eaten

allergy: immune system reaction against substances that are otherwise harmless

hemoglobin: the iron-containing molecule in red blood cells that carries oxygen

oxygen: O$_2$, atmospheric gas required by all animals

anemia: low level of red blood cells in the blood

phosphorus: element essential in forming the mineral portion of bone

vitamin D: nutrient needed for calcium uptake and therefore proper bone formation

temperate zone: region of the world between the tropics and the arctic or Antarctic

Vitamin and mineral supplements are popular with more than 50 percent of parents of preschoolers and toddlers. Most use a multivitamin/mineral supplement with iron. Parents should be aware, however, that such supplements do not necessarily fulfill the needs for marginal or deficient nutrients. For example, although calcium is often a nutrient that is low in children, most multivitamin/mineral supplements do not include it, or include it in very low doses. The American Academy of Pediatrics does not support routine supplementation for normal, healthy kids. Although there is no harm in giving children a standard children's supplement, megadoses should always be avoided, and caution should be used when supplementing the fat-soluble **vitamins** (vitamins A, D, E, and K).

Potential Feeding Problems

As young children develop their likes and dislikes and learn to feed themselves, parents need to allow them to become more independent. As a result of these changes, potential concerns arise. Common feeding problems among preschoolers and toddlers are: **obesity**, nursing bottle mouth syndrome, food jags, and iron-deficiency anemia.

According to the national Pediatric Nutrition Surveillance System, 10.2 percent of children in the United States under the age of five were **overweight** in 1998. These rates have been increasing steadily since the 1960s. Prevention education is the key to lowering the **incidence** of obesity in children. Success has been shown in programs that include family involvement, nutritional information and modification, activity planning, and behavior therapy.

Most often seen in children under age three, nursing bottle mouth syndrome (or baby bottle tooth decay) results from extended bottle feeding. It occurs when a child is routinely given a bottle with sweetened beverages (such as milk or juice) at bedtime. As the child sleeps, the liquid pools around the teeth. The result is severe **caries** on the **incisors** and cheek surfaces of **molars**. Parents should avoid giving a bottle at bedtime and begin serving beverages in a cup as early as possible.

Most children undergo a normal part of development know as a *food jag*. Food jags occur when children either refuse to eat a previously accepted food, or when they insist on eating one particular food all the time. A food jag is generally a case of a child testing his or her independence. Although annoying for most parents, food jags are rarely a reason for concern. The best strategy is to continue offering a variety of foods every day, while keeping the favorite food available. Most children will eventually return to a normal eating pattern. Letting a food jag take its course is the best plan of action; force will accomplish little.

Despite the wide availability of iron-rich foods, iron-deficiency anemia is the most common nutrient deficiency in the world. Reasons for this deficiency in toddlers may be the consumption of large quantities of milk, and thus limited intake of solids and iron-fortified foods. In addition, many young children do not like the best sources of iron, such as meats and seafoods. Parents should pay special attention to include good dietary sources of iron in their children's diet. When meat or seafood sources are limited, the availability of iron from plant sources can be increased with the consumption of ascorbic acid (vitamin C).

vitamin: necessary complex nutrient used to aid enzymes or other metabolic processes in the cell

obesity: the condition of being overweight, according to established norms based on sex, age, and height

overweight: weight above the accepted norm based on height, sex, and age

incidence: number of new cases reported each year

caries: cavities in the teeth

incisor: chisel-shaped tooth used for cutting; one of the types of primary teeth

molar: grinding tooth toward the rear of the mouth

Feeding Strategies for Parents

- Allow kids to eat five to six small meals per day.
- Allow them to eat when they are hungry and do not force them to eat when they are not.
- Do not use food as a reward or punishment.
- Be aware of the risk of choking in these age groups. Avoid foods that are round, hard, or do not easily dissolve in saliva (such as hot dogs, grapes, raw vegetables, popcorn, nuts, peanut butter, and hard candy).
- Avoid feeding too many sweetened beverages (especially in the bottle); encourage them to drink plenty of water.

The preschool and toddler years often create anxiety in parents as food likes, dislikes, and requirements may change continuously. Understanding that these changes are a normal part of development, and understanding the nutritional requirements for this age group, will help parents make educated decisions. Parents should also be aware of the potential feeding problems of this group, and of the ways to prevent them. SEE ALSO BABY BOTTLE TOOTH DECAY; CHILDHOOD OBESITY.

Kirsten Herbes

Bibliography

Ballabriga, Angela, ed. (1996) *Feeding from Toddlers to Adolescence*. Philadelphia, PA: Lippincott-Raven.

Duyff, Roberta L. (1998). *The American Dietetic Association's Complete Food & Nutrition Guide*. Minneapolis, MN: Chronimed Publishing.

Herbest, Victor, and Subak-Sharpe, Genell J., eds. (1995). *Total Nutrition: The Only Guide You'll Ever Need*. New York, NY: St. Martin's Griffin.

Hovasi Cox, Jance, ed. (1997) *Nutrition Manual for At-Risk Infants and Toddlers*. Chicago, IL: Precept Press.

Mahan, L. Kathleen, and Escott-Stump, Sylvia, eds. (2000). *Krause's Food, Nutrition, and Diet Therapy*, 10th ed. Philadelphia, PA: W. B. Saunders Company.

McWilliams, Margaret (1986). *Nutrition for the Growing Years*. New York, NY: Macmillan Publishing Company.

Queen Samor, Patricia; King Helm, Kathy; and Lang, Carol E. (1999). *Handbook of Pediatric Nutrition*, 2nd ed. Gaithersburg, MD: Aspen Publishers, Inc.

Tamborlane, William V., ed. (1997). *The Yale Guide to Children's Nutrition*. New Haven, CT: Yale University Press.

Wardlaw, Gordon M. (1999). *Perspectives in Nutrition*, 4th ed. New York, NY: WCB/McGraw-Hill.

Internet Resources

American Dietetic Association. "Child Feeding." American Dietetic Association. Available from <http://www.eatright.com/healthy/child/>

American Dietetic Association. "Position of the ADA: Dietary Guidance for Healthy Children Aged 2 to 11 years." Available from <http://www.eatright.com/adap0199.html>

American Dietetic Association. "Food Guide Pyramid for Young Children." Available from <http://www.usda.gov/cnpp/kidspyra>

Probiotics

nonpathogenic: not promoting disease

microorganisms: bacteria and protists; single-celled organisms

gastrointestinal: related to the stomach and intestines

microflora: microscopic organisms present in small numbers

allergy: immune system reaction against substances that are otherwise harmless

eczema: skin disease causing itching and flaking

candidal: related to the yeast Candida

cancer: uncontrolled cell growth

gastric: related to the stomach

acidity: measure of the tendency of a molecule to lose hydrogen ions, thus behaving as an acid

bile: substance produced in the liver which suspends fats for absorption

functional food: food whose health benefits are claimed to be higher than those traditionally assumed for similar types of foods

Probiotics are live, **nonpathogenic microorganisms** that may interact with **gastrointestinal** and vaginal **microflora**. Clinical studies indicate that certain probiotics may be useful in treating some diarrheal disorders, respiratory **allergies**, and **eczema**, as well as in controlling inflammation and reducing the risk of **candidal** vaginitis and colon **cancer**.

Dietary sources of probiotics are usually found in dairy products. Yogurt, for example, contains intestinal species of lactobacilli and bifidobacteria, two groups of probiotic bacteria. **Gastric** survival rates of probiotics are estimated at 20 to 40 percent, with the main obstacles to survival being gastric **acidity** and the action of **bile** salts. Investigations into different modes of administering probiotics may expand their applications in **functional foods**. SEE ALSO FUNCTIONAL FOODS.

M. Elizabeth Kunkel
Barbara H. D. Luccia

Bibliography

Gibson, G. R., and Roberfroid, Marcel B. (1999). *Colonic Microbiota, Nutrition, and Health*. Boston: Kluwer Academic.

Protein

Proteins are compounds composed of carbon, hydrogen, **oxygen**, and **nitrogen**, which are arranged as strands of **amino acids**. They play an essential role in the cellular maintenance, growth, and functioning of the human body. Serving as the basic structural molecule of all the tissues in the body, protein makes up nearly 17 percent of the total body weight. To understand protein's role and function in the human body, it is important to understand its basic structure and composition.

Amino Acids

Amino acids are the fundamental building blocks of protein. Long chains of amino acids, called *polypeptides*, make up the multicomponent, large complexes of protein. The arrangement of amino acids along the chain determines the structure and chemical properties of the protein. Amino acids consist of the following elements: carbon, hydrogen, oxygen, nitrogen, and, sometimes, sulfur. The general structure of amino acids consists of a carbon center and its four substituents, which consists of an amino group (NH_2), an organic acid (carboxyl) group (COOH), a hydrogen atom (H), and a fourth group, referred to as the R-group, that determines the structural identity and chemical properties of the amino acid. The first three groups are common to all amino acids. The basic amino acid structure is R-CH(NH2)-COOH.

There are twenty different forms of amino acids that the human body utilizes. These forms are distinguished by the fourth variable substituent, the R-group, which can be a chain of different lengths or a carbon-ring structure. For example, if hydrogen represents the R-group, the amino acid is known as *glycine*, a **polar** but **uncharged** amino acid, while methyl (CH_3) group is known as *alanine*, a **nonpolar** amino acid. Thus, the chemical components of the R-group essentially determine the identity, structure, and function of the amino acid.

The structural and chemical relatedness of the R-groups allows classification of the twenty amino acids into chemical groups. Amino acids can be classified according to optical activity (the ability to polarize light), **acidity** and basicity, polarity and nonpolarity, or hydrophilicity (water-loving) and hydrophobicity (water-fearing). These categories offer clues to the function and **reactivity** of the amino acids in proteins. The **biochemical** properties of amino acids determine the role and function of protein in the human body.

Of the twenty amino acids, eleven are considered *nonessential* (or *dispensable*), meaning that the body is able to adequately synthesize them, and nine are *essential* (or *indispensable*), meaning that the body is unable to adequately synthesize them to meet the needs of the cell. They must therefore be supplied through the **diet**. Foods that have protein contain both nonessential and essential amino acids, the latter of which the body can use to synthesize some of the nonessential amino acids. A healthful diet, therefore, should

protein: complex molecule composed of amino acids that performs vital functions in the cell; necessary part of the diet

oxygen: O_2, atmospheric gas required by all animals

nitrogen: essential element for plant growth

amino acid: building block of proteins, necessary dietary nutrient

polar: containing regions of positive and negative charge; likely to be soluble in water

uncharged: neither positively nor negatively charged

nonpolar: without a separation if charge within the molecule; likely to be hydrophobic

acidity: measure of the tendency of a molecule to lose hydrogen ions, thus behaving as an acid

reactivity: characteristic set of reactions undergone due to chemical structure

biochemical: related to chemical processes within cells

diet: the total daily food intake, or the types of foods eaten

THE TWENTY AMINO ACIDS

Name	Abbreviation	Linear structure formula (atom composition and bonding)
Alanine	ala	$CH_3\text{-}CH(NH_2)\text{-}COOH$
Arginine	arg	$HN\text{=}C(NH_2)\text{-}NH\text{-}(CH_2)3\text{-}CH(NH_2)\text{-}COOH$
Asparagine	asn	$H_2N\text{-}CO\text{-}CH_2\text{-}CH(NH_2)\text{-}COOH$
Aspartic acid	asp	$HOOC\text{-}CH_2\text{-}CH(NH_2)\text{-}COOH$
Cysteine	cys	$HS\text{-}CH_2\text{-}CH(NH_2)\text{-}COOH$
Glutamine	gln	$H2N\text{-}CO\text{-}(CH_2)2\text{-}CH(NH_2)\text{-}COOH$
Glutamic acid	glu	$HOOC\text{-}(CH_2)2\text{-}CH(NH_2)\text{-}COOH$
Glycine	gly	$NH_2\text{-}CH_2\text{-}COOH$
Histidine	his	$NH\text{-}CH\text{=}N\text{-}CH\text{=}C\text{-}CH_2\text{-}CH(NH_2)\text{-}COOH$ (nitrogen bonded to carbon)
Isoleucine	ile	$CH_3\text{-}CH2\text{-}CH(CH_3)\text{-}CH(NH_2)\text{-}COOH$
Leucine	leu	$(CH_3)2\text{-}CH\text{-}CH_2\text{-}CH(NH_2)\text{-}COOH$
Lysine	lys	$H_2N\text{-}(CH_2)4\text{-}CH(NH_2)\text{-}COOH$
Methionine	met	$CH_3\text{-}S\text{-}(CH_2)2\text{-}CH(NH_2)\text{-}COOH$
Phenylalanine	phe	$Ph\text{-}CH_2\text{-}CH(NH_2)\text{-}COOH$
Proline	pro	$NH\text{-}(CH_2)3\text{-}CH\text{-}COOH$
Serine	ser	$HO\text{-}CH_2\text{-}CH(NH_2)\text{-}COOH$
Threonine	thr	$CH_3\text{-}CH(OH)\text{-}CH(NH_2)\text{-}COOH$
Tryptophan	trp	$Ph\text{-}NH\text{-}CH\text{=}C\text{-}CH_2\text{-}CH(NH_2)\text{-}COOH$
Tyrosine	tyr	$HO\text{-}Ph\text{-}CH_2\text{-}CH(NH_2)\text{-}COOH$
Valine	val	$(CH_3)2\text{-}CH\text{-}CH(NH_2)\text{-}COOH$

SOURCE: Institute for Chemistry

consist of a sufficient and balanced supply of both essential and nonessential amino acids in order to ensure high levels of protein production.

Protein Quality: Nutritive Value

The quality of protein depends on the level at which it provides the nutritional amounts of essential amino acids needed for overall body health, maintenance, and growth. Animal proteins, such as eggs, cheese, milk, meat, and fish, are considered *high-quality*, or *complete*, *proteins* because they provide sufficient amounts of the essential amino acids. Plant proteins, such as grain, corn, nuts, vegetables and fruits, are *lower-quality*, or *incomplete*, *proteins* because many plant proteins lack one or more of the essential amino acids, or because they lack a proper balance of amino acids. Incomplete proteins can, however, be combined to provide all the essential amino acids, though combinations of incomplete proteins must be consumed at the same time, or within a short period of time (within four hours), to obtain the maximum nutritive value from the amino acids. Such combination diets generally yield a high-quality protein meal, providing sufficient amounts and proper balance of the essential amino acids needed by the body to function.

Protein Processing: Digestion, Absorption, and Metabolism

Protein digestion begins when the food reaches the stomach and stimulates the release of hydrochloric acid (HCl) by the parietal cells located in the **gastric mucosa** of the GI (**gastrointestinal**) tract. Hydrochloric acid provides for a very acidic **environment**, which helps the protein digestion process in two ways: (1) through an acid-catalyzed *hydrolysis* reaction of breaking peptide bonds (the chemical process of breaking peptide bonds is referred to as a hydrolysis reaction because water is used to break the bonds); and (2) through conversion of the gastric **enzyme** pepsinogen (an inactive precursor) to pepsin (the active form). Pepsinogen is stored and secreted by the "chief cells" that line the stomach wall. Once converted into the active form, pepsin attacks the peptide bonds that link amino acids together, breaking the long polypeptide chain into shorter segments of amino acids known as dipeptides and tripeptides. These protein fragments are then further broken down in the duodenum of the small **intestines**. The *brush border enzymes*, which work on the surface of **epithelial cells** of the small intestines, **hydrolyze** the protein fragments into amino acids.

The cells of the small intestine actively absorb the amino acids through a process that requires **energy**. The amino acids travel through the hepatic portal vein to the liver, where the **nutrients** are processed into **glucose** or **fat** (or released into the bloodstream). The tissues in the body take up the amino acids rapidly for glucose production, growth and maintenance, and other vital cellular functioning. For the most part, the body does not store protein, as the metabolism of amino acids occurs within a few hours.

Amino acids are metabolized in the liver into useful forms that are used as building blocks of protein in tissues. The body may utilize the amino acids for either **anabolic** or *catabolic reactions*. Anabolism refers to the chemical process through which digested and absorbed products are used to effectively build or repair bodily tissues, or to restore vital substances broken down through metabolism. **Catabolism**, on the other hand, is the process that results in the release of energy through the breakdown of nutrients, stored materials, and cellular substances. Anabolic and catabolic reactions work hand-in-hand, and the energy produced in catabolic processes is used to fuel essential anabolic processes. The vital biochemical reaction of **glycolysis** (in which glucose is oxidized to produce carbon dioxide, water, and cellular energy) in the form of adenosine triphosphate, or ATP, is a prime example of a catabolic reaction. The energy released, as ATP, from such a reaction is used to fuel important anabolic processes, such as protein synthesis.

The metabolism of amino acids can be understood from the dynamic catabolic and anabolic processes. In the process referred to as **deamination**, the nitrogen-containing amino group (NH_2) is cleaved from the amino acid unit. In this reaction, which requires vitamin B6 as a cofactor, the amino group is transferred to an acceptor **keto-acid**, which can form a new amino acid. Through this process, the body is able to make the nonessential amino acids not provided by one's diet. The keto-acid intermediate can also be used to synthesize glucose to ultimately yield energy for the body, and the cleaved nitrogen-containing group is transformed into urea, a waste product, and excreted as urine.

---

gastric: related to the stomach

mucosa: moist exchange surface within the body

gastrointestinal: related to the stomach and intestines

environment: surroundings

enzyme: protein responsible for carrying out reactions in a cell

intestines: the two long tubes that carry out the bulk of the processes of digestion

epithelial cell: sheet of cells lining organs throughout the body

hydrolyze: to break apart through reaction with water

energy: technically, the ability to perform work; the content of a substance that allows it to be useful as a fuel

nutrient: dietary substance necessary for health

glucose: a simple sugar; the most commonly used fuel in cells

fat: type of food molecule rich in carbon and hydrogen, with high energy content

anabolic: promoting building up

catabolism: breakdown of complex molecules

glycolysis: cellular reaction that begins the breakdown of sugars

deamination: removal of an NH2 group from a molecule

keto-acid: an acid compound containing the reactive CO group

Vital Protein Functions

Proteins are vital to basic cellular and body functions, including cellular regeneration and repair, tissue maintenance and regulation, **hormone** and enzyme production, fluid balance, and the provision of energy.

Cellular and tissue provisioning.
Protein is an essential component for every type of cell in the body, including muscles, bones, organs, tendons, and ligaments. Protein is also needed in the formation of enzymes, **antibodies**, hormones, blood-clotting factors, and blood-transport proteins. The body is constantly undergoing renewal and repair of tissues. The amount of protein needed to build new tissue or maintain structure and function depends on the rate of renewal or the stage of growth and **development**. For example, the intestinal tract is renewed every couple of days, whereas blood cells have a life span of 60 to 120 days. Furthermore, an infant will utilize as much as one-third of the dietary protein for the purpose of building new connective and muscle tissues.

Hormone and enzyme production.
Amino acids are the basic components of hormones, which are essential chemical signaling messengers of the body. Hormones are secreted into the bloodstream by endocrine glands, such as the thyroid gland, adrenal glands, pancreas, and other ductless glands, and regulate bodily functions and processes. For example, the hormone **insulin**, secreted by the pancreas, works to lower the blood glucose level after meals. Insulin is made up of forty-eight amino acids.

Enzymes, which play an essential **kinetic** role in **biological** reactions, are composed of large protein **molecules**. Enzymes facilitate the rate of reactions by acting as *catalysts* and lowering the activation energy barrier between the reactants and the products of the reactions. All chemical reactions that occur during the digestion of food and the **metabolic** processes in tissues require enzymes. Therefore, enzymes are vital to the overall function of the body, and thereby indicate the fundamental and significant role of proteins.

Fluid balance.
The presence of blood protein molecules, such as *albumins* and *globulins*, are critical factors in maintaining the proper fluid balance between cells and extracellular space. Proteins are present in the capillary beds, which are one-cell-thick vessels that connect the arterial and venous beds, and they cannot flow outside the capillary beds into the tissue because of their large size. Blood fluid is pulled into the capillary beds from the tissue through the mechanics of oncotic pressure, in which the pressure exerted by the protein molecules counteracts the **blood pressure**. Therefore, blood proteins are essential in maintaining and regulating fluid balance between the blood and tissue. The lack of blood proteins results in clinical **edema**, or tissue swelling, because there is insufficient pressure to pull fluid back into the blood from the tissues. The condition of edema is serious and can lead to many medical problems.

Energy provision.
Protein is not a significant source of energy for the body when there are sufficient amounts of **carbohydrates** and fats available, nor is protein a storable energy, as in the case of fats and carbohydrates. However, if insufficient amounts of carbohydrates and fats are ingested, protein is used for energy needs of the body. The use of protein for energy is

---

hormone: molecules produced by one set of cells that influence the function of another set of cells

antibody: immune system protein that protects against infection

development: the process of change by which an organism becomes more complex

insulin: hormone released by the pancreas to regulate level of sugar in the blood

kinetic: related to speed of reaction

biological: related to living organisms

molecule: combination of atoms that form stable particles

metabolic: related to processing of nutrients and building of necessary molecules within the cell

blood pressure: measure of the pressure exerted by the blood against the walls of the blood vessels

edema: accumulation of fluid in the tissues

carbohydrate: food molecule made of carbon, hydrogen, and oxygen, including sugars and starches

PROTEIN CONTENT OF REPRESENTATIVE FOODS IN THE HUMAN DIET	
Food	Protein (grams)
Milk, 244 g (8 oz)	8.0
Cheddar Cheese, 84 g (3 oz)	21.3
Egg, 50 g (1 large)	6.1
Apple, 212 g (1, 3 ¼ in. diameter)	0.4
Banana, 74 g (1, 8 ¾ in. long)	1.2
Potato, cooked, 136 g (1 potato)	2.5
Bread, white, slice, 25 g	2.1
Fish, cod, poached, 100 g (3 ½ oz)	20.9
Oyster, 100 g (3 ½ oz)	13.5
Beef, pot roast, 85 g (3 oz)	22.0
Liver, pan fried, 85 g (3 oz)	23.0
Pork chop, bone in, 87 g (3.1 oz)	23.9
Ham, boiled, 2 pieces, 114 g	20.0
Peanut butter, 16 g (1 tablespoon)	4.6
Pecans, 28 g (1 oz)	2.2
Snap beans, 125 g (1 cup)	2.4
Carrots, slicked, 78 g (½ cup)	0.8

SOURCE: U.S. Department of Agriculture

not necessarily economical for the body, because tissue maintenance, growth, and repair are compromised to meet energy needs. If taken in excess, protein can be converted into body fat. Protein yields as much usable energy as carbohydrates, which is 4 kcal/gm (kilocalories per gram). Although not the main source of usable energy, protein provides the essential amino acids that are needed for adenine, the nitrogenous base of ATP, as well as other nitrogenous substances, such as creatine phosphate (nitrogen is an essential element for important compounds in the body).

Protein Requirement and Nutrition

The recommended protein intake for an average adult is generally based on body size: 0.8 grams per kilogram of body weight is the generally recommended daily intake. The recommended daily allowances of protein do not vary in times of strenuous activities or exercise, or with progressing age. However, there is a wide range of protein intake which people can consume according to their period of development. For example, the recommended allowance for an infant up to six months of age, who is undergoing a period of rapid tissue growth, is 2.2 grams per kilogram. For children ages seven through ten, the recommended daily allowance is around 36 total grams, depending on body weight. Pregnant women need to consume an additional 30 grams of protein above the average adult intake for the nourishment of the developing fetus.

Sources of protein. Good sources of protein include high-quality protein foods, such as meat, poultry, fish, milk, egg, and cheese, as well as prevalent low-quality protein foods, such as **legumes** (e.g., navy beans, pinto beans, chick peas, soybeans, split peas), which are high in protein.

legumes: beans, peas and related plants

Protein–Calorie Malnutrition

The nitrogen balance index (NBI) is used to evaluate the amount of protein used by the body in comparison with the amount of protein supplied from daily food intake. The body is in the state of nitrogen (or protein) equilibrium

adipose tissue: tissue containing fat deposits

immune system: the set of organs and cells, including white blood cells, that protect the body from infection

plasma: the fluid portion of the blood, distinct from the cellular portion

anemia: low level of red blood cells in the blood

infectious diseases: diseases caused by viruses, bacteria, fungi, or protozoa, which replicate inside the body

kwashiorkor: severe malnutrition characterized by swollen belly, hair loss, and loss of skin pigment

when the intake and usage of protein is equal. The body has a *positive nitrogen balance* when the intake of protein is greater than that expended by the body. In this case, the body can build and develop new tissue. Since the body does not store protein, the overconsumption of protein can result in the excess amount to be converted into fat and stored as **adipose tissue**. The body has a *negative nitrogen balance* when the intake of protein is less than that expended by the body. In this case, protein intake is less than required, and the body cannot maintain or build new tissues.

A *negative nitrogen balance* represents a state of protein deficiency, in which the body is breaking down tissues faster than they are being replaced. The ingestion of insufficient amounts of protein, or food with poor protein quality, can result in serious medical conditions in which an individual's overall health is compromised. The **immune system** is severely affected; the amount of blood **plasma** decreases, leading to medical conditions such as **anemia** or edema; and the body becomes vulnerable to **infectious diseases** and other serious conditions. Protein malnutrition in infants is called **kwashiorkor**, and it poses a major health problem in developing countries, such as Africa, Central and South America, and certain parts of Asia. An infant with kwashiorkor suffers from poor muscle and tissue development, loss of appetite, mottled skin, patchy hair, diarrhea, edema, and, eventually, death (similar symptoms are present in adults with protein deficiency). Treatment or prevention of this condition lies in adequate consumption of protein-rich foods. SEE ALSO AMINO ACIDS.

Jeffrey Radecki
Susan Kim

Bibliography

Berdanier, Carolyn D. (1998). *CRC Desk Reference for Nutrition.* Boca Raton, FL: CRC Press.

Briggs, George M., and Calloway, Doris Howes (1979). *Bogert's Nutrition and Physical Fitness,* 10th edition. Philadelphia, PA: W. B. Saunders.

Johnston, T. K. (1999). "Nutritional Implications of Vegetarian Diets." In *Modern Nutrition in Health and Disease,* 9th edition. M. E. Shills, et al, eds. Baltimore, MD: Williams & Wilkins.

Robinson, Corrinne H. (1975). *Basic Nutrition and Diet Therapy.* New York: Macmillan.

U.S. Department of Agriculture (1986). *Composition of Foods.* (USDA Handbooks 8–15.) Washington, DC: U.S. Government Printing Office.

Wardlaw, Gordon M., and Kesse, Margaret (2002). *Perspectives in Nutrition,* 5th edition. Boston: McGraw-Hill.

Internet Resources

Institute for Chemistry. "Amino Acids." Available from <http://www.chemie.fuberlin.de>

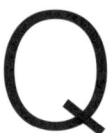

Quackery

Quackery is a type of health fraud that promotes products and services that have questionable and unproven scientific bases. Quackery is short for quacksalver, which is derived from two Middle Dutch terms that mean "healing with unguents." However, quacken means "to boast," so a kwakzalver might be a healer who boasts about his power or products.

Quacks, the people who promote these products, have been around for years. One of the most enduring images of nineteenth-century medicine is the charlatan or quack. These individuals sold primarily patent medicines that promised to cure everything from **cancer** to the common cold. Patent medicines were concoctions (elixirs, salves, balms, etc.) for which individuals received exclusive rights to sell for a given period of time. Patent medicines were available by mail or over the counter at chemists' shops, general stores, and even seed stores. Most patent medicines contained alcohol, and many also contained opium or morphine. Virtually none contained the "healing" ingredients they claimed to have, and none healed.

Some quacks were called "snake oil" salesmen. These individuals traveled from town to town, sometimes with a carnival, selling their products. Today, quacks have more sophisticated ways to sell their products. The products are now promoted on the Internet, TV, and radio; in magazines, newspapers, and infomercials; by mail; and even by word-of-mouth. Many consider quackery to be a pejorative term and now use the term *alternative medicine*. However, this term is used in a variety of ways. The physician Stephen Barrett suggests that "alternative" methods be classified as genuine, experimental, or questionable, whereas *quackery* refers solely to questionable and unproven methods.

Claims and Promises

Fraudulent products are designed solely to make money. They often use paid actors in the infomercials and advertisements to make their products sound and look convincing. They also may use celebrities to endorse the products. Fraudulent products usually:

- Promise quick, painless cures or results.
- Claim to be effective for a wide range of ailments.
- Promise weight loss without dieting or exercise.
- Claim to be made from a special, secret ingredient.
- Guarantee all results.
- Use testimonials or undocumented case histories from satisfied patients.
- Offer an additional amount of the product as a "special promotion."

Nutrition Quackery

Nutrition quackery is one of the most profitable types of quackery. Dietary supplements, weight loss products, **herbal** remedies, and "sports" foods are not registered with the Food and Drug Administration (FDA). Federal law allows certain claims to be made on the labels of food and dietary supplements. These include claims that show a strong scientific link between a food substance and a disease or health condition. These approved claims can state only that the product may reduce the risk of certain health problems, not cure them. The labels of dietary supplements must state that the claim "has not been evaluated by the FDA," and that the "product is not intended to diagnose, treat, cure, or prevent any disease." Yet, the infomercials and ads for many products do not include these warnings.

One of the basic premises of many dietary supplements is that most individuals have vitamin and mineral deficiencies. In addition, the promoters of supplements often assert that the soil in which food is grown is often

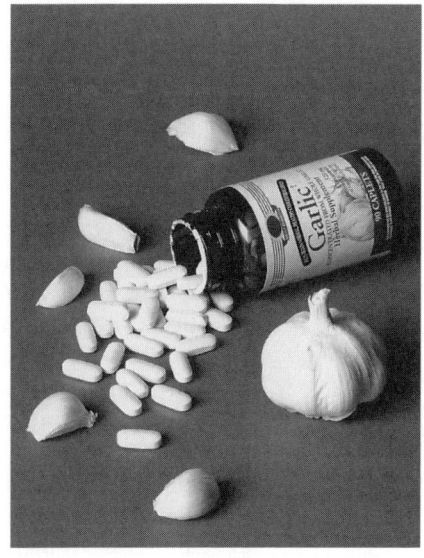

Garlic is frequently touted as a remedy for high blood pressure, blood sugar imbalances, and arterial plaque. Some advocates even claim that garlic can prevent or cure cancer. But according to the National Center for Complimentary and Alternative Medicine, although garlic may have some health benefits, its reputation as a miracle remedy is not supported by available research. *[Octane Photographic. Reproduced by permission.]*

cancer: uncontrolled cell growth

herbal: related to plants

> ## Patent Medicines
>
> The term "patent medicine" originated before the American Revolution, when members of European royal families granted "letters patent" allowing the use of their endorsements to advertise products. As patent medicines became increasingly popular during the nineteenth century, traveling "medicine shows," featuring musclemen and other entertainers, were organized to pitch products that were alleged to miraculously cure cancer, venereal disease, tuberculosis, cholera, leprosy, arthritis, or other ailments. The pitchmen touted their products' exotic origins (such as "Kickapoo Indian Sagwa," supposedly based on a Native American recipe) or their basis in scientific breakthroughs (such as "Bonnore's Electro Magnetic Bathing Fluid" and products containing radium and uranium). The medicines, which frequently combined narcotics such as cocaine in an alcohol base, were both toxic and addictive. During the early twentieth century, newspapers began to publicize the hazards of patent medicines. In 1906 Congress took the first steps toward outlawing the most fradulent and dangerous claims by passing the Pure Food and Drug Act, and in 1938 patent medicines were prohibited entirely.
>
> —*Paula Kepos*

vitamin: necessary complex nutrient used to aid enzymes or other metabolic processes in the cell

mineral: an inorganic (non-carbon-containing) element, ion or compound

heart disease: any disorder of the heart or its blood supply, including heart attack, atherosclerosis, and coronary artery disease

hypertension: high blood pressure

obesity: the condition of being overweight, according to established norms based on sex, age, and height

chronic: over a long period

nutritional deficiency: lack of adequate nutrients in the diet

diet: the total daily food intake, or the types of foods eaten

fortified: altered by addition of vitamins or minerals

nutrient: dietary substance necessary for health

processed food: food that has been cooked, milled, or otherwise manipulated to change its quality

fiber: indigestible plant material which aids digestion by providing bulk

food additive: substance added to foods to improve nutrition, taste, appearance or shelf-life

arthritis: inflammation of the joints

nutritionally depleted in **vitamins** and **minerals**, and that the food supply cannot, therefore, adequately nourish the population. However, very few individuals in industrially developed countries suffer from specific vitamin and mineral deficiencies. They are more likely to suffer from **heart disease**, **hypertension**, **obesity**, and other **chronic** diseases. In lesser-developed countries, deficiencies are due to inadequate food intake. **Nutritional deficiencies** can be corrected with a well-balanced **diet**. In addition, most manufactured products are **fortified** with specific vitamins and minerals. The body recognizes and utilizes these **nutrients** as effectively as the ones sold in health food stores, though **processed foods** can be lacking in other nutrients, such as **fiber**.

Another claim is that **food additives** and pesticide residues are poisoning the food supply. This claim is usually used to promote organic and other "health" foods. The United States government has very strict standards for the use of additives, preservatives, and pesticide residues. The United States Department of Agriculture has approved standards for organic foods, but it makes no claim that organic foods are safer or more nutritious than conventionally grown foods.

Victims

Quacks primarily target older adults, the health conscious, the beauty conscious, and those with chronic diseases such as cancer and AIDS. Older people have more chronic illnesses than younger people, so they are likely targets for fraud. Most people are susceptible to quackery because they are frightened, in pain, and desperate for relief. Common products that are targeted to these populations include:

- *Anti-aging products.* In a youth-oriented society, a wide variety of products are advertised. No product can stop the aging process, however, and any "results" that are seen are temporary.

- *Arthritis remedies.* There is no cure for most forms of arthritis, but some products can temporarily reduce pain and increase flexibility.

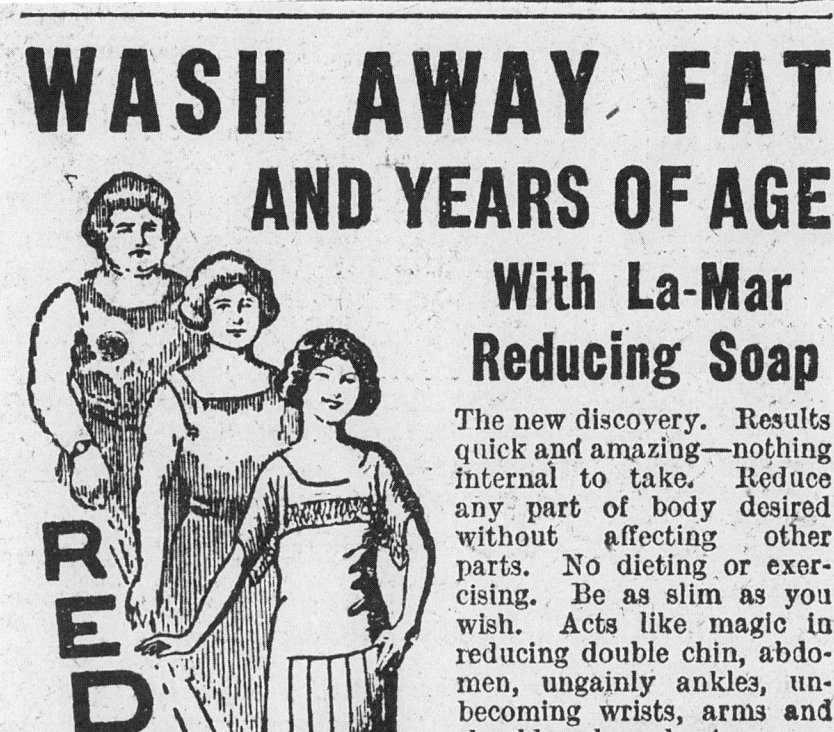

A 1920s advertisement for weight-loss soap promises quick, painless results and offers a money-back guarantee. Both claims are frequently made by quacks about the fraudulent health products or services they sell. [Bettmann/Corbis. Reproduced by permission.]

- *Cancer cures.* Quacks prey on people's fear of cancer. Cancer treatment is specific for the type of cancer, and common treatments include surgery, radiation, and chemotherapy. Some cancers go into remission and reappear later. No food or supplements have been proven to "cure" cancer.
- *HIV/AIDS cures.* There is no known cure for this disease. Legitimate scientific treatments can, however, extend life and improve the quality of life for people with AIDS.

Quackery is big business. Individuals spend billions of dollars every year looking for the next miracle cure. Consumers must learn to protect themselves by questioning what they see or hear in ads. The media that promote these products usually do not regularly screen their ads for truth or accuracy. Prescription **drugs** undergo rigorous testing for safety and effectiveness before they are sold, and **over-the-counter** medicines also are subject to a drug review process. Dietary supplements are not required to undergo government testing or review before they are marketed, yet these products may have harmful effects that could present risks for people on certain

drugs: substances whose administration causes a significant change in the body's function

over-the-counter: available without a prescription

medicines or with certain medical conditions. Individuals who are aware of a questionable health product can contact the Federal Trade Commission or their state attorney general's office. SEE ALSO ALTERNATIVE MEDICINES AND THERAPIES; CANCER; DIETARY SUPPLEMENTS; FAD DIETS; HIV/AIDS; WEIGHT LOSS DIETS.

Delores C. S. James

Internet Resources

National Institute on Aging. "Health Quackery: Spotting Health Scams." Available from <http://www.nia.nih.gov/health/agepages/healthqy.html/>

Barrett, Stephen. "Be Wary of Alternative Health Methods." Available from <http://www.quackwatch.org/01QuackeryRelatedTopics/altwary.html>

Federal Trade Commission. "Medical Health Claims: Add a Dose of Skepticism." Available from <http://www.ftc.gov/bcp/conline/pubs/health/frdheal.htm>

James Cook University, Multimedia and Print Services. "Pictures of Health: Quack and Quackery." Available from <http://www.maps.jcu.edu.au/hist/quack>

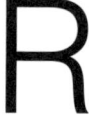

Recommended Dietary Allowances

Recommended Dietary Allowances: nutrient intake recommended to promote health

nutrient: dietary substance necessary for health

Dietary Reference Intakes: set of guidelines for nutrient intake

chronic: over a long period

The **Recommended Dietary Allowances** (RDAs) are **nutrient** intake levels that meet the needs of most healthy Americans. They were originally developed by the National Academy of Sciences, and were based on nutrient levels that would prevent nutrient deficiencies. Since the mid-1990s, RDAs have been developed as one component of nutrient intake standards called **Dietary Reference Intakes** (DRIs). RDAs, developed as part of DRIs, target nutrient levels needed not only to prevent nutrient deficiencies, but also to reduce the risk of **chronic** disease. They are meant to be intake goals averaged over several days, rather than daily requirements. RDAs can help people establish eating habits that promote health and reduce disease risk. SEE ALSO DIETARY REFERENCE INTAKE (DRI); NATIONAL ACADEMY OF SCIENCES (NAS).

Linda Benjamin Bobroff

Bibliography

Insel, Paul; Turner, R. Elaine; and Ross, Don (2001). *Nutrition*. Sudbury, MA: Jones and Bartlett.

National Research Council (1989). *Recommended Dietary Allowances*, 10th edition. Washington, DC: National Academy Press.

Internet Resources

U.S. Department of Agriculture. "Dietary Reference Intakes (DRI) and Recommended Dietary Allowances (RDA)." Available from <http://www.nal.usda.gov/fnic>

Refugee Nutrition Information System

Every year, thousands of individuals are displaced from their homes and homelands because of wars, political conflicts, and natural disasters. The Refugee Nutrition Information System (RNIS) was established in 1993 to collect data and report on the nutrition, health, and survival status of the most nutritionally vulnerable people in the world, including refugees, internally displaced populations, and those who are forced to migrate.

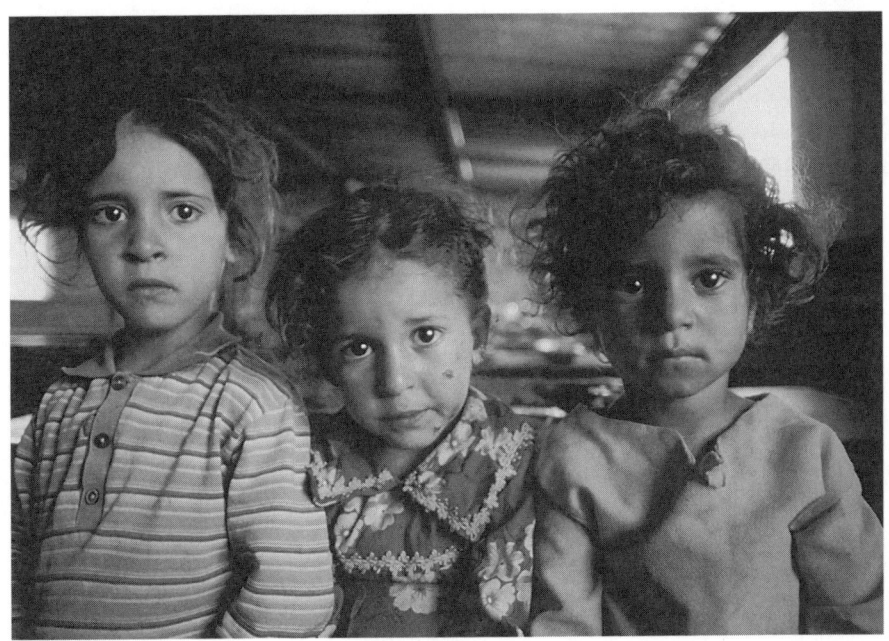

These girls are among more than four million Palestinian refugees in Gaza Strip and the West Bank. A recent report from the Refugee Nutrition Information System found Palestinian refugees to be satisfactorily coping with the nutritional impacts of the latest Intifada. *[Corbis. Reproduced by permission.]*

The RNIS publication, *Report on the Nutrition Situation of Refugees and Displaced Populations,* is published every three months, with interim updates as needed. The United Nations (UN) Administration Committee on Coordination Sub Committee on Nutrition (ACC/SCN) compiles this report. Information is obtained from a variety of UN agencies and nongovernmental organizations.

The report focuses primarily on sub-Saharan Africa, with some information provided on Asia. The report gives an estimate of the total number of refugees and displaced persons, and of the returning population, broken down by risk category. Refugees and displaced populations are classified by country of origin and country of asylum. The report also shows trends over time in total numbers and risk categories.

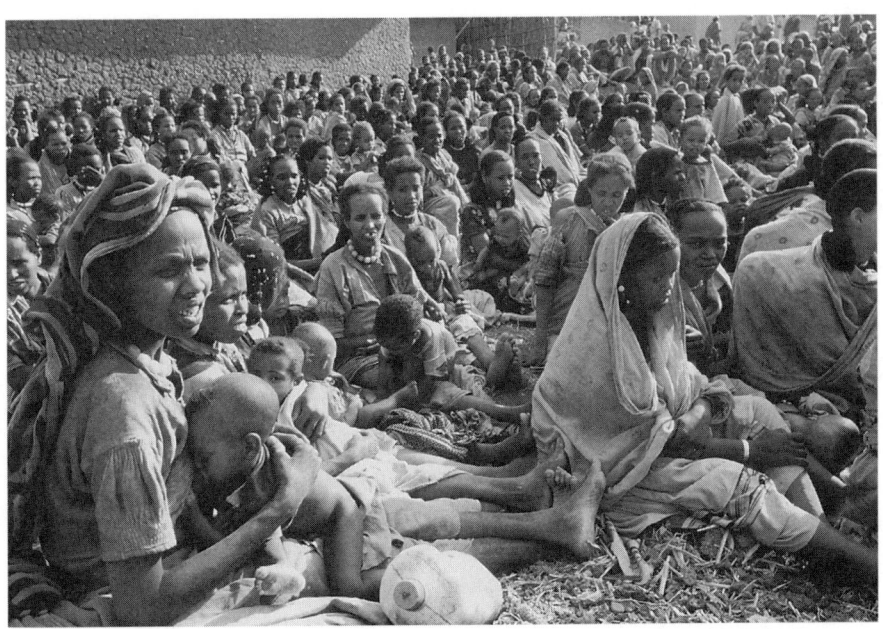

These refugees were displaced by years of warfare in their own countries. In the 1980s they came to Sudan from Ethiopia and Chad, only to find a famine awaiting them. *[Photograph by Chris Rainier. Chris Rainier/Corbis-Bettmann. Reproduced by permission.]*

The report is organized by "situation," a category that crosses national boundaries, and it includes a section that highlights the most pressing humanitarian needs. Recommendations are made by agencies or individuals directly involved in assessments or humanitarian response. Nutritional surveys are used to assess populations that are in a critical situation. Populations at high risk are identified either on the basis of indicators that are approaching crisis levels or through subjective information collected when security and logistical issues prevent rigorous data collection. SEE ALSO DISASTER RELIEF ORGANIZATIONS.

Delores C. S. James

Internet Resources

United Nations (2000). "About RNIS." Available from <http://www.unsystem.org/accscn/page6.html>

World Health Organization. "Nutrition in Emergencies." Available from <http://www.who.int/nut/index.htm>

Regional Diet, American

It is quite clear that nutritional intake is associated with common health conditions such as **obesity**, **hypertension** (**high blood pressure**), **cancer**, **diabetes** (high blood sugar), and **cardiovascular** disease. People in the United States make daily decisions related to grocery purchases, meal choices, food preparation, and other factors influencing their consumption of food and **nutrients**, and, thus, likely affecting their health. However, much of the current knowledge and most published works are based on studies or other information that concern the general population. This information is important in influencing dietary patterns, but additional information is needed regarding specific regional and minority populations. Additionally, more detailed information is necessary to determine if there are any differences or similarities between these subpopulations. What follows is a general literature review related to minority groups in the United States.

African-American Influences

As might be surmised, the daily **diet** can be greatly influenced by cultural variables related to a specific ethnic group, as well as differences within an ethnic group. The **socioeconomic status** of a group is also relevant when considering decisions about dietary intake.

The **prevalence** of hypertension, cardiovascular disease, and diabetes is greater among African Americans than other groups. Dietary intake has been strongly associated with both of these conditions for many years. Therefore, it seems prudent to focus on diet in an attempt to reduce the number of premature disabilities and deaths as the result of these conditions.

However, the researchers Christian Lindquist, Barbara Gower, and Michael Goran found that African-American children and white children had similar dietary intake patterns. The small differences in consumption were found to be more favorable for African-American children. The researchers found, for example, that African-American children ate more fruits and vegetables than white children. Both groups, however, do not meet the national

obesity: the condition of being overweight, according to established norms based on sex, age, and height

high blood pressure: elevation of the pressure in the bloodstream maintained by the heart

cancer: uncontrolled cell growth

diabetes: inability to regulate level of sugar in the blood

cardiovascular: related to the heart and circulatory system

nutrient: dietary substance necessary for health

diet: the total daily food intake, or the types of foods eaten

socioeconomic status: level of income and social class

prevalence: describing the number of cases in a population at any one time

> ### U.S. Regional Cooking
>
> Regional cuisine in the United States has been influenced by the ingredients native to each region as well as by the culinary heritage of the groups that first settled there. Characteristic ingredients of New England cooking include seafood, cranberries, rhubarb, and apples. Heavily influenced by British settlers, cooking techniques in New England rely on roasting and boiling to produce such dishes as clam chowder, baked beans, and salt cod. The Southern states were influenced by French, English, and Spanish colonists and by African slaves, who often served as household cooks and who introduced okra, black-eyed peas, and eggplant to the menu. The region is fertile ground for rice, which is featured in the classic Southern rice pudding; other typical dishes include fried green tomatoes, squash casserole, fried chicken, cornbread, and grits. The Midwest is known for corn, beef, and dairy products, and the region's cooking techniques reflect the influence of German and Scandinavian settlers. Traditional dishes include beef pot roast, bratwurst, sauerkraut, and corn on the cob. In the Southwest, where Spanish and Mexican influences predominate, typical ingredients include chiles, cumin, cinnamon, tortillas, and tomatoes. Barbecuing is the best-known cooking technique, and common dishes include chili, burritos, flan, and other Tex-Mex interpretations of Mexican cooking. The Pacific Northwest is known for seafood, game, and berries. Dishes identified with the Pacific Northwest include salmon, venison, pumpkin soup, and gooseberry relish.
>
> —*Paula Kepos*

standards for recommended daily intake. African-American children have a lower **insulin** sensitivity and higher **acute** insulin response than white children, suggesting a higher risk of diabetes.

Socioeconomic status (SES) has been connected to diabetes. African-American women are more likely to be diabetic if they have low SES. This association was not found to be evident in African-American men, however. While it is possible that a condition such as diabetes causes a reduction in or loss of income, and thus has a negative impact on SES, there is little evidence to support this theory.

Diets with a high **fat** content have been associated with various cancers. Brown and colleagues found that African Americans have higher frequency of being **overweight** and **obese** (20 percent or more above the recommended weight), while Caucasians use more vitamin C supplements. This may explain part of the higher **incidence** of multiple myeloma, a type of cancer, in African Americans. It is also congruent with literature that suggests vitamin C consumption may decrease the risk of some cancers.

African Americans generally have greater rates of hypertension and the associated complications, such as cerebrovascular accidents (**strokes**) and renal (kidney) disease. In 1996, Frederick Brancati and colleagues found that potassium supplements reduce **blood pressure** in African Americans who eat foods low in potassium. This phenomenon could be due to a distinct sensitivity to potassium, or because the diets are low in potassium, or a combination of both.

From a sociological standpoint, Kaja Perina reported in 2001 that African-American television stations show more food (especially junk food) and beverage commercials during prime time than other stations. To compound the emphasis on weight management, Perina highlights that 27 percent of

insulin: hormone released by the pancreas to regulate level of sugar in the blood

acute: rapid-onset and short-lived

fat: type of food molecule rich in carbon and hydrogen, with high energy content

overweight: weight above the accepted norm based on height, sex, and age

obese: above accepted standards of weight for sex, height, and age

incidence: number of new cases reported each year

stroke: loss of blood supply to part of the brain, due to a blocked or burst artery in the brain

blood pressure: measure of the pressure exerted by the blood against the walls of the blood vessels

nutrition: the maintenance of health through proper eating, or the study of same

calorie: unit of food energy

vitamin: necessary complex nutrient used to aid enzymes or other metabolic processes in the cell

energy: technically, the ability to perform work; the content of a substance that allows it to be useful as a fuel

calcium: mineral essential for bones and teeth

protein: complex molecule composed of amino acids that performs vital functions in the cell; necessary part of the diet

iron: nutrient needed for red blood cell formation

cholesterol: multi-ringed molecule found in animal cell membranes; a type of lipid

actors on African American networks are overweight, compared to 2 percent of actors on other networks.

Another obstacle to satisfactory daily **nutrition** may be the inability to access ethnic foods in the inner city. Monique Brown suggests that quality comprehensive grocery stores are frequently missing from African American communities. Instead, smaller convenience marts provide limited foods and goods, severely limiting dietary choices, in addition to being more expensive than supermarkets.

The elderly population in the United States does not regularly follow dietary recommendations. Typically, not enough **calories** are consumed, as well as inadequate amounts of some **vitamins** and nutrients. Insufficient income, disability, inadequate knowledge, and lack of transportation contribute to poor dietary habits. The diets of elderly African Americans have been found to be deficient in **energy**, **calcium**, and vitamin B_6, **protein**, thiamine, riboflavin, and **iron**. Black men tend to consume more energy, fat, and **cholesterol** than black women, but less vitamins C, B_6, and thiamine.

Hispanic Influences

Mexican-American children who participated in a San Diego study related to children's activity and nutrition were more likely than non-Hispanic white children to be overweight, to eat more fat, and to exercise less. Those who watched more television were more likely to consume excess fat. However, children who ate less sodium were more knowledgeable about food and more likely to avoid fat consumption. Study participants who were identified as being in lower socioeconomic levels tended to consume more sodium. Accordingly, education has been a valuable tool in behavior modification programs for a variety of different target areas related to health.

Likewise, there is some evidence that Mexican-American children over fifteen years of age have smaller statures, but weigh more, than white children. This may have a negative effect on future health risks related to diabetes, cancer, and cardiovascular disease.

The economics of a family greatly influence choices related to food intake. If one family of four allocates $150 per week for groceries and another budgets $100, there is a wide disparity in the quantity of food eaten by these two families. Economically disadvantaged Hispanics in twelve counties in southern Colorado were found to focus on their children's nutritional habits and on avenues to preparing quick, healthy menus. Socioeconomic status and geographic isolation due to the mountains have a negative effect on the food availability of this cultural group, who frequently earn a living as migrant farm workers. Barriers to changing eating habits included lack of finances, limited education and cooking abilities, customs, and confusion related to communication from nutrition professionals.

Research by Judith A. Beto, Gopali Sheth, and Patricia Rewers suggests that a broad supply of basic foods are readily available to low-income families. For example, sugar, flour, eggs, pasta, and vegetables are commonly eaten by such families. However, the way in which the food is prepared varies, accounting for a wide difference in fat consumption. This data implies that education related to healthful food preparation can assist in reducing fat intake.

In addition to studies that investigate the Hispanic population in general, there are also some reports concentrating on nutrition that investigate individual sectors of this population. Indeed, researchers Carlos Crespo, Catherine Loria, and Vicki Burt note that Hispanics have lower or equal rates of hypertension, but higher prevalence rates of obesity and diabetes than non-Hispanic whites. Hispanic females appear to have increased awareness of treatment and control of hypertension than Hispanic males. In addition, Cuban-American women were more aware of their hypertensive state than Mexican-American and Puerto Rican females. The vast majority of Hispanic men with high blood pressure do not keep it under control. Moreover, Mexican-American and Puerto Rican women have higher rates of being overweight than other female and male Hispanics. In addition, people who are overweight are commonly diagnosed with hypertension.

Food purchasing practices also affect dietary intake. Geoffrey Paulin found that there are differences in the purchasing power of Hispanics compared to other groups, as well as within the subpopulations of the general group. Hispanics only have about two-thirds the income of non-Hispanics, and they are more likely to have participated in a food stamp program. Furthermore, Hispanics have fewer years of education and are less likely to live in rural areas. Hispanics usually purchase more meats, fruits, and vegetables than non-Hispanics, while purchasing fewer potatoes, sweets, and dairy products. This food purchasing pattern may reflect the origin of certain immigrant groups. For example, citrus fruits are commonly grown in Mexico, and bananas are grown in Central and South America. It is also noted that Hispanics spend less on snack foods, such as potato chips, candy, and cakes, and may view these foods as unnecessary or as a luxury.

There are also important differences within the specific Hispanic population. For example, Cubans spend twice as much money on coffee as Mexicans do. Such spending differences suggest that consumption habits are also different within Hispanic subpopulations.

There may also be changes in diets as the result of relocation. For example, Laura McArthur, Ruben Anguiano, and Diego Nocetti studied Hispanic immigrants in North Carolina who had resided in the United States for 10 years or less. They found that these immigrants did not generally maintain their dietary habits. Children were found to be greatly influenced by school meals. Foods high in fat and sugar were consumed in larger quantities than in the countries of origin of these immigrants. This type of change due to relocation is known as *acculturation* and is common in immigrant groups.

The need for continued research related to dietary intake patterns and influences is apparent. The majority of studies have historically investigated dietary behavior within the general population. However, it appears that cultural differences can affect the daily diet, and, thus, impact certain health conditions. SEE ALSO DIETARY TRENDS, AMERICAN.

Katherine E. W. Will

Bibliography

Beto, Judith A.; Sheth, Gopali; and Rewers, Patricia (1997). "Assessing Food Purchase Behavior among Low-Income Black and Hispanic Clients Using a Self-Reported Shelf Inventory." *Journal of American Dietetic Association* 97(1):69–70.

Brancati, Frederick L.; Appel, Lawrence J.; Seidler, Alexander J.; and Whelton, P. K. (1996). "Effect of Potassium Supplementation on Blood Pressure in African Americans on a Low-Potassium Diet." *Archives of Internal Medicine* 156(1):61–67.

Brown, Linda M.; Gridley, Gloria; Pottern, Linda; et al. (2001). "Diet and Nutrition as Risk Factors for Multiple Myeloma among Blacks and Whites in the United States." *Cancer Causes and Control* 12(2):117–125.

Brown, Monique R. (1999). "Supermarket Blackout: There Are Few Supermarkets in Cities, Meaning That Blacks Pay More for Food, Lose Out on Jobs and Go Elsewhere for Quality Goods." *Black Enterprise* 29(12): 81–94.

Cohen, Nancy L.; Ralston, Penny A.; Laus, Mary J.; et al. (1998). "Food Practices, Service Use, and Dietary Quality in Elderly Blacks." *Journal of Nutrition for the Elderly* 17(4):17–34.

Crespo, Carlos J.; Loria, Catherine M.; and Burt, Vicki L. (1996). "Hypertension and Other Cardiovascular Disease Risk Factors among Mexican Americans, Cuban Americans, and Puerto Ricans from the Hispanic Health and Nutrition Examination Survey." *Public Health Reports*, 3(2):7–10.

Lindquist, Christine H.: Gower, Barbara A.; and Goran, Michael I. (2000). "Role of Dietary Factors in Ethnic Differences in Early Risk of Cardiovascular Disease and Type 2 Diabetes." *American Journal of Clinical Nursing* 71(3):725–732.

McArthur, Laura H.; Anguiano, Ruben P; and Nocetti Diego (2001). "Maintenance and Change in the Diet of Hispanic Immigrants in Eastern North Carolina." *Family and Consumer Sciences Journal* 29(4):307–335.

Palmeri, Denise; Auld, Gary W.; Taylor, T.; et al. (1998). "Multiple Perspectives on Nutrition Education Needs of Low-Income Hispanics." *Journal of Community Health* 23(4):301-316.

Paulin, Geoffrey D. (2001). "Variation in Food Purchases: A Study of Inter-Ethnic and Intra-Ethnic Group Patterns Involving the Hispanic Community." *Family and Consumer Sciences Research Journal* 29(4):336–381.

Perina, Kaja (2001). "Obesity: Watch What You Watch." *Psychology Today* 34(5):32.

Robbins, Jessica; Vaccarino, Viola; Zhang, Heping; and Kasl, Stanislav V. (2001). "Socioeconomic Status and Type 2 Diabetes in African American and Non-Hispanic White Women and Men: Evidence from the Third National Health and Nutrition Examination Survey." *American Journal of Public Health* 91(1):76–83.

Ryan, Alan. S.; Roche, Alex F.; and Kuczmarski, Robert J. (1999). "Weight, Stature, and Body Mass Index Data for Mexican Americans from the Third National Health and Nutrition Examination Survey (NHANES III, 1988–1994)." *American Journal of Human Biology* 11:673–686.

Zive, Michelle M.; Frank-Spohrer, Gail C.; Sallis, James F.; et al. (1998). "Determinants of Dietary Intake in a Sample of White and Mexican-American Children." *Journal of American Dietetic Association* 98(11):1282–1289.

Regulatory Agencies

At the beginning of the twenty-first century, increased levels of terrorist activities and a higher **incidence** of food-borne illness made regulation and protection of the food supply a worldwide concern. The goal of food regulatory agencies is to ensure that the public food supply is safe from disease caused by infection from human handling or by contamination from chemical or other hazardous substances. Such contamination can occur during all phases of food production, including cultivation, harvesting, processing, packaging, storage, and cooking.

United States Agencies

In the United States, the regulation and safety of the food supply has received attention since the mid-nineteenth century. Today, many of the U.S. federal agencies serve as regulators or advisors for the food supply in the United States and throughout the world. There are four major U.S. federal agencies involved in food regulation and safety.

incidence: number of new cases reported each year

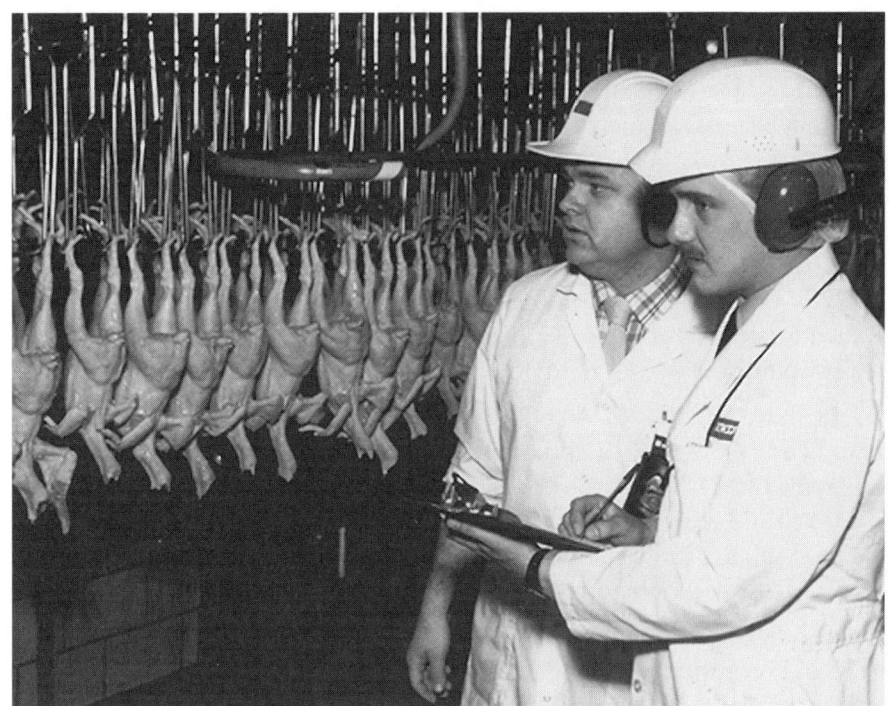

USDA staff working in the Food Safety and Inspection Service inspect more than eight billion birds annually. They ensure that raw meats are processed according to health standards, and help prevent and investigate outbreaks of food-borne illness. [USDA. Reproduced by permission.]

The U.S. Department of Agriculture (USDA) is the oldest federal agency that monitors the food supply in the United States; it was established in 1862 by President Abraham Lincoln. In its earlier years, the agency worked with farmers, who were the country's main source of food. Today, the mission of the USDA includes a goal that ensures people a safe, affordable, nutritious, and accessible food supply. USDA accomplishes this goal through the administration of a variety of food-related programs, all of which either assist suppliers or protect consumers.

Consumers are protected by USDA programs that regulate and monitor soil, water, and wildlife on privately owned property; drinking water for rural Americans; and meat, poultry, and egg products for all Americans. Federal antihunger efforts, such as the Food Stamp Program, the National School Lunch Program, the School Breakfast Program, and the Special Supplemental Nutrition Program for Women, Infants, and Children (WIC) also serve a regulatory purpose by providing recipients access to safe food products. Other USDA services include programs for food suppliers, such as small-business owners and farmers, who can receive assistance in growing and merchandising safe foods. The USDA also runs the Food and Nutrition Information Center, which provides information to the public on a variety of topics related to food safety and healthy food choices.

The Food and Drug Administration (FDA) is an operating division of the U.S. Department of Health and Human Services (DHHS). While the responsibility of DHHS is to protect the overall health of Americans, the FDA has a more specialized role in the oversight of food, **drugs**, and related products. The FDA was established after the passage of the Pure Food and Drugs Act of 1906. This act was the first nationwide consumer protection law, and it made the distribution of misbranded or adulterated foods, drinks, and drugs across state lines illegal. Today, the FDA is mandated by federal law to protect public health by ensuring the safety of the

drugs: substances whose administration causes a significant change in the body's function

food additive: substance added to foods to improve nutrition, taste, appearance or shelf-life

production, processing, packaging, storing, and holding of all domestic and imported foods, except for those products that are under the jurisdiction of the U.S. Department of Agriculture. FDA is also responsible for safeguarding all ingredients used in food products, approving new **food additives**, monitoring ingredients and foods to see that they are contaminant free, and monitoring dietary supplements, infant formulas, and medical foods for safety. The FDA oversees food labeling and requires that food product labels be informative, truthful, and useful to the consumer. The Hazard Analysis Critical Control Point (HACCP) system, one of the most well-known food safety monitoring programs in use today in the United States, is also sponsored by the FDA.

In July 2003, the FDA submitted a ten-point program to DHHS that would ensure the safety and security of the nation's food supply. Under this program, the FDA will work with the Department of Homeland Security (DHS) to add more staff, develop bioterrorism regulations, assess threats to the food supply, and train food service workers and the public in emergency preparedness and how to respond to a crisis.

Another operating division of DHHS is the Centers for Disease Control and Prevention (CDC). Established in 1946, the CDC collaborates with state agencies, private organizations, and other federal agencies such as the FDA, the Environmental Protection Agency (EPA), and the USDA to provide credible health information, primarily in the area of disease prevention. CDC's Food Safety Initiative Activity focuses solely on the prevention of food-borne illness by improving systems for disease surveillance and outbreak response, as well as through research, training, and education.

environment: surroundings

The Environmental Protection Agency (EPA) is a separate agency dedicated to the regulation of pesticide usage and the establishment of water quality standards for the United States. The agency has been in existence since 1970 and it develops and enforces regulations that implement federal laws written to protect the **environment**. The agency accomplishes this by collaborating with the states and Native American tribes, which have been given the responsibility for monitoring and enforcing compliance, and by issuing sanctions if the regulations are not followed. The EPA also provides financial assistance to states, nonprofit organizations, educational institutions, and small businesses to support research, education, and public awareness programs. Voluntary efforts, cosponsored by industries, businesses, nonprofit organizations, and state and local governments can also receive assistance from the EPA.

Worldwide Agencies

Although not a regulator in the truest sense, the World Health Organization (WHO) establishes policy and makes recommendations regarding the safety of the world food supply through its Food Safety Department (FOS). A primary focus of the FOS is the reduction of the negative impact of food-borne disease worldwide. Recently, a resolution was adopted by WHO to recognize food safety as an essential public health function, and to develop a global strategy to reduce the burden of food-borne diseases. Because the responsibility for food safety is often divided among several agencies with overlapping authority, there have been many challenges in solving the problems of worldwide food-borne disease. To address these challenges, the FOS is developing an integrated production-to-consumption approach to food safety for its 192 member states. The approach is patterned after the FDA-sponsored HACCP program.

Other activities of the FOS include monitoring food, air, and water-supply pollution; observing food manufacturing and processing for the presence of additives and contaminants; conducting research on the safety of genetically modified foods; amassing larger food and supply inventories for countries to access in times of disaster; and assisting with the management of malicious contamination of food for terrorist purposes.

Other international agencies include:

- The Food and Agriculture Organization of the United Nations (FAO)
- The World Health Organization (WHO)
- The Codex Alimentarius Commission
- European Union Food Safety Policy Committee
- The World Food Safety Organization.

In conclusion, various aspects of the U.S. food supply are monitored by the USDA, FDA, CDC, and EPA. These federal agencies collaborate with state and local governments, as well as with nonprofit organizations, private businesses, and individuals to oversee the safety of the food supply for the United States. While each of these agencies also works with foreign countries to assist in the quest for a safe food supply worldwide, the WHO functions in a policymaking capacity for its 192 members, and provides a greater overall international presence in this effort. The importance of securing the safety and security of food for all countries of the world will continue to be of great importance, as commerce becomes more global and more new products are introduced through bioengineering and other means. The regulation and monitoring of the continuum from grower to consumer will require a great deal of collaboration among all countries of the world in order to be successful. SEE ALSO FOOD SAFETY; HEALTH CLAIMS.

Claire D. Schmelzer

Internet Resources

Centers for Disease Control and Prevention. "About CDC." Available from <http://www.cdc.gov/>

Centers for Disease Control and Prevention. "Food Safety Office." Available from <http://www.cdc.gov/foodsafety>

U.S. Department of Agriculture. "Welcome to the United States Department of Agriculture." Available from <http://www.usda.gov/>

U.S. Department of Agriculture, National Agriculture Library. "Food and Nutrition Information Center." Available from <http://www.nal.usda.gov/fnic/>

U.S. Department of Health and Human Services. "HHS: What We Do." Available from <http://www.hhs.gov/>

U.S. Environmental Protection Agency. "About EPA." Available from <http://www.epa.gov/>

U.S. Food and Drug Administration. "About the U.S. Food and Drug Administration." Available from <http://www.fda.gov/>

U.S. Food and Drug Administration (2003). "Progress Report to Secretary Tommy G. Thompson: Ensuring the Safety and Security of the Nation's Food Supply." Available from <http://www.fda.gov/>

U.S. Food and Drug Administration, Center for Food Safety and Applied Nutrition. "Hazard Analysis Critical Control Point." Available from <http://www.cfsan.fda.gov/>

World Health Organization. "Food Safety." Available from http://www.who.int/foodsafety/en/>

Religion and Dietary Practices

Since the beginning of time, dietary practices have been incorporated into the religious practices of people around the world. Some religious sects abstain, or are forbidden, from consuming certain foods and drinks; others restrict foods and drinks during their holy days; while still others associate dietary and food preparation practices with **rituals** of the faith. The early biblical writings, especially those found in Leviticus, Numbers, and Deuteronomy of the Old Testament (and in the Torah) outlined the dietary practices for certain groups (e.g., Christians and Jews), and many of these practices may still be found among these same groups today. Practices such as fasting (going without food and/or drink for a specified time) are described as tenets of faith by numerous religions.

Religious Belief Expressed as Food Customs

To understand the reasons for nutritional and dietary customs in any religion requires a brief orientation of the rationale for such practices and laws. Many religious customs and laws may also be traced to early concerns for health and safety in consuming foods or liquids. In the past, preservation techniques for food were limited. Modern conveniences such as electricity were unavailable, and the scholars of the day did not understand theories of health promotion, disease prevention, and illness as they do today.

Therefore, religious leaders of the day developed rules about the consumption of foods and drinks, and religious practices, restrictions, and laws evolved. Specific laws about what can be consumed remain in most religions today. The lack of mechanisms to refrigerate or preserve foods led to certain rituals, such as the draining of blood from slaughtered animals, while restrictions on the eating of foods known to spoil easily, such as eggs, dairy products, and meats, were devised for safety reasons.

Attention to specific eating practices, such as overeating (gluttonous behaviors), use of strong drink or oral stimulants, and vegetarian diets, were also incorporated into the doctrine of religious practice. In addition to laws about the ingestion of foods or drinks, the practice of fasting, or severely restricting intake of food and/or drink, became prevalent, and is still practiced by many religions today.

The Role of Fasting

Many religions incorporate some element of fasting into their religious practices. Laws regarding fasting or restricting food and drink have been described as a call to holiness by many religions. Fasting has been identified as the mechanism that allows one to improve one's body (often described as a "temple" created by God), to earn the approval of Allah or Buddha, or to understand and appreciate the sufferings of the poor.

Fasting has also been presented as a means to acquire the discipline required to resist temptation, as an act of atonement for sinful acts, or as

ritual: ceremony or frequently repeated behavior

the cleansing of evil from within the body. Fasting may be undertaken for several hours, at a specified time of the day (e.g., from sunrise to sunset, as practiced by modern Jews), for a specified number of hours (e.g., twelve, twenty-four, or more, as observed by Catholics or Mormons who fast on designated days), or for consecutive days, such as during the month of Ramadan for certain Muslims. Regardless of the time frame or rationale, religious groups observe the practice of fasting worldwide.

Health Benefits and Risks Associated with Specific Practices

Certain groups of people must necessarily be excused from fasting and restrictive practices. These groups include pregnant or nursing women; individuals with **diabetes** or other **chronic** disorders; those engaged in very strenuous work; **malnourished** individuals; young children; and frail elderly or disabled persons. Recognition of these exceptions has been addressed by each religious group. Most fasting practices allow certain intakes of liquid, particularly water. In fasting regimes where water is restricted, a danger of **dehydration** exists, and those fasting should be monitored.

diabetes: inability to regulate level of sugar in the blood

chronic: over a long period

malnourished: lack of adequate nutrients in the diet

dehydration: loss of water

Those who fast without liquids increase their risk of a number of health problems. Symptoms of dehydration include headache, dry mouth, **nausea**, fever, sleepiness, and, in extreme cases, coma. When these symptoms occur, it is important to end the fast or add water to the fast. Depending on the extent of the symptoms, ending the fast may be the only alternative. In severe dehydration cases, medical care should be sought as soon as possible to restore proper health.

nausea: unpleasant sensation in the gut that precedes vomiting

Some negative health consequences have been observed as a result of fasting practices, however, especially those carried out over longer periods, such as the Muslim fast during Ramadan. For example, excess acids can build up in the digestive system during a prolonged fast. This **gastric acidity** results in a sour taste in the mouth, a burning in the stomach, and other symptoms of illness.

gastric: related to the stomach

acidity: measure of the tendency of a molecule to lose hydrogen ions, thus behaving as an acid

The structure and outward appearance of each person's body is, in part, a reflection of the food and drink he or she consumes. All the organs of the body, as well as the skin, bones, muscles, and nerves, need **nutrition** to survive, regenerate, maintain function, and develop structural foundations. The vital organs, such as the liver, heart, brain, and kidneys, depend upon essential **nutrients** from food and drink to sustain life, increase strength, and improve health. Throughout life, the body constantly breaks down the food products that are ingested, using some components to rebuild the tissues that contribute to good health. Similarly, the body also disposes of the waste products of food through excretory processes or in storage centers (**fat** deposits, for instance) in the body.

nutrition: the maintenance of health through proper eating, or the study of same

nutrient: dietary substance necessary for health

fat: type of food molecule rich in carbon and hydrogen, with high energy content

The restriction of, or abstention from, certain foods may have a direct impact on the health of those engaged in such practices. Some effects have been found to be positive, as in the case of vegetarian diets, which are eaten by many Seventh-day Adventists, Hindus, Buddhists, and Rastafarians. Research results have documented a 50 percent reduction in **heart disease** and longer life expectancy in people who eat a well-planned vegetarian **diet**. There are a number of religious rationales for a vegetarian diet. According to the Book of Genesis in the Bible, humans were given a plant-based diet

heart disease: any disorder of the heart or its blood supply, including heart attack, atherosclerosis, and coronary artery disease

diet: the total daily food intake, or the types of foods eaten

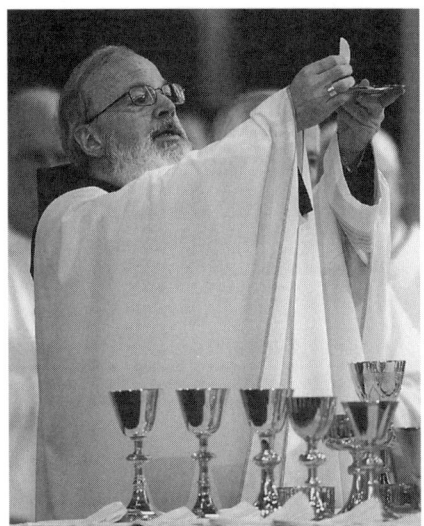

An archbishop leads communion at a Catholic mass. The importance of the ceremony, which calls for ritual consumption of bread and wine, shows how food traditions and religion have evolved together. *[Photograph by Stephen Senne. AP/Wide World Photos. Reproduced by permission.]*

nervous system: the brain, spinal cord, and nerves that extend throughout the body

physiology: the group of biochemical and physical processes that combine to make a functioning organism, or the study of same

drugs: substances whose administration causes a significant change in the body's function

malignant: spreading to surrounding tissues; cancerous

cancer: uncontrolled cell growth

high blood pressure: elevation of the pressure in the bloodstream maintained by the heart

proscription: prohibitions, rules against

wellness: related to health promotion

at the creation of the world. There are also ethical issues that involve the killing of animals for food, and environmental issues regarding the raising of livestock and the safety of the food supply.

Use of, and Abstention from, Stimulants

A stimulant is a product, food, or drink that excites the **nervous system** and changes the natural **physiology** of the body, such as **drugs** and consumable products that contain caffeine, such as tea, coffee, or chocolate. The use of caffeine is prohibited or restricted by many religions because of its addictive properties and harmful physical effects. Many also restrict spices and certain condiments, such as pepper, pickles, or foods with preservatives, because they are injurious by nature and flavor the natural taste and effect of foods.

The use of wine in religious ceremonies is regarded as acceptable by certain groups. For example, Roman Catholics, Eastern Orthodox Christians, and certain Protestant denominations use wine as a sacramental product to represent the blood of Christ in communion services. According to the writings of the apostle Paul, wine used in moderation may be consumed for the soothing effect it has upon an upset stomach. Mormons, however, specifically forbid wine or any alcoholic drinks because of their stimulant properties. Jews regard grapes as a fruit of idolatry, and therefore forbid the use of wine or products made from grapes except under special conditions.

Many religious leaders and health care experts regard tobacco, another stimulant, as a **malignant** poison that affects the health of its users. Research continues to support the harmful and deleterious effects of the use of cigarettes and tobacco products. **Cancer**, **high blood pressure**, and heart disease have all been linked to tobacco use.

Although marijuana has been shown to control pain in advanced diseases such as cancer, it has been considered a restricted drug by all but those practicing Rastafarianism. Rastafarians introduced marijuana into their religious rites because they consider it the "weed of wisdom," and because they believe it contains healing ingredients.

Major Religions with Food Proscriptions

Although no two religions hold exactly the same ideology about diet, health, and spiritual **wellness**, many do embrace similar practices.

Buddhism. Many Buddhists are vegetarians, though some include fish in their diet. Most do not eat meat and abstain from all beef products. The birth, enlightenment, and death of Buddha are the three most commonly recognized festivals for feasting, resting from work, or fasting. Buddhist monks fast completely on certain days of the moon, and they routinely avoid eating any solid foods after the noon hour.

Eastern Orthodox Christianity. An essential element of practicing an Orthodox life includes fasting, since its intrinsic value is part of the development of a spiritual life. To practicing Orthodox believers, fasting teaches self-restraint, which is the source of all good.

Hinduism. Hindus do not consume any foods that might slow down spiritual or physical growth. The eating of meat is not prohibited, but pork, fowl, ducks, snails, crabs, and camels are avoided. The cow is sacred to Hindus,

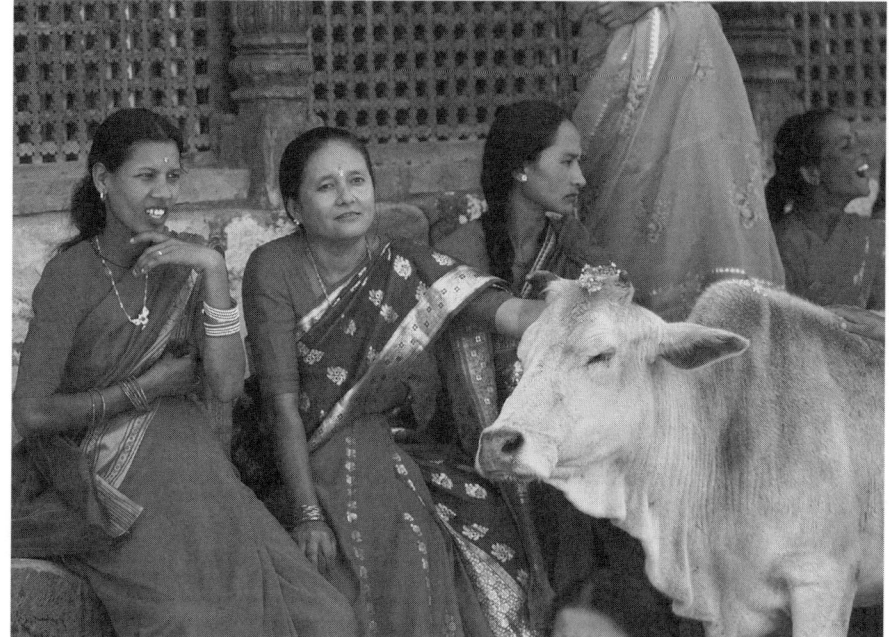

Many Hindus are strict vegetarians. Those who do eat meat are forbidden from eating beef, because cows occupy a sacred place in the Hindu religion. [Photograph by Craig Lovell. Corbis. Reproduced by permission.]

and therefore no beef is consumed. Other products from the cow, however, such as milk, yogurt, and butter are considered innately pure and are thought to promote purity of the mind, spirit, and body.

Many devout Hindus fast on the eighteen major Hindu holidays, as well as on numerous personal days, such as birthdays and anniversaries of deaths and marriages. They also fast on Sundays and on days associated with various positions of the moon and the planets.

Islam. To the Muslims, eating is a matter of faith for those who follow the dietary laws called *Halal*, a term for all permitted foods. Those foods that are prohibited, such as pork and birds of prey, are known as *Haram*, while the foods that are questionable for consumption are known as *Mashbooh*. Muslims eat to preserve their good health, and overindulgence or the use of stimulants such as tea, coffee, or alcohol are discouraged. Fasting is practiced regularly on Mondays and Thursdays, and more often for six days during Shawwal (the tenth month of the Islamic year) and for the entire month of Ramadan (the ninth month). Fasting on these occasions includes abstention from all food and drink from sunrise to sunset.

Judaism. The Jewish dietary law is called *Kashrut*, meaning "proper" or "correct." The term *kosher* refers to the methods of processing foods according to the Jewish laws. The processing laws and other restrictions regarding to the preparation of food and drink were devised for their effects on health. For example, rules about the use of pans, plates, utensils, and separation of meat from dairy products are intended to reduce contamination. Other rules include:

1. A Jewish person must prepare grape products, otherwise they are forbidden.
2. Jewish laws dictate the slaughter and removal of blood from meat before it can be eaten.
3. Animals such as pigs and rabbits and creatures of the sea, such as lobster, shrimp, and clams, may not be eaten.

Ramadan

In the Muslim faith, the holy month of Ramadan is the ninth month of the Islamic year and is devoted to prayer, fasting, and charity. Muslims believe that it was during this month that God first began to reveal the holy book of Islam, the Quran, to the prophet Muhammad. Most Muslims are required to refrain from food and drink during daylight hours for the entire month. The fast is broken in the evening by a meal called the *iftar,* which traditionally includes dates and water or sweet drinks, and is resumed again at sunrise. Fasting during Ramadan is one of the five Pillars of Faith, which are the most important religious duties in Islam. The practice is meant to remind Muslims of the poor, to cleanse the body, and to foster serenity and spiritual devotion. Ramadan ends with Eid al-Fitr, the "Festival of Breaking the Fast."

—Paula Kepos

4. Meat and dairy products cannot be eaten at the same meal or served on the same plate, and kosher and nonkosher foods cannot come into contact with the same plates.

Mormonism. The law of health—the Word of Wisdom—contains the laws for proper eating and the rules of abstinence for tobacco, alcohol, coffee, tea, chocolate, and illegal drugs. Mormons must choose foods that build up the body, improve endurance, and enhance intellect. Products from the land, such as grains, fruits, vegetables, and nuts, are to take the place of meats; meats, sugar, cheeses, and spices are to be avoided. Reason and self-control in eating is expected in order to stay healthy.

Rastafarianism. Members of this group are permitted to eat any food that is *I-tal* food, meaning that it is cooked only slightly. Therefore, meats are not consumed, canned goods are avoided, and drinks that are unnatural are not allowed. Fish under twelve inches long may be eaten, but other types of seafood are restricted.

Roman Catholicism. The dietary practices of devout Catholics center around the restriction of meat or fasting behaviors on specified holy days.

WORLD RELIGIONS, FOODS PRACTICES AND RESTRICTIONS, AND RATIONALE FOR BEHAVIOR

Type of religion	Practice or restriction	Rationale
Buddhism	• Refrain from meat, vegetarian diet is desirable • Moderation in all foods • Fasting required of monks	• Natural foods of the earth are considered most pure • Monks avoid all solid food after noon
Eastern Orthodox Christianity	• Restrictions on Meat and Fish • Fasting Selectively	• Observance of Holy Days includes fasting and restrictions to increase spiritual progress
Hinduism	• Beef prohibited • All other meat and fish restricted or avoided • Alcohol avoided • Numerous fasting days	• Cow is sacred and can't be eaten, but products of the "sacred" cow are pure and desirable • Fasting promotes spiritual growth
Islam	• Pork and certain birds prohibited • Alcohol prohibited • Coffee/tea/stimulants avoided • Fasting from all food and drink during specific periods	• Eating is for good health • Failure to eat correctly minimizes spiritual awareness • Fasting has a cleansing effect of evil elements
Judaism	• Pork and shellfish prohibited • Meat and dairy at same meal prohibited • Leavened food restricted • Fasting practiced	• Land animals that do not have cloven hooves and that do not chew their cud are forbidden as unclean (e.g., hare, pig, camel) • Kosher process is based upon the Torah
Mormonism	• Alcohol and beverages containing caffeine prohibited • Moderation in all foods • Fasting practiced	• Caffeine is addictive and leads to poor physical and emotional health • Fasting is the discipline of self-control and honoring to God
Protestants	• Few restrictions of food or fasting observations • Moderation in eating, drinking, and exercise is promoted	• God made all animal and natural products for humans' enjoyment • Gluttony and drunkenness are sins to be controlled
Rastafarianism	• Meat and fish restricted • Vegetarian diets only, with salts, preservatives, and condiments prohibited • Herbal drinks permitted; alcohol, coffee, and soft drinks prohibited • Marijuana used extensively for religious and medicinal purposes	• Pigs and shellfish are scavengers and are unclean • Foods grown with chemicals are unnatural and prohibited • Biblical texts support use of herbs (marijuana and other herbs)
Roman Catholicism	• Meat restricted on certain days • Fasting practiced	• Restrictions are consistent with specified days of the church year
Seventh-day Adventist	• Pork prohibited and meat and fish avoided • Vegetarian diet is encouraged • Alcohol, coffee, and tea prohibited	• Diet satisfies practice to "honor and glorify God"

On the designated days, Catholics may abstain from all food, or they may restrict meat and meat products. Water or nonstimulant liquids are usually allowed during the fast.

Seventh-day Adventists. The Seventh-day Adventist Church advocates a lacto-ovo vegetarian diet, including moderate amounts of low-fat dairy products and the avoidance of meat, fish, fowl, coffee, tea, alcohol, and toboaccoo products (though these are not strictly prohibited). The church's beliefs are grounded in the Bible, and in a "belief in the wholistic nature of people" (Seventh-day Adventist General Conference Nutrition Council).

While the dietary practices of different religions vary, and the rationale for each practice is based upon different texts, there is also much commonality. The practice of fasting is almost universal across religious groups, and most regard it as a mechanism to discipline the followers in a humbling way for spiritual growth. Many fasting practices are connected with specific holy days. The variation in consumption of meat and vegetables has a much wider variation. SEE ALSO EATING HABITS; FASTING.

Ruth A. Waibel

Bibliography

Brown, Linda Keller, and Mussell, Kay, eds. *Ethnic and Regional Foodways in the United States: The Performance of Group Identity.* Knoxville: University of Tennessee Press.

Desai, Anita (2000). *Fasting, Feasting.* New York: Houghton Mifflin.

Fishbane, Michael (1992). *The Garments of Torah: Essays in Biblical Hermaneutics.* Bloomington, MN: Indiana University Press.

Gordon, Lewis, ed. (1997). *Existence in Black: An Anthology of Black Existential Philosophy.* New York: Routledge.

Landman-Bouges, J. (1997). "Rastafarian Food Habits." *Cajanus* 9(4):228–234.

Siregar, Susan Rogers (1981). *Adat, Islam, and Christianity in a Batak Homeland.* Athens, OH: Center for International Studies at Ohio University.

Internet Resources

Church of Jesus Christ of the Latter-Day Saints. "The Word of Wisdom." Available from <http://www.mormon.org>

"Judaism 101." Available from <http://www.jewfaq.org>

Orthodox Christian Information Center. "Living an Orthodox Life." Available from <http://orthodoxinfo.com>

"The Rastafarian Religion." Available from <http://www.aspects.net/~nick/religions.html>

"Rastafarianism." Available from <http://hem1.passagen.se/perdavid/rastafar.htm>

Seventh-day Adventist General Conference Nutrition Council. "GCNC Position Statements." Available from <http://www.andrews.edu/NUFS/resources.html>

Rice-based Diets

Rice is the most important cereal crop for human consumption. It is the staple food for over 3 billion people (most of them poor) constituting over half of the world's population. All of the world's great civilizations developed only after the domestication of various cereal grains, which provided an adequate food supply for large populations. These have included corn in the Americas, wheat in the Near East and southern Europe (Greece and Rome), and rice in China and India. The use of rice spread rapidly from

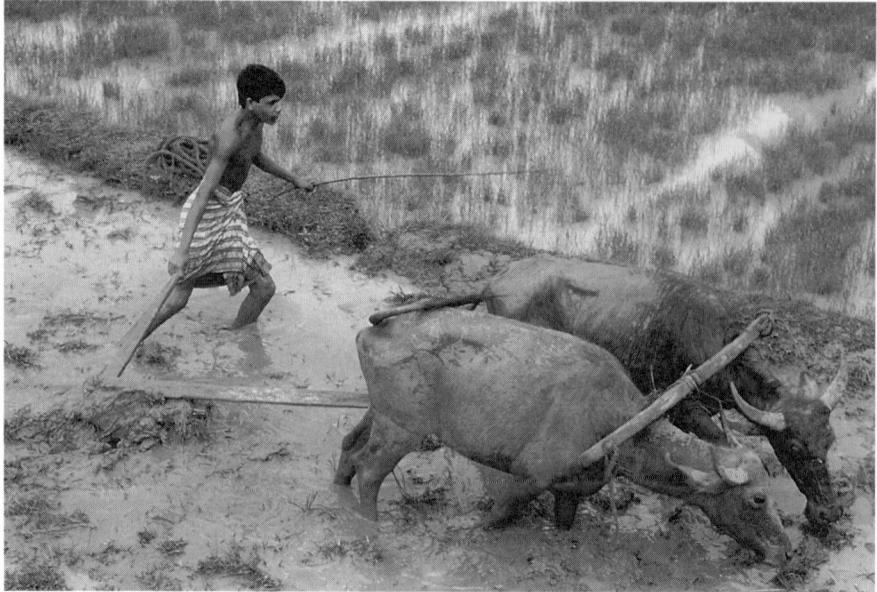

The people of Sri Lanka get about 40 percent of their calories from rice. Though rice is the most important crop in Sri Lanka, the per-capita consumption of imported wheat is increasing. *[Photograph by Tim Page. Corbis. Reproduced by permission.]*

China, India, and Africa, and at the present time it is used as a principal food throughout the world. After the discovery of the Americas, the use of rice took hold in both continents. The national dish of Belize in Central America, for example, is composed of rice and beans. There are now hundreds of rice recipes, with each ethnic cuisine having developed individual recipes. Almost all cookbooks have rice recipes, including recipes for risottos and pilafs. Vegetarians, in particular, cherish rice because it is such an excellent food and can be prepared in so many different and appetizing ways. Rice, delicious in itself, readily takes on any flavor that is added. Long-grain rice, when cooked, becomes separate and fluffy, while medium-grain rice is somewhat chewier. Short-grain rice tends to clump together and remains sticky with its starchy sauce. Arborio is an example of a short-grained rice. Wehani rice has a nutty flavor. Basmati rice (aromatic) is very popular, as is jasmine rice.

Rice is the only subsistence crop grown in soil that is poorly drained. It also requires no **nitrogen** fertilizer because soil microbes in the rice roots fix nitrogen and promote rice growth. Rice adapts itself to both wetlands and dry soil conditions.

Nutritional Properties

Rice is a high-carbohydrate food with 85 percent of the **energy** from carbohydrate, 7 percent from **fat**, and 8 percent from **protein**. However, rice also has a considerable amount of protein, with an excellent spectrum of **amino acids**. The protein quality of rice (66%) is higher than that of whole wheat (53%) or corn (49%). Of the small amount of fat in brown rice, much is **polyunsaturated**. White rice is extremely low in fat content.

A cup of cooked rice has approximately 5 grams of protein, which is sufficient for growth and maintenance, provided that a person receives adequate **calories** to maintain body weight or to increase it, if full growth has not yet occurred. Asiatic children for whom rice is the chief food source have not developed protein deficiency disorders such as **kwashiorkor**, as have infants

nitrogen: essential element for plant growth

energy: technically, the ability to perform work; the content of a substance that allows it to be useful as a fuel

fat: type of food molecule rich in carbon and hydrogen, with high energy content

protein: complex molecule composed of amino acids that performs vital functions in the cell; necessary part of the diet

amino acid: building block of proteins, necessary dietary nutrient

polyunsaturated: having multiple double bonds within the chemical structure, thus increasing the body's ability to metabolize it

calorie: unit of food energy

kwashiorkor: severe malnutrition characterized by swollen belly, hair loss, and loss of skin pigment

THE NUTRITIONAL COMPOSITION OF ONE CUP OF COOKED RICE		
	Brown Rice	White Rice
Calories	218	266
Protein (grams)	4.5	5.0
Carbohydrate (g)	45.8	58.6
Fiber (g)	3.5	0.5
Fat (g)	1.6	0.4
Polyunsaturated fatty acids (g)	0.6	0.1
Cholesterol (mg)	0	0
Thiamin (mg)*	0.20	0.34**
Vitamin A	0	0

*Daily requirement of thiamin is 1.2 mg for an adult man
**Enriched or parboiled rice

that are fed corn or cassava as a chief staple after weaning. Growth and development are normal on a rice **diet**. Due to its easy digestibility, rice is a good transition food after the cessation of breast or formula feeding.

diet: the total daily food intake, or the types of foods eaten

Rice and Thiamine Deficiency

In Asiatic populations, rice has been, and still is, a main source of **nutrition**. Thiamine, or vitamin B_1, is contained in the outer husk and coating of the rice kernel. When the technology for polishing rice became available, people took to eating white rice in preference to brown rice, but that process removed thiamine, causing beriberi, or thiamine deficiency, in many people, as well as heart and nerve diseases.

nutrition: the maintenance of health through proper eating, or the study of same

Dutch physicians in Java and Japanese physicians particularly noted the occurrence of beriberi with **edema**, heart failure, **neuropathy**, and many deaths. Thiamine, of course, was an unknown substance at that time. The history of rice is of interest in illustrating how the technology to make a food more appetizing (i.e., white rice versus brown rice) led to an epidemic of a new disease for those populations whose food intake was largely based upon rice. Studies by physicians in Japan and in Indonesia led to a cure for beriberi that included a more varied diet, plus the use of rice husks and the outer coatings of rice, which contained thiamine.

edema: accumulation of fluid in the tissues

neuropathy: malfunction of nerve cells

Today, much of the rice consumed is either enriched with thiamine or parboiled, which leads to retention of thiamine in the matrix of the white rice kernel. Beriberi, as a disease from the consumption of white rice, is now rare if the rice is parboiled or enriched. However, some varieties of polished (white) rice may not be enriched with thiamine. Thus, when thiamine intake from other food sources is limited, thiamine deficiency could still occur. In the United States, thiamine deficiency typically occurs in **chronic** alcoholics.

chronic: over a long period

Rice for Medical Therapy and Prevention

Rice has been the mainstay of treatment for a number of conditions, particularly for **hypertension** at a time when few effective drug therapies were available. In the 1940s, Walter Kempner developed a treatment for mild, and even **malignant**, hypertension at Duke University. His hypothesis was that a low-protein diet, free of salt, would be an effective treatment. He devised the "rice diet," which consisted of rice, fruits, and vegetables. This treatment had good results: the **blood pressure** of his patients fell, and even malignant hypertension was partially reversed. In addition, blood **cholesterol** levels also fell.

hypertension: high blood pressure

malignant: spreading to surrounding tissues; cancerous

blood pressure: measure of the pressure exerted by the blood against the walls of the blood vessels

cholesterol: multi-ringed molecule found in animal cell membranes; a type of lipid

allergy: immune system reaction against substances that are otherwise harmless

Since this was a cholesterol-free and low-fat diet, it was one of the first to document a cholesterol-lowering effect from diet.

The other therapeutic role of rice is in the treatment of **allergies**. Rice seems to be nonallergenic, and rice milk has been fed to infants allergic to cow's milk. Rice proteins have also been incorporated into standard infant formulas.

Genetic Engineering of Rice

enzyme: protein responsible for carrying out reactions in a cell

mucosa: moist exchange surface within the body

"Golden rice" was genetically engineered to contain beta-carotene, not present in standard rice, to combat the widespread vitamin A deficiency and ensuing blindness in the children of the developing world. Beta-carotene is a vitamin A precursor that is converted to the vitamin by **enzymes** of the intestinal **mucosa**. Vitamin A, or retinol, is then absorbed and transported to the tissues, including the structures of the eye. Golden rice would thus seem to be an advance in the fight against vitamin A deficiency in rice-eating populations. However, there are some concerns about golden rice and other genetically engineered foods. Genetically engineered products have not necessarily been proven safe, and environmental or social risks may outweigh potential benefits that they may bring about.

Clinical trials of golden rice are needed before it is accepted universally. Only when it is clearly determined that it can prevent vitamin A deficiency in experimental animals, and that it presents no hazards, will this genetically engineered food be considered safe for use in human nutrition. Further, society itself must also decide if genetically created foods are acceptable, a point currently in dispute.

Sequencing the Rice Genome

Since the 1960s, the "green revolution" has improved the yield of rice, and now the "green genome revolution" may bring about further improvements. The rice genome has now been sequenced, an achievement of great importance. The sequence of the rice genome will provide the template for the sequencing of other grasses (maize, barley, wheat, etc.). The genome sequences are now known for the *japonica* rice favored in Japan and other countries with a temperate climate, and for the *indica* subspecies of rice grown in China and most other parts of Asia. This knowledge will permit a future harnessing of **genes** for disease prevention, drought resistance, nutritional improvement, and many other possible modifiable features of rice. As a recent issue of *Science* suggested, a "green gene revolution" is needed to meet the challenge of "population growth, loss of arable land and climate changes."

gene: DNA sequence that codes for proteins, and thus controls inheritance

In summary, rice is an inexpensive, easily prepared, and delicious food. It is also a very nutritious food that benefits humans all over the world. SEE ALSO ASIAN AMERICANS, DIETS OF; ASIANS, DIET OF; BERIBERI; BETA-CAROTENE; CORN- OR MAIZE-BASED DIETS; DIETARY SUPPLEMENTS; FORTIFICATION; KWASHIORKOR; NUTRITIONAL DEFICIENCY.

William E. Connor
Sonja L. Connor

Bibliography

Beyer, P.; Al-Babili, S.; Ye, X.; et al. (2002). "Golden Rice: Introducing the B-Carotene Bisosynthesis Pathway into Rice Endosperm by Genetic Engineering to Defeat Vitamin A Deficiency." *Journal of Nutrition* 132:506S–509S.

Cantral, R. P., and Reeves, T. G. (2002). "The Cereal of the World's Poor Takes Center Stage." *Science* 296:53:

Chang, Te-Tzu (2000). "Rice" in *The Cambridge World History Food*, Vol. 1. Cambridge, England: Cambridge University Press.

Committee on Amino Acids Food and Nutrition Board National Research Council (1974). *Improvement of Protein Nutriture*. Washington, DC: National Academic of Sciences.

Davidson, A. (1999). *The Oxford Companion to Food*. New York: Oxford University Press.

Davidson, S.; Passmore, R.; Brock, J. F.; and Truswell, A. S. (1979). *Human Nutrition and Dietetics*, 7th edition. New York: Livingstone, Churchill.

Pennington, J. A. T. (1998). *Bowes and Church's Food Values of Portions Commonly Used*, 17th edition. Philadelphia: Lippincott.

Rickets

Rickets was once considered an extremely common disorder of childhood. The term itself is derived from the old English word for "twist," or "wrick," and throughout history children with rickets could be identified by their bowed legs and knock knees, which gave them a twisted appearance.

Rickets is caused by a deficiency in **vitamin D**. During growth, human bone is made and maintained by the interaction of **calcium**, **phosphorus**, and vitamin D. Calcium is deposited in immature bone (osteoid) in a process called calcification, which transforms immature bone into its mature and familiar form. However, in order to absorb and use the calcium available in food, the body needs vitamin D. In rickets, the lack of this important vitamin leads to low calcium, poor calcification, and deformed bones.

Vitamin D is the only vitamin that can be both acquired through food and made by the body itself. Although vitamin D can be absorbed through foods rich in animal **fat**, such as milk, cheese, fish, and meat, this **absorption** constitutes only about 10 percent of what the body needs in a single day. The remaining 90 percent is created by the body. Ultraviolet radiation from the sun converts 7-dihydrocholesterol in the skin to vitamin D_3. This is then converted to the **hormone** calcitriol (the active form of vitamin D) in the kidney. Calcitriol allows absorption of calcium and phosphorus in the gut, primarily in the small intestine, and maintains the body's balance of calcium and phosphate through the kidney and bone. Without adequate vitamin D, the body can only absorb 10 to 15 percent of the calcium available in food. This balance of vitamin D, calcium, and phosphate is essential to the growth and maintenance of bones, especially in children. Deficiencies can also occur in elderly adults, a condition called **osteomalacia**.

Historically, rickets plagued the populations of European countries in the northern latitudes—at one time it was called "the English disease." During the Industrial Revolution and into the early 1900s, **smog** filled the developing cities of Europe, diminishing the amount of sunlight to which children were exposed and causing an epidemic of rickets. Some researchers estimate that prior to 1915, almost 85 percent of children in these industrialized areas of Europe and North America suffered from rickets. With research into the sources and function of vitamin D in the 1920s, however, the use of cod-liver oil, **fortified** cow's milk, and fortified formula virtually eliminated rickets in Europe and North America.

rickets: disorder caused by vitamin D deficiency, marked by soft and misshapen bones and organ swelling

vitamin D: nutrient needed for calcium uptake and therefore proper bone formation

calcium: mineral essential for bones and teeth

phosphorus: element essential in forming the mineral portion of bone

fat: type of food molecule rich in carbon and hydrogen, with high energy content

absorption: uptake by the digestive tract

hormone: molecules produced by one set of cells that influence the function of another set of cells

osteomalacia: softening of the bones

smog: air pollution

fortified: altered by addition of vitamins or minerals

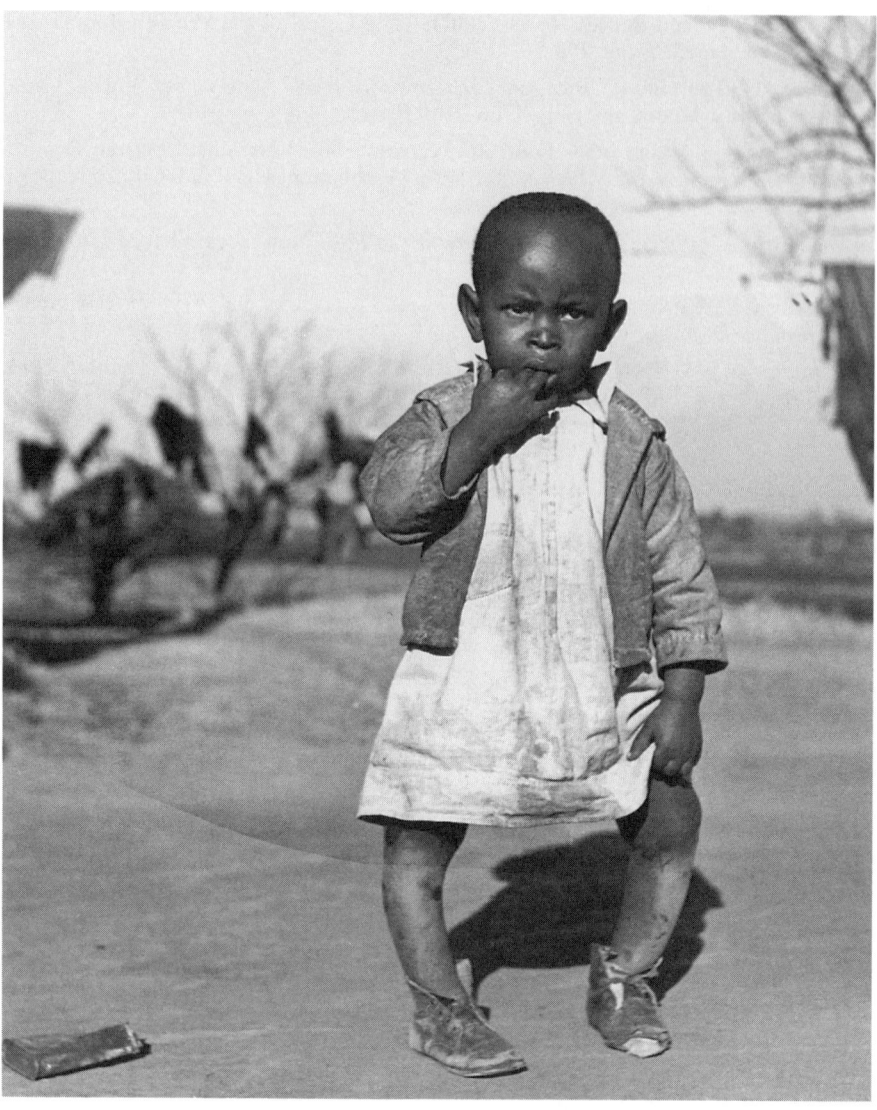

This child's bowed legs are a symptom of rickets, a disease resulting from vitamin-D deficiency. Because their skin absorbs less sunlight, dark-skinned people need more sun exposure to synthesize the recommended daily amount of vitamin-D. *[photograph by Marion Post Wolcott. Corbis. Reproduced by permission.]*

diet: the total daily food intake, or the types of foods eaten

nutrition: the maintenance of health through proper eating, or the study of same

As vitamin D can either be consumed in small quantities through the **diet** or made in the skin, there are two main groups of risk factors for developing rickets. Dietary risk factors include diets low in vitamin D–rich foods, such as eggs, cow's milk, meat, and fish. Breast milk, a primary source of childhood **nutrition**, contains very little vitamin D, and infants who are exclusively breastfed are more likely to develop the disease. While human milk does contain sufficient amounts of calcium and phosphorus for an infant, its vitamin D content is only 4-60 IU/L (international units per liter), while the full-term infant requires approximately 400 IU daily. Infants and children who are not exposed to sunlight, like those in smog-filled cities or those who remain indoors or covered for cultural or religious reasons, are also at increased risk of developing rickets. In children with darkly pigmented skin, melanin acts in a similar way to block sunlight's ability to help the skin make vitamin D. Dark-skinned people require almost six times as much sunlight exposure to make the same amount of vitamin D as those with lighter skin.

Populations that remain at risk today include people with darkly pigmented skin, those who live in industrialized northern cities, and children in certain Arab countries where covering clothing and staying indoors during early childhood are cultural norms. Even in tropical and sunny climates, rickets remains a problem in dense city centers like Calcutta and Johannesburg, and it is still diagnosed in mostly African-American children in the United States. Children who consume vegetarian or **vegan** diets, as well as infants of lactating mothers who have chronically low levels of vitamin D, may also be at increased risk for rickets. Although rare, diets directly deficient in calcium and/or phosphorus may also lead to rickets.

vegan: person who consumes no animal products, including milk and honey

One of the earliest signs of rickets in the infant is craniotabes (a softening of the skull) and delayed closing of the anterior fontanelle (the soft spot on the head). The infant's skull becomes large and thick (though soft), and muscle tone is poor. Poor calcification of osteoid at the ends of bones makes the bone spread in that area. At the ends of ribs, these splayed areas create a knobby-looking chain called the "rachitic rosary" on the front of the chest. In other areas, the pressure of a child's weight bends poorly mineralized bones, creating shortness, bow legs, and knock knees. Poor calcification also creates weakness, making bones prone to fracture. Children can also have delayed **dentition**, pelvic abnormalities, and enlarged joints, along with a curved spine and a forward projected breastbone. Rickets also lowers a child's immune defenses. For those with severe and untreated disease, bone bowing, short stature, and fractures can lead to long-term pain and immobility and require bracing and/or surgery.

dentition: formation of the teeth

Luckily, rickets is a very treatable and preventable disorder. Researchers have found that as little as twenty to thirty minutes of sun exposure per week in children in temperate climates is sufficient to maintain adequate levels of vitamin D in the blood. Other studies have found that oral supplements of 400 IU of vitamin D daily, often in the form of fish-liver oil, can prevent the disease in at-risk populations. Supplementation can also aid in the healing process. A single dose of 600,000 IU, or gradual treatment with 5,000–10,000 IU daily for two to three months, can be a sufficient treatment. And although some bony deformities may remain, many will repair themselves, and most growth parameters will return to near normal. Treatment can prevent grave complications, including developmental delays, waddling gait, and seizures.

Once a widespread scourge of childhood, rickets is now a preventable and treatable disease. It is necessary to understand the roles of vitamin D, calcium, and phosphorus in bone growth, as well as the mechanism of the disease in order to appropriately diagnose and treat it. When addressing the global impact of this disease, it is especially important to understand local environments, community diets, and cultural beliefs. SEE ALSO CALCIUM; MINERALS; OSTEOMALACIA; OSTEOPENIA; OSTEOPOROSIS.

Seema P. Kumar
Neelima Pania

Bibliography

Hartman, J. J. "Vitamin D Deficiency Rickets in Children: Prevalence and Need for Community Education." *Orthopedic Nursing* 19(1):63–66.

Joiner, T. A.; Foster, C.; and Shope, T. "The Many Faces of Vitamin D Deficiency Rickets." *Pediatrics in Review* 21(9):296–302.

McCafree, J. "Rickets on the Rise." *Journal of the American Dietetic Association* 101(1):16–17.

Specker, B. L., and Tsang, R. C. "Cyclical Serum 25-Hydroxyvitamin D Concentrations Paralleling Sunshine Exposure in Exclusively Breast-Fed Infants." *Journal of Pediatrics* 110:744–747.

Internet Resources

Finberg, Laurence (2002). "Metabolic Bone Disease." Available from <http://www.emedicine.com>

Finberg, Laurence (2002). "Rickets." Available from <http://www.emedicine.com>

Latham, Michale C. (1997). "Rickets and Osteomalacia." In *Food and Nutrition in the Developing World*. Rome, Italy: Food and Agricultural Organization of the United Nations (FAO). Available from <http://www.fao.org>

Roth, Karl S. "Hypophosphatemic Rickets." Available from <http://www.emedicine.com>

Rosenstein, Nils Rosén von

Nils Rosén von Rosenstein (1706–1773) was a Swedish physician, born in the city of Gothland. He is considered a founder of modern pediatrics, primarily because of a systematic treatise he wrote on the treatment of children and infants. This work, entitled *The Diseases of Children and Their Remedies*, was the first modern pediatric textbook, and it encouraged progress in the area of child health.

Rosenstein's writings were first disseminated as parts of calendars issued by the Swedish Royal Academy of Sciences, the oldest learned society in Sweden. In 1764, the academy compiled all the parts and put them in book form. According to Nigel Philips, a contemporary of Rosenstein, his book was considered "the most progressive which had yet to be written." The book contained chapters on such topics as **smallpox** and smallpox inoculation, teething, and measles. Also included were suggestions on the frequency of breastfeeding and information on how breastfeeding affects an infant's health. *The Diseases of Children and Their Remedies* was written so intelligibly and with such universal appeal that the average person of the time could read it.

Rosenstein was particularly interested in infant feeding. He was ahead of his time when he recommended feeding young children with diluted cow's milk by means of a bottle for sucking. He also advised that children's foods be covered to avoid contact with insects, along with other hygienic precautions. Rosenstein had an extensive medical practice that allowed him to make frequent practical observations. He laid the foundation of pediatrics as a specialty, and he gave direction to future pediatrics. Using his own notes he was also able to accurately describe and prescribe care for scarlet fever, whooping cough, diarrhea, and other illnesses. In his day, he was the most eminent physician in Sweden. He became a world famous professor of practical medicine at Uppsala University, and he was knighted by Queen Lovisa of Sweden. By the time the last Swedish edition of Rosenstein's book was published, in 1851, there existed at least twenty-five editions published in eight different languages.

Slande Celeste

smallpox: deadly viral disease

The title page to Nils Rosén von Rosenstein's *The Diseases of Children and Their Remedies*. The book includes advice for feeding infants, preventing disease in children, and curing some common illnesses. Its publication established Rosenstein as a pioneer in pediatrics. *[Eskind Library, Vanderbilt University.]*

Bibliography

Knipe, K. (2001). "Paediatrics: The Individuals and External Influences Involved in Forming this Special Branch of Medicine, from Hippocrates to the Present Day." Proceedings of the Royal College of Physicians Edinburgh 31:339–341.

Internet Resources

Rosenstein, Nils Rosén von (1776). *The Diseases of Children and Their Remedies*. Available from <http://www.collphyphil.org> and <www.mc.vanderbilt.edu/biolib/hc/nh6.html>

Satiety

Satiety is a feeling of fullness and satisfaction after eating. It is the opposite of hunger or appetite. The mechanisms and events that lead to a state of satiety are numerous, complex, and not well understood. It is believed that the release of certain **hormones** and the firing of certain nerves when food enters the intestine sends messages to the brain to signal that it is time to stop eating. **Genetic** predisposition and **learned behaviors** may affect at what point satiety occurs in an individual. Learning to stop eating when satiety is reached is an important component of weight control. SEE ALSO APPETITE; CRAVINGS; WEIGHT MANAGEMENT.

Beth Fontenot

hormone: molecules produced by one set of cells that influence the function of another set of cells

genetic: inherited or related to the genes

learned behaviors: actions that are acquired by training and observation, in contrast to innate behaviors

Scandinavians, Diet of

Scandinavia is a peninsula in northern Europe that is occupied by Norway and Sweden. Denmark is also generally considered to be part of Scandinavia because of its historical, political, and cultural ties to Norway and Sweden. These three countries are also part of the Nordic countries, which also include Finland and Iceland. With the exception of Denmark and Iceland, these countries are located north of the Baltic and North Seas and share common borders with each other and Russia. All of these countries are part of the Nordic Council. The Nordic countries have historical and cultural ties, and during the Viking era they had a common language and religion. They are also predominantly Protestant countries.

Nutrition and Health Status

There is a high **prevalence** of **cardiovascular** disease (**coronary heart disease, stroke, hypertension**) in this area, mainly due to the high intake of saturated fats, **cholesterol**, and sodium. Stomach **cancer** is also very common due to the high intake of salt and salt-cured foods, especially salted fish. Accidental injuries are the largest cause of death for individuals under forty-five years of age. Suicide and alcoholism are also prevalent, and **obesity** is on the rise.

Food-borne diseases such as **tularemia** are endemic in the Scandinavian region. These diseases are transmitted through the handling of undercooked, infected meat. "Mad cow disease" was also identified in cows in this region, and an outbreak of human *Salmonella* infections in the summer of 2000 was traced to hedgehogs.

Eating Habits and Dietary Patterns

The descendants of the Vikings continue to eat many of the foods of their ancestors, and they often prepare them in the same way. Preserved food are very common and include dried, smoked, salted, or pickled fish; dried fruits and jams; and fermented milk. Fresh fruits and vegetables are only available for a few months a year and are dried and stored for the fall and winter months. Strawberries, blueberries, and raspberries abound in the summer. Potatoes are an important staple of the **diet** and are served in a variety of

prevalence: describing the number of cases in a population at any one time

cardiovascular: related to the heart and circulatory system

coronary heart disease: disease of the coronary arteries, the blood vessels surrounding the heart

stroke: loss of blood supply to part of the brain, due to a blocked or burst artery in the brain

hypertension: high blood pressure

cholesterol: multi-ringed molecule found in animal cell membranes; a type of lipid

cancer: uncontrolled cell growth

obesity: the condition of being overweight, according to established norms based on sex, age, and height

tularemia: bacterial infection by Francisella tularensis, causing fever, skin lesions, and other symptoms

diet: the total daily food intake, or the types of foods eaten

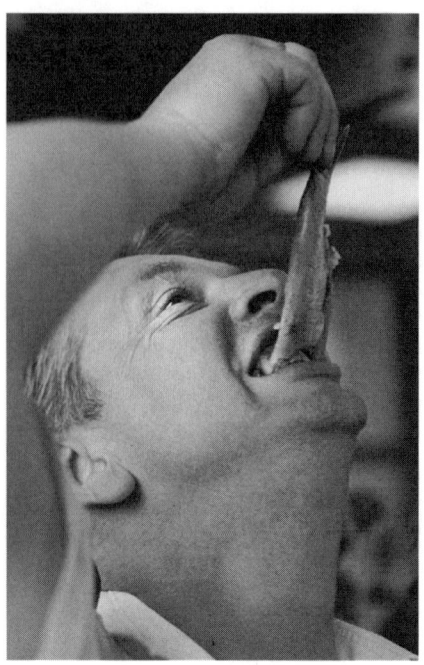

A Dutch man eats raw herring, which is a delicacy in the Netherlands. Seafood is an important part of the Scandinavian diet, but it is not always eaten raw. Popular preparations include smoking, drying, pickling, and salting. [AP/Wide World Photos. Reproduced by permission.]

staples: essential foods in the diet

fat: type of food molecule rich in carbon and hydrogen, with high energy content

ways, including as pancakes. Other **staples** include fish, seafood, mutton, cheese, cabbage, apples, onions, berries, nuts, and bread. Bread is often made with rye, and both leaven and unleavened varieties are common.

Scandinavians eat simple, hearty meals. They generally eat three meals a day, plus a coffee break. Breakfast is light and usually includes bread or oatmeal porridge, fruit, eggs, cheese, herring, or potatoes. Fruit soup is a popular breakfast item in the winter and is topped with cream and served with bread and cheese.

Smorgasbords (bread and butter buffet tables) are popular at lunch in Scandinavia. In Denmark, open-faced sandwiches are made from the buffet table and eaten with a knife and fork. Buttered bread is topped with items such as sausage, herring, smoked salmon, boiled potatoes, cheese, and tomatoes. Such sandwiches are also served as a late-afternoon or bedtime snack. In Sweden, the buffet table offers a large variety of both hot and cold dishes. The Swedes eat herring first, followed by other fish dishes. Meats, salads, and hot dishes then follow (in that order), and dessert is eaten last. Dinner usually has several courses, including appetizer, soup, entrée, vegetables, and dessert. Pea soups served with pancakes are popular dinner items in the winter.

Desserts are rich but not overly sweet. Popular desserts include pancakes with preserves, fruit pies, and pastries. Danes are internationally known for their pastries, and Swedes are known for their butter cookies. Beverages served with meal include milk, coffee, tea, beer, schnapps, dry sherry, sweet Madeira, port, or *aquavit* (water of life). Aquavit (also called akavit, aquavite and akvavit) is an alcoholic beverage made from a grain or potato mash that is double-distilled. The second distillation features the addition of various flavorings such as caraway (most common), cumin, cardamom, lemon peel, aniseed, or fennel. Aquavit is generally not aged, and it is usually drunk straight and chilled, from a small chilled glass. It is a popular drink at smorgasbords.

Dairy products (from cows, goats, and reindeer) are heavily consumed. In addition to drinking milk, Scandanavians also have a high intake of sour cream, buttermilk, and cheese. Cheese is generally served at every meal. Cheese from this region of the world is popular internationally and includes Danish Blue and Havarti from Denmark, Herrgardsost and Svecia from Sweden, and Gammelost and Gjeitost (brown goats cheese) from Norway.

Fish is a major staple in the diet, and Scandinavia is the largest supplier of fish in Europe. The region is one of the largest exporters of dried salt cod in the world. Sweden is famous for its crayfish, Denmark for its oysters, and Norway for its lobsters and prawns. Smoked and cured fish (e.g., herring, mackerel, cod, salmon, and eel) are produced commercially for both the domestic market and for exporting. Cured cod is traditionally prepared for Christmas in Norway and Sweden and served with pork **fat** and bacon.

Historically, meat was in limited supply, so it was often combined with other ingredients. The famous Swedish meatballs and the Danish *fricadeller* (patties made of ground beef, lamb, and pork) came out of this tradition. Today, the Scandinavians are hearty meat eaters. Pork is the favorite meat in Denmark, a country that has as many pigs as people. Scandinavians also hunt wild birds, elk, deer, and bear, just as their Viking ancestors did. Even a few

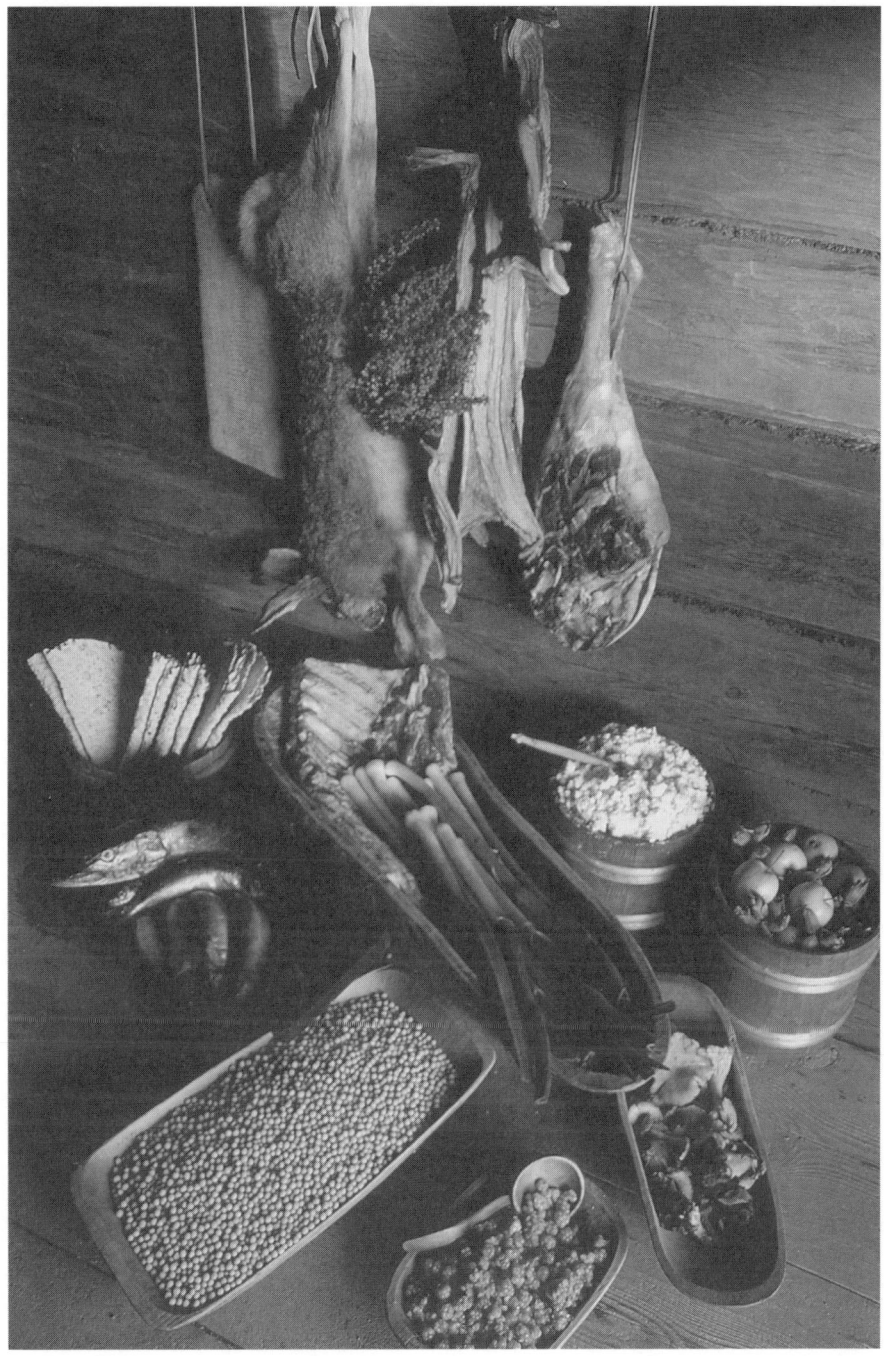

Long winters and short summers limit the fruits and vegetables available to Scandinavians. Their diet tends to be high in fat and salt, and includes such exotic fare as reindeer milk, whale steak, and lutefisk. *[Photograph by Ted Spiegel. Corbis. Reproduced by permission.]*

of the more esoteric tastes of the Vikings live on. Norwegians love whale steak and claim that it tastes as good as beef. Smoked horseflesh is also popular with the Swedes—they call it "hamburger" and buy it thinly sliced.

Special Meals

Christmas is a welcome holiday during the long Scandinavian winter. Traditional foods eaten on Christmas Eve are rice porridge, fresh cod, and lutefisk. Rice porridge is served with cinnamon and sugar and has one hidden blanched almond. The person who finds the almond is believed to be blessed with good luck for the following year. Lutefisk is boiled cod (treated in a lye solution); it is served with a white sauce, melted butter, green peas, boiled potatoes, and mustard. Christmas Day dinner features ham or pork served with red cabbage or sauerkraut. The Danes usually serve goose on Christmas Day.

In Norway, Christmas festivities begin weeks before the holiday. Most families brew a Christmas beer called *juleol.* They also cook traditional pork dishes, bake biscuits, cookies, cakes, and *julekake,* a sweet bread filled with raisins, candied peel, and cardamom. Swedes have a month-long Christmas celebration that begins on December 13, the feast of St. Lucia. Christmas is celebrated on December 24 with rice pudding and ginger cookies. In Denmark, the Christmas feast is held at midnight on Christmas Eve.

Midsummer's Day (June 24) is another popular holiday in Scandinavia. It features maypole dancing, feasting, and bonfires. Fish, such as herring and cured salmon (*gravlax*), along with boiled new potatoes are common. In Norway, a cream pudding (*rommegrot*) is served with cinnamon and sugar. In Sweden, wild strawberries are eaten.

Delores C. S. James
Ranjita Misra

Bibliography

Haas, Elson M. (1992). *Staying Healthy with Nutrition: The Complete Guide to Diet and Nutritional Medicine.* Berkeley, CA: Celestial Press.

Kittler, Pamela G., and Sucher, Kathryn P. (2001). *Food and Culture,* 3rd edition. Stamford, CT: Wadsworth/Thomson Learning.

Ojakangas, Beatrice (2001). *Scandinavian Feasts: Celebrating Traditions throughout the Year.* Minneapolis, MN: University of Minnesota Press.

Internet Resources

"Explore Denmark." Available from <http://www.geocities.com/denmark1.geo/explor10.htm>

World Health Organization (2000). "Disease Outbreaks." Available from <http://www.who.int/disease-outbreak-news>

School-Aged Children, Diet of

The category of school-aged children includes children three to four years old who are preschoolers; elementary school children (kindergarten to fourth grade), who may be between four and ten years of age; middle school children between eleven and thirteen (grades five to eight); and high school children fourteen to eighteen (grades nine to twelve). Often, the **nutrients** their bodies need for optimal functioning and growth are different for each of these age groups.

Nutritional Needs

The **Recommended Dietary Allowances** (RDAs) represent levels of intake of essential nutrients that, on the basis of scientific knowledge, are judged by the Food and Nutrition Board of the National Academy of Sciences to be adequate to meet the nutrient needs of practically all healthy persons. In the United States, the National School Lunch Program (NSLP) and the School Breakfast Program (SBP), which provide free and reduced-priced meals for children in schools, are required to provide one-third of the RDAs

nutrient: dietary substance necessary for health

Recommended Dietary Allowances: nutrient intake recommended to promote health

at lunch and one-fourth of the RDAs at breakfast, thus ensuring that children eating at school consume adequate amounts of essential nutrients.

The *Dietary Guidelines for Americans* (DGA), published by the U.S. Department of Agriculture (USDA), is also used to help determine the nutritional needs of American children. Through the DGA, the USDA recommends using the Food Guide Pyramid (FGP) as a tool for healthful food choices. Some key guidelines include not exceeding 30 percent of total **energy** intake from **fat** and getting less than 10 percent from saturated fats. The FGP for young children (two to six years old) identifies recommended portions of foods from grains (six servings), vegetables (three servings), fruit (two servings), milk (two servings), and meat (two servings), as well as recommending limiting the intake of fats and sweets. The nutrient needs of teens can be determined using the FGP for adults. The DGA also provide guidance in determining the number of servings of foods from each group, depending on total energy need.

Dietary Patterns

While school-food service personnel attempt to provide healthful meals and food choices, children do not always eat the food they receive. The dietary patterns of children are determined by social, **psychological**, and economic factors.

Toddlers and preschoolers spend more time eating at home than they do in school. Their food choices and food preferences are thus largely dependent on what their parents and caregivers provide. When children are young, their parents and families have greater control over what they eat. As they get older, however, what their friends eat in the school **environment**, and what is available to them in school and elsewhere, will have an impact on what they eat. According to Kweethai Neill, Tom Dinero, and Diane Allensworth, what children eat at school is dependent on many factors, including the cafeteria environment, peer pressure, administrative support, teacher participation, cafeteria staff, and the quality of food choices offered.

At the beginning of the twenty-first century, more families are headed by single parents than ever before, and a greater number of two-parent families have both parents in the workforce. As a result, toddlers and preschoolers often have to depend on their schools to feed them. If they are eligible for the SBP and NSLP at school, they can have free or reduced-priced breakfasts and lunches. Even so, there is no guarantee they will eat what they are given.

Children need nutritious foods to grow and to function. Many American adolescents skip breakfast by choice either because they do not have the time to eat or in order to lose weight. In addition, many school-aged children depend on **junk foods** for their nourishment. Studies on American adolescents show that, in general, they have inadequate intake of fruit, vegetables, and whole grains. More than one-third of their daily intake comes from eating snacks between meals. These snacks include high-fat **fast-food** items such as cheeseburgers and potato chips. American teens consume more than a third of their **calories** from saturated fats. Krebs-Smith and colleagues found that one-fourth of the vegetables that children consume are frenchfried potatoes. The Centers for Disease Control and Prevention has reported that 70.7 percent of high school students do not eat five or more servings of fruits and vegetables during the day, that 72.6 percent do not attend

---

Junk Food in Schools

In recent years, public health officials and school administrators have come to realize that schools are frequently working against the cause of sound nutrition in children and adolescents. Many school districts have negotiated exclusive contracts with fast food and beverage companies to provide their products to students, with a portion of the revenues going to the schools. As a result, cafeteria and vending machine lunches commonly include pizza, burgers, chips, soda, candy, and ice cream. Exacerbating the situation, approximately twelve thousand schools (with eight million students) show Channel One, which features commercials promoting junk food. The United States Department of Agriculture and five major medical associations have called for school administrators to reverse this trend and foster better nutrition in schools. The movement has begun to take hold, as school systems including Los Angeles, New York, and Texas have taken steps to ban junk food from vending machines and cafeterias.

—*Paula Kepos*

---

energy: technically, the ability to perform work; the content of a substance that allows it to be useful as a fuel

fat: type of food molecule rich in carbon and hydrogen, with high energy content

psychological: related to thoughts, feelings, and personal experiences

environment: surroundings

junk food: food with high fat and sugar content, without correspondingly high amounts of protein, vitamins, or minerals

fast food: food requiring minimal preparation before eating, or food delivered very quickly after ordering in a restaurant

calorie: unit of food energy

obesity: the condition of being overweight, according to established norms based on sex, age, and height

physical education class daily. It is not surprising, given such findings, that childhood **obesity** is increasing.

Vending machines in schools also contribute to the obesity problem of school children. Many schools have signed contracts with beverage companies to place vending machines in schools. Schools receive huge amounts of "kickback" money for these contracts. In return, vending machines offer high-calorie non-nutritious sodas to students. Many vending machines in schools also provide snacks that are high in calories, fats, and sugars.

Snacking

Snacking is fast becoming the main eating style among children in America. According to Jans and colleagues, there was a significant increase in snacking among children between the years 1977 to 1996. They found that the number of snacking occasions increased, thus increasing the total energy consumption for these children. They also reported that the proportion of energy consumption from fat increased.

globalization: development of worldwide economic system

Worldwide, adolescents consume more fat than they need to. **Globalization** and free trade have brought fast-food eating establishments to most countries, especially to developing nations. McDonalds, Pizza Hut, Burger King, and places like these are commonly found in Europe, Asia, Australia, the Caribbean, and Latin America. Vegetable oils and fats are cheap and easily available, and more food products high in fats are accessible even to those of low-income persons in developing countries. Consequently, even poorer nations are no longer immune to the ills of Westernization, including obesity.

convenience food: food that requires very little preparation for eating

The shrinking world brought about by satellite television and the Internet has created a popular culture among teens around the world—a culture inundated by junk snacks, sodas, pizzas, and **convenience foods**. Eating a meal at the table is no longer a tradition, as nuclear families are more rare. Teens are used to "grab and run" eating styles, as are many adults. Food manufacturers and franchisers take advantage of this profit-making opportunity to produce more convenience foods, snacks, and beverages that are high in fats and calories. Teens prefer popular, tasty, and easy-to-find junk foods. The average American consumes more than forty-two gallons of soda a year. Many teens are included in this group.

Obesity

While adolescents around the world are eating more calories, they are not necessarily eating healthier food. High fats and more calories, combined with a decrease in physical activity, have created an obesity problem among adolescents around the world. The increase in popularity of television viewing and video games, better public and private transportation, and the urbanization of cities account for adolescents adopting more **sedentary** lifestyles. In addition, children have fewer safe neighborhoods to walk, run, play and ride their bicycles in.

sedentary: not active

overweight: weight above the accepted norm based on height, sex, and age

Between 1980 and 1994, the percentage of children who are **overweight** increased from 11 percent to 24 percent. The trend is also evident in Brazil, Chile, Britain, Ireland, Spain, Sweden, China (among children of high-income parents), Taiwan, Thailand, and Australia. American adolescents, although they are eating more in calories, have diets that are low in many important nutrients. Because of this, many are at risk for **hyperlipidemia**, **cardiovascular** problems, **diabetes**, and obesity. Sixty-one percent of children between five and fifteen who are overweight have one or more risk factors for cardiovascular disease, and 27 percent of these children have two or more risk factors. Increasing numbers of children are being diagnosed with type 2 diabetes, which was once considered an adult-onset disease related to obesity.

Overweight children have a 70 percent chance of becoming overweight adults. Obesity in childhood, leading to obesity in adulthood, multiplies the health risks for these individuals. Obesity in childhood also brings with it emotional pain from being teased, isolated, and discriminated against. Overweight children also suffer from low self-esteem, which may affect their ability to succeed at school.

While more adolescents become overweight, the media and peer pressure demand that girls look thinner and boys get bulkier. These societal pressures lead many teens to engage in disordered eating behaviors, such as extreme dieting. Consequently, many suffer from some form of **eating disorder**. Teens face a dilemma in a society that values youthfulness and thinness but encourages a **lifestyle** of sedentary convenience. Such a lifestyle includes a decrease in physical activity, and therefore energy expenditure, as well as fast foods full of fat and high in calories, making it difficult for adolescents to escape a sentence of obesity and ill health.

It is therefore important to encourage children, teenagers, and adults to adopt a physically active lifestyle and healthful eating habits, and to try to motivate young people to become healthier individuals. In addition, public policy to limit junk foods in schools and to encourage families to make healthful food choices for their children can also play a role. SEE ALSO ADOLESCENT NUTRITION; DIETARY GUIDELINES; FAST FOODS; FOOD GUIDE PYRAMID; PRESCHOOLERS AND TODDLERS, DIET OF; SCHOOL FOOD SERVICE.

Kweethai C. Neill

hyperlipidemia: high levels of lipids (fats or cholesterol) in the blood

cardiovascular: related to the heart and circulatory system

diabetes: inability to regulate level of sugar in the blood

eating disorder: behavioral disorder involving excess consumption, avoidance of consumption, self-induced vomiting, or other food-related aberrant behavior

lifestyle: set of choices about diet, exercise, job type, leisure activities, and other aspects of life

Bibliography

Drenowski, A., and Popkin, B. M. (1997). "The Nutrition Transition: New Trends in the Global Diet." *Nutrition Reviews* 55:31–34.

Freedman, D. S.; Dietz, W. H.; Srinavasan, S. R.; and Berenson, G. S. (1999). "The Relation of Overweight to Cardiovascular Risk Factors among Children and Adolescents: The Bogalusa Heart Study." *Pediatrics* 103:1175–1182.

Jahns, L.; Siega-Riz, A. M.; and Popkin, B. M. (2001). "The Increasing Prevalence of Snacking among U.S. Children from 1977 to 1996." *Journal of Pediatrics* 138(4):493–498.

Krebs-Smith, S. M.; Cooke, A.; Subar, A. F.; Cleveland, L.; Friday, J.; and Kahle, L. (1996). "Fruit and Vegetable Intakes of Children and Adolescents in the United States." *Archives of Pediatric and Adolescent Medicine* 150:81–86.

Neill, K. C.; Dinero, T. E.; and Allensworth, D. (1997). "School Cafeteria: A Culture for Promoting Child Nutrition Education." *The Health Education Monograph Series* 15(3):40–48.

Popkin, B. M. (1994). "The Nutrition Transition in Low-Income Countries: An Emerging Crisis." *Nutrition Reviews* 52:285–298.

Popkin, B. M. (1998). "The Nutrition Transition and Its Health Implications in Lower–Income Countries." *Public Health Nutrition* 1(1):5–22.

Scneider, D. (2000). "International Trends in Adolescent Nutrition." *Social Science and Medicine* 51(6):955–967.

U.S. Department of Agriculture (2000). *Nutrition and Your Health: Dietary Guidelines for Americans*, 5th edition. Washington, DC: U.S. Government Printing Office.

National Research Council (1989). *Recommended Dietary Allowances*, 10th edition.

National Center for Health Statistics. (2000). *The Adolescent Chart Book.* Washington, DC: U.S. Government Printing Office.

School Food Service

There are 48 million school children who are served by school food services in the United States everyday. Many of these children participate in the National School Lunch Program (NSLP), which was established by Congress in 1946 to provide low-cost or free nutritionally sound lunches to public school children. By 1946, about 7.1 million children were being served. This grew to 22 million by 1970, and by 2000 more than 27.4 million children were fed through the NSLP. Since 1946 more than 180 billion lunches have been served. School food service and the NSLP play a very important role in children's learning.

The NSLP is administered by the Food and Nutrition Service of the U.S. Department of Agriculture (USDA) at the federal level and by state educational agencies at the local level. Most school districts have a food service or child nutrition service director who oversees the work of cafeteria managers and staff in individual school cafeterias. In many school districts, meals are prepared from scratch by kitchen staff, while many districts contract commercial caterers to provide the food. **Fast-food** companies are also competing to get into school cafeterias.

School districts that participate in the NSLP receive cash subsidies and food commodities from the USDA. They serve lunches to eligible students (who may receive the meals free or at a reduced price) and are then reimbursed for the meals. In addition to the NSLP, the School Breakfast Program (SBP) was begun in 1966. By 2001, 7.7 million students were served free or reduced-price breakfasts through the SBP.

Children from families with incomes at or below 130 percent of the poverty level (as described by the U.S. Department of Health and Human Service) are eligible for free meals. Those from families with incomes between 130 and 185 percent of the poverty level are eligible for reduced-priced meals. Usually these children pay no more than forty cents for lunch and thirty cents for breakfast. School food-service programs must operate their business as nonprofit programs.

To qualify for federal reimbursements, school lunches must meet the Dietary Guidelines for Americans (DGAs) which recommend that no more than 30 percent of an individual's total caloric intake come from **fat**, and no more than 10 percent from **saturated fat**. Federal regulations also mandate that school lunches provide one-third of the Recommended Dietary Allowance (RDA) for **protein**, vitamin A, vitamin C, **iron**, **calcium**, and **calories**. The SBP provides breakfasts that meet the Dietary Guidelines for Americans, and provide one-fourth of the RDA for the above **nutrients**. RDAs vary for children of different ages. Elementary schools, middle schools, and high schools should therefore serve meals that meet the age-appropriate RDAs. Table 1 shows the school lunches that meet the RDA requirements of children at different grade levels.

---

fast food: food requiring minimal preparation before eating, or food delivered very quickly after ordering in a restaurant

fat: type of food molecule rich in carbon and hydrogen, with high energy content

saturated fat: a fat with the maximum possible number of hydrogens; more difficult to break down that unsaturated fats

protein: complex molecule composed of amino acids that performs vital functions in the cell; necessary part of the diet

iron: nutrient needed for red blood cell formation

calcium: mineral essential for bones and teeth

calorie: unit of food energy

nutrient: dietary substance necessary for health

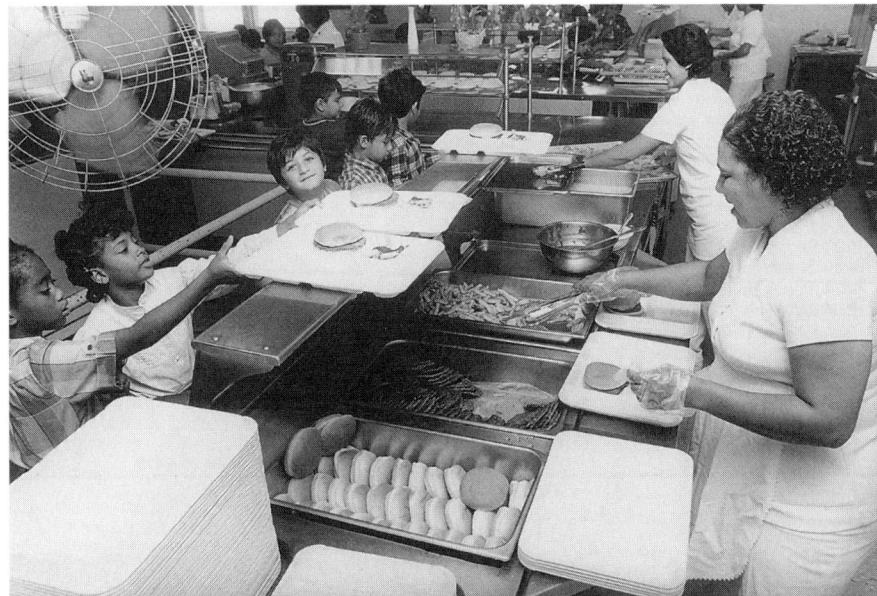

With the help of the American School Food Service Association, school cafeterias around the nation provide balanced meals, which are crucial to growing children's bodies and minds. *[Photograph by Martha Tabor. Working Images Photographs.]*

Plate Waste

Children do not always eat everything on their lunch or breakfast trays. While the USDA attempts to mandate compliance in nutrition integrity of meals provided by school food service, there is no guarantee that children will actually consume everything. G. Richard Jansen and Judson M. Harper, in their 1978 study of the consumption and plate waste of food in the NSLP of fifty-eight elementary schools and high schools, reported that of the 23,000 lunches measured, students tended not to eat all items in the meals. High school students tended to waste less food than elementary students. In 2001, Shanklin found that while students chose meals that were healthful, many did not finish their meals. Vegetables were the least popular item in the meals. While 64 percent of the students selected green peas, most of the students discarded half of what they chose.

The issue of plate waste is an important one. Parents and teachers may help by educating students about nutrition and the importance of eating healthful meals, while school-food service personnel can strive to offer nutritious choices in ways that students will find more appealing.

Competitive Foods

According to the USDA, competitive foods are foods "sold to children in food service areas during meal periods in competition with the federal meal programs." The USDA divides competitive foods into two categories. The first is *foods of minimal nutritional value* (FMNV). USDA regulations prohibit the sale of FMNV in school-food service areas during mealtimes. FMVN include carbonated drinks (such as sweetened soft drinks), chewing gum, and candy. These items may be sold in other areas at anytime during the school day. States and local school districts may have their own restrictions on the sale of FMNV.

The second category includes other foods offered for individual sale in food service or other areas on a school campus. These foods may include

MINIMUM NUTRIENT AND CALORIE LEVELS FOR SCHOOL LUNCHES (SCHOOL WEEK AVERAGES)

	Preschool	Grades K–6	Grades 7–12
Calories	517	664	825
Total fat (percentage of total food energy)	*1	*1, 2	*2
Saturated fat (percentage of actual total food energy)	*1	*1, 3	*3
RDA for protein (g)	7	10	16
RDA for calcium (mg)	267	286	400
RDA for iron (mg)	3.3	3.5	4.5
RDA for vitamin A (RE)	150	224	300
RDA for vitamin C (mg)	14	15	18

*1. The Dietary Guidelines for Americans recommends that after 2 years of age, children should gradually adopt a diet, that by about 5 years of age, contains no more than 30 percent of calories from fat.
2. Not to exceed 30 percent over a school week
3. Less than 10 percent over a school week.
"RE" refers to "retinol equivalent," a measure of the vitamin A activity in foods.

second servings of foods from the NSLP, a la carte items, and other foods and beverages from vending machines, school stores, or snack bars that students buy in addition to or in place of the NSLP.

FMNV items include snacks that are high in fat and sugar, as well as sodas, which are dense with empty calories. Most of these items are offered in vending machines, snack bars, school stores, and sometimes as fund raisers that occur during mealtimes at school. These foods have certain characteristics. First, they have minimal nutritional value and have no regulated nutrition standards. Second, these foods usually contain high amounts of fat, calories, and sugar. In many schools, the lunch period does not offer sufficient time for students to stand in line, get their food and to eat it. In cases where lines are long at the school cafeteria, many students choose to buy snacks from vending machines. Often students spend all their lunch money in the vending machines before they get to the cafeteria.

School food service (SFS) personnel face many problems when it comes to providing quality service to children. For one thing, they are not allowed to make a profit. Yet, they have to compete with commercial food caterers for staff and customers. They also have to provide meals that are appealing, low cost, and that follow the DGA and federal regulations for RDAs in order to qualify for reimbursements for free and reduced-price lunches. While most parents do not mind giving their children as much as five dollars to spend at fast-food restaurants, they complain about spending $2.75 for a well- prepared nutritious school meal for their children.

SFS personnel have to please the school administrators, parents, teachers, children, and the public in order to be successful. The public is often not aware that cafeteria workers work very hard, often get no benefits because most of them are part-time workers, get paid less than their counterparts in commercial operations, and do not get much appreciation for their work. Strangely, many cafeteria workers remain in their jobs for long periods. Many of America's school cafeterias are staffed by dedicated individuals who love children.

The American School Food Service Association maintains that their mission goes beyond traditional school meal programs to better their schools and communities. They are committed to the health and well-being of the children served by their programs. SEE ALSO ADOLESCENT NUTRITION; SCHOOL-AGED CHILDREN, DIET OF.

Kweethai C. Neill

Bibliography

Jansen, G. R. and Harper, J. M. (1978). "Consumption and Plate Waste of Menu Items Served in the National School Lunch Program." *Journal of the American Dietetic Association* 73 (4), 395–400.

Shanklin, C. "Kids Choose Healthy Lunches, But Don't Eat Them." *Journal of the American Dietetic Association* 101, 1060–1063.

Internet Resources

U.S. Department of Agriculture. "National School Lunch Program." Available from <http://www.fns.usda.gov>

U.S. Department of Agriculture. "School Breakfast Program." Available from <http://www.fns.usda.gov>

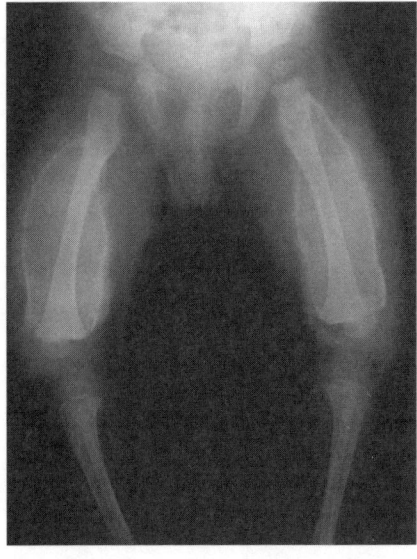

This X-ray of an infant afflicted by scurvy shows some of the skeletal effects of the disease, including bowed legs, stunted bone growth, and swollen joints. Infants who are fed only cow's milk are at risk of developing scurvy, since cow's milk is not an adequate source of vitamin C. [Photograph by Lester V. Bergman. Corbis Images. Reproduced by permission.]

Scurvy

Scurvy is a condition characterized by hemorrhages around the hair follicles of the arms and legs, generalized weakness, **anemia**, and gum disease (gingivitis) resulting from a lack of ascorbic acid (vitamin C) in the **diet**. Early epidemics of scurvy occurred during the Renaissance (1600–1800s) among explorers and seafaring men. In 1746, James Lind, a British naval surgeon, established that eating lemons and oranges cured the disease.

Vitamin C is destroyed by heat, and thus not present in pasteurized and commercially **processed foods**. Children and teenagers who consume too many processed foods and few fresh fruits and vegetables may be getting inadequate amounts of vitamin C. (In 1914, an increased **incidence** of scurvy among infants was attributed to consumption of heated (pasteurized) milk and vitamin C–deficient commercially processed foods.) Though rare, scurvy is now frequently observed among elderly persons, alcoholics, and **malnourished** adults. In addition, smokers have higher requirements for vitamin C, and are therefore more at risk.

Kiran B. Misra

scurvy: a syndrome characterized by weakness, anemia, and spongy gums, due to vitamin C deficiency

anemia: low level of red blood cells in the blood

diet: the total daily food intake, or the types of foods eaten

processed food: food that has been cooked, milled, or otherwise manipulated to change its quality

incidence: number of new cases reported each year

malnourished: lack of adequate nutrients in the diet

Small for Gestational Age

Small for gestational age, also known as intrauterine growth retardation, is defined as an infant or fetus smaller in size than expected, meaning a weight in the bottom tenth percentile for a particular age. Small for gestational age is believed to be related to placental insufficiency, infectious disease, **congenital** malformations, drug and alcohol abuse, and cigarette smoking. Other risk factors include maternal **hypertension**, first pregnancies, and exposure to environmental **toxins**. It is considered to be one cause of low birth weight (less than twenty-five hundred grams, or five pounds eight ounces). It is not synonymous with prematurity, which is defined as birth before thirty-seven-weeks gestation. SEE ALSO INFANT MORTALITY RATE; LOW BIRTH WEIGHT INFANT; PREGNANCY.

Mary Cowley Parke

congenital: present from birth

hypertension: high blood pressure

toxins: poison

Bibliography

Strauss, R. S. (2000). "Adult Functional Outcome of Those Born Small for Gestational Age: Twenty-Six Year Follow-Up of the 1970 British Birth Cohort." *Journal of the American Medical Association* 283:625–632.

Internet Resources

Centers for Disease Control and Prevention (1994). "Low Birth Weight and Intrauterine Growth Retardation." In *From Data to Action: Public Health Surveillance for Women, Infants, and Children.* Available from <http://www.cdc.gov/nccdphp>

"Small-for-Gestational-Age Infant." *Merck Manual.* Available from <http://www.merck.com>

Smoking

Smoking is an important and preventable cause of death and illness. However, as more money has been spent on smoking cessation programs, the **incidence** of cigarette smoking has risen. In 2002, 48 percent of men and 12 percent of women in the world were smokers (World Health Organization). Tobacco consumption increased from 1,100 million individuals during the early 1990s to 1,300 million by the year 2000 (United Nations Economic and Social Council). At this rate, the number of tobacco-related deaths is projected to reach more than 9 million by the year 2020. The number of tobacco-related deaths increased from 4.2 million to 4.9 million between 2000 and 2002, meaning that more than nine people die due to smoking-related illnesses every minute.

Research indicates that tobacco causes more than twenty categories of fatal and disabling diseases, including lung **cancer**, **cardiovascular** disease, and respiratory diseases. However, tobacco is very addictive, and the majority of smokers have difficulty quitting even when they have a medical condition. For example, a 2000 study of 15,660 adults by the Agency for Healthcare Research and Quality found that 38 percent of people with emphysema, 25 percent of people with **asthma**, 20 percent of people with **hypertension** and cardiovascular problems, and 19 percent of people with **diabetes** continue to smoke. Although smoking was responsible for their health conditions, they perceived that, since their health conditions already exist, quitting would not have an affect on their future health and well-being.

A recent area of concern related to tobacco use has been nonsmokers' exposure to second-hand smoke. Parental smoking has been proven to contribute to increased rates of sudden infant death syndrome (SIDS) in addition to **chronic** illnesses in children such as asthma, bronchitis, colds, and **pneumonia**. Pregnant women who chew tobacco, smoke, or are exposed to second-hand smoke have a higher risk of miscarriage and of giving birth to low birth weight babies, who are prone to infection. Women who smoke are more likely to be victims of primary and secondary infertility, to have delays in conceiving, and to have an increased risk of early **menopause** and low bone density ("Current Issues and Forthcoming Events"). Most women are unaware of these dangers. Not only can the expectant mother place her unborn fetus in danger, but she can also place herself at risk for future smoking-related diseases and early mortality.

---

incidence: number of new cases reported each year

cancer: uncontrolled cell growth

cardiovascular: related to the heart and circulatory system

asthma: respiratory disorder marked by wheezing, shortness of breath, and mucus production

hypertension: high blood pressure

diabetes: inability to regulate level of sugar in the blood

chronic: over a long period

pneumonia: lung infection

menopause: phase in a woman's life during which ovulation and menstruation end

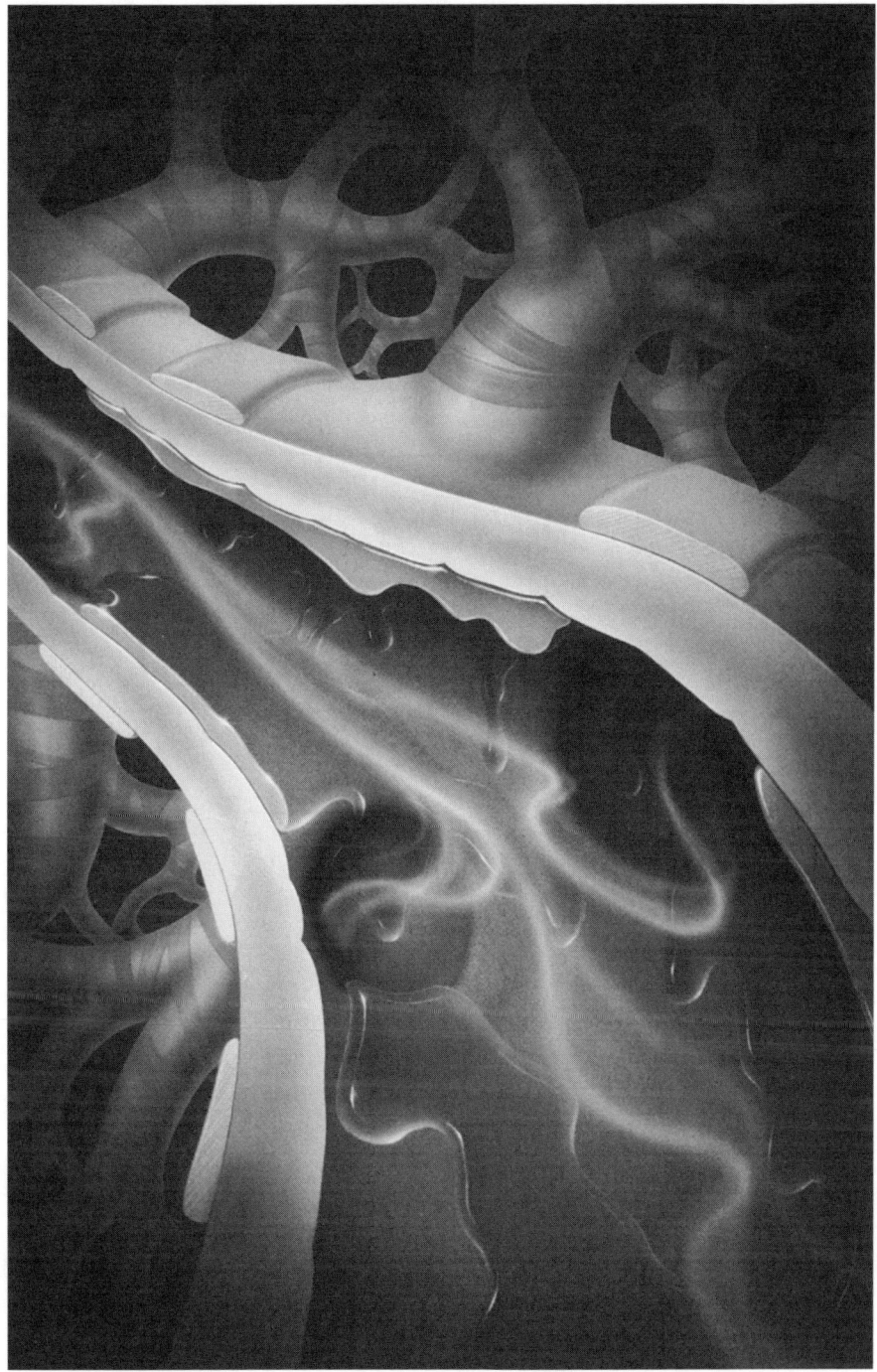

An illustration of cigarette smoke entering the lungs. Cigarette smoke contains over 4,000 chemicals, many of which are toxic or carcinogenic. Repeated inhalation of the smoke causes permanent damage to internal organs and reduces the body's ability to fight infection. [Todd Buck/Custom Medical Stock Photo, Inc. Reproduced by permission.]

Quitting smoking at any age improves life expectancy. The 2002 Cancer Prevention Study examined the benefits of smoking cessation in 877,243 men and women in the United States. Life expectancy of smokers who quit before age thirty-five was extended by 8.5 years in men and by 7.7 years in women. The study found that smokers who quit at any age are subjected to meaningful life extensions (Taylor, et al.). In addition to a life free from smoking-related diseases, an individual who quits smoking can experience increased longevity. SEE ALSO CANCER; HEART DISEASE; LOW BIRTH WEIGHT INFANT; NUTRITIONAL DEFICIENCY; PREGNANCY.

Daphne C. Watkins

BIBLIOGRAPHY

"Current Issues and Forthcoming Events" (2001). *Journal of Advanced Nursing*, 36(5).

Taylor, Donald H., Jr., et al. "Benefits of Smoking Cessation for Longevity." *American Journal of Public Health* 92(6).

World Health Organization (2002). *World Health Report 2002—Reducing Risks, Promoting Healthy Life.* Geneva: Author.

Internet Resources

United Nations Economic and Social Council (2002). "Secretary General's Report to the Economic and Social Council (ECOSOC) on the activities of the United Nations Ad-Hoc Interagency Task Force on Tobacco Control." Available from <http://www.un.org/esa/coordination/ecosoc/SG_UNTF_ECOSOC.pdf>

Society for Nutrition Education

The Society for Nutrition Education (SNE) is an organization of nutrition professionals whose aim is to be involved in nutrition education and health promotion. The organization represents professional interests in nutrition education within the United States and worldwide. SNE is dedicated to promoting healthy, sustainable food choices and has a vision of healthy people in healthy communities.

The organization was founded in July 1968, and, according to its mission statement, is "the premier association linking the fields of food, nutrition, and education. The society enhances members' ability to help the public make informed food choices."

The society also publishes the *Journal of Nutrition Education and Behavior* (formerly know as the *Journal of Nutrition Education*).

Susan Himburg

BIBLIOGRAPHY

Ullrich, Helen D. (1992). *The SNE Story: 25 Years of Advancing Nutrition Education.* Berkeley, CA: Nutrition Communications Associates.

Internet Resources

Society for Nutrition Education. "SNE Membership." Available from <http://www.sne.org/>

South Americans, Diet of

South America is the fourth largest continent on the planet, making up 12 percent of the earth's surface. It contains twelve independent nations: Argentina, Brazil, Bolivia, Chile, Colombia, Ecuador, Guyana, Paraguay, Peru, Suriname, Uruguay, and Venezuela. In addition, it contains three territories: The Falkland Islands (Great Britain), French Guiana (France), and the Galapagos Islands (Ecuador). The continent has a very diverse population. There are small pockets of native Indian groups and significant numbers of descendents of Spanish, Portuguese, Italian, German, West African, and East Indians settlers. There also are considerable numbers of Chinese and Japanese. Approximately 90 to 95 percent of South Americans are Roman Catholic.

Nutritional Status

A high percentage of South Americans live in extreme poverty. **Parasitic** infection, **protein-calorie malnutrition**, iron-deficiency **anemia**, iodine deficiency, and vitamin-A deficiency are common nutritional problems in the rural and urban areas in many South American countries. **Heart disease**, **hypertension**, and **obesity** are also on the rise.

Eating Habits and Meal Pattern

South Americans typically eat three meals and one or two snacks daily. Milk is usually not consumed as a beverage but used in fruit-based drinks and coffee, and milk-based desserts are popular. Fruits, vegetables, and nuts are eaten in abundance. Cassava flour and meal are common in many areas.

Coffee is a major beverage throughout the continent, and South American countries now produce most of the coffee consumed worldwide; Brazil alone produces about a third of the world's coffee. Coffee usually is served concentrated, then diluted with evaporated milk or water. Coffee is consumed heavily in Argentina, Colombia, Ecuador, and Brazil, while tea is popular in Chile and Uruguay. **Herbal** teas are used as remedies throughout the continent.

Yerba maté (pronounced "yerba mahtay") is a caffeinated, tea-like beverage that is consumed for its "medicinal" properties. Its many health claims include energizing the body, stimulating mental alertness, strengthening the **immune system**, and aiding weight loss. Maté is consumed mainly in Argentina, Uruguay, Paraguay, and southern Brazil. It is brewed from the dried leaves and stemlets of the perennial tree *Ilex paraguarensis*. The *bombilla* is a special metal straw used to drink this brew.

Breakfast is normally a light meal with coffee or tea; bread with butter and jam; and sometimes fruit or fruit juice. Meat and cheese are usually eaten in Brazil and Chile. Lunch is traditionally a heavy meal, and it is followed by a *siesta* (nap), which helps one recover from both the food and the heat. The *siesta* is still common among many locals, but the tradition is disappearing from the business day. Appetizers such as fritters and turnovers may start the lunch meal, followed by grilled meat, rice, beans, cassava, and greens. Dinner is another heavy meal, and it often lasts several hours. Dinner usually begins late in the evening, sometimes as late as 9:00 P.M. Desserts are usually simple. Typical desserts are fresh or canned fruits with cheese, a custard called *flan*, and a milk cake called *tres leches*. Snacks are readily available from street vendors and bakeries. Popular snacks include turnovers filled with spicy meats, seafood, and vegetables; hot dogs; and steak or meat sandwiches.

Traditional Cooking Methods and Food Habits

The cuisine of South America varies from country to country and region to region. The cuisine tends to be a blend of cultural backgrounds, available foods, cooking styles, and the foods of colonial Europeans. Some regions have a largely maize-based **diet** (often spiced with chili peppers), while other regions have a rice-based diet. Grilled meats are popular. Traditionally, sides of beef, hogs, lamb, and goats are grilled slowly for hours. Another cooking method is to steam foods in a pit oven. For example, in Peru, a *pachamanca*

Coffee Comes to Brazil

Coffee was first brought to the Americas by French colonists in the early eighteenth century. According to legend, the emperor of Brazil dispatched Lieutenant Colonel Francisco de Mello Palheta to obtain seeds of the precious crop from the governor of French Guiana, sending him to the country under the pretext of mediating a border dispute. When the governor refused de Mello's request for seeds, the colonel turned his attentions to the governor's wife, who seems to have launched the entire Brazilian coffee industry by slipping him a few seedlings in a bouquet. Three hundred years later, Brazil produces one-third of the world's coffee.

—*Paula Kepos*

---

parasitic: feeding off another organism

protein: complex molecule composed of amino acids that performs vital functions in the cell; necessary part of the diet

calorie: unit of food energy

malnutrition: chronic lack of sufficient nutrients to maintain health

anemia: low level of red blood cells in the blood

heart disease: any disorder of the heart or its blood supply, including heart attack, atherosclerosis, and coronary artery disease

hypertension: high blood pressure

obesity: the condition of being overweight, according to established norms based on sex, age, and height

herbal: related to plants

immune system: the set of organs and cells, including white blood cells, that protect the body from infection

diet: the total daily food intake, or the types of foods eaten

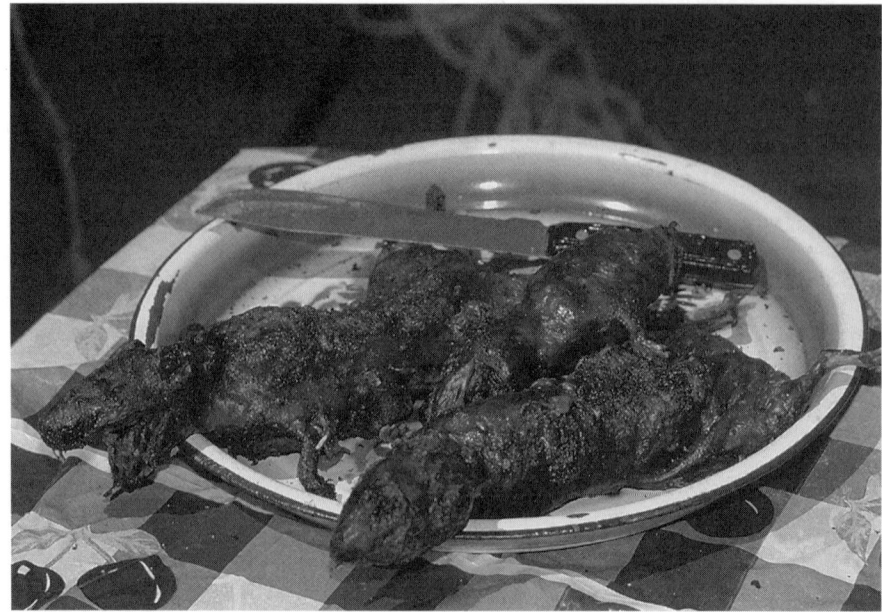

Some of the delicacies found on South American menus are toasted fire ants from Columbia, called *hormiga,* and these barbecued guinea pigs, or *cuy,* from Ecuador. [Photograph by Owen Franken. Corbis. Reproduced by permission.]

typically includes a young pig or goat (as well as chicken, guinea pig, tamales, potatoes, and corn) cooked under layers of hot stones, leaves, and herbs. Clambakes are popular in Chile.

Quinoa, the seed of the *Chenopodium,* or goosefoot plant, has been a staple food of millions of native inhabitants, but production declined for centuries after the Spanish conquest in the 1500s. It is used as a grain and substituted for grains because of its cooking characteristics. It became a minor crop due to its decline, and at times it has been grown only by peasants in remote areas for local consumption. In Peru, Chile and Bolivia, quinoa is widely cultivated for its nutritious seeds, which are used in creating various soups and bread, and it is also fermented with millet to make a beer-like beverage. A sweetened concoction of quinoa is used medicinally.

Regional Food Habits

Brazil. Brazilian foods have a heavy Portuguese, African, and native influence. The Portuguese contributed dried salt cod, *linguiça* (Portuguese sausage), spicy meat stews, and desserts such as corn and rice pudding. Africans brought to the area as slaves contributed okra, *dendê* oil (palm oil), and peppercorns. The national dish of Brazil is *feijoda completa,* which consists of black beans cooked with smoked meats and sausages served with rice, sliced oranges, boiled greens, and hot sauce. It is topped with toasted cassava meal. Coffee, rum, and beer are common beverages.

Colombia and Venezuela. Venezuelan and Colombian foods have Spanish influences. Many foods are cooked or served with olive oil, cheese, parsley, cilantro, garlic, and onions. Hot chile peppers are served on the side of most dishes. Local fruits and vegetables are abundant, and tropical fruits are often dried to make fruit leather. In Columbia, chicken stew and *sancocho* (a meat stew with starchy vegetables) are popular. One of the most unusual specialties of Columbia is *hormiga,* a dish made from fire ants. Toasted ants are also a favorite treat during the insect season in June. In Venezuela, cornmeal bread, or *arepa*, is a staple food. *Arepa* is cooked on a griddle and is sometimes stuffed with meat or cheese before it is fried. *Pabellón caraqueño* is also popular. This dish consists of flank steak served on rice with black beans, topped with fried eggs and garnished with plantain chips. Coffee, rum, and beer are common beverages.

Argentina, Chile, Bolivia, Uruguay, and Paraguay.

These southern countries are major beef producers. Argentineans eat more beef per capita than any other country in the world. Argentina is famous for *asados*, restaurants specializing in barbecued and grilled meat dishes—mainly beef, but also pork, lamb, and chicken. The national dish of Argentina is *matambre*, which is herb-seasoned flank steak rolled around a filling of spinach, whole hard-boiled eggs, and whole or sliced carrots. It is then tied with a string and either poached in broth or baked.

Citizens of these southern states enjoy hearty soups and stews daily. Fish soups and stews are popular in coastal Chile. Stews in Argentina often combine meats, vegetables, and fruits. The soups of Paraguay have heavy European influences and include *bori-bori*, which is a beef soup with cornmeal and cheese dumplings. Pizza, pasta, and meat dishes are popular in these countries. Wines from the midlands of Chile are considered to be some of the best produced on the continent.

Guyana, French Guiana, and Suriname.

Guyanese cuisine is a culinary hybrid with African, East Indian, Portuguese, and Chinese influences. Guyanese usually cook three full meals every day. Rice and *roti* (flat bread) are **staples** at lunch and dinner. Fresh cow's milk may be part of the morning or evening meal. A favorite dish is *pepper pot*, a stew made with bitter cassava juice, meat, hot pepper, and seasoning. Other popular foods are *roti* and curry, garlic pork, cassava bread, chow mein, and "cook up," a one-pot meal that can include any favorite meats or vegetables. Popular homemade drinks are *mauby*, made from the bark of a tree, *sorrel*, made from a leafy vegetable used in salads, and ginger beer. People in French Guiana enjoy an international cuisine, as well as Chinese, Vietnamese, and Indonesian dishes. Imported soft drinks and alcoholic drinks are popular but expensive. Suriname's cuisine has heavy Javanese, Dutch, Creole, Chinese, and Hindustani influences. Beer and rum are popular alcoholic drinks.

staples: essential foods in the diet

Peru and Ecuador.

The cuisine of Peru and Ecuador is typically divided into the highland foods of the Andes and the lowland dishes of the tropical coastal regions. The cuisine in the mountain areas is the most unique in South America, preserving many dishes of the Inca Indians. Potatoes are eaten at nearly every meal, including snacks. More than 200 varieties of potato can be found in the Lake Titicaca region. They range in color from purple to blue, and from yellow to brown. Size and texture vary as well—some are as small as nuts, while others can be as large as oranges. The foods of Peru and Ecuador feature an abundant use of chile peppers. *Salsa de ají*, a mixture of chopped chile, onion, and salt is served at most meals. The coastal region is famous for its *cerviches*, a method for preparing seafood in which the main ingredient is marinated in lime or sour orange.

The natural beauty of South America makes it a popular ecotourism destination. Food-borne and water-borne diseases are the number one cause of illness in travelers. Visitors are therefore advised to wash their hands often and to drink only bottled or boiled water or carbonated drinks in cans or bottles. They also should avoid tap water, fountain drinks, and ice cubes. SEE ALSO CARIBBEAN ISLANDERS, DIET OF; CENTRAL AMERICANS AND MEXICANS, DIETS OF.

Delores C. S. James

Bibliography

Kittler, P. G., and Sucher, K. P. (2001). *Food and Culture*, 3rd edition. Stamford, CT: Wadsworth.

Internet Resources

U.S. Centers for Disease Control and Prevention. "Health Information for Travelers to Temperate South America." Available from <http://www.cdc.gov/travel/temsam.htm>

Hamre, Bonnie. "South America for Visitors." Available from <http://gosouthamerica.about.com/cs/cuisin1/>

Southern Europeans, Diet of

Italy, Spain, Portugal, Greece, and southern France make up the region known as southern Europe. Southern France is included because it is culturally similar to the rest of southern Europe. Greece is often grouped with eastern Europe; however, it is included here because Greek food has greatly influenced the cuisine of southern Europe.

Italy is a boot-shaped country that protrudes into the Mediterranean Sea. The Alps separate it from the rest of Europe. The island of Sicily is part of Italy and is famous for its cuisine. Spain lies to the west of France and occupies most of the Iberian peninsula. It is separated from France by the Pyrenees Mountains. The remainder of the peninsula is taken up by Portugal, which lies to the west of Spain. Portugal also includes the Azore and Madeira Islands, which are located in the Atlantic Ocean.

Influences on Traditional Foods

diet: the total daily food intake, or the types of foods eaten

The **diet** of southern Europeans differs from that of northern and eastern Europeans mainly due to the regions that influenced it. The ancient Greeks brought the olive tree to southern Europe, and Spain is now the world's largest producer of olives. Chickpeas and fish stew were also introduced by the Greeks. Different adaptations of this fish stew are now popular dishes in France (*boullabaisse*) and in Italy (*zuppa di pesce alla marinara*).

Muslim culture also played a role in the food traditions of southern Europe. Spices (in particular, saffron), oranges, lemons, rice, sugar cane, and several types of sweetmeats were brought to the area by Muslims. Spanish cuisine reflects Muslim tradition in its use of saffron-colored rice and the addition of nuts to sauces and desserts. The Italians often use a sweetened almond paste called *marzipan*, which came from the Muslims, in their desserts. Italians add saffron to their rice to create dishes such as *risotto alla Milanese*, popular in northern Italy.

Asia has also added to southern Europe's food traditions, mainly affecting the cuisine of Portugal. Spices (such as pepper and nutmeg) as well as fruits (such as mangoes and bananas) came from Asia. Lastly, the discovery

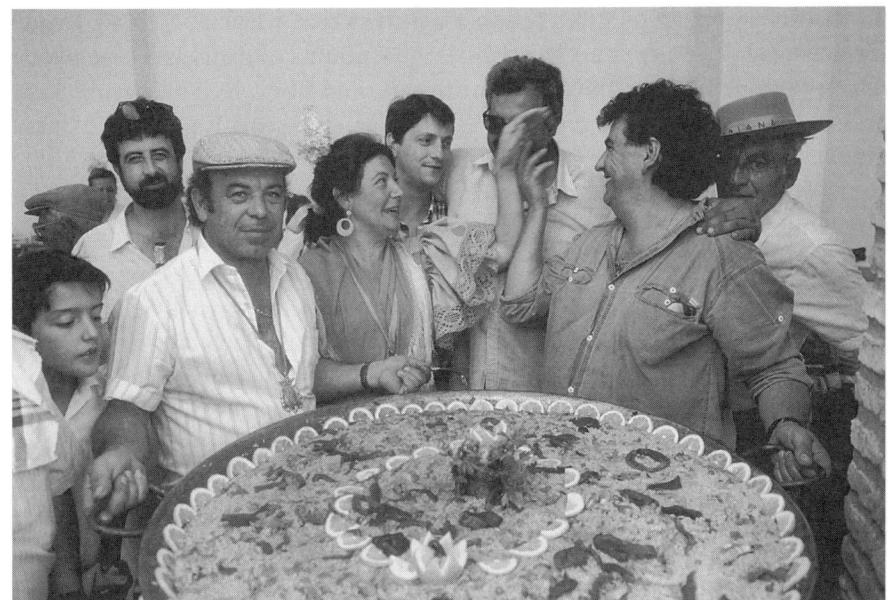

A Spanish celebration featuring *paella,* a rice and seafood dish served here in a giant *paellera.* Saffron, a spice from the Muslim countries to the south and east, gives the dish its yellow color. [Photograph by Owen Franken. Corbis. Reproduced by permission.]

of the Americas brought new fare to southern Europe, including vanilla, chocolate, pineapple, tomatoes, white potatoes, corn, turkey, and squash.

Similar foods are used across southern Europe. It is mainly the method of preparation and presentation that differs from country to country. Italian cuisine can generally be divided into that of northern and southern Italy. In the north, pasta is made with eggs and shaped in ribbons, while in the south, which is generally poorer, it is made without eggs and in hollow tubes, like macaroni. Northern dishes are served with cream sauces and stuffed with meats and cheeses, while southern dishes are served unstuffed with tomato sauce. People in the north use more meats, dairy, and rice than those in the south, which is known for its use of olive oil, vegetables, and little meat.

The Spanish include a lot of seafood in their diet. Meats are served alongside plenty of vegetables. Soups and stews are **staples** and are flavored with garlic and tomatoes. Red wine and crusty bread accompany each meal. Portuguese dishes are very similar to those of Spain, but generally include more spices.

staples: essential foods in the diet

Dietary Benefits, Deficits, and Changes

The International Conference on Nutrition (ICN) was convened in Rome in 1992 and established the food-based dietary guidelines (FBDG) for Europe. The purpose of the FBDG is to provide dietary guidance to the public. They are based on scientific knowledge, but are presented in a way that assists people in reaching nutritional goals. The southern European diet is fairly representative of these guidelines (see accompanying figure).

Southern Europeans experience less **heart disease**, stomach and lung cancers, **strokes**, **high blood pressure**, **diabetes**, and **obesity** than other Western nations. This lower rate of **chronic** disease has been attributed to diet. The diet of people in this area is similar to that recommended in the American Food Guide Pyramid. It differs mainly in the amount of meat and dairy consumed.

heart disease: any disorder of the heart or its blood supply, including heart attack, atherosclerosis, and coronary artery disease

stroke: loss of blood supply to part of the brain, due to a blocked or burst artery in the brain

high blood pressure: elevation of the pressure in the bloodstream maintained by the heart

diabetes: inability to regulate level of sugar in the blood

obesity: the condition of being overweight, according to established norms based on sex, age, and height

chronic: over a long period

vitamin: necessary complex nutrient used to aid enzymes or other metabolic processes in the cell

mineral: an inorganic (non-carbon-containing) element, ion or compound

fiber: indigestible plant material which aids digestion by providing bulk

fatty acids: molecules rich in carbon and hydrogen; a component of fats

fast food: food requiring minimal preparation before eating, or food delivered very quickly after ordering in a restaurant

overweight: weight above the accepted norm based on height, sex, and age

sedentary: not active

Meals are based on grain products, such as rice, pasta, and bread. In addition, southern Europeans consume large amounts of fruits and vegetables, which provide plenty of **vitamins**, **minerals**, and **fiber**. Red meats, chicken, and eggs are used sparingly. Fish is popular and provides omega-3 **fatty acids**. A moderate intake of red wine also provides health benefits. Additionally, southern Europeans tend to lead a more relaxed, stress-free life. They often have a post-lunch siesta, which aids proper digestion. They also tend to be physically active.

Although the dietary habits described above are traditionally true, recent trends show that the southern European diet now also includes elements of the Western **fast-food** craze. A study by Eurostat, the European Commission's statistical branch, found that southern Europeans are getting fatter. Thirty-five percent of Greek males are **overweight**, as are 32 percent of Spanish males. Thirty-one percent of Greek and Portuguese women are overweight. Rates of high blood pressure, heart disease, and diabetes are increasing.

Southern Europeans have not abandoned their traditional foods; rather, they have added hamburgers and fries to them. In addition, **sedentary** jobs are on the rise, as fewer people are earning their money through manual labor. Governments of southern Europe don't have the finances to fight this trend. Michele Carruba of the Research Center on Obesity at the University of Milan says that "the advertising budget of Coke alone is more than Italy spends on food research."

Influences on the American Diet

The influence of the southern European diet can be seen in many dishes in the United States. Italian pasta dishes have become a mainstay. *Fettuccine Alfredo*, *lasagne Bolognese*, and *tortellini* can be found in many American restaurants. Soups like *pasta e fagiole* and cheeses like *gorgonzola*, *parmesan*, and *mozzarella* are popular. Many meals are accompanied by Italian wines, such as *chianti*, and crusty bread.

Dishes of Spain's southern region can be found in American cooking. Plenty of seafood and vegetables characterize these dishes (such as *paella*). Fruits and desserts such as rice pudding and *flan* are also popular in the United States. The influence of Portuguese foods is more subtle, but often characterized by exotic fruits. SEE ALSO CENTRAL EUROPEANS AND RUSSIANS, DIETS OF; FOOD GUIDE PYRAMID; NORTHERN EUROPEANS, DIET OF; SCANDINAVIANS, DIET OF.

Kirsten Herbes

Bibliography

Goyan Kittler, Pamela, and Sucher, Kathryn P. (2001). *Food and Culture*. Belmont, CA: Wadsworth.

Wardlaw, Gordon M. (1999). *Perspectives in Nutrition*, 4th edition. New York, NY: WCB/McGraw-Hill.

Internet Resources

British Heart Foundation (2000). "Diet: Mortality and Morbidity Attributable to Poor Diets." Available from <http://www.dphpc.ox.ac.uk/bhfhprg/>

"The Fat of the Land." *Time Europe*. 157(1). Available from <http://www.time.com/time/europe>

Food and Agricultural Organization of the United States. "Food-Based Dietary Guidelines." Available from <http://www.fao.org>

Oldways Preservation and Exchange Trust. "The Mediterranean Diet Pyramid." Available from <http://www.oldwayspt.org>

Peanut Institute. "Mediterranean Diet Found to be More Effective than Strict Low-fat Option." Available from <http://www.peanut-institue.org>

Soy

A member of the legume family, the soybean is rich in omega-3 **fatty acids**, **fiber**, folic acid, **calcium**, magnesium, potassium, and the **B vitamins** and is also **cholesterol** free and low in **saturated fat**. The **protein** in soybeans is complete, containing all the essential **amino acids** found in animal sources (4 ounces of **tofu** [soybean curd] contain the same amount and quality of protein as a similar-size hamburger). For individuals who want to include more plant-based protein in their **diet** and particularly for those on a vegetarian diet, soy products provide a way to add nonmeat protein to the diet.

Soy and Your Heart

Among the many benefits of soy are the potential for lowering one's risk of **heart disease**, **menopausal** bone loss, breast and **prostate cancer**, and **osteoporosis**. The results of a 1995 meta-analysis (combining results from separate but related studies) published in the *New England Journal of Medicine* found that consuming an average of 47 grams of soy protein a day, rather than animal protein, significantly decreased LDL cholesterol in people with moderately elevated or elevated cholesterol levels (low-density **lipoproteins** (LPLs) are the "bad" type of cholesterol and have been associated with clogged **arteries** and heart attacks). The study also found that high-density lipoprotein **HDL** cholesterol (the beneficial, or "good," cholesterol) was not affected by the consumption of soy protein.

Scientists suggest that soy protein and **isoflavones** are the active substances helping to keep blood vessels flexible and preventing deadly blood clots. Isoflavones are **phytochemicals** (naturally occurring compounds) found in plants, and they have potentially strong **biological** activity, meaning they exert a **physiological** effect, in the body. Phytochemicals give plants their color, flavor, and odor, and they have benefits to the body beyond basic **nutrition**. The U.S. Food and Drug Administration (FDA) has approved a health claim stating that consuming 25 grams of soy protein per day, along with a diet low in saturated fat and cholesterol, may reduce the risk for heart disease. The FDA also suggests that four servings of soy foods per day can lower LDL cholesterol by 10 percent. To use this claim, a food product must contain 6.25 grams of soy protein per serving. The claim does not include a recommendation for isoflavone level, which remains an issue of debate. The 25 gram recommendation applies to all ages.

Soy sources	Amount of soy protein
1 cup (8 ounces) soymilk	10 grams
4 ounces tofu	13 grams
1 soy burger	10–12 grams
1 soy protein bar	14–gram average
1 soy sausage link	6 grams
¼ cup roasted soy nuts	18–20 grams

fatty acids: molecules rich in carbon and hydrogen; a component of fats

fiber: indigestible plant material which aids digestion by providing bulk

calcium: mineral essential for bones and teeth

B vitamins: a group of vitamins important in cell energy processes

cholesterol: multi-ringed molecule found in animal cell membranes; a type of lipid

saturated fat: a fat with the maximum possible number of hydrogens; more difficult to break down that unsaturated fats

protein: complex molecule composed of amino acids that performs vital functions in the cell; necessary part of the diet

amino acid: building block of proteins, necessary dietary nutrient

tofu: soybean curd, similar in consistency to cottage cheese

diet: the total daily food intake, or the types of foods eaten

heart disease: any disorder of the heart or its blood supply, including heart attack, atherosclerosis, and coronary artery disease

menopausal: related to menopause, the period during which women cease to ovulate and menstruate

prostate: male gland surrounding the urethra that contributes fluid to the semen

cancer: uncontrolled cell growth

osteoporosis: weakening of the bone structure

lipoprotein: blood protein that carries fats

artery: blood vessel that carries blood away from the heart toward the body tissues

HDL: high density lipoprotein, a blood protein that carries cholesterol

isoflavones: estrogen-like compounds in plants

phytochemical: chemical produced by plants

biological: related to living organisms

physiological: related to the biochemical processes of the body

nutrition: the maintenance of health through proper eating, or the study of same

lifestyle: set of choices about diet, exercise, job type, leisure activities, and other aspects of life

calorie: unit of food energy

fat: type of food molecule rich in carbon and hydrogen, with high energy content

polyunsaturated: having multiple double bonds within the chemical structure, thus increasing the body's ability to metabolize it

Many of today's common diseases are not diseases of aging, but of **lifestyle**, and they can take twenty to thirty years to develop. Typically, when soy protein replaces animal protein, the consumption of saturated fat and cholesterol goes down. About 40 percent of the soybean's **calories** come from **fat**, with the majority (54 %) being unsaturated. The **polyunsaturated** fat in the soybean includes omega-3 fatty acids, which are not frequently found in plants.

Soy and Cancer

Soybeans and soy foods in the diet may provide strong anticancer activity because they are natural sources of isoflavones. A specific isoflavone called genistein, which is found is soy, appears to help block tumor-cell growth. Current studies indicate that consuming soy may reduce the risk of developing prostate cancer, while isoflavone supplements may help physicians stabilize prostate cancer by decreasing the prostate-specific antigen (PSA) level used to measure how well the cancer is being controlled.

estrogen: hormone that helps control female development and menstruation

hormone: molecules produced by one set of cells that influence the function of another set of cells

There has been much debate and disagreement about soy consumption and its role in breast cancer. Similar in chemical structure to **estrogen**, isoflavones are in fact, weak estrogens, and they may act as such in the body. **Hormone** replacement therapy (HRT) has been shown to increase breast density, a factor in breast-cancer risk (as breast density increases, so does the risk for breast cancer), while recent soy studies have found that soy use in both premenopausal and postmenopausal women did not affect breast density.

Soy and Menopause

The popularity of soy-based foods is also due to their potential for reducing the symptoms of menopause. In a study published in *Obstetrics and Gynecology*, researchers found that women who consumed 60 grams of isolated soy protein daily reported a reduction in moderate to severe hot flashes. Other studies have contradicted this finding, however, Japanese women, who typically have a soy-rich diet, do experience a lower **incidence** of most postmenopausal symptoms than women in Western countries, including hot flashes, hormone-related cancers, and osteoporosis.

incidence: number of new cases reported each year

Soy and Osteoporosis

metabolism: the sum total of reactions in a cell or an organism

absorption: uptake by the digestive tract

Another area with conflicting studies is the link between soy and osteoporosis. One method for determining your bone health and changes in bone density over time is calcium **metabolism** (a process where a substance, necessary for life, is synthesized or broken down). For bone density to increase, more calcium must be kept in the bones. This retention is measured by tests that look at calcium **absorption** versus calcium loss as measured in the urine. In studies that have compared a soy diet to a calcium/whey diet, calcium loss through the urine was much lower on the soy diet. Some researchers suggest that the amino-acid content of soy protein, as compared to that of animal protein, is the reason for less calcium loss in the urine.

The versatile soybean remains a popular food choice, and adding soy to the diet is one component of a healthful eating program. Even the soybean

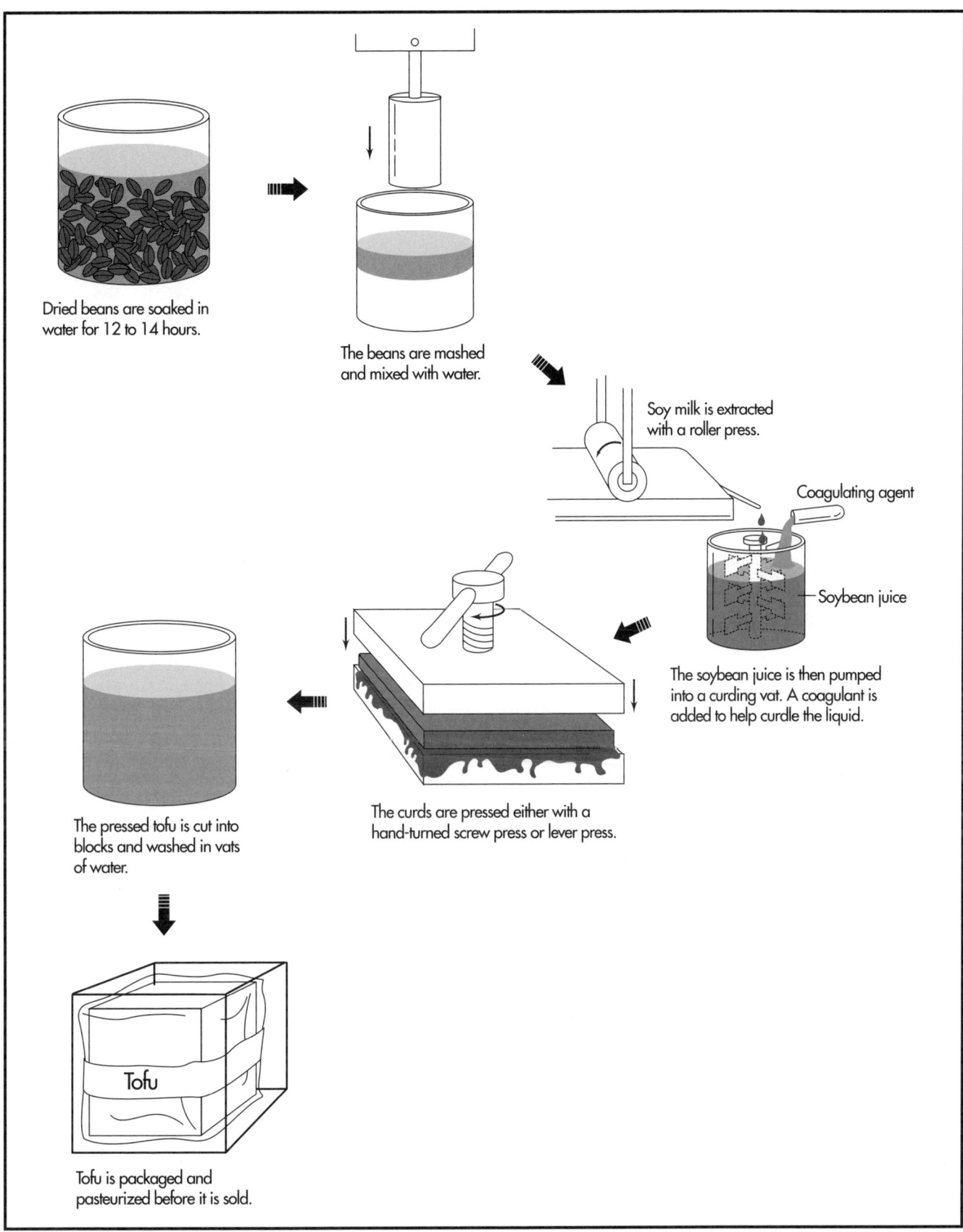

Soybeans are soaked, mashed, mixed with water, and then pressed to extract soy milk, which is curdled to make tofu. Combining 25 grams of soy protein per day with a low-fat diet can have significant health benefits. *[Hans & Cassidy. The Gale Group. Reproduced by permission.]*

pod itself, called edamame, is sometimes eaten as a snack food. SEE ALSO Functional Foods; Legumes; Meat Analogs; Plant-Based Diets; Vegetarianism.

Susan Mitchell

Bibliography

Anderson, James W., et al. (1995). "Meta-Analysis of the Effects of Soy Protein Intake on Serum Lipids." *New England Journal of Medicine* 333:276–82.

Albertazzi P., et al. (1998). "The Effect of Dietary Soy Supplementation on Hot Flashes." *Obstetrics and Gynecology* 91:6–11.

Internet Resources

Messina, Mark (2002). "Symposium Highlights Significant Research On Soy and Human Health." *The Soy Connection*, Winter. Chesterfield, MO: United Soybean Board. Also available from <http://www.talksoy.com>

Stevens and Associates (2002). "The U.S. Soyfoods Directory." Available from <http://www.soyfoods.com>

United States Department of Agriculture, Agricultural Research Service (2002). "USDA-Iowa State University Database on the Isoflavone Content of Foods." Available from <http://www.nal.usda.gov/fnic/foodcomp/Data/isoflav/isoflav.html>

Space Travel and Nutrition

Nutrition has played a critical role throughout the history of exploration, and space exploration is no exception. While a one- to two-week flight aboard the Space Shuttle might be analogous to a camping trip, adequate nutrition is absolutely critical when spending several months aboard the International Space Station or several years on a mission to another planet. To ensure adequate nutrition, space-nutrition specialists must know how much of various individual **nutrients** astronauts need, and these nutrients must be available in the spaceflight food system. To complicate matters, spaceflight **nutritional requirements** are influenced by many of the **physiological** changes that occur during spaceflight.

Space Physiology

Spacecraft, the space **environment**, and weightlessness itself all impact human physiology. Clean air, drinkable water, and effective waste collection systems are required for maintaining a habitable environment. Without the Earth's atmosphere to protect them, astronauts are exposed to a much higher level of radiation than individuals on the Earth. Weightlessness impacts almost every system in the body, including those of the bones, muscles, heart and blood vessels, and nerves.

Bone. Bone loss, especially in the legs, is significant during spaceflight. This is most important on flights longer than thirty days, because the amount of bone lost increases as the length of time in space increases. Weightlessness also increases excretion of **calcium** in the urine and the risk of forming **kidney stones**. Both of these conditions are related to bone loss.

Many nutrients are important for healthy bone, particularly calcium and **vitamin D**. When a food containing calcium is eaten, the calcium is absorbed by the **intestines** and goes into the bloodstream. **Absorption** of calcium from the intestines decreases during spaceflight. Even when astronauts take extra calcium as a supplement, they still lose bone.

---

nutrition: the maintenance of health through proper eating, or the study of same

nutrient: dietary substance necessary for health

nutritional requirements: the set of substances needed in the diet to maintain health

physiological: related to the biochemical processes of the body

environment: surroundings

calcium: mineral essential for bones and teeth

kidney stones: deposits of solid material in kidney

vitamin D: nutrient needed for calcium uptake and therefore proper bone formation

intestines: the two long tubes that carry out much of the processes of digestion

absorption: uptake by the digestive tract

On Earth, the body can produce vitamin D after the skin is exposed to the sun's ultraviolet light. In space, astronauts could receive too much ultraviolet light, so spacecraft are shielded to prevent this exposure. Because of this, all of the astronauts' vitamin D has to be provided by their **diet**. However, it is very common for vitamin D levels to decrease during spaceflight.

diet: the total daily food intake, or the types of foods eaten

Sodium intake is also a concern during spaceflight, because space diets tend to have relatively high amounts of sodium. Increased dietary sodium is associated with increased amounts of calcium in the urine and may relate to the increased risk of kidney stones. The potential effect of these and other nutrients on the maintenance of bone health during spaceflight highlights the importance of optimal dietary intake.

Bone is a living tissue, and is constantly being remodeled. This remodeling is achieved through breakdown of existing bone tissue (a process called resorption) and formation of new bone tissue. Chemicals in the blood and urine can be measured to determine the relative amounts of bone resorption and formation. During spaceflight, bone resorption increases significantly, and formation either remains unchanged or decreases slightly. The net effect of this imbalance is a loss of bone mass.

It is not clear whether bone mass lost in space is fully replaced after returning to Earth. It is also unclear whether the quality (or strength) of the replaced bone is the same as the bone that was there before a spaceflight. Preliminary data seem to show that some crew members do indeed regain their preflight bone mass, but this process takes about two or three times as long as their flight. The ability to understand and counteract weightlessness-induced bone loss remains a critical issue for astronaut health and safety.

The changes in bone during spaceflight are very similar to those seen in certain situations on the ground. There are similarities to **osteoporosis**, and even **paralysis**. While osteoporosis has many causes, the end result seems to be similar to spaceflight bone loss. Paralyzed individuals have **biochemical** changes very similar to those of astronauts. This is because in both cases the bones are not being used for support. In fact, one of the ways spaceflight bone loss is studied is to have people lie in bed for several weeks. Using this approach, scientists attempt to understand the mechanisms of bone loss and to test ways to counteract it. If they can find ways to successfully counteract spaceflight bone loss, doctors may be able to use similar methods to treat people with osteoporosis or paralysis.

osteoporosis: weakening of the bone structure

paralysis: inability to move

biochemical: related to chemical processes within cells

Muscle. Loss of body weight (mass) is a consistent finding throughout the history of spaceflight. Typically, these losses are small (1 percent to 5 percent of body mass), but they can reach 10 percent to 15 percent of preflight body mass. Although a 1 percent body-weight loss can be explained by loss of body water, most of the observed loss of body weight is accounted for by loss of muscle and adipose (**fat**) tissue. Weightlessness leads to loss of muscle mass and muscle volume, weakening muscle performance, especially in the legs. The loss is believed to be related to a **metabolic** stress associated with spaceflight. These findings are similar to those found in patients with serious diseases or trauma, such as burn patients.

fat: type of food molecule rich in carbon and hydrogen, with high energy content

metabolic: related to processing of nutrients and building of necessary molecules within the cell

Exercise routines have not succeeded in maintaining muscle mass or strength of astronauts during spaceflight. Most of the exercises performed have been **aerobic** (e.g., treadmill, stationary bicycle). Use of resistance

aerobic: designed to maintain adequate oxygen in the bloodstream

exercise, in which a weight (or another person) provides resistance to exercise against, has been proposed to aid in the maintenance of both muscle and bone during flight. Ground-based studies (not done in space) of resistance exercise show that it may be helpful, not only for muscle but also for bone. Studies being conducted on the International Space Station are testing the effectiveness of this type of exercise for astronauts.

Blood. A decrease in the mass of red blood cells (i.e., the total amount of blood in the body) is also a consistent finding after short- and long-term spaceflight. The actual composition of the blood changes little, because the amount of fluid (blood **plasma**) decreases as well. The net result is that the total volume of blood in the circulatory system decreases. While this loss is significant (about 10 percent to 15 percent below preflight levels), it seems to be simply an adaptation to spaceflight, with no reported effect on body function during flight.

The initial loss of red blood cells seems to happen because newly synthesized cells (which are not needed in a smaller blood volume) are destroyed until a new steady state is reached. One consequence of the increased destruction of red blood cells is that the **iron** released when they are destroyed is processed for storage in the body. Too much iron may be harmful, and is thus a concern for long space missions.

plasma: the fluid portion of the blood, distinct from the cellular portion

iron: nutrient needed for red blood cell formation

Space Food Systems

Historically, space food systems have evolved as U.S. space programs have developed. The early Mercury program (1961–1963) included food packaged in bite-sized cubes, freeze-dried powders, and semiliquid foods (such as ham salad) stuffed into aluminum tubes.

The Gemini program (1965–1966) continued using bite-sized cubes, which were coated with plain gelatin to reduce crumbs that might clog the air-handling system. Freeze-dried foods were put into a special plastic container to make rehydrating easier.

The Apollo program (1968–1972) was the first to have hot water. This made rehydrating foods easier, and also improved taste and quality. Apollo astronauts were the first crew members to use the *spoonbowl*, a utensil that eliminated having to consume food into the mouth directly from the package.

The quality, taste, and variety of foods improved even more during the Skylab program (1973–1974), the only program to have refrigerators and freezers for storage of fresh foods. The menu contained seventy-two different food items.

The Shuttle program, which began in 1981, includes food prepared on Earth from grocery store shelves. With the help of a dietitian, crew members plan individual three-meal-per-day menus that contain a balanced supply of the nutrients needed for living and working in space. Crew members are allowed to add a few of their own personal favorite foods (which may require special packaging to withstand the rigors of spaceflight). Freeze-dried foods are rehydrated using water that is generated by the Shuttle's fuel cells. Foods are eaten right from the package (on individual food trays), or they may be heated in a convection oven in the Shuttle galley.

Space Travel and Nutrition

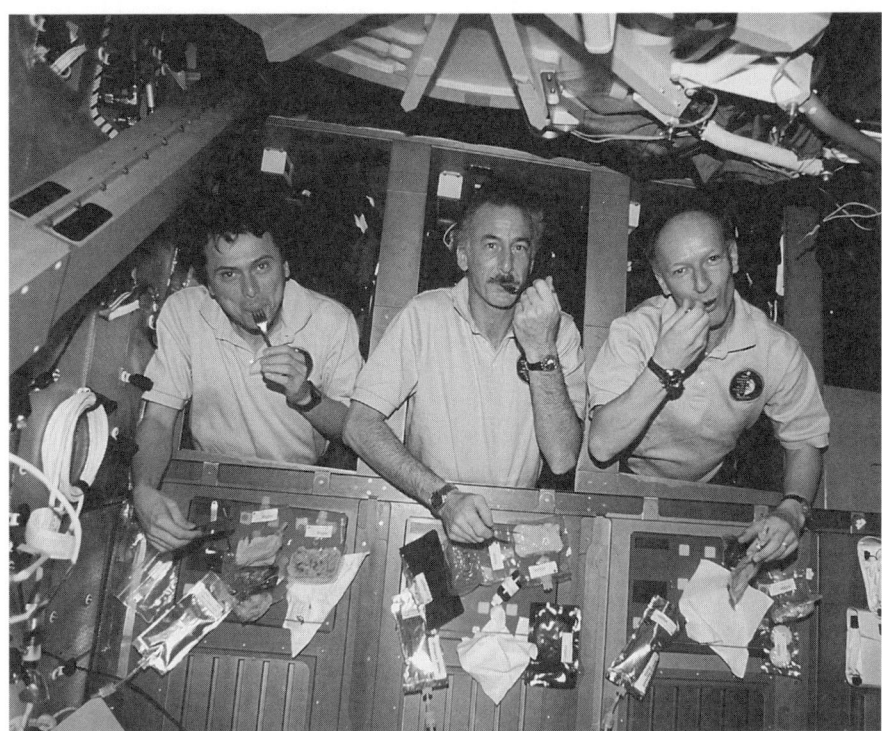

Astronauts on the International Space Station prepare to share a meal. The quality of their menu contrasts sharply with those of the early space explorers, whose meals were either semi-liquids—squeezed from a tube—or bite-sized cubes. [NASA. Reproduced by permission.]

During the Shuttle-Mir program (1995–1998), a joint menu was used that contained half Russian and half U.S. Shuttle foods. These had to meet the nutritional needs established by technical committees representing both space programs. The Russian four-meal-per-day menu was used, with each space program providing two of the meals. Three larger meals were designed to be eaten as scheduled meals; the fourth meal was composed of foods that could be eaten at any time throughout the day.

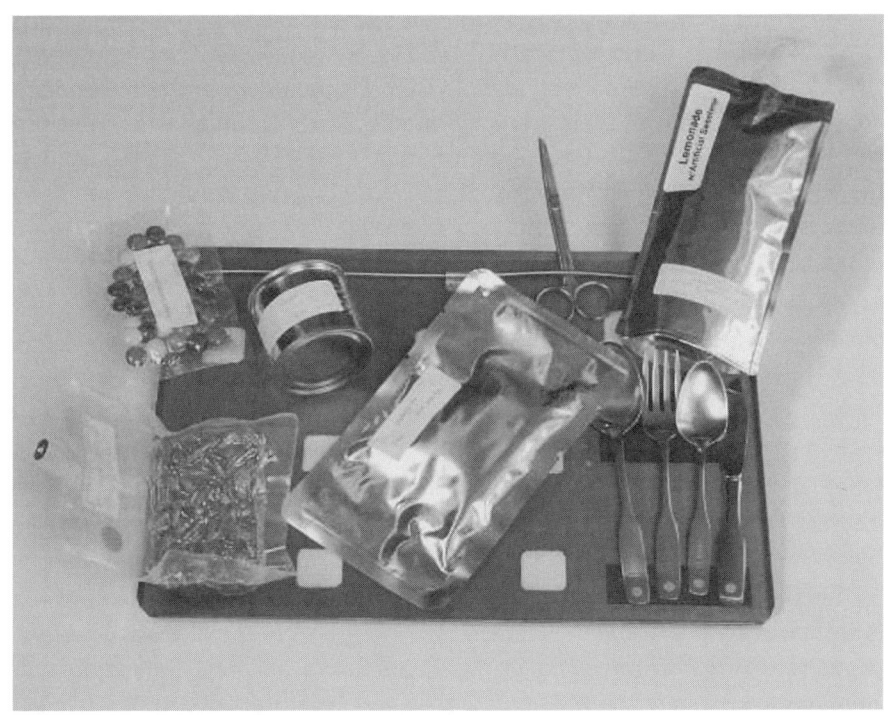

A Space Shuttle meal tray includes scissors to cut open food packages and Velcro to hold them in place. The tray itself is secured to the wall or to an astronaut's lap to keep it from drifting away. [NASA. Reproduced by permission.]

The current food system for the International Space Station, which started in 2000, is similar to the system used in the Shuttle-Mir program. The four-meal-per-day menu plan is used, with equal provision of foods by the U.S. and Russian space programs. The menu is composed mainly of packaged foods that are freeze-dried and thermostabilized (canned), with very few fresh foods. The crew members plan their own menus with the assistance of a dietitian, and an effort is made to include all of the nutrients needed for working in the space environment. After the habitation module galley is equipped with refrigerators, freezers, and a microwave-convection oven, a more extensive menu, including a variety of fresh foods, will be available.

Dietary Intake during Spaceflight

Dietary intake has been monitored on select Apollo, Skylab, Shuttle, and Shuttle-Mir flights as a part of scientific studies. Preflight and postflight intakes are determined using conventional methods for **dietary assessment**. Crew members are provided a diet-record logbook and digital scale, or the foods are weighed by the research dietitian and provided during each of the five- to eighteen-day data collection sessions. A variety of nutrient-analysis software programs are used. Crew members record their intake during spaceflight by writing it in a log or, more frequently, they use a barcode reader that scans the food package label and then record the amount consumed. The amounts of certain nutrients in each meal are calculated from the record of how much of each type of food was eaten, plus knowledge of the amount of each nutrient in each type of food. Nutrient calculations using chemical analysis data for each spaceflight food item are performed after the flight. On the International Space Station, crew members complete a food-frequency questionnaire each week, and the data is down-linked for analysis. Dietary intake can thus be assessed in real time. Changes in diet may then be suggested to the crew members to prevent nutrient deficiencies.

A primary concern is that astronauts consume enough **energy** (**calories**) for optimal work performance and good health. Of the flight crews that have been monitored, only the Skylab crew members consumed enough energy—99 percent of their predicted intake. Most of the crew members in other flight programs consumed about 70 percent of what was planned. On the Skylab flights, much time and attention was given to eating and food preparation, and the crew members' extensive exercise program may have stimulated their appetite. On all other flights, the crew members have had a very busy schedule, with little time and attention devoted to eating.

Crew members' dietary intakes on Skylab, Shuttle, and Shuttle-Mir flights have tended to be higher in **carbohydrate** and lower in fat than their preflight intakes. This change may have been related to an abundance of foods high in carbohydrates, especially sugar-sweetened beverages, or perhaps these items are more easily prepared during a busy work schedule. Ample fat sources are available in the Shuttle food inventory—more than half of the main dish items contain greater than 30 percent of their calories as fat.

Intake of fluid should be about 2,000 milliliters (2 liters) per day, which is sufficient to prevent **dehydration** and kidney stone formation. Fluid intakes have varied from 1,000 to 4,000 milliliters per day, indicating that some crew members are getting less than the recommended amount.

---

dietary assessment: analysis of nutrients in the diet

energy: technically, the ability to perform work; the content of a substance that allows it to be useful as a fuel

calorie: unit of food energy

carbohydrate: food molecule made of carbon, hydrogen, and oxygen, including sugars and starches

dehydration: loss of water

Inflight sodium intakes of all crew members have exceeded the recommendation of less than 3,500 milligrams per day. Sodium intake is high because many of the "off-the-shelf" food items used have a high sodium content.

Calcium intakes have been below the recommended range of 1,000 to 1,200 milligrams per day. This level is estimated to minimize the bone mineral loss that occurs during spaceflight.

Iron intakes have been 50 to 60 percent greater than the recommendation of ten milligrams per day. As with sodium, iron intakes are high because the food items have already been iron-fortified. Too much iron in the body may cause tissue damage.

Nutrition is critical for health, both on Earth and during spaceflight. Specific nutrition concerns for spaceflight include adequate consumption of calories for energy, adequate fluid intake to prevent dehydration and renal stones, adequate calcium to minimize bone loss.

There seems to be an excess of both sodium and iron in the inflight diet, compared to predicted requirements. A food delivery system needs to be designed to include foods that will provide nutrients at the recommended levels, while providing variety and palatability to make eating more pleasant.

The International Space Station represents the beginning of an era of humans living and working in space, with the potential for a permanent human presence in space. Nutrition will play a vital role in ensuring the health and safety of spacefaring individuals, whether they are in low Earth orbit or on journeys to the moon, Mars, or beyond. A more complete understanding of the effects of spaceflight will not only help humans to explore the universe, but will provide information needed to maintain human health and treat diseases here on Earth. SEE ALSO NUTRITIONAL DEFICIENCY; OSTEOPOROSIS.

Scott M. Smith
Barbara L. Rice

Bibliography

Bourland, Charles T. (1998). "Advances in Food Systems for Space Flight." *Life Support and Biosphere Science* 5:71–77.

Lane, Helen W., and Smith, Scott M. (1998). "Nutrition in Space." In *Modern Nutrition in Health and Disease*, 9th edition, eds. M. E. Shils, J. A. Olson, M. Shike, and A. C. Ross. Baltimore: Williams & Wilkins.

Smith, Scott M.; Davis-Street, Janis E.; Rice, Barbara L.; Nillen, Jeannie L; Gillman, Patricia L.; and Block, Gladys (2001). "Nutritional Status Assessment in Semi-Closed Environments: Ground-Based and Space Flight Studies in Humans." *Journal of Nutrition* 131:2053–2061.

Smith, Scott M., and Lane, Helen W. (1999). "Gravity and Space Flight: Effects on Nutritional Status." *Current Opinion in Clinical Nutrition and Metabolic Care* 2:335–338.

Smith, Scott M., and Lane, Helen W. "Nutritional Support." In *Principles of Clinical Medicine for Space Flight*, ed. Michael R. Barratt and Sam L. Pool. New York: Springer-Verlag (2002).

Sports Nutrition

Aside from training, **nutrition** is the most important influence on sports performance. To reach one's highest potential, all of the body's systems

nutrition: the maintenance of health through proper eating, or the study of same

calorie: unit of food energy

carbohydrate: food molecule made of carbon, hydrogen, and oxygen, including sugars and starches

protein: complex molecule composed of amino acids that performs vital functions in the cell; necessary part of the diet

fat: type of food molecule rich in carbon and hydrogen, with high energy content

vitamin: necessary complex nutrient used to aid enzymes or other metabolic processes in the cell

mineral: an inorganic (non-carbon-containing) element, ion or compound

energy: technically, the ability to perform work; the content of a substance that allows it to be useful as a fuel

fortified: altered by addition of vitamins or minerals

glycogen: storage form of sugar

fatigue: tiredness

diet: the total daily food intake, or the types of foods eaten

fiber: indigestible plant material which aids digestion by providing bulk

processed food: food that has been cooked, milled, or otherwise manipulated to change its quality

legumes: beans, peas and related plants

absorption: uptake by the digestive tract

must be working optimally. The best way to achieve this is to eat a variety of nutritious foods. **Calories**, **carbohydrate**, **protein**, **fat**, **vitamins**, **minerals**, and fluids all play a unique and crucial role.

Calories

To have enough **energy** for exercise (and for life), an adequate number of calories must be consumed. The amount of calories needed depends on many different factors, such as age, sex, height, weight, muscle mass, and fat mass. Too few calories can negatively affect workouts and energy levels, as well as cause the breakdown of muscle and bone, increasing the risk of injury.

It is important to nourish the body after several hours with no food (such as during sleep), so breakfast is an important part of adequate calorie intake. Choosing high-nutrient foods—such as **fortified** cereals with milk, peanut butter with whole grain bread, yogurt, cheese, or fruit—gives the body the right fuel to start the day. Nutritious meals and snacks can also help the body stays fueled throughout the day.

Carbohydrates

Carbohydrates are the body's main energy source for all types of exercise. Carbohydrate is stored as **glycogen** in the body, and the amount of glycogen stored in the body affects stamina and endurance. When muscle cells run out of glycogen, **fatigue** sets in and performance will suffer, though the effects will vary among different sports. Training and eating properly, with particular attention to carbohydrates, can increase and maintain glycogen stores, which is particularly important for endurance athletes.

A large part of an athlete's **diet** should be carbohydrate. Foods high in carbohydrate include pasta, rice, cereals, starchy vegetables (e.g., potatoes, carrots, corn, sweet potatoes), fruit, and bread. Not all carbohydrates are equal in providing needed nutrients, however. Focusing on carbohydrate from whole grains, fruits, and vegetables will make sure vitamins, minerals, **fiber**, and other important nutrients are part of one's diet, while filling up on too many sweets and **processed foods** can negatively impact sports performance.

Protein

Protein is essential to build and repair muscle tissue. Protein allows muscles to contract, gain in size, and increase in strength. Loading up on protein does not guarantee larger muscles. Protein in excess of the body's needs is stored as fat, not protein. Muscle growth comes from hard work, proper training, and balanced nutrition. Food sources of protein include lean meat and poultry (fish and chicken), fish, **legumes** (dried beans and peas), nuts, seeds, and dairy products. Protein needs for active athletes, especially endurance sports, are higher than for non-athletes. The maximum recommended amounts of protein is 1.2 to 1.4 g/kg of body weight. This requirement can be met through diet alone.

Fat provides energy, protects the body's organs and helps with the **absorption** of some vitamins. When fats are eaten as part of healthful foods, they provide an important energy source for athletes in training. Good choices include the fats from nuts, seeds, vegetable oils (canola, olive, peanut), and avocados.

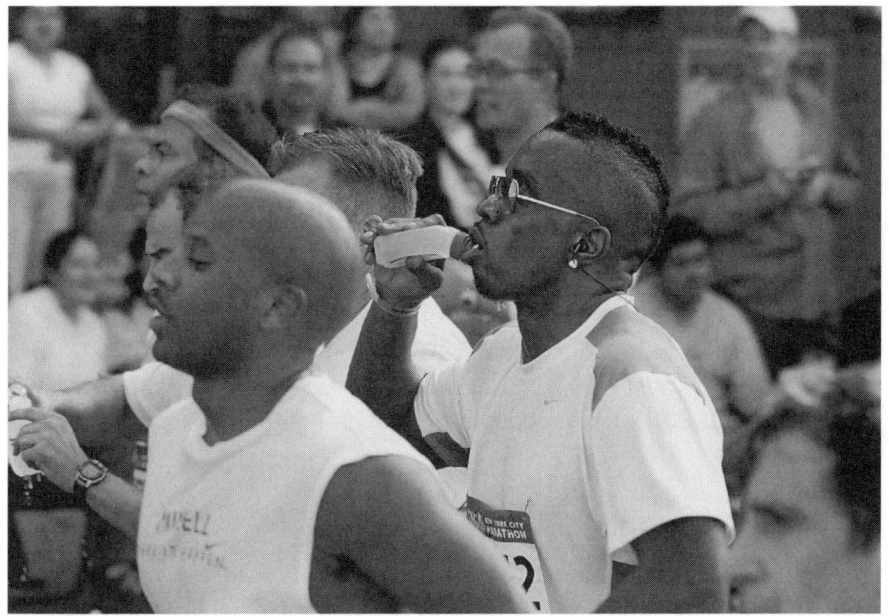

When the body is dehydrated, blood circulation decreases and the muscles do not receive enough oxygen for maximum performance. Thirst is an indication that dehydration has already occurred, so it is important to drink frequently during exercise, before thirst sets in. Here, Sean "P. Diddy" Combs drinks from a water bottle during the 2003 New York City Marathon. [Photograph by Richard Cohen. Corbis. Reproduced by permission.]

Vitamins and Minerals

All vitamins and minerals are important. Two that deserve special attention from athletes are **iron** and **calcium**. Iron is important to carry **oxygen** in blood, and it plays a key role in sports performance. The best sources of iron are lean red meats, shrimp, iron-fortified cereals, and bread products.

Calcium keeps bones strong. Foods from the dairy group, including milk, yogurt, and cheese are excellent sources of calcium. Non-dairy sources of calcium include dark leafy green vegetables, but the calcium may not be absorbed as well. There are also many calcium-fortified juices and foods that can help boost calcium intake. In addition, weight-bearing exercises increase bone density. Calcium needs for female teenage athletes is 1300 mg daily.

iron: nutrient needed for red blood cell formation

calcium: mineral essential for bones and teeth

oxygen: O_2, atmospheric gas required by all animals

Fluids

Water is critical to all body functions and makes up about 60 percent of a person's body weight. Water helps move nutrients throughout the body and helps remove waste from the body. Replacing the fluids lost during exercise is essential to sustaining performance, preventing **dehydration**, and avoiding injury. Even mild dehydration can cause muscle and body fatigue, which will reduce athletic performance. Since thirst is not always a reliable indicator of fluid loss, athletes should drink fluids before they get really thirsty.

Eight to ten cups a water a day is the recommended daily intake for most people. However, extra fluids are needed by athletes to replenish what is lost during exercise. Drinks with caffeine or alcohol should be avoided, as they are dehydrating. Exercising in extreme heat increases fluid needs even more, since more is lost through sweat. Taking in too much water can be just as dangerous as not taking in enough. Athletes should experiment with different fluid intakes to determine the best amounts for optimal performance.

Sports drinks can be helpful, especially for events lasting sixty minutes or longer. In addition to fluid, they provide the advantage of quick replacement of carbohydrate and minerals and also replace **electrolytes** lost

dehydration: loss of water

electrolyte: salt dissolved in fluid

FLUID INTAKE GUIDELINES	
Time in reference to event	Ounces of fluid (oz.)
24 hours before	Drink freely
2 hours before	8–16 oz.
15 minutes before	8–16 oz.
During	4 to 8 oz. every 15–20 minutes
After	Drink freely

in sweat. Another advantage is taste. Athletes may be more likely to drink more fluid if the beverage has a desirable flavor. The ideal carbohydrate solution is 4 to 8 percent carbohydrate, which is typically found in sports drinks.

Sports Supplements

Sports supplements are advertised widely and promise increased power and strength, improved athletic performance, and better overall health. However, in addition to being potentially dangerous, they can be extremely expensive.

The majority of supplements have not been researched thoroughly, especially on teenage athletes. In addition, long-term studies on safety are not extensively available. Stimulating herbs such as guarana and yohimbine can cause **anxiety** and dizziness. One dangerous example is ephedra, which can have adverse effects such as nervousness, irregular heartbeat, and can be deadly in some cases. Creatine supplements may negatively affect kidney function and promote dehydration. **Amino acid** and protein supplements, while not dangerous, are an unnecessary expense when diet alone can meet protein needs. No supplement is the world can take the place of hard training and proper nutrition, and food should be the first priority in an athlete's nutrition program.

The Timing of Meals

The importance of what foods are eaten is matched only by when they're eaten. Proper nutrition is important not just on the day of competition, but on a daily basis. Eating a meal or snack an hour or so before athletic activity will provide energy without having a full stomach. It is also important to replenish the body's stores after athletic activity. A meal or snack within one hour of activity will assure this. Carbohydrates should be the main focus, along with protein in smaller amounts.

Female Athlete Triad

In females, three associated medical conditions form the female athlete triad: disordered eating, **amenorrhea** (suppression of the menstrual cycle), and **osteoporosis** (weakening of the bones). A female athlete can have one, two, or all of these conditions.

Disordered eating is a medical term that includes a broad spectrum of eating disorders. Girls may feel pressured to "lose a few pounds" to increase performance. The intentions may be good at the start, but it can escalate to serious health problems. Heavy exercise and low calorie intake can cause a drop in **estrogen** (a **hormone**), which has a protective effect on bone. Low-

---

anxiety: nervousness

amino acid: building block of proteins, necessary dietary nutrient

amenorrhea: lack of menstruation

osteoporosis: weakening of the bone structure

estrogen: hormone that helps control female development and menstruation

hormone: molecules produced by one set of cells that influence the function of another set of cells

ered estrogen can also lead to irregular menstrual periods, or to the complete cessation of periods. Amenorrhea is not a normal response to high levels of physical activity, but a sign of serious potential problems.

With lowered estrogen levels, the female athlete can experience bone loss similar to that seen in **menopause**. Unfortunately, the lost bone is never replaced. This has both short- and long-term consequences on bone health. The increased risk of bone damage, for example, can lead to **stress** fractures and osteoporosis.

Athletes spend many hours training so their body can perform at its best. It is important that proper nutrition also be a focus so the hours aren't spent in vain. An adequately nourished body provides the proper fuel to maximize athletic effort. SEE ALSO DEHYDRATION; ERGOGENIC AIDS; FEMALE ATHLETE TRIAD.

Kim Schenck

menopause: phase in a woman's life during which ovulation and menstruation end

stress: heightened state of nervousness or unease

Bibliography

American Dietetic Association (2000). "Nutrition and Athletic Performance: Position of the American Dietetic Association, Dietitians of Canada, and the American College of Sports Medicine." *Journal of American Dietetic Association* 100:1543–1566.

Clark, Nancy (2003). *Nancy Clark's Sports Nutrition Guidebook.* Champaign, IL: Human Kinetics.

Coleman, Ellen (2003). *Eating for Endurance.* Boulder, CO: Bull Publishing.

Sizer, Frances, and Whitney, Eleanor (2003). *Nutrition Concepts and Controversies.* Belmont, CA: Wadsworth/Thomson Learning.

Internet Resources

University of Illinois Extension. "Sports and Nutrition: The Winning Connection." Available from <http://www.urbanext.uiuc.edu/hsnut>

Stark, William
British physician
1747–1770

William Stark (1741–1770) was born in Birmingham, England, of Scottish parentage. He obtained his medical degree at Leiden, Netherlands, in 1769. Upon returning to London in June 1769, Stark began a series of dietary studies in which he was his own subject. At the start of his twenty-four experiments, he described himself as being a healthy, six-foot tall young man.

These experiments were performed in an effort to prove that a "pleasant and varied **diet**" was as healthful as simpler strict diets. Stark kept accurate measures of temperature and weather conditions, the weights of all food and water he consumed, and the weight of all daily excretions. Stark also recorded how he felt on a daily basis.

In his first experiment, Stark ate bread and water with a little sugar for thirty-one days. This experiment left Stark dull and listless. He consumed a more varied diet for a few weeks. When he felt better, however, the experiments resumed. Gradually, he added other foods to this regimen, one at a time. He added olive oil, milk, roast goose, boiled beef, **fat**, figs, and veal. After the first two months, his gums were red and swollen, and they bled when pressure was put on them. This was a symptom of **scurvy**, a disease

diet: the total daily food intake, or the types of foods eaten

fat: type of food molecule rich in carbon and hydrogen, with high energy content

scurvy: a syndrome characterized by weakness, anemia, and spongy gums, due to vitamin C deficiency

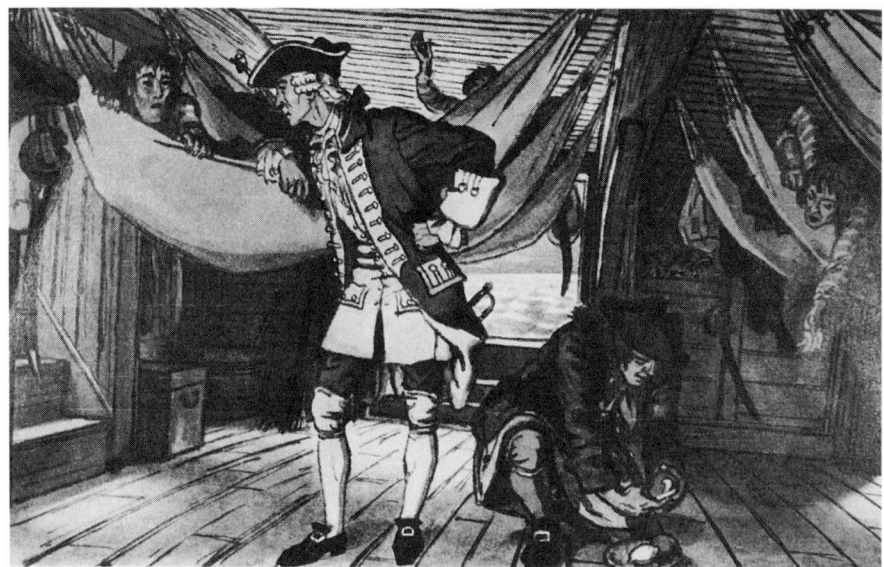

William Stark's self-sacrificing dietary research ended in his death from scurvy, a disease caused by vitamin C deficiency. Had he heeded the recent discoveries of James Lind, pictured here giving lemons to sailors, Stark would have known to include citrus fruits in his experimental diet. [© Bettman/Corbis. Reproduced by permission.]

caused by a lack of vitamin C that was fairly common at the time. By November, he was living on nothing but pudding, except for a pint of black currants in celebration of Boxing Day (the day after Christmas). Stark did consider testing the effects that fresh fruits and vegetables would have on his health, but decided instead on honey puddings and Cheshire cheese.

After eight months of experimenting, Stark died on February 23, 1770, at the age of twenty-nine. He did not discover anything new about scurvy, but, through his experiments and record-keeping skills, he showed to what extent human scurvy is caused by a lack of vitamin C in the diet. Stark showed that simple diets that do not include fruits and vegetables are not conducive to health. He thus showed the value of a pleasant and varied diet by clearly demonstrating the consequences of a dietary regime lacking variety. James Carmichael Smyth published Stark's experiments eighteen years after his death. SEE ALSO SCURVY.

Slande Celeste

Bibliography

Saunders, Alan. "Martyrs of Nutrition." Australian Broadcasting Corporation. Available from <http://www.abc.net.au/science/sweek/bites/comfy.htm>

Vanderbilt University Medical Center. "Scurvy and Vitamin C." Available from <http://www.mc.vanderbilt.edu>

Sustainable Food Systems

A *food system* is a process that aims to create a more direct link between the producers (farmers) of food and **fiber** and the consumers of the food. This system consists of several components, including production, processing, distribution, consumption, and waste disposal.

A food system can be characterized as being local, regional, national, or global. The word *sustainable* is often associated with the sustainable agriculture movement, which had its beginnings in North America in the 1980s. This period was characterized by a wave of bank foreclosures of farm oper-

fiber: indigestible plant material which aids digestion by providing bulk

ations, particularly small and family-owned farms. Many were unable to compete with the large national and international farming corporations and were forced to sell their farms and go out of business. **Globalization**, through international trade agreements, were also viewed by some in the agriculture community as another reason for the demise of many small and family-owned farms.

Misuse and overuse of chemical fertilizers and pesticides contributed heavily to the degradation of many farms and waterways throughout the United States, Canada, and other developing countries. Out of this "farm crisis" came national and international institutions and organizations of concerned citizens, producers, community organizations, and environmental groups. They agitated for the creation of policies and laws that supported new environmentally safe approaches to producing food and fiber and that would ensure the livelihood of farmers and vibrant rural communities. Thus, a sustainable food system is a system that sustains people as well as the land.

globalization: development of world-wide economic system

Why Are Sustainable Food Systems Important?

A sustainable food system, whether it is local or regional, brings farmers closer to consumers by producing fruits and vegetables or raising livestock or fish closer to the places they are sold. Advocates of this system believe that when it comes to food security, the closer producers are to homes and neighborhoods, the greater the access to more nutritious and affordable food.

Globally, crop production is a highly intensive operation in both inputs and **energy** consumption. Of the 10 to 20 percent of the fossil-fuel energy that is used by agricultural operations, 40 percent is indirect energy used in the development of chemical pesticides and fertilizers. There is thus a need to work with natural processes to conserve all resources, minimize waste, and lessen the impact on the **environment**. In theory, this usually means limited use of synthetic fertilizers, pesticides, growth regulators, and livestock feed additives. Instead, it means more reliance on methods such as crop rotations, animal manures, **legumes**, mechanical cultivation, mineral-bearing rocks to maintain soil fertility and productivity; and on natural, cultural, and **biological** controls to manage insects, weeds, and other pests. The emphasis is on prevention of problems and the use of curative interventions, such as pesticides, as last resorts.

energy: technically, the ability to perform work; the content of a substance that allows it to be useful as a fuel

environment: surroundings

legumes: beans, peas and related plants

biological: related to living organisms

Urban growth and infrastructure development has reduced the amount of prime agricultural land. The United States, for example, loses two acres of farmland every minute to urban growth between 1992 and 1997. According to the United Nations projections, 4.9 billion people or 60 percent of the world population will be living in urban areas by 2030. It is not clear how this population can be adequately fed and nourished. Increasing population also means increased quantities of food to be distributed, which increases the amount of trucks used to transport the food, thereby contributing to traffic congestion and air pollution.

Promoting Sustainable Local Food Systems

Consumers around the world can make a difference by choosing to vote with their dollars to support local and regional food systems. There are a

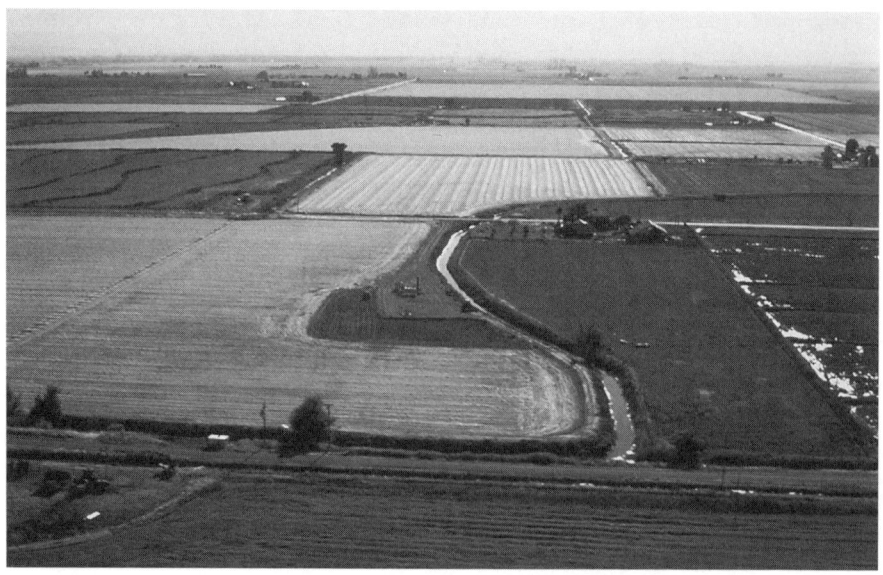

Sustainable agriculture is a method of farming that minimizes environmental damage and depletion of resources. To be successful, sustainable agriculture requires a commitment from food producers as well as food consumers. [JLM Visuals. Reproduced by permission.]

number of ways that individuals can support and help to sustain food systems in their area.

Farmers markets. Buying fresh food from local farmers markets supports family farms and circulates money within the community. Organic foods should be purchased, if possible, since they are grown with little or no artificial pesticides or fertilizers.

Community and school gardens. These gardens provide fresh produce, particularly for underserved populations in low-income and poverty-stricken neighborhoods. This increases the dietary quality and ensures a measure of food security.

Community-supported agriculture (CSA). In this type of arrangement, individuals buy shares the harvest of a farm before the crops are planted. In return, individuals receive fresh fruits and vegetables and sometimes local meats, cheeses, flowers, and eggs, on a weekly or prearranged basis.

Pick-your-own farms (U-Pick-It) and roadside stands. At some rural farms, consumers are allowed to pick their own fresh fruits and vegetables. This can serve as a social outing for urban families who drive to rural roadside stands.

These practices help consumers choose foods grown using agricultural practices that keep water sources clean, support healthy soil, and encourage wildlife conservation. A healthy and successful food system emphasizes support for local sources of food production and processing, encourages and supports environmental responsibility, and provides economic stability all within the context of a local or regional area. Sustainable food systems also encompass and emphasize such larger issues as stable farm families, food security and access, community self-reliance, and even entrepreneurship. Sustainable food systems provide hope for a sustainable future. SEE ALSO FAMINE; FOOD INSECURITY; ORGANIC FOODS; PESTICIDES.

Carlos Robles

Internet Resources

American Farmland Trust. "Farming on the Edge: Sprawling Development Threatens Americas Best Farmland." Available from <http://www.farmland.org/farmingontheedge>

Deumling, D.; Wackernagel, M.; and Monfreda C. "Eating Up the Earth: How Sustainable Food Systems Shrink Our Ecological Footprint." *Agriculture Footprint Brief*, July 2003. Available from <http://www.RedefiningProgress.org>

Food and Agricultural Organization (FAO) of the United Nations. *Studying Food Supply and Distribution Systems to Cities in Developing Countries and Countries in Transition: Methodological and Operational Guide*, revised edition. Available from <http://www.fao.org>

Wilkins, J. "Community Food Systems: Linking Food, Nutrition, and Agriculture." Cornell Cooperative Extension, Food and Nutrition Available from <http://www.cce.cornell.edu/food>

Toxemia

Toxemia is the presence of abnormal substances in the blood, but the term is also used in reference to a condition in pregnancy also known as *preeclampsia*. This refers to pregnancy-induced hypertension (**high blood pressure**) and any possible accompanying symptoms, such as quick or sudden weight gain, water retention, and excessive swelling of the feet, hands, and face. The condition is most common among first pregnancies, with multiple births (e.g., twins), in younger or older women, and in women who had preeclampsia in previous pregnancies. It generally occurs near the due date, but it can also occur earlier in pregnancy. When monitoring a female with toxemia, the **blood pressure** and urine **protein** are checked often and bed rest may be prescribed. Toxemia can be mild or severe. When severe, it is dangerous for both the pregnant female and her child, especially if the mother's blood pressure gets too high. SEE ALSO PREGNANCY.

Judith C. Rodriguez

high blood pressure: elevation of the pressure in the bloodstream maintained by the heart

blood pressure: measure of the pressure exerted by the blood against the walls of the blood vessels

protein: complex molecule composed of amino acids that performs vital functions in the cell; necessary part of the diet

Bibliography

Sizer, Frances, and Whitney, Eleanor (2003). *Nutrition Concepts and Controversies*, 9th edition. Belmont, CA: Thomson.

Internet Resources

Hill, D. Ashley. "Issues and Procedures in Women's Health: Pre-eclampsia." Available from http://www.obgyn.net

Tulp, Nicolaas

Dutch physician
1593–1674

The Dutch physician Nicolaas Tulp was born on October 11, 1593, in Amsterdam, Holland, the fourth child of a prominent merchant family. He was originally named Claes (Nicolas) Pieterz, but he later adopted the name Tulp, meaning "tulip." Tulp attended Leiden University in Holland, receiving his medical degree in 1614. He then returned to Amsterdam, opening a practice in surgery and general medicine. In 1628, Tulp was appointed as a lecturer of the Suregon's Guild, a position he held until 1652. His duties were to lecture in anatomy and surgery, to apprentice surgeons, and to

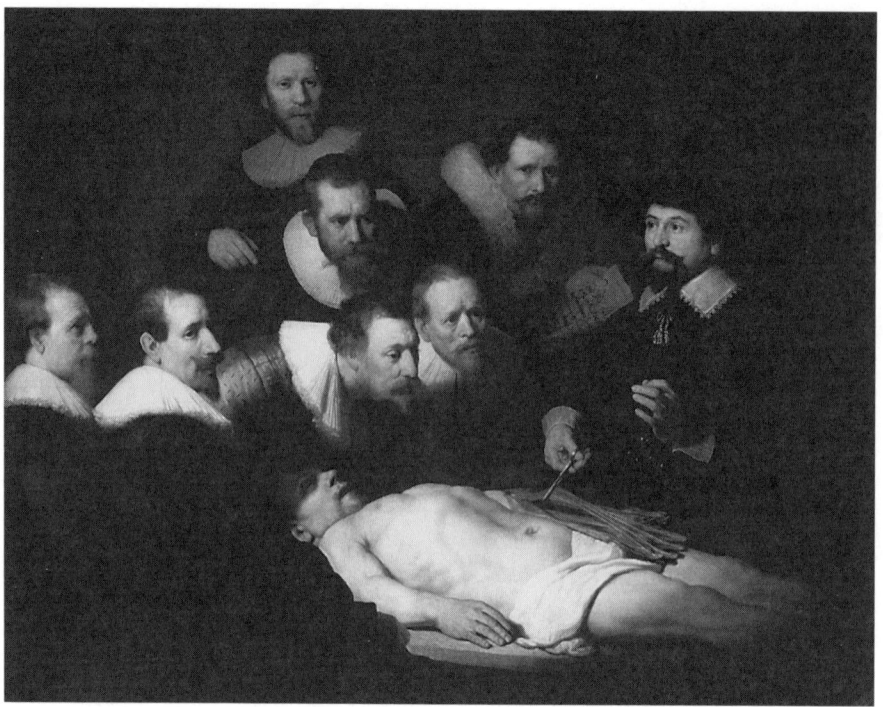

Rembrandt's "The Anatomy Lecture of Dr. Nicolaes Tulp." Dr. Tulp was a lecturer for the Amsterdam Surgeon's Guild, and among his duties was the presentation of public dissections. [© Francis G. Mayer/Corbis. Reproduced by permission.]

deliver public dissections. The most famous of these, held on January 31, 1632, was depicted by the artist Rembrandt in his famous painting "The Anatomy Lesson of Dr. Tulp," now in Holland's Mauritshuis museum.

Tulp's best-known medical work, published in Latin in 1641, is titled *Observationes Medicae*. Tulp believed that all medical publications should be published in Latin, which the public could not read, to prevent people from treating their own illnesses. In his book, Tulp summarized his own cases and observations, including his description of beriberi, a disease caused by vitamin B1 (thiamine) deficiency. This is one of the first known descriptions of beriberi. Tulp had treated a Dutchman who was brought back to Holland from the East Indies, suffering from what the natives of the Indies called beriberi or "the lameness." Although Tulp described beriberi in detail, he was unaware that it was caused by a dietary deficiency. It was more than two hundred years later that Dutch physicians discovered the cause of beriberi. Tulp also described the ileocecal valve at the junction of the large and small **intestines**, still known as Tulp's valve.

intestines: the two long tubes that carry out the bulk of the processes of digestion

During the plague epidemic of 1635, Tulp supported quarantine as a means to control the spread of the disease. At the same time, Tulp suggested that local pharmacists be placed under municipal control, because he viewed them as inefficient. This resulted in the formation of the first local medical authority in Holland. Another result of Tulp's concern was the publication of the first Dutch pharmacopoeia, a book describing **drugs**, chemicals, and medicinal preparations.

drugs: substances whose administration causes a significant change in the body's function

In addition to his scientific endeavors, Tulp was an active public servant. He served four times as mayor of Amsterdam, was treasurer of the city for twenty-seven years, and was elected several times as a city councilor. Tulp also served as a judge, trustee of the city orphanage, and curator of two local schools. Tulp was married to Aagfe Van der Vogh in 1617; unfortunately, she died in 1628. Tulp died in the The Hague in 1674, at the age of eighty-one. SEE ALSO BERIBERI.

Karen Bryla

Bibliography

Gillispie, Charles Coulston, ed. (1976). *Dictionary of Scientific Biography*. Vol. XIII. New York: Scribners.

Spencer, Frank, ed. (1997). *History of Physical Anthropology: An Encyclopedia*, Vol. 2. New York: Garland.

Todhunter, E. Neige (1967). "Biographical Notes from the History of Nutrition." *Journal of the American Dietetic Association* 50:200.

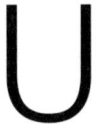

Underweight

A person is considered underweight if his or her **body mass index** (BMI) falls below a certain threshold (body mass index is a measure determined by a person's age, height, and weight). For infants and children, a BMI below the 10th percentile for a specific age indicates an individual who is underweight. For adults, a BMI below 19.1 for females and 20.7 for males is considered underweight. A BMI of 17.5 indicates an individual is very underweight.

Individuals who are underweight are at high risk for **malnutrition**. Being underweight can affect growth and **development**, and it can cause infertility or delayed menstruation. It can also result in **fatigue**, irritability, and a lack of concentration, as well as impairing the body's ability to **thermoregulate** itself. Due to a decreased immune response, underweight individuals are less resistant to infections and disease.

It is recommended that underweight individuals gain one pound per week until an appropriate weight is reached. This can be accomplished by consistently (daily) increasing one's intake of calorically denser foods (i.e., nuts instead of pretzels), eating more frequently, and drinking fluids between meals rather than with meals. SEE ALSO BODY MASS INDEX; MALNUTRITION; NUTRITIONAL DEFICIENCY; WEIGHT MANAGEMENT.

Leslie Bonci

body mass index: weight in kilograms divided by square of the height in meters; a measure of body fat

malnutrition: chronic lack of sufficient nutrients to maintain health

development: the process of change by which an organism becomes more complex

fatigue: tiredness

thermoregulate: regulate temperature

Bibliography

Duyff, Roberta L. (1996). *The American Dietetic Association's Complete Food and Nutrition Guide*. Minneapolis, MN: Chronimed.

Internet Resources

American Dietetic Association. Available from <http://www.eatright.org>

United Nations Children's Fund (UNICEF)

The United Nations International Children's Emergency Fund (UNICEF) was created in 1946. It was renamed the United Nations Children's Fund in 1953, when the fund's focus changed from emergency aid to on going support of children's needs. The acronym UNICEF was retained, however. With eight regional offices and 125 country offices, UNICEF strives to create a world where all children share in the joy and promise of childhood with dignity, security, and self-fulfillment.

Administration of UNICEF

The United Nations, headquartered in New York, hosts the world center for UNICEF operations. Thirty-six members of an executive board report to the Economic and Social Council of the United Nations. The Board oversees implementation of policies; monitoring of worldwide activities; and the consistency and acceptability of UNICEF strategies and programs, as well as the organization's financial budget, administrative plans, and reports.

Resources for UNICEF Operations

National governments and other United Nations organizations support UNICEF efforts in 161 sites around the world. The United States provides the greatest annual contribution ($248 million in 2000), while combined funds from the United Kingdom, Japan, Sweden, Norway, the Netherlands, Denmark, Australia, Canada, and Italy ($335 million) add significant governmental support. One-third of UNICEF's resources are received through Private Sector Division partnerships with social organizations, celebrities, and businesses.

Mission

The goal of UNICEF is to give every child a brighter future. The organization's pledge, "we will continue the same unwavering support for children that we have maintained," remains, as partners allocate resources for basic childhood needs of food, security, and shelter. The partnerships further support education for all children and enforcement of child labor practices. UNICEF's staff and volunteers must combat the enormous challenges facing children in war-torn countries, where poverty is rampant, as they try to control infection and disease, provide safe food and water, and fight discrimination.

UNICEF Accomplishments Since 1990

During the 1990s, there were many successful efforts by UNICEF to improve health, **nutrition**, and survival for women and children around the world. In 1990, UNICEF members, who held voting rights, supported the formation of the Convention on the Rights of the Child. During 1991, UNICEF and the World Health Organization (WHO) initiated efforts to improve the health and nutritional status of pregnant women, mothers with babies, and infants, through the Ten Steps to Successful Breastfeeding program. In response, health centers around the world adopted the "ten steps," and became "baby-friendly" hospitals and birthing centers. By 2002, more than 15,000 sites in 136 counties were educating women and promoting healthful behaviors to improve the nutritional status of babies.

The first International Children's Day of Broadcasting began in 1992 to promote excellence in radio and television programming for children. Since then, more than two thousand media groups have provided wholesome and child-sensitive programs around the world. In 1993, twenty-five years of success with oral rehydration therapy (ORT) was celebrated. ORT provides a simple solution of sugar, salt, and water, and has saved millions of children in developing countries where safe water and sanitary conditions are unavailable. The highlight of 1994 was the Global Girls' Education Pro-

---

UNICEF in Bam, Iran

In December 2003, the city of Bam in southeastern Iran was hit by an earthquake that measured 6.3 on the Richter scale. It was estimated that 30,000 people were killed and 40,000 others injured. More than 100,000 people were affected, with more than 90 percent of homes heavily damaged or destroyed. Within 48 hours, UNICEF had sent two major shipments of emergency supplies and gone to work to provide safe water and sanitation. The organization created a tracing system utilizing a digital camera to help document missing children and reunite them with their families. Within one month, the first children returned to temporary schools established by UNICEF.

—*Paula Kepos*

---

nutrition: the maintenance of health through proper eating, or the study of same

gramme in which education for young girls was a priority. UNICEF research efforts on the status of young girls began in 1994 with household surveys administered in sixty countries. This provided a baseline for a vast database about the status of health, nutrition, security, and other programs.

During 1995, UNICEF strengthened the initiatives to make issues of gender for women and the impact of war on children less of a problem. UNICEF sought support from nations through a 20/20 initiative—asking them to allocate 20 percent of their budgets for 20 percent of UNICEF's social services programs. By 1996, UNICEF had expanded its programs in AIDS awareness, prevention, and assistance to families and children in need of support for AIDS-related resources, and the Voices of Youth, a website where children can share information and insights on AIDS and other topics of interest, had begun. In 1997, a UNICEF document signed by 123 nations sought to protect children from weapons of destruction, and the International Conference on Child Labour met to support the elimination of employment for children where exploitation or hazardous conditions exist.

UNICEF, with the WHO and others, increased their efforts to address **malaria** prevention efforts in 1998, and by 1999 had formed a partnership with Global Alliance for **Vaccines** and Immunizations (GAVI) to supply vaccines against measles, mumps, **hepatitis** B, **diphtheria** and other preventable communicable conditions. During 2000 and 2001, the Say Yes for Children program received pledges of financial support from government and private sources in the ongoing effort to fund the improvement of health, education, nutrition, and safety of children.

malaria: disease caused by infection with Plasmodium, a single-celled protozoon, transmitted by mosquitoes

vaccine: medicine that promotes immune system resistance by stimulating pre-existing cells to become active

hepatitis: liver inflammation

diphtheria: infectious disease caused by Cornybacterium diphtheriae, causing damage to the heart and other organs

Programs and Operations of UNICEF

UNICEF and partners worldwide provide programs and oversee operations that have been directed either toward specific causes or generally to improve health, nutrition, security, or other needs. These programs include:

- The Oneworld Alliance for UNICEF, which is a partnership with airline companies who show in-flight UNICEF videos, collect donations from passengers, and ship emergency supplies.

- Rotary International supports and funds the Global Polio Eradication Initiative and National Immunization Days, a program of the United States Centers for Diseases Control and Prevention.

- The Kiwanis Worldwide Service Project focuses on iodine deficiency disorders. As a result, 70 percent of all households worldwide have iodized salt, a significant step toward improvement of the nutritional and health status of children.

- Check Out for Children is a program in place in hotels outside of North America where guests are invited to donate $1 to UNICEF. In celebration of the success of this program and the five million dollars contributed since inception, a Give Me Five (for $5 donations) program has been launched in Europe, Africa, India, and the Middle East.

- The Federation Internationale de Football Association (FIFA) has partnered with UNICEF to support implementation of the Convention

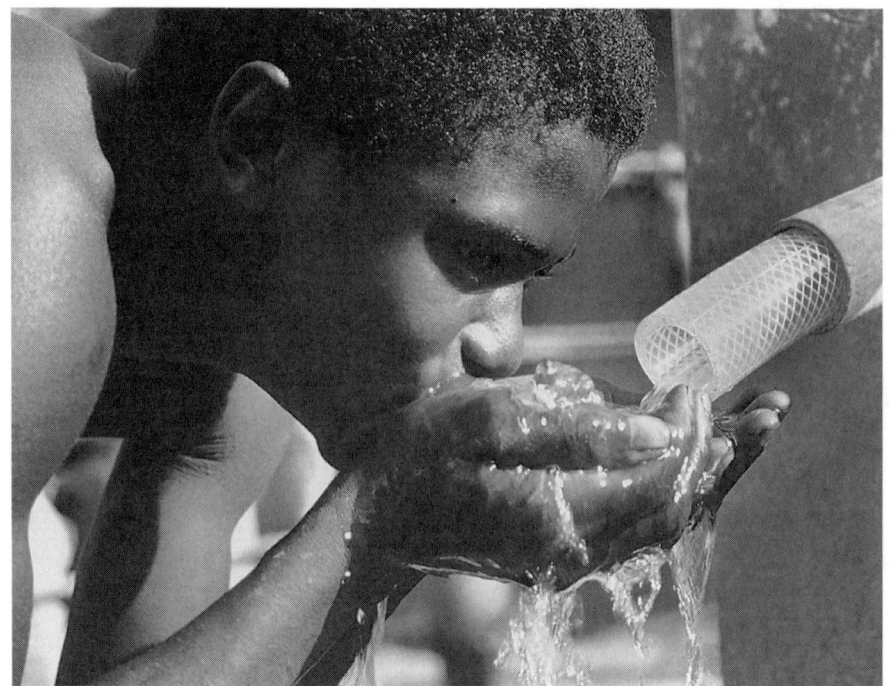

Six thousand people, many of them children, die every day from infections caused by contaminated water. UNICEF responds to this situation by educating people about water safety and helping people secure their water supplies. *[Photograph by Liba Taylor. Corbis. Reproduced by permission.]*

on the Rights of the Child. FIFA projects include the sale of notebooks, t-shirts, backpacks, and other items with FIFA and UNICEF logos that focus on children's rights to education, health care, and play.

- UNICEF greeting card and product sales have accounted for over $1 billion in revenues to support UNICEF programs.
- Global Movement for Children is a program to assist children in war-torn areas and to protect at-risk children from sexual exploitation and violence.
- Trick or Treat for UNICEF, on National UNICEF Day (October 31), raises awareness of UNICEF programs and the importance of ongoing support through volunteerism and contributions.

In summary, UNICEF funds programs and provide unique partnerships to eradicate disease, improve the health and nutritional status of children, and to make the world a better place for children to grow and develop. Other efforts to educate girls, improve children's working conditions, and establish housing and security in impoverished and war-torn environments have been addressed and supported. More work is needed, however, as the future of the global community depends, in part, on the health and well-being its children. SEE ALSO ORAL REHYDRATION THERAPY; WORLD HEALTH ORGANIZATION (WHO).

Ruth A. Waibel

Internet Resources

UNICEF. "Annual Report, 2000." Available from <http://www.unicef.org/ar00>

UNICEF. "The Progress of Nations, 2000." Available from <http:www.unicef.org/pon00>

UNICEF. "The State of the World's Children, 2001." Available from <http://www.unicef.org/sowc01>

Vegan

A **vegan** (pronounced VEE-gun) is a vegetarian who does not eat any animal products, including eggs and dairy products. A well-planned vegan **diet** can be nutritionally adequate, even for children and pregnant and lactating women. However, it is important that wise food selections are made. These selections include soymilk **fortified** with vitamin B_{12}, **vitamin D**, and **calcium**. Also important are whole grains, nuts, and seeds, which are rich sources of **zinc** and other **nutrients**. Foods high in vitamin C will help to increase **iron absorption**. SEE ALSO PLANT-BASED DIETS; VEGETARIANISM.

Cheryl Flynt

vegan: person who consumes no animal products, including milk and honey

diet: the total daily food intake, or the types of foods eaten

fortified: altered by addition of vitamins or minerals

vitamin D: nutrient needed for calcium uptake and therefore proper bone formation

calcium: mineral essential for bones and teeth

zinc: mineral necessary for many enzyme processes

nutrient: dietary substance necessary for health

iron: nutrient needed for red blood cell formation

absorption: uptake by the digestive tract

Bibliography

Seventh-day Adventist Dietetic Association (1997). *The Vegetarian/Vegan Resource: An Annex to Diet Manuals.* Roseville, CA: Author.

Internet Resources

Vegetarian Nutrition Resource Group. Available from <http://www.vegetariannutrition.net>

Vegetarian Resource Group. Available from <http://www.vrg.org>

Vegetarianism

A vegetarian eating plan, also known as plant-based eating, is based on a diet of grains, fruits, vegetables, nuts, and seeds, with occasional use of dairy and egg products. This style of eating has existed since the beginning of recorded history. As early as 600 B.C.E., a vegetarian movement was founded in ancient Rome. Vegetarian eating became popular in England and the United States in the mid-nineteenth century. For many individuals, their whole **lifestyle** is defined by their vegetarian eating. In 1998, 7 percent of American adults considered themselves to be vegetarians.

lifestyle: set of choices about diet, exercise, job type, leisure activities, and other aspects of life

Types of Vegetarians

There are several vegetarian eating styles. Most vegetarians consider themselves lacto-ovo vegetarians, meaning they generally eat dairy and egg products, but do not include meat, poultry, or fish in their diet. Lacto vegetarians eliminate all animal foods except dairy products. Total vegetarians, or vegans (pronounced VEE-guns), eliminate all animal products. Individuals who occasionally eat meat, poultry, or fish consider themselves semi-vegetarian.

Most individuals who choose a vegetarian eating style want to be healthier and lower their risk for disease. Others are concerned about the **environment** and the cost of raising animals for food. Some do not agree with the inhumane treatment and killing of animals for food. There are also a number of individuals who choose vegetarian eating for religious purposes.

environment: surroundings

heart disease: any disorder of the heart or its blood supply, including heart attack, atherosclerosis, and coronary artery disease

high blood pressure: elevation of the pressure in the bloodstream maintained by the heart

diabetes: inability to regulate level of sugar in the blood

obesity: the condition of being overweight, according to established norms based on sex, age, and height

osteoporosis: weakening of the bone structure

Benefits of Vegetarianism

Research has shown a number of health benefits related to vegetarian eating. **Heart disease**, **high blood pressure**, adult-onset **diabetes**, **obesity**, **osteoporosis**, and certain cancers occur less often in people who are vegetarian. Science has demonstrated that these health benefits are related to healthful

saturated fat: a fat with the maximum possible number of hydrogens; more difficult to break down than unsaturated fats

protein: complex molecule composed of amino acids that performs vital functions in the cell; necessary part of the diet

fortified: altered by addition of vitamins or minerals

calcium: mineral essential for bones and teeth

tofu: soybean curd, similar in consistency to cottage cheese

iron: nutrient needed for red blood cell formation

absorption: uptake by the digestive tract

calorie: unit of food energy

nutrient: dietary substance necessary for health

vitamin: necessary complex nutrient used to aid enzymes or other metabolic processes in the cell

mineral: an inorganic (non-carbon-containing) element, ion or compound

fiber: indigestible plant material which aids digestion by providing bulk

vitamin D: nutrient needed for calcium uptake and therefore proper bone formation

food choices. Eating whole grains, fruits, vegetables, nuts, and seeds provides the body with the ammunition needed to fight disease and illness. A diet high in meat, **saturated fat**, milk, cheese, and butter does not provide the same health benefits.

Nutritional Adequacy

Almost every food contains **protein**. Even though animal foods are high in protein, they are not the only foods able to supply protein, which is necessary for the growth and maintenance of the body. Sources of protein in the vegetarian diet include cooked dried beans, nuts, seeds, and soy products.

Dairy and egg products provide vitamin B_{12}. For the vegetarian, foods such as **fortified** cereals and soymilk can provide the vitamin B_{12} needed by the body. Dairy products are also an excellent source of **calcium**, along with calcium-fortified soymilk, **tofu** processed with calcium, broccoli, nuts, collard greens, and calcium-fortified orange juice. High-calcium foods are important for strong bones and should be consumed early in life to build the body's calcium stores.

Although red meat is a major source of **iron** in Western diets, vegetarians actually have higher iron intakes than nonvegetarians. Plant sources of iron include beans, fortified cereals, whole grain products, tofu, dark green leafy vegetables, seeds, prune juice, and blackstrap molasses. Including a vitamin C–rich food with meals will help to increase the body's **absorption** of iron.

The American Dietetic Association has stated that "appropriately planned vegetarian diets are healthful, are nutritionally adequate, and provide health benefits in the prevention and treatment of certain diseases" (*Journal of the American Dietetic Association*, 1317).

Vegetarianism at Different Ages

When choosing vegetarian eating, it is important to be aware that there are special nutritional needs at different stages of life. Pregnancy and breast-feeding require additional **calories** and **nutrients**. A well-planned vegetarian diet can provide these in the amounts needed for a healthy mother and baby.

During infancy, childhood, and the teenage years, adequate calories to sustain proper growth are necessary. This usually is not a problem for infants because they are either breastfed or on formula. During childhood and the teenage years, meals should consist of high-calorie, high-nutrient (good sources of protein, **vitamins**, and **minerals**) foods. Because many plant foods are low in calories and high in **fiber**, it is easy for the child or teenager to feel full before eating an adequate amount of calories. Moderate amounts of high-fat foods can help to increase calorie intake. In-between-meal snacks are useful, as they also provide needed calories. Healthy snacks include items like peanut-butter sandwiches and milk (or soy milk), a melted cheese and bagel sandwich, fruit smoothies, and, after three years of age, dried fruits, nuts, and seeds.

Older adults may have difficulty obtaining vitamins D and B_{12}, as well as calories. Many people do not get enough sunlight for their bodies to produce the recommended amount of **vitamin D**, which is essential for

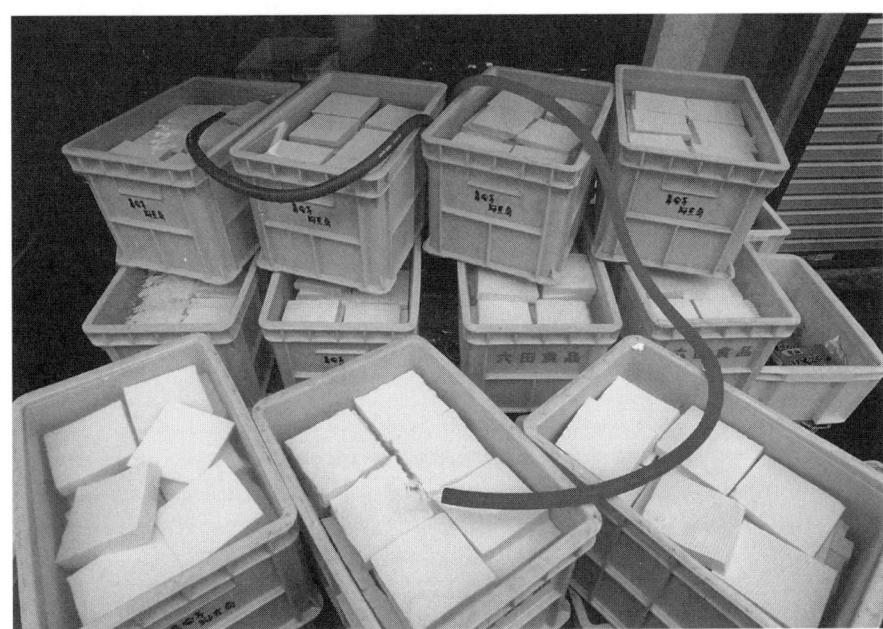

Fresh tofu is packed in water for shipping, which helps it retain its flavor and form. Tofu is made from soybean curds. It provides all the excellent nutritive properties of soy, including high-quality protein. [© *Michael S. Yamashita/Corbis. Reproduced by Corbis Corporation.*]

absorbing calcium and preventing osteoporosis. Using breakfast cereals and soy products fortified with vitamin D is important, though it may also be necessary to take a supplement because the absorption of vitamin B_{12} decreases as people get older.

It is important to eat foods that are fortified with B_{12}, such as soymilk, or to take a B_{12} supplement. Older adults are also at risk for not getting enough calories, because the appetite tends to decrease with age. Eating foods that are low in calories and high in fiber makes it difficult to get the needed **energy** intake to stay healthy. Eating high-calorie, nutrient-dense foods and in-between-meal snacks is important.

Careful planning ensures that vegetarian eating will provide the **nutrition** needed to stay healthy. One helpful tool is the Vegetarian Food Guide Pyramid, which provides guidelines for selecting foods and the appropriate portion sizes.

Using a variety of foods is essential to good health when following the Food Guide Pyramid. One single food cannot provide the body with all the nutrition it needs. Five portions of fruits and vegetables should be consumed daily, including a citrus fruit and a dark green leafy vegetable. Whole grains should be eaten whenever possible; these have more nutrients and fiber than processed grains such as white bread and white rice. Proteins should be chosen wisely. While dairy products and eggs are good protein sources, they are also high in saturated fats and **cholesterol**. Nuts, seeds, beans, and soy products should be part of the diet.

A carefully planned vegetarian diet can provide the nutrients needed for health at any time during the life cycle. Most individuals who choose this eating style do so because of the many health benefits associated with vegetarian eating, including reduced risk for heart disease, diabetes, and some cancers. SEE ALSO MEAT ANALOGS; PLANT-BASED DIETS; SOY; VEGAN; WHOLE FOODS DIET.

Cheryl Flynt

energy: technically, the ability to perform work; the content of a substance that allows it to be useful as a fuel

nutrition: the maintenance of health through proper eating, or the study of same

cholesterol: multi-ringed molecule found in animal cell membranes; a type of lipid

Bibliography

American Dietetic Association. "Position of the American Dietetic Association: Vegetarian Diets." *Journal of the American Dietetic Association* 97(11):1317–1321.

Duyff, Roberta Larson (1996). *The American Dietetic Association's Complete Food and Nutrition Guide.* Minneapolis, MN: Chronimed.

Seventh-day Adventist Dietetic Association (1997). *The Vegetarian/Vegan Resource: An Annex to Diet Manuals.* Roseville, CA: Author.

Vitamins, Fat-Soluble

fat: type of food molecule rich in carbon and hydrogen, with high energy content

vitamin: necessary complex nutrient used to aid enzymes or other metabolic processes in the cell

intestines: the two long tubes that carry out much of the processes of digestion

malabsorption: decreased ability to take up nutrients

absorption: uptake by the digestive tract

adipose tissue: tissue containing fat deposits

water-soluble: able to be dissolved in water

carotenoid: plant-derived molecules used as pigments

Because they dissolve in **fat**, **vitamins** A, D, E, and K are called *fat-soluble* vitamins. They are absorbed from the small **intestines**, along with dietary fat, which is why fat **malabsorption** resulting from various diseases (e.g., cystic fibrosis, ulcerative colitis, Crohn's disease) is associated with poor **absorption** of these vitamins. Fat-soluble vitamins are primarily stored in the liver and **adipose tissues**. With the exception of vitamin K, fat-soluble vitamins are generally excreted more slowly than **water-soluble** vitamins, and vitamins A and D can accumulate and cause toxic effects in the body.

Vitamin A

Vitamin A was the first fat-soluble vitamin identified (in 1913). Vitamin A comprises the preformed retinoids, plus the precursor forms, the provitamin A **carotenoids**. *Preformed retinoids* is a collective term for retinol, retinal, and retinoic acid, all of which are biologically active. The *provitamin A carotenoids* include beta-carotene and others, which are converted to retinoids with varying degrees of efficiency. Retinoids are sensitive to heat, light, and oxidation by air. Beta-carotene is relatively more stable. Vitamin E helps protect vitamin A from oxidation. There is some loss of vitamin A with cooking, but only after boiling for a comparatively long period.

protein: complex molecule composed of amino acids that performs vital functions in the cell; necessary part of the diet

Retinoids are converted to retinol in the intestines and transported with dietary fat to the liver, where it is stored. A special transport **protein**, retinol-binding protein (RBP), transports vitamin A from the liver to other tissues. Carotenoids are absorbed intact at a much lower absorption rate than retinol. Of all the carotenoids, beta-carotene has the highest potential vitamin-A activity. The active forms of vitamin A have three basic functions: vision, growth and **development** of tissues, and immunity.

development: the process of change by which an organism becomes more complex

- *Vision.* Vitamin A combines with a protein called *opsin* to form *rhodopsin* in the rod cells of the retina. When vitamin A is inadequate, the lack of rhodopsin makes it difficult to see in dim light.

- *Growth and development of tissues.* Vitamin A is involved in normal cell differentiation—a process through which embryonic cells transform into mature tissue cells with highly specific functions. Vitamin A supports male and female reproductive processes and bone growth.

- *Immunity.* Vitamin A is essential for immune function and vitamin-A deficiency is associated with decreased resistance to infections. The severity of some infections, such as measles and diarrhea, is reduced by vitamin-A supplementation among those who suffer from vitamin-A deficiency.

FAT SOLUBLE VITAMINS

Vitamin	Functions	Deficiency symptoms	People at risk	Sources	Daily recommended intakes	Toxicity
Vitamin A Preformed retinoids and provitamin A carotinoids	Vision in dim light and color vision, cell differentiation and growth, immunity	Poor growth, night blindness, blindness, dry skin, Xerophthalmia	Rare in United States but common in preschool children living in poverty in developing countries, alcoholics	Preformed vitamin A: liver, fortified milk, fish liver oils. Provitamin A: red, orange, dark green, and yellow vegetables, orange fruits	Infants: 400–500 mg RAE Children: 300–400 mg RAE Adolescents: 600–900 mg RAE Adult men & women: 700–900 mg RAE Pregnant women: 750–770 mg RAE Lactating women: 1200–1300 mg RAE	Headache, vomiting, double vision, hair loss, dry mucous membranes, bone and joint pain, fractures, liver damage, hemorrhage, coma, teratogenic effects: spontaneous abortions, birth defects. Upper level is 3000 mg of preformed vitamin A based on risk of birth defects and liver toxicity.
Vitamin D Cholecalciferol Ergocalciferol	Maintainence of intracellular and extracellular calcium concentrations	Rickets in children, osteomalacia in older adults	Dark skinned individuals, older adults, breastfed infants from vitamin D deficient mother	Vitamin D fortified milk, fish oils	0–50 years: 5 mg, 51–70 years: 10 mg, >70 years: 15 mg	Calcification of soft tissues, growth restriction, excess calcium excretion via the kidney. Upper level is 50 mg based on the risk of elevated blood calcium.
Vitamin E Tocopherols Tocotrienols	Antioxidant, prevention of propagation of free radicals	Hemolysis of red blood cells, degeneration of sensory neurons	Patients with fat malabsorption syndromes, smokers [overt deficiency is rare]	Plant oils, seeds, nuts, products made from oils	Infants: 4–5 mg Children: 6–7 mg Adolescents:11–15 mg Adult men & women: 15 mg Pregnant women: 15 mg Lactating women: 19 mg	Inhibition of vitamin K metabolism. Upper level is 1000 mg based on the risk of hemorrhage.
Vitamin K Phylloquinone Menaquinone	Synthesis of blood clotting factors and bone proteins	Hemorrhage, fractures	Those taking antibiotics for a long period of time; older adults with scant green vegetable intake	Green vegetables, liver synthesis by intestinal microorganisms	Infants: 2–2.5 mg Children: 30–55 mg Adolescents: 60–75 mg Adult men: 90 mg Adult women: 120 mg Pregnant/lactating women: 75–90 mg	No upper level has been set

SOURCE: Wardlaw, Gordon M.; Hampl, Jeffrey S.; and Disilvestro, Robert A. (2004). *Perspectives in Nutrition*, 6th edition. New York: McGraw-Hill.

phytochemical: chemical produced by plants

antioxidant: substance that prevents oxidation, a damaging reaction with oxygen

free radical: highly reactive molecular fragment, which can damage cells

molecule: combination of atoms that form stable particles

DNA: deoxyribonucleic acid; the molecule that makes up genes, and is therefore responsible for heredity

chronic: over a long period

cancer: uncontrolled cell growth

macular degeneration: death of cells of the macula, part of the eye's retina

cataract: clouding of the lens of the eye

cardiovascular: related to the heart and circulatory system

infectious diseases: diseases caused by viruses, bacteria, fungi, or protozoa, which replicate inside the body

clinical: related to hospitals, clinics, and patient care

It has been suggested that beta-carotene and other carotenoids (also called **phytochemicals**) may function as **antioxidants** by neutralizing **free radicals**. Free radicals are unstable, highly reactive **molecules** that damage **DNA**, cause cell injury, and increase the risk of **chronic** disease. Beta-carotene has also been associated with reducing the risk of lung **cancer**. Lutein and zeaxanthin, yellow carotenoid pigments in corn and dark green leafy vegetables, may reduce the risk of **macular degeneration** and age-related **cataracts**. Lycopene, a red carotenoid pigment in tomatoes, may help reduce the risk of prostrate cancer, **cardiovascular** disease, and skin damage from sunlight.

Deficiency. Dietary deficiency of vitamin A is rare in North America and western Europe, but it is the leading cause of blindness in children worldwide. Newborn and premature infants, the urban poor, older adults, people with alcoholism or liver disease, and those with fat malabsorption syndrome are all at increased risk.

One of the earliest symptoms of vitamin-A deficiency is night blindness. It is a temporary condition, but if left untreated it can cause permanent blindness. This degeneration is called xerophthalmia, and it usually occurs in children after they are weaned. Symptoms include dryness of the cornea and eye membranes due to lack of mucus production, which leaves the eye vulnerable to surface dirt and bacterial infections. Vitamin-A deficiency can cause follicular hyperkeratosis, a condition in which hair follicles become plugged with keratin, giving a bumpy appearance and a rough, dry texture to skin.

In developing countries, the severity of **infectious diseases** such as measles is often correlated to the degree of vitamin-A deficiency. Providing large doses of vitamin A reduces the risk of dying from these infections. The age range of the target population for vitamin-A intervention programs is usually from birth to seven years. Administration of high-potency doses in the range of 15,000 to 60,000 micrograms (µg) are distributed to young children in targeted areas of the world to build up liver stores for up to six months. However, consumption of adequate food sources is the most important long-term solution to vitamin-A deficiency.

Toxicity. Vitamin-A toxicity, called *hypervitaminosis A*, can result from long-term supplementation of two to four times the RDA for preformed vitamin A. Excess intake of preformed vitamin A is a teratogen, meaning it can cause birth defects. Birth defects associated with vitamin-A toxicity include cleft palate, heart abnormalities, and brain malfunction. Acute excess intake during pregnancy can also cause spontaneous abortions. Pregnant women should avoid prenatal supplements containing retinal, as well as medications made from retinoids, such as Accutane and Retin-A. Prolonged and excessive consumption of carotene-rich foods can lead to hypercarotenemia, a **clinical** condition characterized by deep orange discoloration of the skin and increased carotene levels in the blood. This condition is usually harmless.

Vitamin D (Calciferol)

In the seventeenth century, vitamin-D deficiency was so common in British children that it came to be known as "children's disease of the English." In the mid-1800s, cod liver oil became well known for treating this disease. In 1925, Elmer McCollum and coworkers determined that the "antirachitic" (antirickets) substance in cod liver oil was vitamin D. Because vitamin D is relatively stable in foods, many countries fortify milk with vitamin D to help prevent rickets. However, significant losses may result from **fortified** milk exposed to light.

Vitamin D from foods is absorbed from the upper part of the small intestine, along with dietary fat, and transported to the liver. In the skin, ultraviolet (UV) radiation from the sun converts a **cholesterol** derivative to cholecalciferol, which enters the blood stream and is transported to the liver. In the liver, vitamin D is converted to calcidiol, an inactive form that circulates in blood. Kidneys take up calcidiol and convert it to an active **hormone** form of vitamin D called calcitriol. People with chronic kidney failure have very low levels of calcitriol and must be routinely treated with this form of the vitamin.

The best-known function of active vitamin D is to help regulate blood levels of **calcium** and phosphorous. Vitamin D increases absorption of these **minerals** from the **gastrointestinal** (GI) tract. In combination with parathyroid hormone, it enhances their reabsorption from the kidneys and their mobilization from bones into the blood. Vitamin D helps maintain calcium levels even if dietary intakes are not optimal. Calcitriol affects growth of normal cells and some cancer cells. Adequate vitamin-D status has been linked to a reduced risk of developing breast, colon, and prostrate cancers.

Deficiency. Long-term deficiency of vitamin D affects the skeletal system. In children, vitamin-D deficiency leads to rickets, a condition in which bones weaken and bow under pressure. Although vitamin-D **fortification** has reduced **incidence** of rickets in North America, it is sometimes seen in children with malabsorption syndrome and is still common in many parts of the world. In adults, vitamin-D deficiency causes **osteomalacia**, or "soft bones," increasing the risk for fractures in hip, spine, and other bones. Vitamin-D deficiency also contributes to **osteoporosis**. In elderly persons, vitamin-D supplementation reduces the risk of osteoporotic fractures.

Infants are born with stores of vitamin D that last about six months. Breast milk contains very little vitamin D, however, and infants beyond six months of age who are exclusively breastfed must obtain vitamin D via exposure to sunlight or a supplement given under the guidance of a physician.

Older adults are especially at risk for vitamin-D deficiency for several reasons. The skin, liver, and kidneys lose their capacity to synthesize and activate vitamin D with advancing age, and older adults typically drink little or no milk, a major dietary source of vitamin D. Older adults also rarely venture outdoors, and when they do, they apply sunscreen to exposed areas of the body, further contributing to the decline in vitamin-D synthesis in the skin.

Sunscreens with a sun protection factor (SPF) of 8 and above prevent vitamin-D synthesis. Sunscreen should be applied only after enough time has elapsed to provide sufficient vitamin-D synthesis. Exposure to the sun does not cause vitamin-D toxicity, and for most people, exposing the hands, face, and arms on a clear summer day for fifteen minutes a few times a week should provide sufficient Vitamin D. Dark-skinned people require longer sunlight exposure because melanin, a skin pigment, is a natural sunscreen.

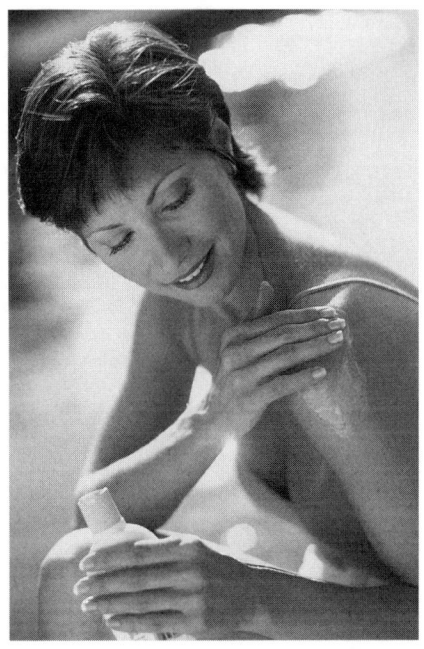

Sunlight stimulates the synthesis of vitamin D, which regulates the body's absorption of calcium and therefore is essential to skeletal health. Just fifteen minutes in the sun several times weekly is sufficient. After that, sunscreen should be applied to avoid ultraviolet damage to the skin. [Photograph by Michael Keller. Corbis. Reproduced by permission.]

fortified: altered by addition of vitamins or minerals

cholesterol: multi-ringed molecule found in animal cell membranes; a type of lipid

hormone: molecules produced by one set of cells that influence the function of another set of cells

calcium: mineral essential for bones and teeth

mineral: an inorganic (non-carbon-containing) element, ion or compound

gastrointestinal: related to the stomach and intestines

fortification: addition of vitamins and minerals to improve the nutritional content of a food

incidence: number of new cases reported each year

osteomalacia: softening of the bones

osteoporosis: weakening of the bone structure

Dietary recommendations assume that no vitamin D is available from exposure to sunlight. Thus, people who do not venture outdoors or who live in northern or predominantly cloudy climates need to pay attention to dietary sources. Plants are poor sources of vitamin D, so strict vegetarians must meet their vitamin-D needs through exposure to sunlight, fortification, or supplementation.

Toxicity. Vitamin D is most likely to have toxic effects when consumed in excessive amounts through supplementation. Excess vitamin D raises blood calcium levels, resulting in calcium precipitation in soft tissues and stone formation in the kidneys, where calcium becomes concentrated in an effort to excrete it.

Vitamin K

In 1929, the Danish researcher Henrik Dam first noted that vitamin K played a critical role in **blood clotting**, and he named it vitamin "K" for "Koagulation." Vitamin K comprises a family of compounds known as *quinones*. These include *phylloquinone* from plants and the *menaquinones* from animal sources. Phylloquinone is the most biologically active form. Menaquinones are also synthesized by **bacteria** in the colon and absorbed, contributing about 10 percent of total vitamin-K needs. Vitamin-K absorption depends on normal consumption and digestion of dietary fat. It is primarily stored in the liver.

Vitamin K helps in the activation of seven blood-clotting-factor proteins that participate in a series of reactions to form a clot that eventually stops the flow of blood. Vitamin K also participates in the activation of bone proteins, which greatly enhances their calcium-binding properties. Low levels of circulating vitamin K have been associated with low bone-mineral density. Thus, an adequate intake of vitamin K may help protect against hip fractures.

Deficiency. A primary deficiency of vitamin K is rare, but a secondary deficiency may result from fat malabsorption syndrome. Prolonged use of **antibiotics** can destroy the intestinal bacteria that produce vitamin K, precipitating deficiency in individuals at risk. Newborn infants are born with a sterile intestinal tract and those who are breastfed, may run the risk of vitamin-K deficiency, since breast-milk production takes a few days to establish and breast milk is naturally low in this vitamin. To prevent hemorrhaging, all infants in North America receive injections of vitamin K within six hours of birth.

Toxicity. High doses of vitamin K can reduce the effectiveness of anticoagulant **drugs** such as warfarin (Coumadin), which is used to prevent blood clotting. People taking these drugs should maintain a consistent daily intake of vitamin K. Megadose supplements of vitamin A and E can pose a risk to vitamin-K status. Vitamin A interferes with absorption of vitamin K, and large doses of vitamin E decrease vitamin K–dependent clotting factors, thus promoting bleeding. Toxicity from food is rare, because the body excretes vitamin K much more rapidly than other fat-soluble vitamins.

Vitamin E

The link between vitamin-E deficiency and reproductive failure in rats was first discovered in 1922 by Herbert Evans and Katherine Scott Bishop. The

---

blood clotting: the process by which blood forms a slid mass to prevent uncontrolled bleeding

bacteria: single-celled organisms without nuclei, some of which are infectious

antibiotic: substance that kills or prevents the growth of microorganisms

drugs: substances whose administration causes a significant change in the body's function

chemical name of vitamin E, tocopherol, is derived from *toco*, meaning "related to childbirth."

Vitamin E comprises a family of eight naturally occurring compounds: four tocopherols and four tocotrienols, of which alpha-tocopherol is the only one to have vitamin-E activity in the human body. It is also the most common form of vitamin E in food. Vitamin E is highly susceptible to destruction by **oxygen**, metals, light, and deep-fat frying. As a result, prolonged food storage lowers the vitamin-E content of food.

oxygen: O_2, atmospheric gas required by all animals

As with other fat-soluble vitamins, absorption of vitamin E requires adequate absorption of dietary fat. In addition, the percentage of absorption declines as the amount consumed is increased. Vitamin E is stored mainly in adipose tissue, while some is stored in the muscle. The remaining vitamin E is found in cell membranes in tissue.

Vitamin E is an antioxidant and one of the body's primary defenders against **oxidative** damage caused by free radicals. Its activity is enhanced by other antioxidants such as vitamin C and the mineral selenium. Vitamin E interrupts free-radical chain reactions by getting oxidized, thus protecting cell membranes from free-radical attack. Scientists have implicated oxidative stress in the development of cancer, **arthritis**, cataracts, **heart disease**, and in the process of aging itself. However, it is not yet known whether supplementation with megadoses of vitamin E offers protection against heart disease and cancer beyond that provided by positive dietary and **lifestyle** changes.

oxidative: related to chemical reaction with oxygen or oxygen-containing compounds

arthritis: inflammation of the joints

heart disease: any disorder of the heart or its blood supply, including heart attack, atherosclerosis, and coronary artery disease

lifestyle: set of choices about diet, exercise, job type, leisure activities, and other aspects of life

Deficiency. Due to the widespread use of vegetable oils, primary vitamin-E deficiency is rare. Most deficiencies occur in people with fat malabsorption syndrome. Smokers and adults on very low-fat diets are at increased risk of developing vitamin-E deficiency. Preterm infants are particularly susceptible to hemolytic **anemia** (anemia caused by the destruction of red blood cells) due to vitamin-E deficiency. These infants are born with limited stores of vitamin E, which are exhausted by rapid growth, and they are inefficient in absorbing vitamin E from the intestinal tract. Without vitamin E to protect against oxidation, the destruction of cell membranes causes red blood cells to burst. To prevent hemolytic anemia, special formulas and supplements containing vitamin E are prescribed for preterm infants.

anemia: low level of red blood cells in the blood

Toxicity. Large doses of vitamin E can counter the actions of vitamin K and decrease the production of vitamin K–dependent clotting factors, thus promoting serious hemorrhaging effects in adults. Individuals who are vitamin-K deficient or who are taking anticoagulant medications such as warfarin or aspirin are especially at risk from megadoses of vitamin E. SEE ALSO VITAMINS, WATER-SOLUBLE.

Kiran B. Misra

Bibliography

Insel, Paul; Turner, Elaine R.; and Ross, Don (2002). *Nutrition*. Sudbury, MA: Jones and Bartlett.

Wardlaw, Gordon M.; Hampl, Jeffrey S.; and Disilvestro, Robert A. (2004). *Perspectives in Nutrition*, 6th edition. New York: McGraw-Hill.

Whitney, Eleanor Noss, and Rolfes, Sharon Rady (2002). *Understanding Nutrition*, 9th edition. Belmont, CA: Wadsworth/Thomson Learning.

Vitamins, Water-Soluble

vitamin: necessary complex nutrient used to aid enzymes or other metabolic processes in the cell

diet: the total daily food intake, or the types of foods eaten

water-soluble: able to be dissolved in water

B vitamins: a group of vitamins important in cell energy processes

niacin: one of the B vitamins, required for energy production in the cell

nervous system: the brain, spinal cord, and nerves that extend throughout the body

Vitamins are essential organic substances that are needed in small amounts in the **diet** for the normal function, growth, and maintenance of body tissues. **Water-soluble** vitamins consist of the **B vitamins** and vitamin C. With exception of vitamin B_6 and B_{12}, they are readily excreted in urine without appreciable storage, so frequent consumption becomes necessary. They are generally nontoxic when present in excess of needs, although symptoms may be reported in people taking megadoses of **niacin**, vitamin C, or pyridoxine (vitamin B_6). All the B vitamins function as coenzymes or cofactors, assisting in the activity of important enzymes and allowing energy-producing reactions to proceed normally. As a result, any lack of water-soluble vitamins mostly affects growing or rapidly metabolizing tissues such as skin, blood, the digestive tract, and the **nervous system**. Water-soluble vitamins are easily lost with overcooking.

Thiamine (Vitamin B_1)

metabolism: the sum total of reactions in a cell or an organism

carbohydrate: food molecule made of carbon, hydrogen, and oxygen, including sugars and starches

edema: accumulation of fluid in the tissues

muscle wasting: loss of muscle bulk

absorption: uptake by the digestive tract

Thiamin functions as the coenzyme thiamin pyrophosphate (TPP) in the **metabolism** of **carbohydrate** and in conduction of nerve impulses. Thiamin deficiency causes beri-beri, which is frequently seen in parts of the world where polished (white) rice or unenriched white flour are predominantly eaten. There are three basic expressions of beriberi: childhood, wet, and dry. Childhood beriberi stunts growth in infants and children. Wet beriberi is the classic form, with swelling due to fluid retention (**edema**) in the lower limbs that spreads to the upper body, affecting the heart and leading to heart failure. Dry beriberi affects peripheral nerves, initially causing tingling or burning sensations in the lower limbs and progressing to nerve degeneration, **muscle wasting**, and weight loss. Thiamine-deficiency disease in North America commonly occurs in people with heavy alcohol consumption and is called Wernicke-Korsakoff syndrome. It is caused by poor food intake and by decreased **absorption** and increased excretion caused by alcohol consumption.

Riboflavin (Vitamin B_2)

Riboflavin is stable when heated in ordinary cooking, unless the food is exposed to ultraviolet radiation (sunlight). To prevent riboflavin breakdown, riboflavin-rich foods such as milk, milk products, and cereals are packaged in opaque containers. Riboflavin is a component of two coenzymes—flavin mononucleotide (FMN) and flavin adenine dinucleotide (FAD)—that act as hydrogen carriers when carbohydrates and fats are used to produce energy. It is helpful in maintaining good vision and healthy hair, skin and nails, and it is necessary for normal cell growth.

cataract: clouding of the lens of the eye

nutrient: dietary substance necessary for health

depression: mood disorder characterized by apathy, restlessness, and negative thoughts

Riboflavin deficiency causes a condition known as ariboflavinosis, which is marked by cheilosis (cracks at the corners of the mouth), oily scaling of the skin, and a red, sore tongue. In addition, **cataracts** may occur more frequently with riboflavin deficiency. A deficiency of this **nutrient** is usually a part of multinutrient deficiency and does not occur in isolation. In North America, it is mostly observed in alcoholics, elderly persons with low income or **depression**, and people with poor eating habits, particularly those who consume highly refined and fast foods and those who do not consume milk and milk products.

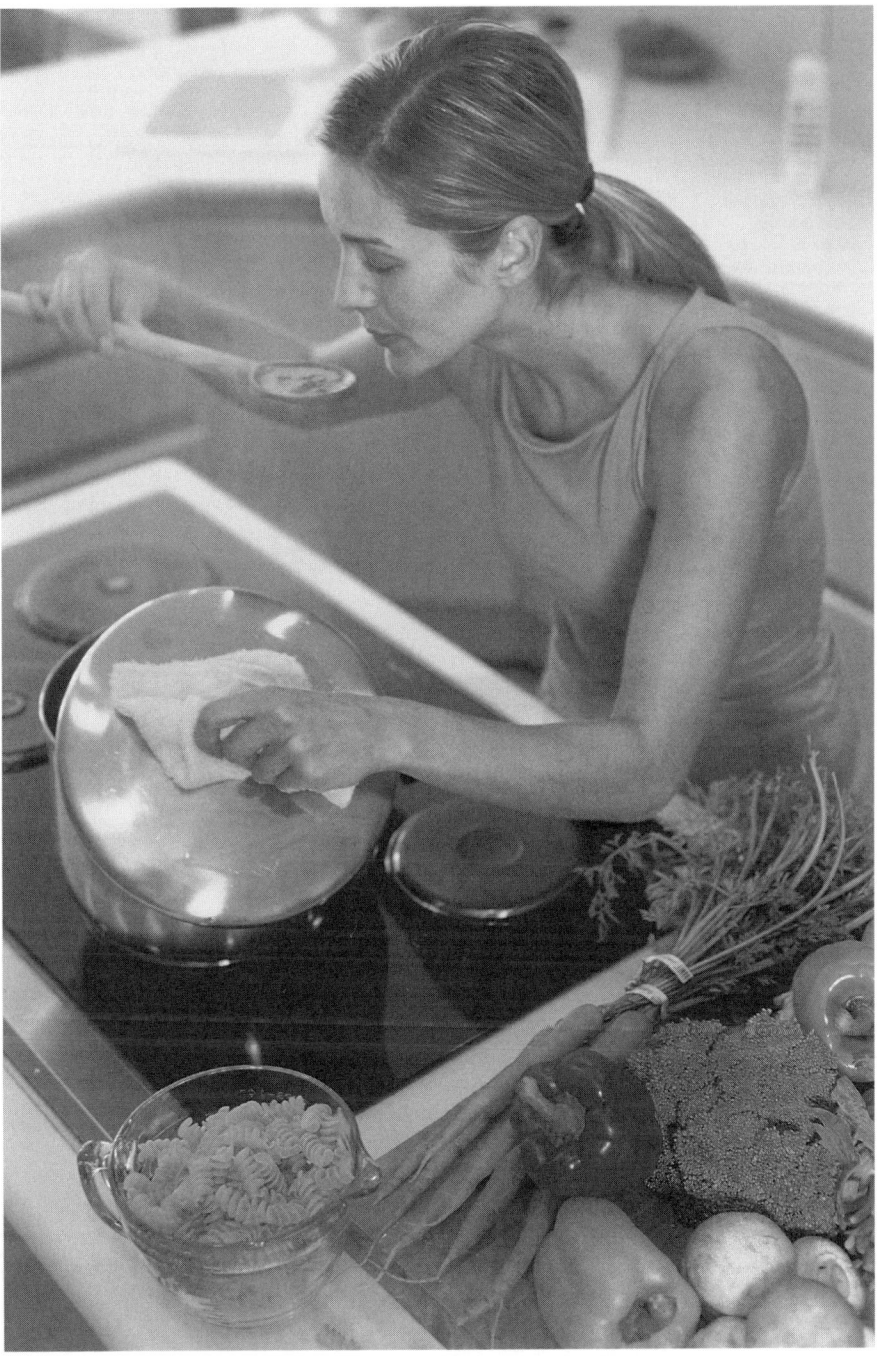

Unlike fat-soluble vitamins, water-soluble vitamins are easily lost during cooking and processing. The body does not store excess quantities of most water-soluble vitamins, so foods bearing them must be consumed frequently. [Photograph by LWA-Stephen Welstead. Corbis. Reproduced by permission.]

Niacin (Vitamin B_3)

Niacin exists in two forms, nicotinic acid and nicotinamide. Both forms are readily absorbed from the stomach and the small intestine. Niacin is stored in small amounts in the liver and transported to tissues, where it is converted to coenzyme forms. Any excess is excreted in urine. Niacin is one of the most stable of the B vitamins. It is resistant to heat and light, and to both acid and alkali environments. The human body is capable of converting the **amino acid** tryptophan to niacin when needed. However, when both tryptophan and niacin are deficient, tryptophan is used for **protein** synthesis.

amino acid: building block of proteins, necessary dietary nutrient

protein: complex molecule composed of amino acids that performs vital functions in the cell; necessary part of the diet

WATER SOLUBLE VITAMINS

Vitamin	Deficiency	Recommended daily intake	Food sources	Toxicity
Thiamine (Vitamin B_1)	Beri Beri: anorexia, weight loss, weakness, peripheral neuropathy Wernicke-Korsakoff syndrome: staggered gait, cross eyes, dementia, disorientation, memory loss	Infants: 0.2 – 0.3 mg Children: 0.5 – 0.6 mg Adolescents: 0.9 – 1.2 mg Men: 1.2 mg Women: 1.1 mg Pregnant/Lactating Women: 1.4 mg	Pork/pork products, beef, liver, yeast/baked products, enriched and whole grain cereals, nuts, and seeds	None reported
Riboflavin	Ariboflavinosis: inflammation of tongue (glossitis), cracks at corners of mouth (cheilosis), dermatitis, growth retardation, conjunctivitis, nerve damage	Infants: 0.3 – 0.4 mg Children: 0.5 – 0.6 mg Adolescents: 0.9 – 1.3 mg Men: 1.3 mg Women: 1.1 mg Pregnant Women: 1.4 mg Lactating Women: 1.6 mg	Milk, eggs, mushrooms, whole grains, enriched grains, green leafy vegetables, yeast, liver, and oily fish	None reported
Niacin	Pellagra: diarrhea, dematitis, dementia, and death	Infants: 2 – 4 mg NE Children: 6 – 8 mg NE Adolescents: 12 – 16 mg NE Men: 16 mg NE Women: 14 mg NE Pregnant Women: 18 mg NE Lactating Women: 17 mg NE	Meat, poultry, fish, yeast, enriched and whole grain breads and cereals, peanuts, mushrooms, milk, and eggs (tryptophan)	Flushing of skin, itching, nausea & vomiting, and liver damage occurs at intake over 35 mg/day from supplements
Pantothenic acid (Vitamin B_5)	Rare	Infants: 1.7 – 1.8 mg Children: 2 – 3 mg Adolescents: 4 – 5 mg Men & Women: 5 mg Pregnant Women: 6 mg Lactating Women: 7 mg	Widely distributed in foods	None reported
Biotin (Vitamin B_8)	Infants: Dermatitis, convulsions, hair loss (alopecia), neurological disorders, impaired growth	Infants: 5 – 6 µg Children: 8 – 12 µg Adolescents: 20 – 25 µg Men & Women: 30 µg Pregnant Women: 30 µg Lactating Women: 35 µg	Whole grains, eggs, nuts and seeds, widely distributed in small amounts	Not known
Vitamin B_6	Dermatitis, anemia, convulsion, depression, confusion, decline in immune function	Infants: 0.1 – 0.3 mg Children: 0.5 – 0.6 mg Adolescents: 1.0 –1.3 mg Men & Women (19 – 50 years): 1.3 mg Men over 50 years: 1.4 mg Women over 50 years: 1.3 mg Pregnant Women: 1.9 mg Lactating Women: 1.2 mg	Meat, fish, poultry, spinach, potatoes, bananas, avocados, sunflower seeds	None from foods, excess intake above 100 mg/day from supplements causes neuropathy (nerve destruction) and skin lesions
Folate	Megaoblastic (macrocytic) anemia, abdominal pain, diarrhea, birth defects	Infants: 65 – 80 µg Children: 150 – 200µg Adolescents: 300 – 400 µg Men & Women: 400 µg/day Pregnant Women: 600 µg Lactating Women: 500 µg	Ready-to-eat breakfast cereals, enriched grain products, green vegetables, liver, legumes, oranges. The use of fortified foods are encouraged for all women of child bearing age (15–45 years).	None (up to 5 mg/day); intake from fortified food and supplements over 1000 µg/day, not including food; folate masks vitamin B_{12} deficiency allowing progression of neurological damage. Supplements containing > 400 µg available by prescription only.

There are two coenzyme forms of niacin: nicotinamide adenine dinucleotide (NAD^+) and nicotinamide adenine dinucleotide phophate ($NADP^+$). They both help break down and utilize proteins, fats, and carbohydrates for energy. Niacin is essential for growth and is involved in **hormone** synthesis.

Pellagra results from a combined deficiency of niacin and tryptophan. Long-term deficiency leads to central nervous system dysfunction manifested as confusion, apathy, disorientation, and eventually coma and death.

hormone: molecules produced by one set of cells that influence the function of another set of cells

WATER SOLUBLE VITAMINS [CONTINUED]				
Vitamin	Deficiency	Recommended daily intake	Food sources	Toxicity
Vitamin B_{12}	Pernicious Anemia: macrocytic anemia, nervous system disturbances; paresthesia (tingling and numbness in limbs), difficulty walking, loss of bowel and bladder control, dementia	Infants: 0.4 – 0.5 µg Children: 0.9 – 1.2 µg Adolescents: 1.8 µg Men & Women: 2.4 µg Pregnant Women: 2.6 µg Lactating Women: 2.8 µg	Meat, fish, poultry, ready-to-eat fortified breakfast cereals, eggs, fermented dairy products (cheese, yogurt, etc). The use of fortified foods and supplements are recommended for adults 51 and over.	None reported
Vitamin C	Scurvy: fatigue, poor wound healing, pinpoint hemorrhages around hair follicles on back of arms & legs, bleeding gums & joints	Infants: 40 – 50 mg Children: 15 – 25 mg Adolescents: 45 – 75 mg Men: 90 mg Women: 75 mg Pregnant Women: 80 – 85 mg Lactating Women: 115 –120 mg Smokers: + 35 mg	Citrus fruits, strawberries, broccoli, greens	Megadoses over 2 g/day causes nausea, abdominal cramps, and diarrhea.

Pellagra is rarely seen in industrialized countries, where it may be observed in people with rare disorder of tryptophan metabolism (Hartnup's disease), alcoholics, and those with diseases that affect food intake.

Recommended intake is expressed as milligrams of niacin equivalents (NE) to account for niacin synthesized from tryptophan. High doses taken orally as nicotinic acid at 1.5 to 2 grams per day can decrease **cholesterol** and **triglyceride** levels, and along with diet and exercise can slow or reverse the progression of **heart disease**. The nicotinamide form of niacin in multivitamin and B-complex tablets do not work for this purpose. Supplementation should be under a physician's guidance.

Pantothenic Acid (Vitamin B_5)

Pantothenic acid is stable in moist heat. It is destroyed by vinegar (acid), baking soda (alkali), and dry heat. Significant losses occur during the processing and refining of foods. Pantothenic acid is released from coenzyme A in food in the small intestine. After absorption, it is transported to tissues, where coenzyme A is resynthesized. Coenzyme A is essential for the formation of energy as adenosine triphosphate (ATP) from carbohydrate, protein, alcohol, and **fat**. Coenzyme A is also important in the synthesis of **fatty acids**, cholesterol, **steroids**, and the **neurotransmitter** acetylcholine, which is essential for transmission of nerve impulses to muscles.

Dietary deficiency occurs in conjunction with other B-vitamin deficiencies. In studies, experimentally induced deficiency in humans has resulted in headache, **fatigue**, impaired muscle coordination, abdominal cramps, and vomiting.

Biotin (Vitamin B_8)

Biotin is the most stable of B vitamins. It is commonly found in two forms: the free vitamin and the protein-bound coenzyme form called biocytin. Biotin is absorbed in the small intestine, and it requires digestion by enzyme biotinidase, which is present in the small intestine. Biotin is synthesized by **bacteria** in the large intestine, but its absorption is questionable. Biotin-containing coenzymes participate in key reactions that produce energy from carbohydrate and synthesize fatty acids and protein.

cholesterol: multi-ringed molecule found in animal cell membranes; a type of lipid

triglyceride: a type of fat

heart disease: any disorder of the heart or its blood supply, including heart attack, atherosclerosis, and coronary artery disease

fat: type of food molecule rich in carbon and hydrogen, with high energy content

fatty acids: molecules rich in carbon and hydrogen; a component of fats

steroids: group of hormones that affect tissue build-up, sexual development, and a variety of metabolic processes

neurotransmitter: molecule released by one nerve cell to stimulate or inhibit another

fatigue: tiredness

bacteria: single-celled organisms without nuclei, some of which are infectious

Avidin is a protein in raw egg white, which can bind to the biotin in the stomach and decrease its absorption. Therefore, consumption of raw whites is of concern due to the risk of becoming biotin deficient. Cooking the egg white, however, destroys avidin. Deficiency may develop in infants born with a **genetic** defect that results in reduced levels of biotinidase. In the past, biotin deficiency was observed in infants fed biotin-deficient formula, so it is now added to infant formulas and other baby foods.

genetic: inherited or related to the genes

Vitamin B_6

Vitamin B_6 is present in three forms: pyridoxal, pyridoxine, and pyridoxamine. All forms can be converted to the active vitamin-B_6 coenzyme in the body. Pyridoxal phosphate (PLP) is the predominant biologically active form. Vitamin B_6 is not stable in heat or in alkaline conditions, so cooking and food processing reduce its content in food. Both coenzyme and free forms are absorbed in the small intestine and transported to the liver, where they are phosphorylated and released into circulation, bound to albumin for transport to tissues. Vitamin B_6 is stored in the muscle and only excreted in urine when intake is excessive.

PLP participates in amino acid synthesis and the interconversion of some amino acids. It **catalyzes** a step in the synthesis of **hemoglobin**, which is needed to transport **oxygen** in blood. PLP helps maintain blood **glucose** levels by facilitating the release of glucose from liver and muscle **glycogen**. It also plays a role in the synthesis of many neurotransmitters important for brain function. This has led some physicians to prescribe megadoses of B_6 to patients with **psychological** problems such as depression and mood swings, and to some women for premenstrual syndrome (PMS). It is unclear, however, whether this therapy is effective. PLP participates in the conversion of the amino acid tryptophan to niacin and helps avoid niacin deficiency. Pyridoxine affects immune function, as it is essential for the formation of a type of white blood cell.

catalyze: cause to happen more rapidly

hemoglobin: the iron-containing molecule in red blood cells that carries oxygen

oxygen: O_2, atmospheric gas required by all animals

glucose: a simple sugar; the most commonly used fuel in cells

glycogen: storage form of sugar

psychological: related to thoughts, feelings, and personal experiences

Populations at risk of vitamin-B_6 deficiency include alcoholics and elderly persons who consume an inadequate diet. Individuals taking medication to treat Parkinson's disease or **tuberculosis** may take extra vitamin B_6 with physician supervision. Carpal tunnel syndrome, a nerve disorder of the wrist, has also been treated with large daily doses of B_6. However, data on its effectiveness are conflicting.

tuberculosis: bacterial infection, usually of the lungs, caused by Mycobacterium tuberculosis

Folic Acid, Folate, Folacin (Vitamin B_9)

Folacin or folate, as it is usually called, is the form of vitamin B_9 naturally present in foods, whereas folic acid is the synthetic form added to **fortified** foods and supplements. Both forms are absorbed in the small intestine and stored in the liver. The folic acid form, however, is more efficiently absorbed and available to the body. When consumed in excess of needs, both forms are excreted in urine and easily destroyed by heat, oxidation, and light.

fortified: altered by addition of vitamins or minerals

All forms of this vitamin are readily converted to the coenzyme form called tetrahydrofolate (THFA), which plays a key role in transferring single-carbon methyl units during the synthesis of **DNA** and **RNA**, and in interconversions of amino acids. Folate also plays an important role in the synthesis of neurotransmitters. Meeting folate needs can improve mood and mental functions.

DNA: deoxyribonucleic acid; the molecule that makes up genes, and is therefore responsible for heredity

RNA: ribonucleic acid, used in cells to create proteins from genetic information

Folate deficiency is one of the most common vitamin deficiencies. Early symptoms are nonspecific and include tiredness, irritability, and loss of appetite. Severe folate deficiency leads to macrocytic **anemia**, a condition in which cells in the **bone marrow** cannot divide normally and red blood cells remain in a large immature form called *macrocytes*. Large immature cells also appear along the length of the **gastrointestinal** tract, resulting in abdominal pain and diarrhea.

Pregnancy is a time of rapid cell multiplication and DNA synthesis, which increases the need for folate. Folate deficiency may lead to **neural** tube defects such as spina bifida (failure of the spine to close properly during the first month of pregnancy) and anencephaly (closure of the neural tube during fetal **development**, resulting in part of the cranium not being formed). Seventy percent of these defects could be avoided by adequate folate status before conception, and it is recommended that all women of childbearing age consume at least 400 micrograms (μg) of folic acid each day from fortified foods and supplements. Other groups at risk of deficiency include elderly persons and persons suffering from alcohol abuse or taking certain prescription **drugs**.

Vitamin B_{12}

Vitamin B_{12} is found in its free-vitamin form, called cyanocobalamin, and in two active coenzyme forms. Absorption of vitamin B_{12} requires the presence of *intrinsic factor*, a protein synthesized by acid-producing cells of the stomach. The vitamin is absorbed in the terminal portion of the small intestine called the ileum. Most of body's supply of vitamin B_{12} is stored in the liver.

Vitamin B_{12} is efficiently conserved in the body, since most of it is secreted into **bile** and reabsorbed. This explains the slow development (about two years) of deficiency in people with reduced intake or absorption. Vitamin B_{12} is stable when heated and slowly loses its activity when exposed to light, oxygen, and acid or alkaline environments.

Vitamin B_{12} coenzymes help recycle folate coenzymes involved in the synthesis of DNA and RNA, and in the normal formation of red blood cells. Vitamin B_{12} prevents degeneration of the myelin sheaths that cover nerves and help maintain normal electrical conductivity through the nerves.

Vitamin-B_{12} deficiency results in *pernicious anemia*, which is caused by a genetic problem in the production of intrinsic factor. When this occurs, folate function is impaired, leading to macrocytic anemia due to interference in normal DNA synthesis. Unlike folate deficiency, the anemia caused by vitamin-B_{12} deficiency is accompanied by symptoms of nerve degeneration, which if left untreated can result in **paralysis** and death.

Since vitamin B_{12} is well conserved in the body, it is difficult to become deficient from dietary factors alone, unless a person is a strict **vegan** and consumes a diet devoid of eggs and dairy for several years. Deficiency is usually observed when B_{12} absorption is hampered by disease or surgery to the stomach or ileum, damage to **gastric mucosa** by alcoholism, or prolonged use of anti-ulcer medications that affect secretion of intrinsic factor. Age-related decrease in stomach-acid production also reduces absorption of B_{12} in elderly persons. These groups are advised to consume fortified foods or take a supplemental form of vitamin B_{12}.

---

anemia: low level of red blood cells in the blood

bone marrow: dividing cells within the long bones that make the blood

gastrointestinal: related to the stomach and intestines

neural: related to the nervous system

development: the process of change by which an organism becomes more complex

drugs: substances whose administration causes a significant change in the body's function

bile: substance produced in the liver which suspends fats for absorption

paralysis: inability to move

vegan: person who consumes no animal products, including milk and honey

gastric: related to the stomach

mucosa: moist exchange surface within the body

Choline

For many years, choline was not considered a vitamin because the body makes enough of it to meet its needs in most age groups. However, research now shows that choline production in the body is not enough to cover requirements. Choline is not considered a B vitamin because it does not have a coenzyme function and the amount in the body is much greater than other B vitamins. Choline not only helps maintain the structural integrity of membranes surrounding every cell in the body, but also can play a role in nerve signaling, cholesterol transport, and energy metabolism. An "adequate intake" is 550 milligrams per day for men and 425 milligrams per day for women. Choline is widely found in foods, so it is unlikely that a dietary deficiency will occur.

Vitamin C (Ascorbic Acid)

In 1746, James Lind, a British physician, conducted the first **nutrition** experiment on human beings in an effort to find a cure for **scurvy**. However, it was not until nearly 200 years later that ascorbic acid, or vitamin C, was discovered. Vitamin C participates in many reactions by donating electrons as hydrogen **atoms**. In a reducing reaction, the electron in the hydrogen atom donated by vitamin C combines with other participating **molecules**, making vitamin C a reducing agent, essential to the activity of many enzymes. By neutralizing **free radicals**, vitamin C may reduce the risk of heart disease, certain forms of **cancer**, and cataracts.

Vitamin C is needed to form and maintain collagen, a fibrous protein that gives strength to connective tissues in skin, cartilage, bones, teeth, and joints. Collagen is also needed for the healing of wounds. When added to meals, vitamin C increases intestinal absorption of **iron** from plant-based foods. High concentration of vitamin C in **white blood cells** enables the **immune system** to function properly by providing protection against **oxidative** damage from free radicals generated during their action against bacterial, viral, or **fungal** infections. Vitamin C also recycles oxidized vitamin E for reuse in cells, and it helps folic acid convert to its active form, (THF). Vitamin C helps synthesize carnitine, adrenaline, **epinephrine**, the neurotransmitter **serotonin**, the thyroid hormone thyroxine, bile acids, and **steroid** hormones.

A deficiency of vitamin C causes widespread connective tissue changes throughout the body. Deficiencies may occur in people who eat few fruits and vegetables, follow restrictive diets, or abuse alcohol and drugs. Smokers also have lower vitamin-C status. Supplementation may be prescribed by physicians to speed the healing of bedsores, skin **ulcers**, fractures, burns, and after surgery. Research has shown that doses up to 1 gram per day may have small effects on duration and severity of the common cold, but not on the prevention of its occurrence. SEE ALSO VITAMINS, FAT-SOLUBLE.

Kiran B. Misra

nutrition: the maintenance of health through proper eating, or the study of same

scurvy: a syndrome characterized by weakness, anemia, and spongy gums, due to vitamin C deficiency

atoms: fundamental particles of matter

molecule: combination of atoms that form stable particles

free radical: highly reactive molecular fragment, which can damage cells

cancer: uncontrolled cell growth

iron: nutrient needed for red blood cell formation

white blood cell: immune system cell that fights infection

immune system: the set of organs and cells, including white blood cells, that protect the body from infection

oxidative: related to chemical reaction with oxygen or oxygen-containing compounds

fungal: of or from fungi

epinephrine: hormone that promotes "fight or flight;" also called adrenaline

serotonin: chemical used by nerve cells to communicate with one another

steroid: class of hormones composed of carbon rings, necessary for sexual development and mineral balance

ulcer: erosion in the lining of the stomach or intestine due to bacterial infection

Bibliography

Insel, Paul; Turner, Elaine R.; and Ross, Don (2002). *Nutrition*. Sudbury, MA: Jones and Bartlett.

Wardlaw, Gordon M.; Hampl, Jeffrey S.; and Disilvestro, Robert A. (2004). *Perspectives in Nutrition*, 6th edition. New York: McGraw-Hill.

Whitney, Eleanor Noss, and Rolfes, Sharon Rady (2002). *Understanding Nutrition*, 9th edition. Belmont, CA: Wadsworth/Thomson Learning.

Waist-to-Hip Ratio

Waist-to-hip ratio is defined as the measurement of waist circumference divided by hip circumference (for example, a waist measurement of 33 and a hip measurement of 44 give a ratio of .75). It is used as a risk-factor assessment tool for **heart disease**, **hypertension**, and type-2 **diabetes**. Excess body fat is considered a risk factor for the degenerative diseases, particularly abdominal fat, and the waist-to-hip ratio is used to determine the risk. A waist circumference of more than 40 inches in men and more than 35 inches in women, or a waist-to-hip ratio of more than 1.0 for men and more than 0.8 for women, indicate an increased risk for the above diseases. SEE ALSO ANTHROPOMORPHIC MEASUREMENTS; WEIGHT MANAGEMENT.

Simin B. Vaghefi

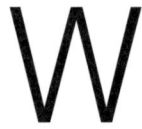

heart disease: any disorder of the heart or its blood supply, including heart attack, atherosclerosis, and coronary artery disease

hypertension: high blood pressure

diabetes: inability to regulate level of sugar in the blood

Water

Water is a colorless and odorless liquid made up of **molecules** containing two **atoms** of hydrogen and one atom of **oxygen**. Water is essential for all life to exist, as it makes up more than 70 percent of most living things. While a human can survive more than a week without food, a person will die within a few days without water.

molecule: combination of atoms that form stable particles

atoms: fundamental particles of matter

oxygen: O_2, atmospheric gas required by all animals

Functions

Water serves as a solvent for **nutrients** and delivers nutrients to cells, while it also helps the body eliminate waste products from the cells. Both the spaces between cells (intercellular spaces) and the spaces inside cells (intracellular spaces) are filled with water. Water lubricates joints and acts as shock absorbers inside the eyes and spinal cord. Amniotic fluid, which is largely water, protects the fetus from bumps and knocks.

nutrient: dietary substance necessary for health

Water also helps the body maintain a constant temperature by acting as a thermostat. When a person is too hot, whether from being in a hot **environment** or from intense physical activity, the body sweats. When sweat evaporates, it lowers the body temperature and restores **homeostasis**.

environment: surroundings

homeostasis: regulation of the proper internal state

Sources of Water

About 70 percent of the earth's surface is covered with water. The amount of water in a human body depends on age, gender, body type, and level of physical activity. The bodies of infants up to about twelve months of age contain about 58 percent water; the bodies of children six to seven years of age are 62 percent water; teenage boys are about 59 percent water; and teenage girls are about 45 percent water. The body of an adult male is approximately 62 percent water, while an adult female is 51 percent water. Physically active individuals generally have more water in their bodies than those who are less physically active. Because they sweat more, active people need to replenish water more often, thus raising their water level. A trained male runner may have up to 71 percent water in his body, while a female gymnast may have 70 percent. **Obese** individuals, on the other hand, have a lower percentage of water in their bodies (about 48%). Morbidly

obese: above accepted standards of weight for sex, height, and age

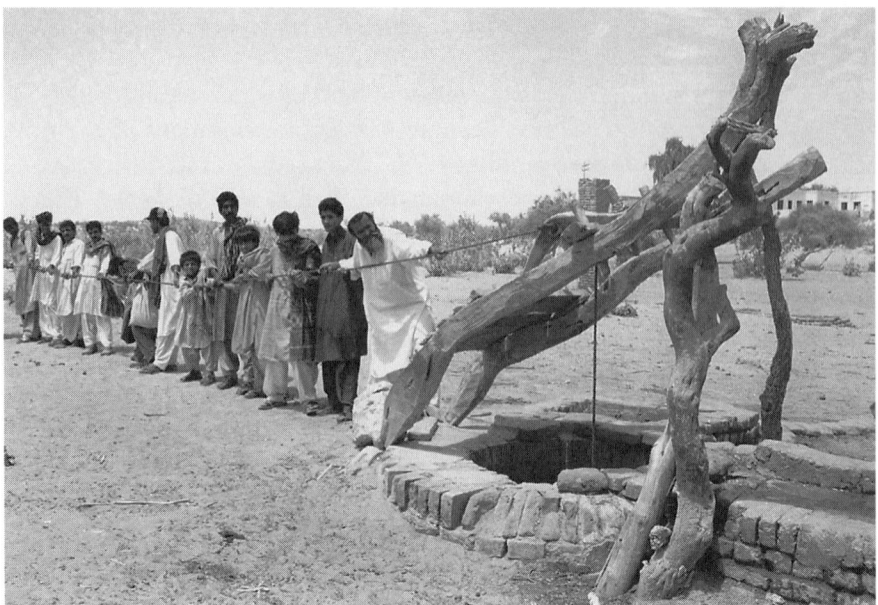

Pakistani villagers pull water from a deep well. Overpumping of groundwater has depleted the water resources of Pakistan and many other nations around the world. [© Reuters NewMedia Inc./Corbis. Reproduced by permission.]

obese individuals are only about 36 percent water. In addition, the older one gets, the less water is retained in one's cells. As a result, old skin looks drier and wrinkles appear.

Recommendations

The most efficient way for the body to get water is for a person to drink water. It is recommended that an adult drink eight to ten eight-ounce glasses of water a day. Athletes and active teens should drink at least ten to twelve glasses of water daily. However, many foods and beverages contain water, which can make up part of this daily intake. Fresh fruits and vegetables, cooked vegetables, canned and frozen fruits, soups, stews, juices, and milk are all sources of water. Most fruits and vegetables contain up to 90 percent water, while meats and cheeses contain at least 50 percent. **Metabolic** processes in the human body generate about 2.5 liters of water daily.

Water Balance

Water balance refers to the balance between the amount of water consumed and the amount of water excreted. The body's water content needs to be constant for optimal functioning. Cells are bathed in **interstitial** fluids (fluids from between cells) that contain nutrients. These fluids also carry metabolic wastes away from the cells. Intracellular fluids facilitate chemical reactions inside the cells, and they help maintain cell structure by adhering to the cell's larger molecules, such as **proteins** and **glycogen**. Body fluids contain solutes (chemical compounds that are soluble in water), which separate into charged particles, or ions, when dissolved in water. Intracellular fluids are high in potassium and phosphate ions, while interstitial fluids are high in sodium and chloride ions. These ions help to maintain the amount of fluids both within and outside the cells. Water molecules follow the solutes moving across cell membranes from a lower to higher solute concentration to maintain homeostasis.

metabolic: related to processing of nutrients and building of necessary molecules within the cell

interstitial: between the tissues

protein: complex molecule composed of amino acids that performs vital functions in the cell; necessary part of the diet

glycogen: storage form of sugar

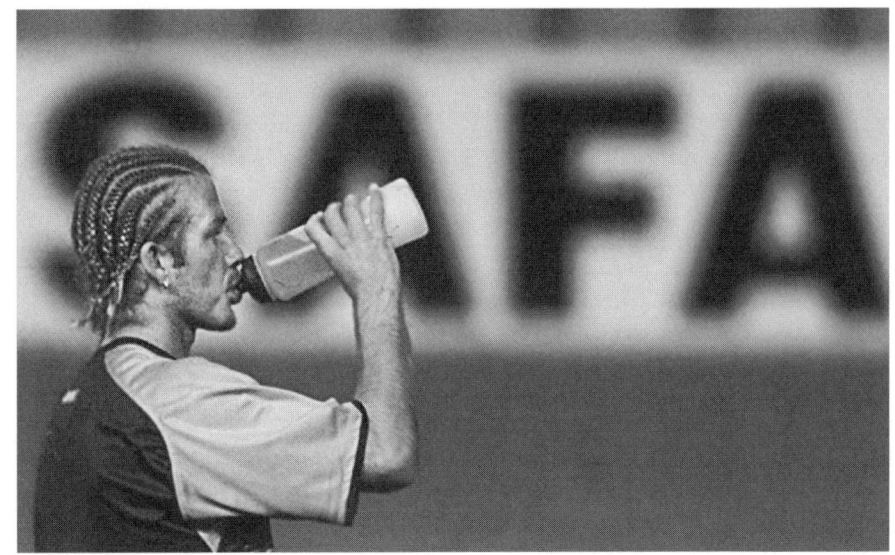

Water facilitates a number of critical body functions, from lubricating joints to carrying away cellular waste. Physical activity speeds fluid loss via perspiration. Athletes who do not drink enough water can easily become dehydrated, which can impair physical and mental functioning. Here, soccer star David Beckham drinks from a water bottle during a practice session. [AP/Wide World Photos. Reproduced by permission.]

Water Intake Regulation

When the body has lost a lot of water, the concentration of solutes in the blood becomes too high. The solutes attract water from the salivary glands, making the mouth dry and causing a person to feel thirsty. The sense of thirst is a craving for water or other fluids. When water loss is slow, a person may have time to feel thirsty enough to replenish the water loss. In cases where the water loss is excessive and **acute**, however, and replenishment is not adequate, a state of dehydration can occur. Dehydration is a state in which the body has lost so much water that normal physiologic functions cannot take place, resulting in symptoms such as fainting and **nausea**.

Heat, intense physical activity (profuse sweating), diarrhea, vomiting, and excessive urination can all cause excessive fluid loss. A runner can sweat off six cups of fluid in an hour. Mild dehydration occurs with a loss of 5 percent or less of a person's bodily fluids, moderate dehydration is a loss of 5 to 10 percent of a person's bodily fluids, and severe dehydration is a loss of 10 to 15 percent of fluids. Severe dehydration can cause death. Some clinical signs of dehydration include dry skin, less frequent urination, **fatigue**, light-headedness, dark-colored urine, dry mouth, and lack of skin elasticity. Often, increased fluid intake and replacement of lost **electrolytes** are sufficient oral rehydration therapy for mild dehydration. However, the cause of dehydration has to be addressed for further improvement. In cases of severe dehydration, it may be necessary to hospitalize the person and restore fluid balance through **intravenous** fluid replacement.

Water Excretion Regulation

The brain and kidneys regulate the amount of water excreted by the body. When the blood volume is low, the concentration of solutes in the blood is high. The brain responds to this situation by stimulating the **pituitary gland** to release an antidiuretic **hormone** (ADH), which signals the kidneys to reabsorb and recirculate water. When the individual needs more water, the kidneys will excrete less and even reabsorb some.

acute: rapid-onset and short-lived

nausea: unpleasant sensation in the gut that precedes vomiting

fatigue: tiredness

electrolyte: salt dissolved in fluid

intravenous: into the veins

pituitary gland: gland at the base of the brain that regulates multiple body processes

hormone: molecules produced by one set of cells that influence the function of another set of cells

When excessive fluid loss occurs, the blood volume will fall, as will **blood pressure**. The kidneys respond by secreting an **enzyme** called rennin. Rennin activates the blood protein angiotensinogen to convert to angiotensin, which causes the blood vessels to constrict and blood pressure to rise. Angiotensin also activates the adrenal glands to release a hormone called aldosterone. Aldosterone causes the kidneys to retain sodium and water. When the body needs water, less is excreted and more is retained.

Water Intoxication

Water intoxication occurs when there is too much fluid in the body. Excess fluid may collect in bodily tissue, particularly in the feet and legs, a condition called **edema**. Excess consumption of fluids, as well as kidney disorders that reduce urine output, may contribute to water intoxication. The symptoms of water intoxication are confusion, convulsions, and, in extreme cases, death. SEE ALSO DEHYDRATION; DIARRHEA; NUTRIENTS; ORAL REHYDRATION THERAPY.

Kweethai C. Neill

Bibliography

Whitney, Eleanor N., and Rolfes, Sharon R. (2002). *Understanding Nutriton*, 9th edition. Belmont, CA: Wadsworth/Thomson Learning.

Shils Maurice, E., and Young, Vernon R. (1988). *Modern Nutrition in Health and Disease*, 7th edition. Philadelphia, PA: Lea and Febinger.

Weight Loss Diets

With over 50 percent of the population of the United States and other industrialized countries being either **overweight** or **obese**, a great number of people want to lose weight. However, weight loss is not easy—and not often successful.

Weight gain is a result of consumed **energy** in the form of high-calorie foods eaten in excess of the body's need for energy. An adult's body needs energy to provide for its **physiological** functions, including heart, kidney, and liver function; blood circulation; respiration; muscle tone; and constant body temperature, called **basal metabolic rate** (BMR), as well as the energy spent in physical activity. An adult woman who is moderately active needs about 2,000 calories per day to meet all her **nutrient** requirements and maintain a healthy weight. She must therefore choose her **diet** carefully, avoiding fast foods and any other high-fat, high-sugar foods, eating a variety of fruits, vegetables, and whole-grain foods, and exercising regularly to avoid depositing excess body fat.

When energy consumption exceeds energy expenditure, excess energy is stored as fat in the body. A person usually gains weight gradually, adding less than a pound per month depending on the level of physical activity and amount and type of food eaten. It is very unusual to gain weight suddenly or at a faster rate than one pound per week. To be successful, the weight loss must also be gradual. Weight loss of one to two pounds per week is recommended, accompanied by a nutrient-dense diet with adequate amounts of high-fiber, whole-grain foods, and exercise.

---

blood pressure: measure of the pressure exerted by the blood against the walls of the blood vessels

enzyme: protein responsible for carrying out reactions in a cell

edema: accumulation of fluid in the tissues

overweight: weight above the accepted norm based on height, sex, and age

obese: above accepted standards of weight for sex, height, and age

energy: technically, the ability to perform work; the content of a substance that allows it to be useful as a fuel

physiological: related to the biochemical processes of the body

basal metabolic rate: rate of energy consumption by the body during a period of no activity

nutrient: dietary substance necessary for health

diet: the total daily food intake, or the types of foods eaten

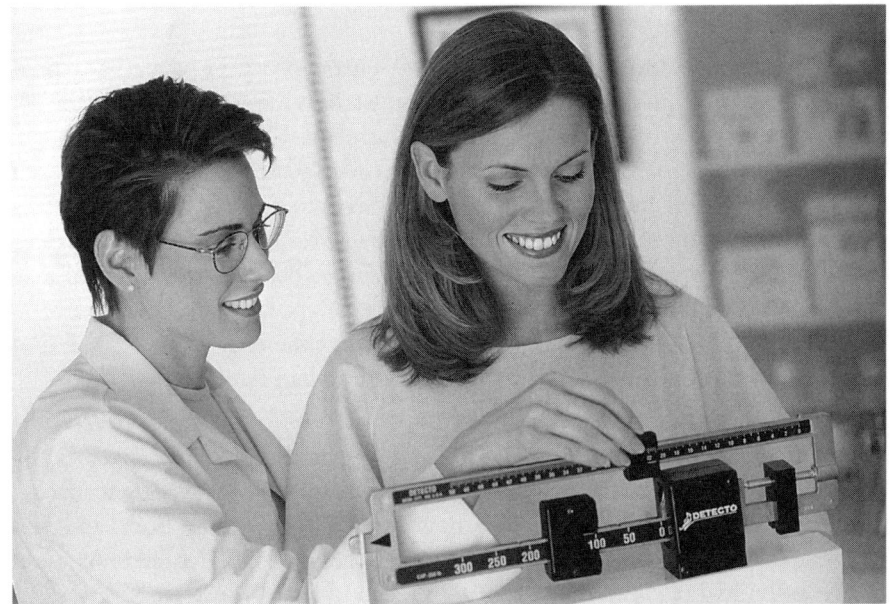

Eating too few calories may cause the loss of lean muscle tissue as the body withdraws glycogen stored in muscles to fuel the nervous system. The ideal weight-loss diet eliminates excess fat but not muscle, which requires moderate diet restriction and increased physical activity. [Photograph by Michael Keller. Corbis. Reproduced by permission.]

In any weight loss attempt the goal is to lose the excess fat that has been accumulated in the body, rather than to lose weight. Therefore, strategies must be chosen carefully to achieve the goal of losing fat. Research has proven that the only long-term way to reduce body fat (and not body **protein** and water, which can be quick but ineffective) is to reduce the intake of high-fat and sugary foods and to exercise regularly. A successful weight loss diet must include adequate amounts of all essential nutrients that the body needs to maintain health. It is important to reduce the fat and concentrated **carbohydrates** (sugar, candy, high-fat and high-sugar desserts, fried foods, fatty meats, and whole-fat dairy products) in the diet, to reduce the intake of red meat and cheese as much as possible, and to avoid soft drinks (soda) and alcohol. However, if such a diet contains less than 1,600 calories per day, health will be compromised. It is also important to exercise regularly (at least thirty minutes per day, or more if the goal is to lose fat faster).

protein: complex molecule composed of amino acids that performs vital functions in the cell; necessary part of the diet

carbohydrate: food molecule made of carbon, hydrogen, and oxygen, including sugars and starches

In spite of reports appearing in popular news magazines and newspapers on high-protein diets, scientific researchers in the field of **nutrition** believe that although high-protein diets may reduce food intake by inducing early satiety and increasing the thermic effect of foods temporarily, the long-term possibility of kidney problems, bone mineral loss, and other unknown long-term risk factors make these diets unsuitable for weight loss.

nutrition: the maintenance of health through proper eating, or the study of same

Losing weight at a rate of about one to two pounds per week is safe and doable. It takes a deficit of about 3,500 calories to lose a pound of weight, which can be accomplished in a week by cutting out 500 Kcalories per day. However, a young girl who eats 2,000 calories a day and cuts back to 1,500 calories per day may end up being deficient in **iron** and **calcium**. A better strategy would be to reduce calorie intake by 250 and burn the other 250 through exercise. That would equal about three miles of race walking or thirty minutes of bicycling each day. With this strategy, a very adequate, balanced, and normal diet can be followed—one that provides all the necessary nutrients. Individuals can vary the foods they eat without getting tired of "being on a diet." Developing a regular exercise habit will not only aid weight loss but will help a person feel better.

iron: nutrient needed for red blood cell formation

calcium: mineral essential for bones and teeth

Fad Diets and Weight Cycling

Many fad diets promise fast weight loss with little effort. However, any program that offers quick and easy results must be viewed with suspicion. If there were any way to easily lose weight there would not be so many overweight and obese people around. Many people fall for these promises and start to lose weight (not fat), but they soon become tired or give themselves a vacation from dieting and gain the lost weight back, plus some more. Remembering their initial weight loss, they then go back on the diet and lose some of the gained weight, but not all of it. Repeating this cycle several times they end up gaining weight because each time they went off the diet they gained a little more weight than what they had lost.

This practice is called "weight cycling" or "yo-yo dieting." As an individual starts reducing his or her food energy intake, body cells sense the reduced energy and nutrients and start economizing in terms of energy expenditure in BMR. Therefore, less heat is produced by the body and less involuntary activity and physiological functioning are performed. As soon as the individual resumes his or her pre diet food habit, more fat is deposited in the body, resulting in a faster rate of weight gain. Repeating this cycle a few times results in a net weight gain rather than weight loss. Under these conditions the body composition also changes, and the percentage of body fat is increased. This increases the risk of degenerative diseases such as **obesity**, **type II diabetes**, **cardiovascular** disease, **hypertension**, and **cancer**.

In order to avoid these problems, an individual interested in losing weight should follow these recommendations:

- Do not believe or follow any of the fad diets that promise easy and quick weight loss, because there is no such thing.
- Combine weight reduction programs with exercise, which not only utilizes more energy, but also increases lean body tissue (muscle fibers), which in turn increases BMR.
- Make sure that one's diet is varied, adequate in all essential nutrients, and includes adequate numbers of servings of fruits, vegetables, and whole-grain products.
- Try to lose body fat rather than body weight by following an exercise program that includes resistance training as well as **aerobic** activity.
- Be patient and lose weight gradually. Remember, weight gain did not happen fast, and neither will weight loss.
- Avoid weight cycling. SEE ALSO DIETING; FAD DIETS; OBESITY; YO-YO DIETING.

Simin B. Vaghefi

Bibliography

Eisenstein, J.; Roberts, S.; Dallal, G.; and Saltzman, E. (2002). "High-Protein Weight-Loss Diets: Are They Safe and Do They Work? A Review of the Experimental and Epidemiological Data." *Nutrition Review* 60:189–197.

Weight Management

Obesity is a **chronic** condition, meaning it is unlikely to be cured, so **behavioral** interventions are needed to help people change their habits and

---

obesity: the condition of being overweight, according to established norms based on sex, age, and height

type II diabetes: inability to regulate the level of sugar in the blood due to a reduction in the number of insulin receptors on the body's cells

cardiovascular: related to the heart and circulatory system

hypertension: high blood pressure

cancer: uncontrolled cell growth

aerobic: designed to maintain adequate oxygen in the bloodstream

obesity: the condition of being overweight, according to established norms based on sex, age, and height

chronic: over a long period

behavioral: related to behavior, in contrast to medical or other types of interventions

improve their quality of life and their **psychological** functioning. The goal of weight management for **obese** people is to help them improve their unhealthful dietary and **sedentary** habits.

Weight-Management Strategies

Behavioral change interventions typically include a number of specific strategies, including self-monitoring, stimulus control, cognitive restructuring, **stress** management, social support, rewards, problem solving, physical activity, and relapse prevention. These interventions make it easier for people to stay on a healthful eating plan and a regular exercise program.

Self-monitoring. The most important behavioral strategy for obese people to follow is self-monitoring—the observing and recording of behavioral patterns, followed by feedback on the behaviors. The obese person should keep a written notebook of all food that is ingested. This is best done on a regular basis, with entries written in a log as soon as possible after the food is eaten. Feedback means looking up and recording the number of **calories** that each food contained. In addition, it is also helpful to record the time of day that food is eaten, as well as one's mood, location, and other people present.

The number of minutes engaged in brisk walking or other physical activity should be recorded in the same notebook. In addition, a bathroom scale should be used to record one's weight on a daily basis. The primary goal of self-monitoring is to serve as a reminder of one's eating and exercise patterns. Results of such record keeping are clear: people who self-monitor lose more weight than those who do not. If a person uses only one weight-management strategy, it should be self-monitoring.

Stimulus control. Stimulus control involves identifying the major barriers that are associated with unhealthful eating habits and sedentary patterns. Modifying these barriers by controlling environmental stimuli can help persons manage their weight-control behaviors. For example, one of the most common barriers to weight loss is a lack of time to exercise. Strategies to help persons find time during the day to exercise, such as setting their alarm clock to wake them up 45 minutes earlier and laying out exercise clothes and shoes before going to bed, are therefore important. When people get up earlier and exercise for even a few days, they tend to feel good about themselves and slowly develop the exercise habit. Other common stimulus-control strategies include avoiding high-risk places (such as a donut shop or **fast-food** restaurant), parking at the far end of the supermarket parking lot, and cleaning out the refrigerator and throwing out all high-calorie foods.

Cognitive restructuring. Cognitive restructuring means changing the way people think about themselves. For example, some people think that they can lose a lot of weight quickly, such as thirty pounds in thirty days. Cognitive restructuring involves helping people set more realistic goals, such as losing about one pound a week and focusing on quality of life and improved health, not just cosmetic goals such as looking better.

Stress management. Stress is one of the major predictors of abandoning a weight-loss or weight-control regimen. It triggers unhealthful eat-

psychological: related to thoughts, feelings, and personal experiences

obese: above accepted standards of weight for sex, height, and age

sedentary: not active

stress: heightened state of nervousness or unease

calorie: unit of food energy

fast food: food requiring minimal preparation before eating, or food delivered very quickly after ordering in a restaurant

Weight Management

One of the most important behavioral changes associated with weight management is the development of a regular, vigorous exercise routine. Not only does such a routine help burn calories, but it can profoundly improve a person's overall sense of well-being.
[William Thomas Cain/Getty Images. Reproduced by Permission.]

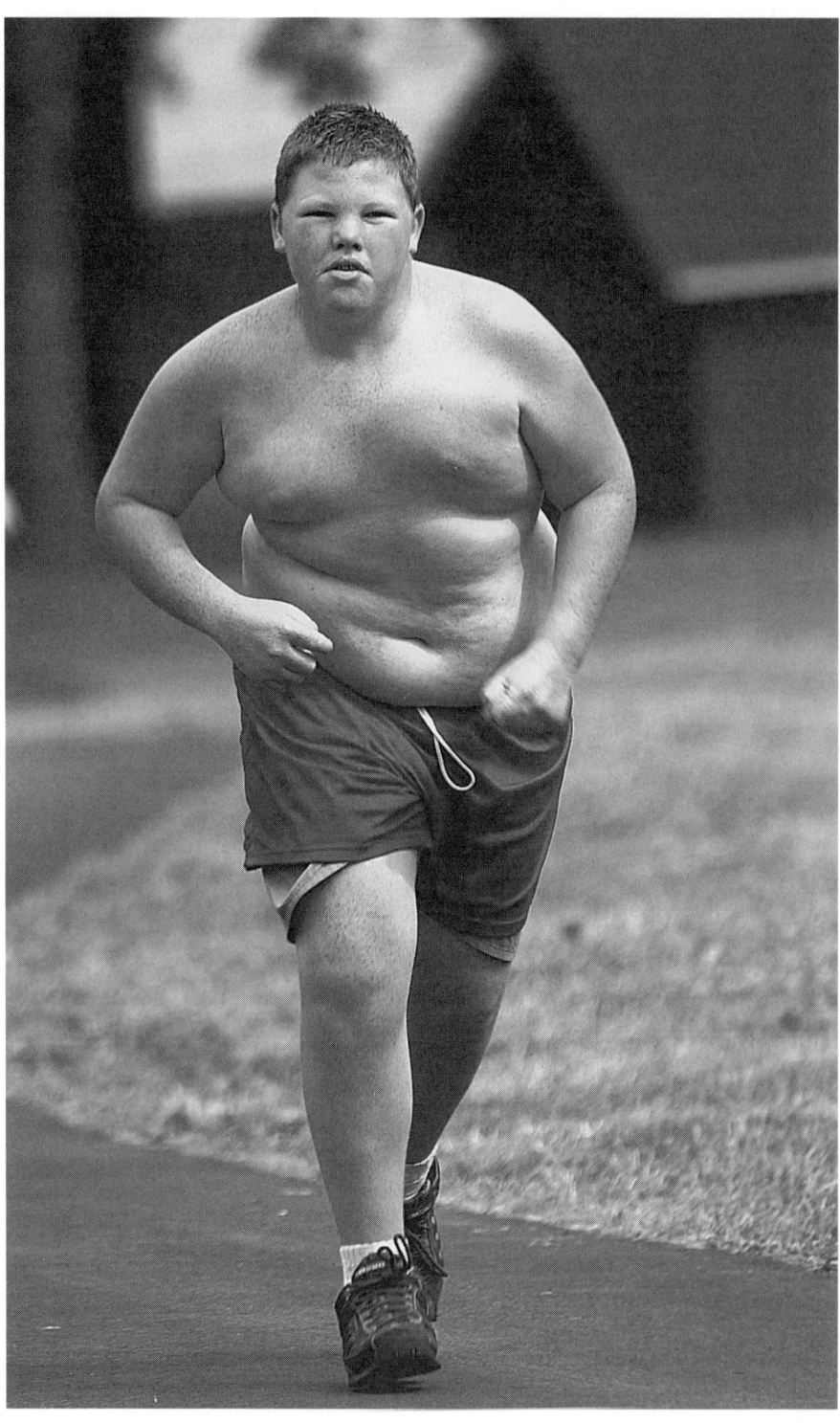

binge: uncontrolled indulgence

ing patterns and is often associated with **binge** eating. Stress management involves teaching people to identify stressful situations and to learn to counteract the stress or tension. Strategies like brisk walking or jogging, meditating, or learning a relaxation response such as deep breathing can help reduce stress and provide distraction from the stress-producing situation.

Social support. Good friends, family members, education classes, community programs, and other social activities can serve as good social-support networks. People with good support networks do better in weight management than people trying to make changes on their own. For example, walking with neighbors in the morning helps build relationships and may help people handle stressful situations in a better way.

Rewards. Rewards for behavior change can help motivate people and reinforce healthful diets and exercise. Rewarding weight loss should be discouraged, however, because some people tend to use unhealthy strategies to achieve their goals. It is better to encourage specific behaviors, such as a certain number of minutes of exercise per day. Small rewards for small behavior changes make good sense for most people.

Problem solving. Problem solving involves identifying and correcting high-risk situations involving one's eating and exercise habits. High-risk situations are usually emotional or social. For example, being invited to a new restaurant may make a person feel anxious. A problem-solving approach may involve calling the restaurant ahead of time and asking for healthful, calorie-controlled suggestions. Bringing a low-calorie vegetable plate to a party may make it easier to stay away from the high-calorie fried chicken wings. Problem solving means planning ahead for high-risk situations. SEE ALSO APPETITE; CRAVINGS; EATING HABITS; EXERCISE; FAD DIETS; WEIGHT LOSS DIETS.

John P. Foreyt

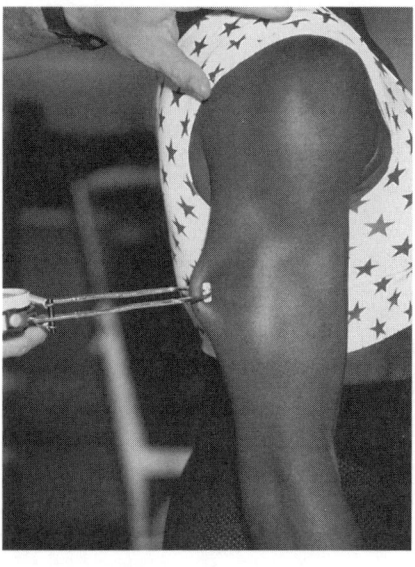

A skin fold test measures the thickness of a fold of skin using calipers. With this data it is possible to estimate what percentage of a person's body mass is fat. *[Photograph by Sean Aidan; Eye Ubiquitous/Corbis. Reproduced by permission.]*

Bibliography

Perri, Michael, and Foreyt, John P. (2003). "Preventing Weight Regain after Weight Loss." In *Handbook of Obesity*, edited by George Bray and Claude Bouchard. New York: Marcel Dekker.

Poston, Walker, S. C.; Hyder, M. L.; O'Bryne, K. K.; and Foreyt, John P. (2000). "Where Do Diets, Exercise, and Behavior Modification Fit in the Treatment of Obesity?" *Endocrine* 13:187–192.

Wadden, Thomas A., and Stunkard, Albert J., eds. (2002). *Handbook of Obesity Treatment*. New York: Guildford Press.

Wellness

Wellness is a state of being in good health, both physically and mentally, and of being free of (and not at risk for) illness. To maintain wellness, individuals need to follow a regimen of periodic risk assessment and adopt behavior changes that lead to a lower risk of acquiring certain diseases. Wellness is the goal behind efforts at health promotion and disease prevention and includes physical fitness, optimal **nutrition**, and spiritual, social, and emotional health.

Wellness exists on a continuum ranging from disease and disability to optimal health (the illness/wellness continuum). The promotion of wellness is intended to encourage people to change their high-risk behaviors in order to enjoy a disease-free and fulfilling life. Prescribed changes in behavior can result in the development of an individual's full potential. SEE ALSO HEALTH.

Simin B. Vaghefi

wellness: related to health promotion

nutrition: the maintenance of health through proper eating, or the study of same

White, Ellen G.

American religious leader and writer
1827–1915

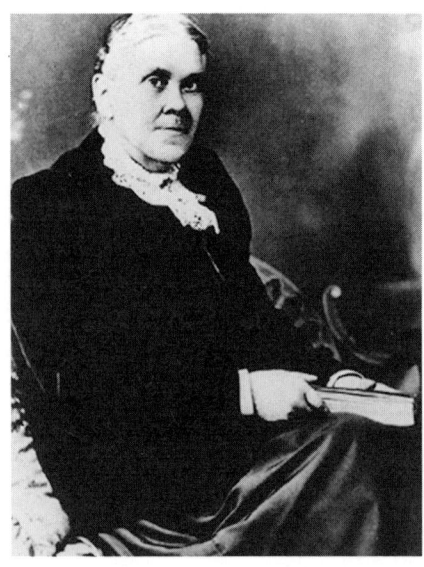

In her 1903 book titled *Education,* Ellen G. White wrote, "Grains, fruits, nuts, and vegetables, in proper combination, contain all the elements of nutrition; and when properly prepared, they constitute the diet that best promotes both physical and mental strength." *[AP/Wide World Photos. Reproduced by permission.]*

nutrition: the maintenance of health through proper eating, or the study of same

diet: the total daily food intake, or the types of foods eaten

drugs: substances whose administration causes a significant change in the body's function

Ellen Gould White was born eight miles east of Portland, Maine, in 1827, during a time characterized by the news analyst and commentator John Harvey as "an era of medical ignorance bordering on barbarism ... when doctors were still bloodletting and performing surgery with unwashed hands." With little education, Ellen White became a prolific writer and a strong advocate of good **nutrition**.

Her parents, Robert and Eunice Harmon, had eight children, including Ellen's twin sister, Elizabeth. They were followers of William Miller, who espoused the second coming of Christ, and part of the Millerite movement, which later led to the founding of the Seventh-day Adventist Church. In 1846, Ellen married James White, who was a preacher and a cofounder of the Seventh-day Adventist Church. The couple had three sons, and they eventually made their home in Battle Creek, Michigan.

Though shy and reluctant, Ellen White was to become a popular lecturer on temperance. Initially unaccustomed to being vegetarian, she became convinced that she should adopt a meatless **diet** (though this was not required by the Church). Other foods, such as coffee and strong cheese, also were eliminated from her table. Not all her books were about health, however. Over her lifetime, she produced a steady amount of work, some devotional, some historical, and some educational in nature.

On June 6, 1863, White had a vision that included instructions on such health-related matters as the use of **drugs**, tobacco, tea, coffee, flesh foods, fresh air, and self-control regarding one's diet. Speaking of this experience, she said, "I saw that it was a sacred duty to attend to our health, and to arouse others to their duty.... We have a duty to speak, to come out against intemperance of every kind.... I saw that we should not be silent upon the subject of health, but should wake up minds to the subject" (Robinson, p. 77–78).

During her prolific lifetime, White produced some 125 books and pamphlets, as well as thousands of articles. While she agreed with other health advocates on many issues, she resolved to write out the principles given to her in her visions. Two of her books, *The Ministry of Healing* (1905), and *Counsels on Diet and Food* (1938), address nutrition, health, and temperance issues.

White promoted the use of natural remedies, advocated dress reform, promoted moderation, and was a strong guiding force in the development of the Western Health Reform Institute, which would become the Battle Creek Sanitarium. In 1903, when John Harvey Kellogg offered his book *The Living Temple* as a means to raise money for the rebuilding of the Battle Creek Sanitarium, she objected to both his plans to rebuild and to pantheistic ideas presented in the book.

In later years she was instrumental in providing vision and inspiration for the building of hospitals in Paradise Valley, Glendale, and Loma Linda, California.

White also traveled and spoke to large gatherings throughout her lifetime, spending ten years in California (1881–1891) and nine years in Australia (1891–1900). She then moved to a home near St. Helena, California, where she lived until her death on July 16, 1915. SEE ALSO BATTLE CREEK SANITARIUM, EARLY, HEALTH SPA; RELIGION AND DIETARY PRACTICES; VEGETARIANISM.

Louise E. Schneider

Bibliography

Coon, Roger (1993). "Reexamining the Adventist Health Message—1: The Good Old Days." *Adventist Review* 10–12.

Graybill, Ron (1992). "The Whites Come to Battle Creek: A Turning Point in Adventist History." *Adventist Heritage*.

Robinson, Dores Eugene (1943). *The Story of Our Health Message*. Nashville, TN: Southern Publishing Association.

Internet Resources

White, Arthur L. "Ellen G. White: A Brief Biography." Available from <http://www.whiteestate.org>

Whole Foods/Diet

The term *whole foods* refers to foods that have not been processed or refined, including whole grains, beans, nuts, seeds, fruits, and vegetables. Whole foods contain compounds known as **phytochemicals** that may reduce the risk for many diseases. In addition, whole grains, such as brown rice and whole wheat, include the whole kernel of the germ, which includes elements such as **fiber** that make them more nutritious than refined grains.

The typical North American **diet**, however, is high in **processed foods** like white bread, potato chips, and desserts made with white flour and white sugar. In these foods, the fiber, **vitamins**, **minerals**, and phytochemicals normally found in whole foods are missing, at least in part. While processed foods used in moderation can be part of a healthful diet, a whole-foods diet provides **nutrients** and health benefits that the typical American diet does not provide. SEE ALSO FIBER; PLANT-BASED DIETS; VEGETARIANISM.

Cheryl A. Flynt

phytochemical: chemical produced by plants

fiber: indigestible plant material which aids digestion by providing bulk

diet: the total daily food intake, or the types of foods eaten

processed food: food that has been cooked, milled, or otherwise manipulated to change its quality

vitamin: necessary complex nutrient used to aid enzymes or other metabolic processes in the cell

mineral: an inorganic (non-carbon-containing) element, ion or compound

nutrient: dietary substance necessary for health

WIC Program

The Special Supplemental Nutrition Program for Women, Infants, and Children (WIC) is funded and administered by the Food and Nutrition Service of the United States Department of Agriculture in partnership with states and local agencies. Its purpose is to serve as an adjunct to good health care during critical times of growth and **development** in order to prevent the occurrence of health problems. It serves pregnant and breastfeeding women, as well as children up to five years of age. Eligibility criteria include poverty and an identified medical or nutritional risk. Program benefits include nutritious foods, nutrition education, and referrals to maternal and child health services.

development: the process of change by which an organism becomes more complex

History

As an amendment to the Child Nutrition Action of 1972, Congress created the Special Supplemental Food Program for Women, Infants, and Children

The WIC program provides aid recipients with checks, much like food stamps, that can be exchanged for certain foods. The foods allowed include cereal, juice, and other nutritious items essential to growing children's health. 45 percent of babies born in the United States get food aid from WIC.

Food Stamp Participation, 1970-1995

Year	Number of Recipients in millions	Cost
1970	4.3 million	$577 million
1975	17.1	4.6 billion
1980	21.1	9.2
1985	19.9	11.7
1990	20.1	15.5
1995	26.6	24.6

malnourished: lack of adequate nutrients in the diet

anemia: low level of red blood cells in the blood

overweight: weight above the accepted norm based on height, sex, and age

iron: nutrient needed for red blood cell formation

fortified: altered by addition of vitamins or minerals

(WIC) as a pilot project. Support came from evidence of the importance of maternal nutrition for positive pregnancy outcomes, and of the potential for permanent physical damage to **malnourished** infants and small children. To further define the intent of the program, nutrition education became a mandated part of the program in 1975. By 1975 the WIC program served approximately 500,000 participants in forty-eight states, Puerto Rico, the Virgin Islands, and two Tribal Organizations. WIC's name was changed under the Healthy Meals for Healthy Americans Act of 1994. Now known as the Special Supplemental Nutrition Program for Women, Infants, and Children, the program serves more than 7 million women and children and covers every state, the District of Columbia, Puerto Rico, the Virgin Islands, American Samoa, Guam, and thirty-three Tribal Indian Organizations, as well as eligible Department of Defense personnel overseas.

How the Program Works

The mission of the WIC program is to safeguard the health of low-income women, infants, and preschool children who are at nutritional risk by providing at no cost: (1) healthful foods to supplement diets, (2) information on healthful eating, and (3) referrals to health care. Income guidelines include those families whose gross income falls at or below 185 percent of the U.S. Poverty Income Guidelines. These guidelines change annually, so that for 2002-2003 a family of two could earn up to $22,089 annually, or $425.00 weekly. Nutritional risk is classified into two major categories: (1) medically based risks, such as **anemia**, underweight or **overweight**, and insufficient growth; and (2) diet-based risks, such as inadequate dietary patterns.

WIC currently serves 45 percent of all babies born in the United States. As the name of the program implies, babies up to twelve months of age are considered infants. They are eligible to receive **iron-fortified** infant formula, infant juice, and dry infant cereals. Children up to five years of age receive iron-fortified cereal, fruit and vegetable juices that are a good source of vitamin C, eggs, milk, cheese, peanut butter, and dried beans and peas. Pregnant women receive larger packages of the same foods that children receive. Following pregnancy, mothers who exclusively breastfeed their babies may receive more foods, including raw carrots and canned tuna, and they are eligible up to one year after the birth of their baby. Those women who do not breastfeed may be eligible up to six months after the birth of their baby. The WIC foods may be obtained at grocery stores. Further, participants can obtain fresh, locally grown fruits, vegetables, and herbs at WIC-authorized Farmers' Markets during the summer and fall harvest months in

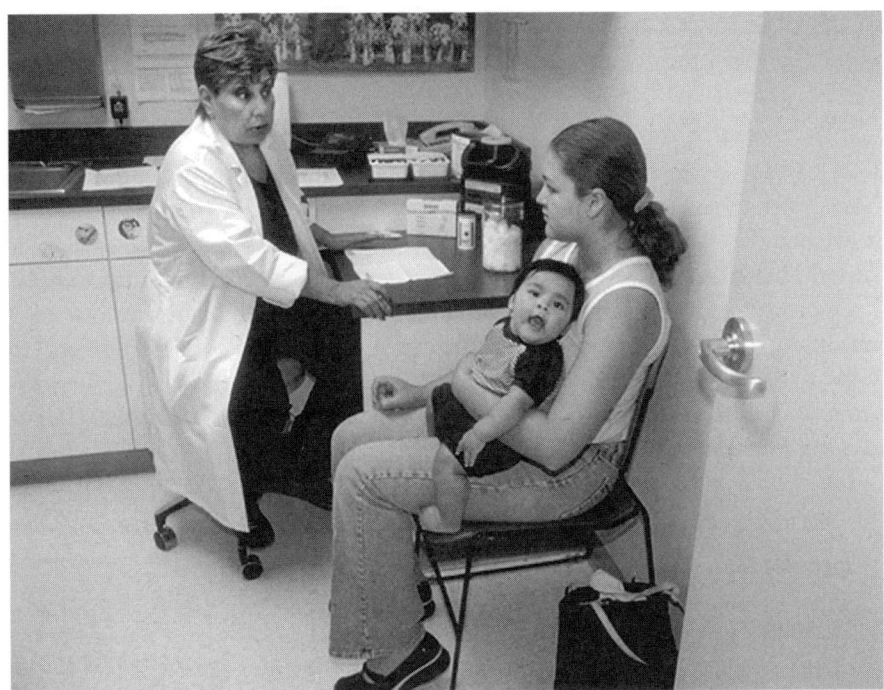

A new mother receives counseling at a WIC clinic. Other services available at the clinics include dental care, immunizations and various health screenings. *[Photo by Ken Hammond. © USDA Photography Center.]*

some locations. WIC foods supply **nutrients** that are generally considered lacking in the diets of low-income populations, such as **protein**, **calcium**, iron, and **vitamins** A and C.

Mandatory provision of nutrition education sets the WIC program apart from other federally funded food programs. The focus of the education is to address participants' specific nutrition needs and to positively affect nutrition and health habits. Education for pregnant women focuses on making food choices that will allow optimal weight gain for good fetal growth. Funding for promotion and support of breastfeeding became a requirement of the program starting in 1989. Parents and caregivers are educated on healthy feeding relationships and the importance of offering age-appropriate, healthful foods to foster proper growth and development. In addition to food and nutrition education, the WIC program encourages the use of prenatal and other medical and social services. Referrals are frequently made to physicians and to other social assistance and health programs, including dental care, alcohol and drug assistance, child care, and housing.

Outcomes and Evaluation

The WIC program has been deemed a success because it has achieved its initial goals, and because other beneficial outcomes have been identified. The initial goals of increasing length of pregnancies, decreasing early births and low birth weights, increasing use of prenatal care and decreasing the **incidence** of iron-deficiency anemia in infants and children have all been achieved. This is partially due to a higher intake of ten nutrients, including the targeted nutrients iron and vitamin C. Increased rates of breastfeeding, as well as improved growth rates, have also been attributed to the WIC program. WIC program enrollment has also significantly improved the nutritional status of pregnant women. Unexpected benefits include a savings in health care costs from $1.77 to $3.13 for each dollar spent on WIC. Further,

nutrient: dietary substance necessary for health

protein: complex molecule composed of amino acids that performs vital functions in the cell; necessary part of the diet

calcium: mineral essential for bones and teeth

vitamin: necessary complex nutrient used to aid enzymes or other metabolic processes in the cell

incidence: number of new cases reported each year

in terms of school achievement, WIC children have improved vocabulary scores and memory of numbers.

New Directions

Due to the success of the program, other issues that affect this population have been added to the services of WIC clinic visits. Participant screening now includes issues such as dental care; lead screening; physical, sexual, or verbal abuse; alcohol, drug, and tobacco use; voter registration; immunizations; and family reading practices. This "melting pot" of health and education initiatives has placed the WIC program in a position of being an important partner in promoting the health and nutritional status of mothers and children. SEE ALSO COMMODITY FOODS; INFANT NUTRITION; PREGNANCY; PRESCHOOLERS AND TODDLERS, DIET OF.

Isabel Parraga
Sharon Doughten

Internet Resources

U.S. Department of Agriculture, Food and Nutrition Service. "The WIC Program." Available from <http: //www.fns.usda.gov/wic>

Wilson, Owen

American pediatrician
1870–1960

development: the process of change by which an organism becomes more complex

heart attack: loss of blood supply to part of the heart, resulting in death of heart muscle

A native of Tennessee, Owen Wilson was a pioneer in pediatric medicine. Born on July 20, 1870, he entered Vanderbilt University in 1884, at the age of fourteen, and graduated with an engineering degree in 1889. He immediately enrolled in Vanderbilt University's Medical School, and graduated two years later. Wilson pursued additional training at New York Polyclinic Medical School and Hospital.

After practicing with a prominent Nashville surgeon for several years, Wilson decided to specialize in children's diseases. He established a large pediatric practice in Nashville and served as Professor of Pediatrics at Vanderbilt University Medical School from 1909 through 1942.

In 1926, Wilson published a book entitled *The Care and Feeding of Southern Babies: A Guide for Mothers, Nurses, and Baby Welfare Workers in the South*. Wilson believed that babies in the southern United States, because of climate and family food habits, required different feeding guidelines than those generally given in the early twentieth century. In his book, Wilson offered instruction on the care and feeding of children from birth until age three, and he included tables of height, weight, and child **development**, as well as some recipes. Only three hundred copies of this book were published. Wilson suffered from a fatal **heart attack** on May 10, 1960. SEE ALSO BEIKOST; BREASTFEEDING; INFANT NUTRITION.

Karen Bryla

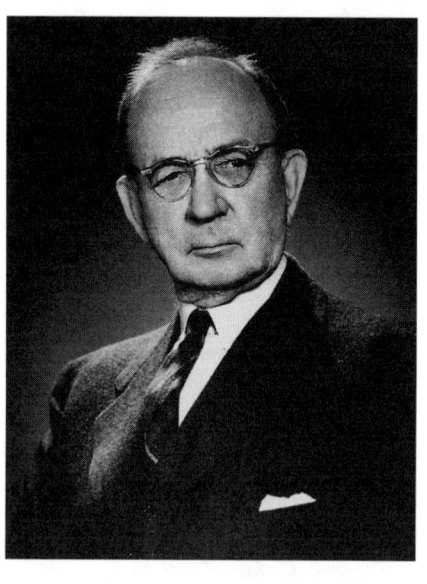

A portrait of Owen Wilson. In the preface of "The Care and Feeding of Southern Babies," Wilson said that other similar works focused on childrearing in cooler climates, and therefore were inapplicable to infants in the southern United States.
[Eskind Library, Vanderbilt University.]

Internet Resources

Vanderbilt University Medical Center. "Infant Feeding." Available from <http://www.mc.vanderbilt.edu/biolib/hc/nh4.html>

Vanderbilt University Medical Center. "Owen Wilson." Available from <http://www.mc.vanderbilt.edu/biolib/hc/Month/october.html>

Women's Nutritional Issues

Women have special nutritional needs due to hormonal changes that occur with menstruation, pregnancy, lactation, and **menopause**, all of which alter the recommended daily intake of **nutrients**. Of the many diseases that affect women, five have a scientific-based connection to **nutrition**: iron-deficiency **anemia**, **osteoporosis**, **heart disease**, type 2 **diabetes**, and some types of **cancer**. In addition, many women look to nutrition for the management of premenstrual and **menopausal** symptoms.

Anemia

Iron-deficiency anemia is a very common nutritional disorder among females following the beginning of the menstrual cycle. Iron deficiency is also common among females with poor diets or very low body weight. The recommended intake of iron for females is 15 to 18 milligrams (mg) per day. Good sources of iron include red meat, dark green leafy vegetables, **legumes**, and **fortified** breads and cereals.

Nutrition for Pregnancy and Breastfeeding

Good nutrition is important during pregnancy and breastfeeding, as there is an increased need for **calories** and for most nutrients. A particularly important nutrient during pregnancy is folic acid, one of the **B vitamins**. Folic acid reduces the chance of having a baby with birth defects of the brain and spinal cord. Experts recommend that women of childbearing age consume 400 micrograms (μg) of folic acid every day. Pregnant women should consume 600 μg per day. Good sources of folic acid include dark green leafy vegetables, oranges and orange juice, dried beans and peas, and fortified breads and cereals.

Adequate **calcium** intake during both pregnancy and breastfeeding is also important, since calcium is drawn from the mother. The recommended intake of calcium during pregnancy and lactation is 1,000 mg a day. A pregnant or lactating teenager needs 1,300 mg of calcium a day. Before becoming pregnant, a woman should discuss folic acid or calcium supplementation with a physician, as well as multivitamin supplementation.

Hormonal changes during pregnancy may trigger a condition called gestational diabetes. Gestational diabetes is characterized by high levels of sugar in the blood. The condition can be diagnosed by a screening test between the twenty-fourth and twenty-eighth week of pregnancy. Changes in **diet** and exercise are often sufficient to keep blood sugar levels in the normal range. For most women, the condition goes away after the birth of the baby. Women who have gestational diabetes are more likely to develop type 2 diabetes later in life.

PMS and Menopause

Many women seek medical help for premenstrual syndrome (PMS). While nutrition advice often varies, there is insufficient scientific evidence that any diet modifications will prevent or relieve PMS symptoms. A combination of good nutrition, exercise, and **stress** management may be the best way to relieve the symptoms of PMS.

---

menopause: phase in a woman's life during which ovulation and menstruation end

nutrient: dietary substance necessary for health

nutrition: the maintenance of health through proper eating, or the study of same

anemia: low level of red blood cells in the blood

osteoporosis: weakening of the bone structure

heart disease: any disorder of the heart or its blood supply, including heart attack, atherosclerosis, and coronary artery disease

diabetes: inability to regulate level of sugar in the blood

cancer: uncontrolled cell growth

menopausal: related to menopause, the period during which women cease to ovulate and menstruate

legumes: beans, peas and related plants

fortified: altered by addition of vitamins or minerals

calorie: unit of food energy

B vitamins: a group of vitamins important in cell energy processes

calcium: mineral essential for bones and teeth

diet: the total daily food intake, or the types of foods eaten

stress: heightened state of nervousness or unease

isoflavones: estrogen-like compounds in plants

Soy has garnered much attention in recent years as a dietary treatment for menopausal symptoms. Soy is a rich source of **isoflavones**, an estrogen-like substance found in plants. Some studies suggest that regularly eating moderate amounts of soy-based food products can help decrease menopausal symptoms; however, other studies do not support the idea. More research is needed to gain a better understanding of the effects of soy on menopausal symptoms.

metabolism: the sum total of reactions in a cell or an organism

During menopause, a woman's **metabolism** slows down and weight gain can occur. The accumulation of body fat around the abdomen also increases. Exercise and careful food choices can minimize both of these occurrences.

Chronic Diseases

overweight: weight above the accepted norm based on height, sex, and age

lifestyle: set of choices about diet, exercise, job type, leisure activities, and other aspects of life

As women age, the risk of developing chronic disease increases. Women over age forty-five who are **overweight**, physically inactive, and have a family history of diabetes are more likely to develop type 2 diabetes. Maintaining a healthy weight, eating a varied and balanced diet, and engaging in an active **lifestyle** can reduce the risk of developing type 2 diabetes. Diabetes carries many risks with it, including eye disease, nerve disease, kidney disease, and heart disease.

genetics: inheritance through genes

hormone: molecules produced by one set of cells that influence the function of another set of cells

vitamin D: nutrient needed for calcium uptake and therefore proper bone formation

protein: complex molecule composed of amino acids that performs vital functions in the cell; necessary part of the diet

Women are at a higher risk of developing osteoporosis as they age than men are. Osteoporosis is an irreversible disease in which the bones become porous and break easily. There are many factors that contribute to this disease, including **genetics**, diet, **hormones**, age, and lifestyle factors. The disease usually has no symptoms until a fracture occurs.

Diets low in calcium, **vitamin D**, or magnesium—or high intakes of caffeine, alcohol, sodium, phosphorous, or **protein**—may increase the chance of developing osteoporosis. Good nutrition and weight-bearing exercise, such as walking, hiking, or climbing stairs, helps to build strong bones.

Good sources of calcium include low-fat dairy products such as cheese, yogurt, and milk; canned fish with bones, such as salmon and sardines; dark green leafy vegetables; and calcium-fortified foods such as orange juice, bread, and cereal. The recommended intake of calcium for women ages nineteen to fifty is 1,000 mg per day. Women over the age of fifty should consume 1,200 mg of calcium per day.

obese: above accepted standards of weight for sex, height, and age

sedentary: not active

Breast cancer is the most common type of cancer among U.S. women other than skin cancer. **Obese, sedentary** women are more likely to develop breast cancer, and dietary factors may possibly play a role in its development. Some studies suggest that excessive fat intake may increase breast-cancer risk, either by raising estrogen levels in a woman or by altering immune function. Diets that include adequate amounts of fruits, vegetables, and other fiber-rich foods may protect against breast cancer. However, controversy exists as to whether diet is actually a contributing factor. Excessive alcohol consumption does appear to raise the risk of breast cancer in women.

antioxidant: substance that prevents oxidation, a damaging reaction with oxygen

The risk of developing heart disease begins to rise once a woman reaches menopause, and it increases rapidly after age sixty-five. Dietary risk factors involved in the cause or prevention of heart disease include dietary **antioxidants**, dietary fiber, and the type and amount of fat in the diet. Antioxidants are non-nutrient compounds in foods that protect the body's cells from damage. They are found in fruits and vegetables. Soluble fiber, such as the fiber

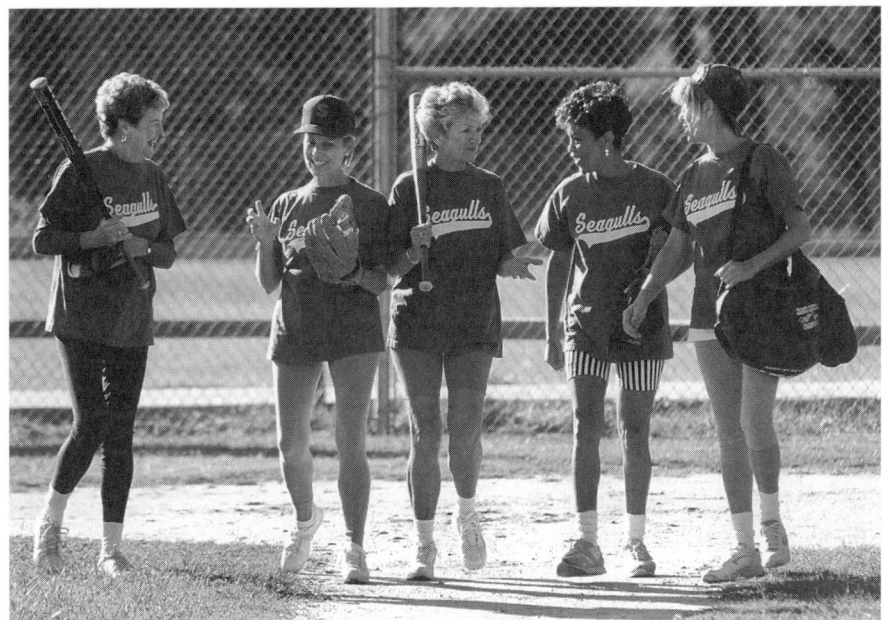

Women over the age of 45 are susceptible to a variety of chronic conditions including type 2 diabetes, osteoporosis, breast cancer, and heart disease. Proper nutrition and physical activity can help prevent these diseases. [Corbis. Reproduced by permission.]

in oatmeal, helps to lower blood **cholesterol** levels, while levels of cholesterol in the blood increase in response to diets high in total fat and/or **saturated fat**. A high level of cholesterol in the blood is a risk factor for heart disease.

Hypertension, or **high blood pressure**, is related to heart disease. After menopause, women with hypertension outnumber men with the condition. Weight control, an active lifestyle, a diet low in salt and fat, and with plenty of fruits and vegetables may help to prevent hypertension.

Good nutrition is the cornerstone of good health for a woman, but the many phases of a woman's life require nutritional adjustments. Learning and following dietary recommendations, and making the appropriate nutritional adjustments, can improve a woman's quality of life and reduce the risk of chronic disease. SEE ALSO ADULT NUTRITION; MENOPAUSE; OSTEOPOROSIS; PREGNANCY; PREMENSTRUAL SYNDROME; WEIGHT MANAGEMENT.

Beth Fontenot

cholesterol: multi-ringed molecule found in animal cell membranes; a type of lipid

saturated fat: a fat with the maximum possible number of hydrogens; more difficult to break down that unsaturated fats

high blood pressure: elevation of the pressure in the bloodstream maintained by the heart

Bibliography

Grosvenor, Mary B., Smolin, Lora A. (2002). *Nutrition: From Science to Life*. Philadelphia, PA: Harcourt College Publishers.

Mitmesser, Susan Hazels (2003). "Nutrition Needs and Cardiovascular Risk in Women." *Today's Dietitian* 5(10):30–33.

Internet Resources

American Dietetic Association. "Women's Health and Nutrition." Available from <http://www.eatright.org>

Food and Nutrition Information Center. "Dietary Reference Intakes (DRI) and Recommended Dietary Allowances (RDA)." Available from <http://www.nal.usda.gov/fnic>

March of Dimes. "Folic Acid FAQ." Available from <http://www.marchofdimes.com>

U.S. Food and Drug Administration, Center for Food Safety and Applied Nutrition. "Information for Pregnant Women." Available from <http://www.cfsan.fda.gov>

WebDietitian. "Nutrition in Women's Health." Available from <http://www.webdietitian.com>

World Health Organization (WHO)

The World Health Organization (WHO), headquartered in Geneva, Switzerland, is an international group of one hundred and ninety-one member states devoted to the maintenance and improvement of the health of all people throughout the world. Member states are divided into six geographic regions: Southeast Asia, the Eastern Mediterranean, the Americas, Africa, the Western Pacific, and Europe. The director general of the organization oversees the mission to preserve, maintain, and improve health through education, nutritional support, health activities, management of disease outbreaks, response to emergencies, and funding programs.

History and Mission

In 1945, three physicians, Drs. Szeming Sze of China, Karl Evang of Norway, and Geraldo de Paula Souza of Brazil, proposed the formulation of a single health organization that would address the health needs of the world's people. Their joint declaration to establish an international health organization was approved when the constitution of the WHO was adopted in 1946.

The preamble to the constitution defines health as "a state of complete physical, mental and social well-being and not merely the absence of disease or infirmity." The initial priorities for world health care included initiatives to address **malaria**, maternal and child health, **tuberculosis**, venereal diseases, **nutrition** and environmental sanitation, public health administration, **parasitic** diseases, **viral diseases**, mental health, and other activities.

WHO Programs

The WHO provides preventive health and improvement of nutritional status through programs that address:

1. Health education
2. Food, food safety, and nutrition
3. Safe water and basic sanitation
4. Immunizations
5. Prevention and control of local endemic diseases
6. Treatment of common diseases and injuries
7. Provision of essential **drugs.**

Special programs include the Applied Nutrition Program, which began in 1960 and attempts to improve the nutritional health of people worldwide. Strategic action plans have been developed to promote breastfeeding, support production of foods that improve local diets, distribute supplementary foods, and provide health education. These plans include multiple factors that address the specific needs of each region. The targets of action to accomplish the plans are nutritonal education, safe diets, and healthy choices for living.

Food safety is another major focus of WHO special programs. Through the Food Safety Program, contaminants of water and food are identified, with efforts targeted at providing clean sources of food and/or water. Environmental health centers serve as the clearinghouse for activities to support

---

WHO and SARS

As Severe Acute Respiratory Syndrome (SARS) broke out in China in 2002, some of the earliest alerts were provided by the Global Public Health Intelligence Network (GPHIN), an automated system that WHO uses to scan Web sites and electronic discussion groups for signs of disease outbreaks that could lead to epidemics. Another WHO system, the Global Outbreak Alert and Response Network (GORAN) links 112 existing networks to monitor and respond to outbreaks of infectious diseases. As SARS came to light, WHO drew on these resources to establish a virtual network of eleven leading laboratories. Using a shared Web site and daily teleconferences to pool information and coordinate activities, they worked to identify the cause of the disease and develop a diagnostic test. WHO's quick response in issuing global alerts and travel advisories and in coordinating international resources have been credited with helping to efficiently contain the spread of the disease.

—*Paula Kepos*

---

malaria: disease caused by infection with Plasmodium, a single-celled protozoon, transmitted by mosquitoes

tuberculosis: bacterial infection, usually of the lungs, caused by Mycobacterium tuberculosis

nutrition: the maintenance of health through proper eating, or the study of same

parasitic: feeding off another organism

viral disease: disease caused by viruses, including flu, colds, AIDS, hepatitis, and others

drugs: substances whose administration causes a significant change in the body's function

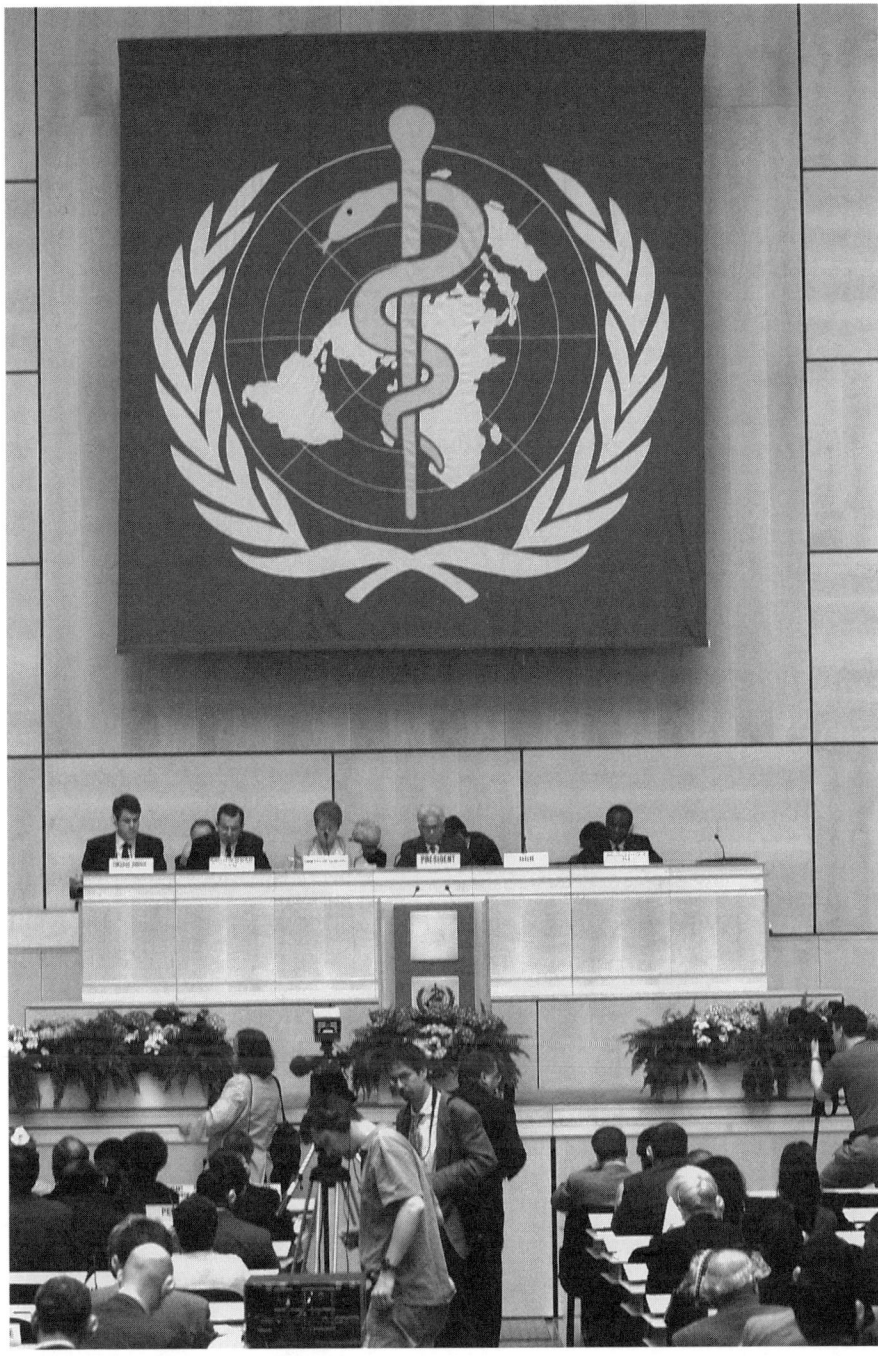

In May 2002, 192 nations gathered as the World Health Organization held its 55th annual World Health Assembly. One of the key resolutions to emerge from the assembly was a commitment to help poorer nations obtain needed medicines at discounted rates. *[Copyright World Health Organization (WHO)/P. Virot]*

improvement of **undernutrition** of infants, deficiencies of iodine, vitamin A, and thiamine; **anemia**, and other nutritional concerns.

Together with UNICEF, the WHO has been successful in overseeing programs to promote breastfeeding and improve the health and nutritional status of pregnant women, infants, and mothers with young children. Hospitals and regional centers have played an important part in the success of this endeavor.

Finally, programs aimed at improving the land and planting crops such as cereals, rice, corn, and potatoes have been introduced in all regions. These programs include production of nutritionally adequate foods to feed those

undernutrition: food intake too low to maintain adequate energy expenditure without weight loss

anemia: low level of red blood cells in the blood

in each region, while also providing education and work opportunities for the people of each region.

Ruth Waibel

Bibliography

Sze, Seming (1982). *The Origins of the World Health Organization: A Personal Memoir 1945–1948.* Boca Raton, FL: LISZ.

Sze, Szeming (1988). "WHO: From Small Beginnings." *World Health Forum* 9(1):29–34.

Internet Resources

World Health Organization (1988). "Fifty Years of the World Health Organization in the Western Pacific." Available from <http://www.wpro.who.int/public policy/50th>

World Health Organization (2001). "Report of the Commission on Macroeconomics and Health 2001." Available from <http://www.cmhealth.org>

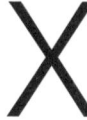

Xerophthalmia

Xerophthalmia is a severe drying of the eye surface caused by a malfunction of the tear glands. Also found in people with immune disorders, it occurs most commonly because of decreased intake or **absorption** of vitamin A. Symptoms include night blindness and eye irritation. In addition to the eyes being very dry, there is a loss of luster on their surface. At later stages, the corneas become soft, with increased **opacity**.

Rarely seen in industrialized countries, xerophthalmia remains the leading cause of childhood blindness in the developing world. Up to ten million cases occur among children every year due to a dietary deficiency of vitamin A, and 5 percent of these children become blind.

Xerophthalmia is treated with artificial eye moisturizers and vitamin A supplementation. In 1999 a genetically engineered form of rice was created that contains up to 20 percent beta-carotene, a rich source of vitamin A. It is hoped that this grain, known as *golden rice*, will alleviate much of the world's vitamin A deficiency. However, critics maintain that the volume of rice needed to reach the daily recommended amount of vitamin A is too excessive to be practical. In addition, lingering concerns about the safety of genetically engineered foods may affect its use. SEE ALSO BETA-CAROTENE; CAROTENOIDS; VITAMINS, FAT-SOLUBLE.

Chandak Ghosh

Internet Resources

National Institutes of Health Clinic Center. "Vitamin A and Carotenoids." Available from <www.cc.nih.gov>

Merck Manual. "Vitamin A Deficiency." Available from <www.merck.com/pubs/mmanual>

absorption: uptake by the digestive tract

opacity: impermeability to light

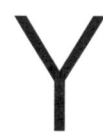

Yo-Yo Dieting

Yo-yo dieting, or weight cycling, is the repeated losing and regaining of weight. This phenomenon is very common in societies that place an emphasis on being thin. People who lose weight through dieting often regain weight in a short time, and they often add more weight than they lost. Yo-yo dieting may increase the risk of developing **heart disease, hypertension**, and **diabetes**. It may also increase emotional distress and contribute to a sense of failure and low self-esteem. SEE ALSO WEIGHT LOSS DIETS; WEIGHT MANAGEMENT.

Frances M. Berg

heart disease: any disorder of the heart or its blood supply, including heart attack, atherosclerosis, and coronary artery disease

hypertension: high blood pressure

diabetes: inability to regulate level of sugar in the blood

Bibliography

Lissner, L.; Odell, P.; D'Agostino, D.; and Stoke, J.; et al. "Variability of Body Weight and Health Outcomes in the Framingham Population." *New England Journal of Medicine* 324:1839–1844.

Brownell, K., and Rodin, J. (1994). "Medical, Metabolic, and Psychological Effects of Weight Cycling." *Archives of Internal Medicine* 154:1325–1330.

Glossary

absorption: uptake by the digestive tract

acid reflux: splashing of stomach acid into the throat

acidity: measure of the tendency of a molecule to lose hydrogen ions, thus behaving as an acid

acidosis: elevated acid level in the blood

acupuncture: insertion of needles into the skin at special points to treat disease

acute: rapid-onset and short-lived

adequate intake: nutrient intake that appears to maintain the state of health

adipose tissue: tissue containing fat deposits

aerobic: designed to maintain adequate oxygen in the bloodstream

allergen: a substance that provokes an allergic reaction

allergic reaction: immune system reaction against a substance that is otherwise harmless

allergy: immune system reaction against substances that are otherwise harmless

amenorrhea: lack of menstruation

Americanized: having adopted more American habits or characteristics

amine: compound containing nitrogen linked to hydrogen

amino acid: building block of proteins, necessary dietary nutrient

anabolic: promoting building up

anaerobic: without air, or oxygen

anaphylaxis: life-threatening allergic reaction, involving drop in blood pressure and swelling of soft tissues especially surrounding the airways

anemia: low level of red blood cells in the blood

angioplasty: reopening of clogged blood vessels

anorexia nervosa: refusal to maintain body weight at or above what is considered normal for height and age

Glossary

anthropometric: related to measurement of characteristics of the human body

antibiotic: substance that kills or prevents the growth of microorganisms

antibody: immune system protein that protects against infection

antioxidant: substance that prevents oxidation, a damaging reaction with oxygen

anxiety: nervousness

appendicitis: inflammation of the appendix

aqueous: water-based

artery: blood vessel that carries blood away from the heart toward the body tissues

arthritis: inflammation of the joints

assisted-living: facility that provides aid in meal preparation, cleaning, and other activities to help maintain independent living

asthma: respiratory disorder marked by wheezing, shortness of breath, and mucus production

asymptomatic: without symptoms

atherosclerosis: build-up of deposits within the blood vessels

atole: a porridge made of corn meal and milk

atoms: fundamental particles of matter

ayurvedic: an Indian healing system

B vitamins: a group of vitamins important in cell energy processes

bacteria: single-celled organisms without nuclei, some of which are infectious

bactericidal: a substance that kills bacteria

bacteriostatic: a state that prevents growth of bacteria

basal metabolic rate: rate of energy consumption by the body during a period of no activity

basal metabolism: level of body energy consumption and chemical processes in the absence of exertion

behavioral: related to behavior, in contrast to medical or other types of interventions

bile: substance produced in the liver which suspends fats for absorption

binge: uncontrolled indulgence

bioavailability: availability to living organisms, based on chemical form

biochemical: related to chemical processes within cells

biodiversity: richness of species within an area

biological: related to living organisms

biotin: a portion of certain enzymes used in fat metabolism; essential for cell function

biotoxin: poison made by living organisms

blood clotting: the process by which blood forms a solid mass to prevent uncontrolled bleeding

blood pressure: measure of the pressure exerted by the blood against the walls of the blood vessels

body mass index: weight in kilograms divided by square of the height in meters times 100; a measure of body fat

bone marrow: dividing cells within the long bones that make the blood

botanical: related to plants

botulism: poisoning from the bacterium Clostridium botulinum

bowel: intestines and rectum

brain allergy: allergy whose symptoms affect brain function

bulimia: uncontrolled episodes of eating (bingeing) usually followed by self-induced vomiting (purging)

calcium: mineral essential for bones and teeth

calorie: unit of food energy

cancer: uncontrolled cell growth

candidal: related to the yeast Candida

candidiasis: a yeast infection

carbohydrate: food molecule made of carbon, hydrogen, and oxygen, including sugars and starches

carbohydrate metabolism: breakdown and use of sugars and starches in the body

carcinogen: cancer-causing substance

cardiovascular: related to the heart and circulatory system

cardiovascular disease: disease affecting the heart and/or circulatory system

caries: cavities in the teeth

carotenoid: plant-derived molecules used as pigments

carrageenan: a thickener derived from red seaweed

catabolism: breakdown of complex molecules

catalyze: cause to happen more rapidly

cataract: clouding of the lens of the eye

cellulose: carbohydrate made by plants; indigestible by humans

chiropractic: manipulation of the spine and other bones for healing

cholera: bacterial infection of the small intestine causing severe diarrhea, vomiting, and dehydration

cholesterol: multi-ringed molecule found in animal cell membranes; a type of lipid

chronic: over a long period

chronic disease: diseases that occur over a long period, in contrast to acute diseases

clinical: related to hospitals, clinics, and patient care

cloning: creation of an exact genetic copy of an organism

congenital: present from birth

Congregate Dining: a support service that provides a meal at a central location on a specified day

constipation: difficulty passing feces

consumerism: reliance on buying, rather than making, items necessary for living

contraindicated: not recommended

convenience food: food that requires very little preparation for eating

coronary heart disease: disease of the coronary arteries, the blood vessels surrounding the heart

cretinism: arrested mental and physical development

crossbreeding: breeding between two different varieties of an organism

cuisine: types of food and traditions of preparation

cytoplasm: contents of a cell minus the nucleus

deamination: removal of an NH2 group from a molecule

dehydration: loss of water

dementia: loss of cognitive abilities, including memory and decision making

dentition: formation of the teeth

deoxyribonucleic acid: DNA, the molecule that makes up genes

dependence: a condition in which attempts to stop use leads to withdrawal symptoms, including irritability and insomnia

depression: mood disorder characterized by apathy, restlessness, and negative thoughts

DETERMINE: checklist used to identify nutritionally at-risk individuals

development: the process of change by which an organism becomes more complex

diabetes: inability to regulate level of sugar in the blood

diet: the total daily food intake, or the types of foods eaten

dietary assessment: analysis of nutrients in the diet

Dietary Reference Intakes: set of guidelines for nutrient intake

diphtheria: infectious disease caused by Cornybacterium diphtheriae, causing damage to the heart and other organs

disaccharide carbohydrate: molecule composed of two linked sugars

diuretic: substance that depletes the body of water

diversity: the variety of cultural traditions within a larger culture

diverticulosis: presence of abnormal small sacs in the lining of the intestine

DNA: deoxyribonucleic acid; the molecule that makes up genes, and is therefore responsible for heredity

drugs: substances whose administration causes a significant change in the body's function

dyslipidemia: disorder of fat metabolism

dysmorphia: the belief that one's body is different (fatter, thinner, etc.) than it really is

eating disorder: behavioral disorder involving excess consumption, avoidance of consumption, self-induced vomiting, or other food-related aberrant behavior

ecological: related to the environment and human interactions with it

eczema: skin disease causing itching and flaking

edema: accumulation of fluid in the tissues

efficacy: effectiveness

electrolyte: salt dissolved in fluid

elemental: made from predigested nutrients

elimination diet: diet in which particular foods are eliminated to observe the effect

endotoxin: toxic substance produced and stored within the plant tissue

enema: substance delivered via the rectum

energy: technically, the ability to perform work; the content of a substance that allows it to be useful as a fuel

enrichment: addition of vitamins and minerals to improve the nutritional content of a food

enteric: pertaining to the intestine; delivered via a tube into the intestine

entrepreneur: founder of a new businesses

environment: surroundings

environmental illness: illness due to substances in the environment

enzymatic: related to use of enzymes, proteins that cause chemical reactions to occur

enzyme: protein responsible for carrying out reactions in a cell

epinephrine: hormone that promotes "fight or flight;" also called adrenaline

epithelial cell: sheet of cells lining organs throughout the body

Escherichia coli: common bacterium found in human large intestine

essential fatty acids: particular molecules made of carbon, hydrogen, and oxygen that the human body must have but cannot make itself

estradiol: female hormone; a type of estrogen

estrogen: hormone that helps control female development and menstruation

etiology: origin and development of a disease

eukaryots: organisms whose cells contain nuclei

failure to thrive: lack of normal developmental progress or maintenance of health

famine: extended period of food shortage

fast food: food requiring minimal preparation before eating, or food delivered very quickly after ordering in a restaurant

fat: type of food molecule rich in carbon and hydrogen, with high energy content

fat-soluble: able to be dissolved in fats, including the membranes of cells

fatigue: tiredness

fatty acids: molecules rich in carbon and hydrogen; a component of fats

fermentation: reaction performed by yeast or bacteria to make alcohol

fiber: indigestible plant material that aids digestion by providing bulk

folate: one of the B vitamins, also called folic acid

food additive: substance added to foods to improve nutrition, taste, appearance, or shelf-life

food poisoning: illness caused by consumption of spoiled food, usually containing bacteria

fortification: addition of vitamins and minerals to improve the nutritional content of a food

fortified: altered by addition of vitamins or minerals

free radical: highly reactive molecular fragment, which can damage cells

functional food: food whose health benefits are claimed to be higher than those traditionally assumed for similar types of foods

fungal: of or from fungi

galactosemia: inherited disorder preventing digestion of milk sugar, galactose

gamma rays: very high energy radiation, more powerful than x rays

gastric: related to the stomach

gastric mucosa: lining of the stomach

gastrointestinal: related to the stomach and intestines

gastrointestinal system: the digestive tract (mouth to anus) plus associated organs

gastrointestinal tract: the continuous tube through which food passes including throat, stomach, and intestines

gene: DNA sequence that codes for proteins, and thus controls inheritance

gene expression: use of a gene to make the protein it encodes

genetic: inherited or related to the genes

genetic engineering: manipulation of genes to change the characteristics of a living organism

globalization: development of world-wide economic system

glucagon: hormone that promotes release of sugar from the liver to raise the level of blood sugar

glucose: a simple sugar; the most commonly used fuel in cells

gluten: a protein found in wheat

glycerol: simple molecule that forms a portion of fats

glycogen: storage form of sugar

glycolysis: cellular reaction that begins the breakdown of sugars

growth factor: protein that stimulates growth of surrounding cells

growth hormone: hormone produced by the pituitary gland that increases the rate of growth

growth spurts: periods of rapid growth

guar gum: a thickener made from a tropical bean

Harris-Benedict equation: a formula for calculating a person's minimum energy expenditure

HDL: high density lipoprotein, a blood protein that carries cholesterol

health-promotion: related to advocacy for better health, preventive medicine, and other aspects of well-being

heart attack: loss of blood supply to part of the heart, resulting in death of heart muscle

heart disease: any disorder of the heart or its blood supply, including heart attack, atherosclerosis, and coronary artery disease

heavy metal: lead, chromium, and other metals found in the middle section of the periodic table of the elements

hemoglobin: the iron-containing molecule in red blood cells that carries oxygen

hemorrhoids: swollen blood vessels in the rectum

hepatitis: liver inflammation

hepatitis B: viral disease affecting the liver

herbal: related to or made from herbs

high blood pressure: elevation of the pressure in the bloodstream maintained by the heart

high potency: a claim about vitamin or mineral content, defined as 100% or more of the Recommended Daily Intake

homeostasis: regulation of the proper internal state

hookworm: parasitic nematode that attaches to the intestinal wall

hormone: molecules produced by one set of cells that influence the function of another set of cells

hydration: degree of water in the body

hydrolyze: to break apart through reaction with water

hygiene: cleanliness

hype: advertising and brash claims

hypercholesterolemia: high levels of cholesterol in the blood

hyperglycemia: high level of sugar in the blood

hyperlipidemia: high levels of lipids (fats or cholesterol) in the blood

hypertension: high blood pressure

hypertrophy: excess increase in size

hypoglycemia: low blood sugar level

hypoglycemic: related to low level of blood sugar

immune system: the set of organs and cells, including white blood cells, that protect the body from infection

immunocompromised: having a weakened immune system

immunologic: related to the immune system, which protects the body from infection

incidence: number of new cases reported each year

incisor: chisel-shaped tooth used for cutting; one of the types of primary teeth

indigestion: reduced ability to digest food

infectious diseases: diseases caused by viruses, bacteria, fungi, or protozoa, which replicate inside the body

informed consent: agreement to a procedure after understanding the risks

injera: spongy flat bread

insoluble: not able to be dissolved in water

insulin: hormone released by the pancreas to regulate level of sugar in the blood

internship: training program

interstitial: between the tissues

intestines: the two long tubes that carry out the bulk of the processes of digestion

intravenous: into the veins

iron: nutrient needed for red blood cell formation

isoflavones: estrogen-like compounds in plants

job sharing: splitting a single job among two or more people

junk food: food with high fat and sugar content, without correspondingly high amounts of protein, vitamins, or minerals

keto-acid: an acid compound containing the reactive CO group

ketoacidosis: accumulation of ketone bodies along with high acid levels in the body fluids

ketones: chemicals produced by fat breakdown; molecule containing a double-bonded oxygen linked to two carbons

ketosis: build-up of ketone bodies in the blood, due to fat breakdown

kidney stones: deposits of solid material in kidney

killer-cell: type of white blood cell that helps protect the body from infection

kinetic: related to speed of reaction

Krebs cycle: cellular reaction that breaks down numerous nutrients and provides building blocks for other molecules

kwashiorkor: severe malnutrition characterized by swollen belly, hair loss, and loss of skin pigment

lactic acid: breakdown product of sugar in the muscles in the absence of oxygen

lactose intolerance: inability to digest lactose, or milk sugar

learned behaviors: actions that are acquired by training and observation, in contrast to innate behaviors

leavening: yeast or other agents used for rising bread

legumes: beans, peas, and related plants

lifestyle: set of choices about diet, exercise, job type, leisure activities, and other aspects of life

lipid: fats, waxes, and steroids; important components of cell membranes

lipoprotein: blood protein that carries fats

listeriosis: infectious disease caused by Listeria bacteria

long-term care facilities: hospitals or nursing homes in which patients remain for a long time for chronic care, rather than being treated and quickly discharged

lymph node: pocket within the lymph system in which white blood cells reside

lymph system: system of vessels and glands in the body that circulates and cleans extracellular fluid

lymphatic system: group of ducts and nodes through which fluid and white blood cells circulate to fight infection

macrobiotic: related to a specific dietary regimen based on balancing of vital principles

macronutrient: nutrient needed in large quantities

macular degeneration: death of cells of the macula, part of the eye's retina

malabsorption: decreased ability to take up nutrients

malaise: illness or lack of energy

malaria: disease caused by infection with Plasmodium, a single-celled protozoon, transmitted by mosquitoes

malignant: spreading to surrounding tissues; cancerous

malnourished: lack of adequate nutrients in the diet

malnutrition: chronic lack of sufficient nutrients to maintain health

marasmus: extreme malnutrition, characterized by loss of muscle and other tissue

meditation: stillness of thought, practiced to reduce tension and increase inner peace

menopausal: related to menopause, the period during which women cease to ovulate and menstruate

menopause: phase in a woman's life during which ovulation and menstruation end

menstrual cycles: the build-up and sloughing off of the lining of the uterus in women commencing at puberty and proceeding until menopause

metabolic: related to processing of nutrients and building of necessary molecules within the cell

metabolic activities: sum total of the body's biochemical processes

metabolism: the sum total of reactions in a cell or an organism

metabolism-free radical: highly reactive molecular fragment, which are created through metabolism, or processing of nutrients

metabolite: the product of metabolism, or nutrient processing within the cell

metabolize: processing of a nutrient

microflora: microscopic organisms present in small numbers

micronutrient: nutrient needed in very small quantities

microorganisms: bacteria and protists; single-celled organisms

mineral: an inorganic (non-carbon-containing) element, ion, or compound

miscarriage: loss of a pregnancy

mitochondria: small bodies within a cell that harvest energy for use by the cell

molar: grinding tooth toward the rear of the mouth

molecule: combination of atoms that form stable particles

monocultural: from a single culture

monoglyceride: breakdown product of fats

morbidity: illness or accident

mucosa: moist exchange surface within the body

muscle wasting: loss of muscle bulk

mycotoxin: poison produced by a fungus

myoglobin: oxygen storage protein in muscle

nandrolone: hormone related to testosterone

nausea: unpleasant sensation in the gut that precedes vomiting

needs assessment: formal procedure for determining needs

nervous system: the brain, spinal cord, and nerves that extend throughout the body

neural: related to the nervous system

neural tube defects: failures of proper development of the spinal cord

neurological: related to the nervous system

neuropathy: malfunction of nerve cells

neurotransmitter: molecule released by one nerve cell to stimulate or inhibit another

NHANES: National Heath and Nutrition Examination Survey

niacin: one of the B vitamins, required for energy production in the cell

nitrite: NO_2, used for preservatives

nitrogen: essential element for plant growth

nonpathogenic: not promoting disease

nonpolar: without a separation if charge within the molecule; likely to be hydrophobic

nutrient: dietary substance necessary for health

nutrient deficiencies: lack of adequate nutrients in the diet

nutrition: the maintenance of health through proper eating, or the study of same

nutritional deficiency: lack of adequate nutrients in the diet

nutritional requirements: the set of substances needed in the diet to maintain health

obese: above accepted standards of weight for sex, height, and age

obesity: the condition of being overweight, according to established norms based on sex, age, and height

opacity: impermeability to light

opportunistic infections: infections not normally threatening, which gain a foothold in people with weakened immune systems

oral-pharyngeal: related to mouth and throat

osteoarthritis: inflammation of the joints

osteoblast: cell that forms bone

osteomalacia: softening of the bones

osteopathic: related to the practice of osteopathy, which combines standard medical therapy with manipulation of the skeleton to correct problems

osteoporosis: weakening of the bone structure

over-the-counter: available without a prescription

overweight: weight above the accepted norm based on height, sex, and age

oxidative: related to chemical reaction with oxygen or oxygen-containing compounds

oxygen: O_2, atmospheric gas required by all animals

paralysis: inability to move

parasite: organism that feeds off of other organisms

parasitic: feeding off another organism

parasitic diseases: diseases caused by parasites, including amebic diseases, Giardia, roundworms, and others

pasteurization: heating to destroy bacteria and other microorganisms, after Louis Pasteur

pathogen: organism that causes disease

pH: level of acidity, with low numbers indicating high acidity

phenylketonuria: inherited disease marked by the inability to process the amino acid phenylalanine, causing mental retardation

phospholipid: a type of fat used to build cell membranes

phosphorus: element essential in forming the mineral portion of bone

physiological: related to the biochemical processes of the body

physiology: the group of biochemical and physical processes that combine to make a functioning organism, or the study of same

phytate: plant compound that binds minerals, reducing their ability to be absorbed

phytochemical: chemical produced by plants

phytoestrogen: plant-derived estrogen compound

pituitary gland: gland at the base of the brain that regulates multiple body processes

plaque: material forming deposits on the surface of the teeth, which may promote bacterial growth and decay

plasma: the fluid portion of the blood, distinct from the cellular portion

plateaus: periods during which growth is greatly reduced

pluralistic: of many different sources

pneumonia: lung infection

polar: containing regions of positive and negative charge; likely to be soluble in water

polyunsaturated: having multiple double bonds within the chemical structure, thus increasing the body's ability to metabolize it

potable: safe to drink

pre-renal: kidney disease caused by change in the blood supply to the kidney

prevalence: describing the number of cases in a population at any one time

preventive medicine: treatment designed to prevent disease, rather than waiting for it to occur before intervening

processed food: food that has been cooked, milled, or otherwise manipulated to change its quality

proscription: prohibitions, rules against

prostaglandin: hormone that helps regulate inflammation and other tissue processes

prostate: male gland surrounding the urethra that contributes fluid to the semen

protein: complex molecule composed of amino acids that performs vital functions in the cell; necessary part of the diet

protein digestion: breakdown of proteins into amino acids in the digestive tract

psoriasis: skin disorder characterized by red, dry, scaly skin

psychological: related to thoughts, feelings, and personal experiences

psyllium: bulk-forming laxative derived from the Plantago psyllium seeds

puberty: time of onset of sexual maturity

reactivity: characteristic set of reactions undergone due to chemical structure

Recommended Dietary Allowances: nutrient intake recommended to promote health

renal failure: inability of the kidneys to cleanse the blood

respiratory system: the lungs, throat, and muscles of respiration, or breathing

rice genome: the set of genes possessed by rice

rickets: disorder caused by vitamin D deficiency, marked by soft and misshapen bones and organ swelling

ritual: ceremony or frequently repeated behavior

RNA: ribonucleic acid, used in cells to create proteins from genetic information

salmonellosis: food poisoning due to Salmonella bacteria

saturated fat: a fat with the maximum possible number of hydrogens; more difficult to break down than unsaturated fats

scurvy: a syndrome characterized by weakness, anemia, and spongy gums, due to vitamin C deficiency

sedentary: not active

serotonin: chemical used by nerve cells to communicate with one another

serum: noncellular portion of the blood

serum estrone: blood level of estrone, a steroid hormone that is one of the estrogens, a type of female hormone

shock: state of dangerously low blood pressure and loss of blood delivered to the tissues

sideroblastosis: condition in which the blood contains an abnormally high number of sideroblasts, or red blood cells containing iron granules

sleep apnea: difficulty breathing while sleeping

smallpox: deadly viral disease

smog: air pollution

social group: tribe, clique, family, or other group of individuals

socioeconomic status: level of income and social class

staples: essential foods in the diet

steroid: class of hormones composed of carbon rings, necessary for sexual development and mineral balance

steroid hormones: class of hormones composed of carbon rings, necessary for sexual development and mineral balance

steroids: group of hormones that affect tissue build-up, sexual development, and a variety of metabolic

sterol: building blocks of steroid hormones; a type of lipid

stillbirth: giving birth to a dead fetus

stress: heightened state of nervousness or unease

stroke: loss of blood supply to part of the brain, due to a blocked or burst artery in the brain

subcutaneous: beneath the skin

sucrose: table sugar

temperate zone: region of the world between the tropics and the arctic or Antarctic

testosterone: male sex hormone

thalassemia: inherited blood disease due to defect in the hemoglobin protein

thermogregulate: regulate temperature

tofu: soybean curd, similar in consistency to cottage cheese

tolerance: development of a need for increased amount of drug to obtain a given level of intoxication

toxicant: harmful substance

toxins: poisons

trace: very small amount

trans-fatty acids: type of fat thought to increase the risk of heart disease

triglyceride: a type of fat

tuber: swollen plant stem below the ground

tuberculosis: bacterial infection, usually of the lungs, caused by Mycobacterium tuberculosis

tularemia: bacterial infection by Francisella tularensis, causing fever, skin lesions, and other symptoms

type II diabetes: inability to regulate the level of sugar in the blood due to a reduction in the number of insulin receptors on the body's cells

typhoid: fever-causing bacterial infection due to Salmonella typhi; transmitted contaminated food or water

typhus: bacterial disease transmitted by infected rodents

ulcer: erosion in the lining of the stomach or intestine due to bacterial infection

uncharged: neither positively nor negatively charged

undernutrition: food intake too low to maintain adequate energy expenditure without weight loss

uric: from urine

vaccine: medicine that promotes immune system resistance by stimulating pre-existing cells to become active

vegan: person who consumes no animal products, including milk and honey

viral disease: disease caused by viruses, including flu, colds, AIDS, hepatitis, and others

virus: noncellular infectious agent that requires a host cell to reproduce

vitamin: necessary complex nutrient used to aid enzymes or other metabolic processes in the cell

vitamin D: nutrient needed for calcium uptake and therefore proper bone formation

wasting: loss of body tissue often as a result of cancer or other disease

water-soluble: able to be dissolved in water

wean: cease breast-feeding

wellness: related to health promotion

white blood cell: immune system cell that fights infection

yeast allergy: allergy to yeasts used in baking or brewing

zinc: mineral necessary for many enzyme processes

Index

*Page numbers in **bold** indicate the main article on a subject. Page numbers in italics indicate illustrations. The number preceding the colon indicates the volume number, and the number after the colon indicates the page number. The letter t after a page number indicates a table.*

A

Absorption
  defined, 1:10
  See also Digestion and absorption
Acesulfame potassium, 1:46
Acetyl coenzyme A, 1:96, 2:55, 56, 57
Acid reflux, defined, 1:256
Acidity, defined, 1:86
Acidosis, defined, 1:149
Acquired immunodeficiency syndrome. *See* HIV/AIDS
Activity disorder, 1:184
Acupuncture, 1:*32*, 2:66
  defined, 1:30
Acute, defined, 1:63
Acute diarrhea, 1:149, 150
Acute rheumatic heart disease, 1:272
ADA. *See* American Dietetic Association (ADA)
Addiction, exercise. *See* Exercise addiction
Addiction, food, **1:1**
  See also Eating disorders
Additives and preservatives, **1:1–4**, 1:*3*
  fat substitutes as additives, 1:212, 213
  and hyperactivity, 1:29
  and quackery, 2:162
  safety regulations, 1:2–4
  uses, 1:2
Adenosine triphosphate (ATP)
  carbohydrate metabolism, 2:55
  catabolism, 2:157
  cellular metabolism, 2:54

  as energy unit, 2:92, 241
  glycolysis, 1:96–97
  protein metabolism, 2:55–56
  thiamine, 1:62
Adequate Intake (AI), 1:155, 2:151, 152
  defined, 2:59
Adipose tissue
  defined, 1:68
  See also Body fat distribution
Administrative dietitians, 1:168
Adolescent nutrition, **1:4–7**
  body image, 1:69
  calcium, 1:84–85
  eating and snacking patterns, 1:5–6
  eating disorders, 2:193
  fat intake, 2:192
  high-risk groups, 1:6–7
  marketing strategies aimed at adolescents, 2:38
  nutritional needs, 1:5, 6, *6*, 2:*103*
  obesity, 2:192–193
  popular culture, 2:192
  pregnancy weight gain, 2:144
  vegetarianism, 2:230
  See also School-aged children, diet of
ADRA (Adventist Development and Relief Agency International), 1:175t
Adult nutrition, **1:7–10**, 1:*9*, 84–85
  See also Aging and nutrition
Adventist Development and Relief Agency International (ADRA), 1:175t
Adverse reaction, 1:26
Advertising, 2:38–40
Advocacy nongovernmental organizations, 2:83
Aerobic, defined, 1:198
African Americans, diet of, **1:10–15**
  cancer, 2:167
  childhood obesity, 1:121

  diabetes, 1:144, 146
  dietary influences, 1:12–13
  elderly, 2:168
  future, 1:14
  hypertension, 1:14, 14t, 290, 2:167
  legacy, 1:*11*, 11–12
  origins, 1:10–11
  poverty and health, 1:13–14, 14t
  regional diet, 1:12, 2:166–168
  and television, 2:167–168
  See also Caribbean Islanders, diet of
Africans, diets of, **1:15–20**
  African diet, 1:16
  and African-American diet, 1:10–11
  biotechnology, 1:17
  early history of Africa, 1:15–16
  East Africa, 1:18
  food security, 1:19
  North Africa, 1:16–17, *17*
  nutrition and disease, 1:19
  Southern Africa, 1:18
  underweight, 2:35
  West Africa, 1:17–18
  See also Caribbean Islanders, diet of
Aging and nutrition, **1:20–23**
  African Americans, 2:168
  body mass index, 1:73
  calcium, 1:85, 86
  commodity foods, 1:129
  dietary problems, 1:21, 21–22
  medical, physical, and functional problems, 1:22–23
  nutrient-drug interactions, 2:89
  Nutrition Screening Initiative, 1:20–21
  social problems, 1:22
  vegetarianism, 2:230–231
  vitamin D, 2:235
  water, 2:50, 246
  See also Meals On Wheels; Recommended Dietary Allowances

283

AHA. *See* American Heart
   Association (AHA)
AI. *See* Adequate Intake (AI)
AIDS. *See* HIV/AIDS
Alanine, 2:155, 156*t*
Albumin, and calcium transport, 1:84
Alcohol and health, **1:23–26**, 1:23*t*,
      25
   absorption, 1:172
   alcoholism, 1:24–25
   cancer, 1:89
   college students, 1:25, 124
   gastric ulcers, 1:172
   heart disease, 1:274
   high-risk groups, 1:25
   hypertension, 1:290
   nutrient-drug interactions, 2:89, 90
   pregnancy, 1:220–221
   Russia, 1:*119*, 120
   Wernicke-Korsakoff syndrome,
      2:238
   wine as functional food, 1:240,
      242*t*
   See also Fetal alcohol syndrome
      (FAS)
Aldosterone, 2:248
Alimentary canal, 1:*171*
Alitame, 1:48
Allergen, defined, 1:26
Allergic reaction, defined, 1:27
Allergies and intolerances, **1:26–30**
   controversies, 1:29
   definitions, 1:26
   food allergy, 1:27, 27–28, *38*
   food intolerance, 1:27, 28
   genetically modified foods, 1:66,
      67, 246
   peanut allergies, 1:29
   rice allergies, 2:182
   treatment, 1:29
Allergy, defined, 1:26
Alliance for Food Security, 1:238
Alpha tocopherol. *See* Vitamin E
Alpha-carotene, as carotenoid, 1:113
Alternative medicines and therapies,
      1:29–34, 2:161
   alternative medicine,
      complementary medicine, and
      integrative medicine, 1:30
   Dietary Supplement Health and
      Education Act (1994), 1:31–32,
      33
   modality selection, 1:33–34
   modality types, 1:30–31, 31*t*, *32*
   supplement facts label, 1:32–33
   See also Dietary supplements;
      Macrobiotic diet
Alzheimer's disease, 2:75

AMA (American Medical
   Association), 1:4, 68, 97
Amalyse, 1:169, 170
Amenorrhea, 1:41, 219, 2:218–219
   defined, 1:41
American Academy of Pediatrics,
   2:112, 153
American Association of Advertising
   Agencies, 2:40
American Association of Diabetes
   Educators, 2:44
American Cancer Society, 1:92
American College of Cardiology, 2:30
American Dental Association,
   2:10–11
American dietary trends. *See* Dietary
   trends, American
American Dietetic Association
      (ADA), **1:34**
   biotechnology, 1:68
   Commission on Accreditation for
      Dietetics Education, 1:105,
      2:44, 105
   Commission on Dietetic
      Registration, 1:106, 168, 2:44,
      105
   fat substitutes, 1:213
   fiber intake, 1:221
   functional foods, 1:243
   medical nutrition therapy
      protocols, 2:45
   vegetarianism, 2:230
American Farm Bureau Federation,
   1:248
American Heart Association (AHA)
   cardiac arrest, 1:273
   fad diets, 1:205–206
   lipid profile, 2:30
   Mediterranean diet, 1:259–260
   men and heart disease, 2:52
American Indians. *See* Native
   Americans
American Institute for Cancer
   Research, 2:117
American Marketing Association,
   2:37
American Medical Association
   (AMA), 1:4, 68, 97
American Psychiatric Association
   anorexia nervosa, 1:70–71
   binge eating disorder, 1:63–64
   bulimia nervosa, 1:71
   eating disorders, 1:176, 177
American Public Health Association
   (APHA), **1:35**
American School Food Service
   Association (ASFSA), **1:35**,
   2:*195*, 196–197
   See also School food service

American School Health Association
   (ASHA), **1:35–36**, 1:130
Americanized, defined, 1:116
Amine, defined, 1:4
Amino acids, **1:36–38**, 1:36*t*
   defined, 1:31
   essential, 1:36, 36*t*, 38, 2:155–156
   food sources, 1:37–38
   functions of proteins, 1:37
   maize, 1:134
   metabolism disorders, 2:5–6
   nonessential, 1:36, 36*t*, 2:155–156
   protein, 2:55–56, 92, 155–156, 156*t*
   structure, 1:36–37
   supplements for sports nutrition,
      2:218
   See also Nutrients; Protein
Amylase, 1:96
Amylopectin, 1:94
Amylose, 1:94
Anabolic, defined, 1:190
Anabolic agents, as ergogenic aids,
   1:190–192, *191*
Anabolism, 2:54, 157
Anaerobic, defined, 1:198
Anaphylaxis, defined, 1:28
"The Anatomy Lesson of Dr.
   Nicolaes Tulp" (Rembrandt),
   2:224, *224*
Andorra, life expectancy in, 2:28
Android fat distribution, 1:68–69
Androstenedione, as ergogenic aid,
   1:191, *191*
Anemia, **1:38–41**
   Asia, 1:56
   defined, 1:5
   hypochromic, 1:38, 39*t*
   iron-deficiency, 1:38–40, 2:153
   macrocytic, 1:38, 39*t*, 2:243
   megaloblastic, 1:40
   microcytic, 1:38, 39*t*
   normochronic, 1:38, 39*t*
   nutritional deficiency, 2:103
   other causes, 1:40
   pernicious, 1:40, 2:243
   sickle-cell, 1:*39*
   treatment, 1:40–41
   types and causes, 1:39*t*
   women, 2:259
Angioplasty, defined, 1:59
Angiotensin, 2:248
Angular cheilosis, 2:111
Animal proteins, 2:156
Animals, biotechnology in, 1:65–66
Anorexia nervosa, **1:41–42**
   binge eating/purging type, 1:177
   body image, 1:*70*, 70–71

defined, 1:41
diagnosis, 1:177
inpatient hospitalization, 1:180
malnutrition, 2:140
medication, 1:181
prevalence, 1:184
restricting type, 1:177
treatment outcomes, 1:181
See also Eating disorders
Anthropometric, defined, 1:42
Anthropometric measurements, **1:42**, 2:35, 99–101, 100*t*
See also Body mass index; Nutritional assessment; Waist-to-hip ratio
Anti-aging products, as quackery, 2:162
Antibacterial soaps, 2:3
Antibiotics
defined, 1:91
nutrient-drug interactions, 2:89
resistance to, 1:246
and vitamin K, 2:236
Antibody, defined, 1:37
Antidepressants
for eating disorders, 1:180–181
nutrient-drug interactions, 2:89
Antigens, 1:37
Antigua, 1:110
Antimicrobial agents, as food additive, 1:2
Antioxidants, **1:42–44**, 1:*43*
and cancer prevention, 1:91
carotenoids as, 1:112
defined, 1:1
as food additive, 1:2, 242*t*
as functional food, 1:242*t*
health benefits and food sources, 1:44*t*
vitamin E as, 2:237
Ants, 2:202, *202*
Anxiety, defined, 1:1
APHA (American Public Health Association), 1:35
Apollo space program, 2:212
Appendicitis, defined, 1:8
Appert, Nicholas, 1:4
Appetite, 1:22, **1:44–45**, 2:89
See also Hunger
Apples/apple juice, glycemic index, 1:251*t*
Aquavit, 2:188
Aqueous, defined, 1:216
Arepa, 2:202–203
Argentina, 2:201, 203
Arginine, 2:156*t*
Ariboflavinosis, 2:238

Arteries, hardening of. *See* Atherosclerosis
Arteriosclerosis, **1:45–46**
See also Atherosclerosis; Cardiovascular disease (CVD)
Artery, 1:99, *101*
defined, 1:45
Arthritis
defined, 1:22
remedies as quackery, 2:162
Artificial colors, 1:2
Artificial flavors and flavor enhancers, 1:2
Artificial sweeteners, **1:46–48**, 1:*47*
American dietary trend, 1:160, *160*
FDA-approved artificial sweeteners, 1:46–47
pending FDA approval, 1:48
sugar alcohols, 1:47
See also Generally recognized as safe; Phenylketonuria
Ascorbic acid. *See* Vitamin C
ASFSA (American School Food Service Association), 1:35, 2:*195*, 196–197
ASHA (American School Health Association), 1:35–36, 130
Asian Americans, diets of, **1:48–52**
childhood obesity, 1:122
fiber, 1:221
food habits, 1:*49*, 49–51
traditional Asian diet, 1:50*t*
See also Asians, diet of
Asian Diet Pyramid, 1:51, *57*
Asian Indians, diet of, 1:50*t*, 55
Asians, diet of, **1:52–59**, 1:*57*
body image, 1:*163*
East Asia, 1:53–54
food security, 1:55
fruit, 1:52–53, *54*
merits and weaknesses, 1:50*t*
micronutrient deficiency, 1:55–56
nutritional transition, 1:56–57
obesity, 1:*163*
osteomalacia, 2:122
other common ingredients, 1:53
rice, 1:52, *53*
South Asia, 1:55
Southeast Asia, 1:54–55
underweight, 2:35
See also Asian Americans, diets of
Asparagine, 2:156*t*
Aspartame, 1:46
Aspirin, 2:88*t*
Assisted-living, defined, 1:22
Asthma, defined, 1:4
Asymptomatic, defined, 1:149

Atherosclerosis, **1:59**, 1:100, 217, 273–274
defined, 1:59
See also Arteriosclerosis; Cardiovascular disease (CVD)
Athletes. *See* Female athlete triad; Sports nutrition
Atkins, Robert, 1:97, *204*
Atkins Diet, 1:97, 203*t*, 204, *204*, 206
Atole, defined, 1:113
Atoms, defined, 1:47
ATP. *See* Adenosine triphosphate (ATP)
Australia
food-borne illness, 2:118
life expectancy, 2:28
skin cancer, 1:88
Avidin, 2:242
Ayurvedic, defined, 1:30

B

B vitamins
defined, 1:115
and oral health, 2:111
See also specific B vitamins by name
Baby bottle tooth decay, **1:59–60**, 2:10–11, 111, 153
See also Oral health
BAC (blood alcohol concentration), 1:23
Bacillus cereus, 2:120*t*
Baciullus thuringiensis, 1:246–247
Bacteria
defined, 1:1
and food-borne illness, 2:119
Bactericidal, defined, 1:1
Bacteriostatic, defined, 1:1
Bad cholesterol. *See* Low-density lipoprotein (LDL)
Bagels, glycemic index, 1:251*t*
Bam (Iran) earthquake, 2:226
Bananas, 1:110, 251*t*
"Bangers and mash," 2:*85*
Banting, William, 1:205
Baraka, Amiri, 1:12
Barbados, 1:110
Barbecue, 1:12
Basal metabolic rate (BMR)
adults, 1:8, *9*
defined, 1:8
menopause, 2:48
and weight loss, 2:248, 250
Battle Creek Sanitarium, **1:60–62**, 1:*61*, 2:16, 17, 254
See also Kellogg, John Harvey; White, Ellen G.
Beauty pageant contestants, 1:69

Beckham, David, 2:247
Behavioral, defined, 1:91
Beikost, **1:62**, 2:9, 10–11
Belize, 1:110
Benign tumors, 1:90
Beriberi, **1:62**
   Funk, Casimir, 1:244
   nutritional deficiency, 2:103
   and rice, 2:181
   and thiamine, 2:238
   Tulp, Nicolaas, 2:224
Berndtson, Keith, 1:279–280
Beta-carotene, **1:62–63**
   as antioxidant, 1:43, 44t
   as carotenoid, 1:113, 2:232, 234
   and golden rice, 2:182, 264
   and lung cancer, 2:234
   risks, 1:157
   supplements during pregnancy, 2:36
   See also Carotenoids; Vitamin A
Beta-hydroxy beta-methylbutyrate (HMB), 1:190
Beta-oxidation, 2:56
Beverages
   with antioxidants, 1:242t
   Caribbean Islands, 1:108
   chocolate, 1:81t
   glycemic index, 1:251t
   nutrient-drug interactions, 2:89, 90
Bezoars, **1:63**
Bile, defined, 1:169
Binge, defined, 1:41
Binge eating, **1:63–64**
   diagnosis, 1:177–178
   as eating disturbance, 1:182, 184
   and malnutrition, 2:140
   medication, 1:181
   prevalence, 1:184
   See also Bulimia nervosa; Eating disorders
Bioavailability, **1:64**, 2:59
   defined, 1:64
   See also Nutrients
Biochemical, defined, 1:152
Biodiversity, defined, 1:67
Biological, defined, 1:45
Biologics Control Act (1902), 2:73
Biotechnology, **1:64–68**
   Africa, 1:17
   in animals, 1:65–66
   food production concerns, 1:66–67
   food safety, 1:67–68, 237
   genetic engineering, 1:65, 66
   and global health, 1:67
   safety and labeling, 1:67–68
   See also Genetically modified foods

Bioterrorism, and food safety, 1:237–238, 2:172
Biotin (vitamin B_8), 2:94, 240t, 241–242
   defined, 1:169
Biotoxin, defined, 2:120
Biphosphanates, 2:124
Birth control pills, 2:88t
Birth defects, 2:142–143, 234, 243
Bleaching agents, as food additive, 1:2
Blood, and space physiology, 2:212
Blood alcohol concentration (BAC), 1:23
Blood clotting, defined, 1:83
Blood pressure, 1:99, 100
   defined, 1:13
Blood proteins, 2:158
Blood soup, 2:80
BMI. See Body mass index (BMI)
BMR. See Basal metabolic rate (BMR)
Body fat distribution, **1:68–69**
   and body mass index, 1:72–73
   measuring with calipers, 2:101, 102, 253
   menopause, 2:48
   nutritional assessment, 2:100–101
   as physical fitness component, 1:200
   See also Waist-to-hip ratio
Body image, **1:69–71**, 1:70, 163, 179, 179
   See also Eating disorders
Body mass index (BMI), **1:71–74**, 1:72, 73t
   and cardiovascular disease, 1:101
   children, 1:121
   defined, 1:42
   in nutritional assessment, 2:100
   and obesity, 2:105, 125, 140
   and overweight, 2:125, 140
   and pregnancy, 2:142, 143, 143t, 146
   and underweight, 2:225
   See also Obesity
Bolivia, 2:202, 203
Bone loss
   and menopause, 2:48
   and space travel, 2:210–211, 215
Bone marrow, defined, 1:40
Boron, as ergogenic aid, 1:190
Botanical, defined, 1:31
Botulism, 2:1, 3–4
   defined, 2:1
Bovine somatotropin (BST), 1:65–66, 262
Bovine spongiform encephalopathy (BSE), 2:118–119, 119, 187
Bowel, defined, 1:91

Brain allergy, defined, 1:29
Brazil, 2:201, 202
Breadfruit, 1:108, 2:127, 130, 130
Breads
   glycemic index, 1:251t
   marketing strategies, 2:38
   Mediterranean diet, 1:257
Breakfast
   School Breakfast Program, 1:284, 2:97, 190–191, 194
   sports nutrition, 2:216
Breast cancer
   and estrogen replacement therapy, 2:48, 49
   and letrozol, 2:75
   and physical activity, 1:92
   and soy, 2:208
   women's nutritional issues, 2:260
   See also Cancer
Breastfeeding, **1:74–78**, 1:77
   benefits, 1:75, 75t, 2:146
   breast implants and breast reduction, 1:76–77
   contraindications, 1:77
   and diarrhea, 1:150, 151
   infant nutrition, 2:8–9, 11
   mastitis, 2:41, 41
   nutrition for, 1:76, 2:259
   physiology, 1:76
   policies and recommendations, 1:77–78
   and rickets, 2:184
   supplementing with formula, 2:38–39
   Ten Steps to Successful Breastfeeding program, 2:226
   trends, 1:75–76
   and vegetarianism, 2:230
   and vitamin D, 2:235
   and vitamin K, 2:236
   WIC program, 2:255, 256, 257
   See also Formula feeding; Infant nutrition
Breastfeeding caries. See Baby bottle tooth decay
Bright-light therapy, 2:149, 149
Brillat-Savarin, Jean Anthelme, 1:78, **1:78–79**
British Virgin Islands, 1:110
Broth, 2:80
Brush border enzymes, 2:157
BSE (bovine spongiform encephalopathy), 2:118–119, 119, 187
BST (bovine somatotropin), 1:65–66, 262
Buddhist food practices, 2:175, 176, 178t

Bulgaria, 1:118
Bulimia, defined, 1:70
Bulimia nervosa, **1:79–80**
　body image, 1:71
　diagnosis, 1:177
　history, 1:181
　inpatient hospitalization, 1:180
　and malnutrition, 2:140
　medication, 1:181
　nonpurging type, 1:177
　prevalence, 1:184
　purging type, 1:177
　treatment outcomes, 1:181
　See also Binge eating; Eating disorders
Burgers, cultural influences on, 1:187–188
Bush, George W., and stem cell research, 2:75
Bush tea, 1:109

C

CACFP (Child and Adult Care Food Program), 1:129, 284
CAD. *See* Coronary artery disease (CAD)
CADE (Commission on Accreditation for Dietetics Education), 1:105, 2:44, 105
Caffeine, **1:80–83**
　effect on body, 1:80
　effect on mood, 2:66
　as ergogenic aid, 1:192
　in food and drugs, 1:81, 81*t*
　and health, 1:*82*, 82–83
　and hypertension, 1:290
　nutrient-drug interactions, 2:*89*
　during pregnancy, 2:145
　religious proscriptions, 2:176
Cajun cooking, 1:12–13
Calcidiol, 2:235
Calciferol. *See* Vitamin D
Calcification, 2:183, 185
Calcitonin, 1:84, 2:124
Calcitriol, 2:183, 235
Calcium, **1:83–87**
　adolescents, 1:5, *6*
　and caffeine, 1:82
　deficiency, 1:84, 2:61
　defined, 1:5
　disease prevention and treatment, 2:61
　functions, 2:60
　and lactose intolerance, 2:22–23
　lead poisoning prevention, 2:24, 26
　in orange juice, 1:242*t*, 243
　and osteomalacia, 2:122
　and osteoporosis, 1:10, 85, *85*, 2:61, 124
　during pregnancy, 2:145
　for premenstrual syndrome, 2:148
　preschoolers and toddlers, 2:152, 153
　requirements and supplementation, 1:84–87, *85*, 86*t*
　and soy, 2:208
　and space travel, 2:210, 215
　sports nutrition, 2:217
　supplements, 2:59
　toxicity, 1:84, 2:61
　in vegetarianism, 2:230
　and vitamin D, 2:235
　women, 2:259, 260
　See also Osteoporosis
Calcium carbonate, 1:86*t*
Calcium citrate, 1:86*t*
Calcium glubionate, 1:86*t*
Calcium gluconate, 1:86*t*
Calcium lactate, 1:86*t*
Calcium phosphate, 1:86*t*
Calipers, skinfold, 2:101, 102, *253*
Calories, **1:87**
　adolescents, 1:5
　alcoholic beverages and mixers, 1:23*t*
　American dietary trends, 1:160, 161
　defined, 1:5
　effect on mood, 2:66*t*
　infant nutrition, 2:8
　international dietary trends, 1:162
　and marasmus, 2:36, 37
　needs of obese, 2:105
　preschoolers and toddlers, 2:151–152, 152*t*
　during space travel, 2:214
　sports nutrition, 2:216
　and vegetarianism, 2:230, 231
　See also Protein-energy malnutrition (PEM)
CAM (complementary and alternative medicine), 1:30, 2:148–149
　See also Alternative medicines and therapies
Cambodians, diet of, 1:50*t*
Campaigning nongovernmental organizations, 2:83
Campylobacter jejuni, 2:1, 119, 120*t*
Canadians, Recommended Nutrient Intakes for, 1:155
Cancer, **1:87–92**
　African Americans, 2:167
　breast, 1:92, 2:48, *49*, 75, 208, 260
　and caffeine, 1:82
　carcinogenesis process, 1:90–91
　causes, 1:88–90, *90*
　colon, 1:91, 92
　cures as quackery, 2:163
　defined, 1:3
　and diet, 1:91, 92
　and food additives, 1:3–4
　growth and spread, 1:88, *89*
　lung, 2:234
　macrobiotic diet, 2:*32*, 33
　men, 2:51, *52*
　nutrition for people with cancer, 1:92
　and pesticides, 2:116, 117
　and physical activity, 1:91
　prevalence, 1:88
　prevention, 1:91, 2:234
　prostate, 1:91, 2:208, 234
　and saccharin, 1:47
　and soy, 2:208
　types, 1:88
　and vitamin C, 2:134, 167
　See also Antioxidants; Phytochemicals
Cancer Prevention Study (2002), 2:199
Candidal, defined, 2:154
Candidiasis, defined, 2:108
Canning, discovery of, 1:4
Capillaries, 1:99
Capsaicin intolerance, 1:28
Carbohydrate-based fat substitutes, 1:*212*, 212*t*, 217–218
Carbohydrates, **1:93–99**
　absorption, 1:172
　carbohydrate-modified diets, 1:97, 98
　chemical structure, 1:93
　complex, 1:94–96, *95*, 2:91
　counting, 1:98
　defined, 1:8
　and diabetes, 1:98
　digestion and absorption, 1:96
　and eating disturbances, 1:184
　effect on mood, 2:66*t*
　exchange system, 1:98
　glycolysis, 1:96–97
　low-carb diets, 1:97
　metabolism, 2:6–7, 54–55
　as nutrient, 2:91–92
　recommended intake, 1:93, 97
　simple, 1:93–94, 94*t*, 2:91
　sports nutrition, 2:216
　See also Glycemic index
Carcinogen, 1:89
　defined, 1:4

Carcinogenesis process, 1:90–91
Carcinoma, 1:88
Cardiac arrest, 1:272, 273, 2:75
Cardiovascular, defined, 1:8
Cardiovascular disease (CVD), **1:99–104,** 1:*102*
  Asia, 1:56, 57
  atherosclerosis, 1:100
  and caffeine, 1:82
  Central Europe and Russia, 1:117–118, 119–120
  coronary artery disease, 1:100, *101*
  hypertension, 1:99–100, *100*, 103
  and lipid profile, 2:28
  and lycopene, 2:234
  preventing, 1:100–103
  stroke, 1:100
  See also Arteriosclerosis; Atherosclerosis; Heart disease
Cardiovascular fitness, 1:200
The Care and Feeding of Southern Babies (Wilson), 2:258, *258*
CARE (Cooperative for Assistance and Relief Everywhere), 1:175t
Careers in dietetics, **1:104–107**
  knowledge and skills, 1:106
  practice roles, 1:104–105
  registration and licensure, 1:106
  training, 1:105–106
  See also Dietetic technician, registered (DTR); Dietitian; Nutritionist
Caribbean Cooperation in Health, 1:111
Caribbean Food and Nutrition Institute (CFNI), 1:111
Caribbean Islanders, diet of, **1:107–112**
  European settlement, 1:107–108, *108*
  foods of the islands, 1:*108*, 108–110, 110t
  health issues, 1:110–111, 112
  public health initiatives, 1:111–112
Caries, 2:110, 111–112, 153
  defined, 1:46
  See also see Baby bottle tooth decay
Carotenoids, 1:43, **1:112–113,** 2:232, 234
  defined, 1:42
  See also Antioxidants; Beta-carotene; Vitamin A
Carpal tunnel syndrome, 2:242
Carrageenan, defined, 1:212
Carrots, glycemic index, 1:251t
Catabolism, 2:54, 157
  defined, 1:150
Catalyze, defined, 2:242

Cataracts, 2:234, 238
  defined, 1:56
Catholic food practices, 2:176, *176*, 178–179, 178t
Cavities, 2:110, 111–112, 153
  See also see Baby bottle tooth decay
CBOs (community-based organizations), 2:83
CCK (cholecystokinin), 1:170, 216
CDC. *See* U.S. Centers for Disease Control and Prevention (CDC)
CDE (Certified Diabetes Educator), 1:105
CDR. *See* Commission on Dietetic Registration (CDR)
Celebrities, in advertising, 2:*39*
Cellulose, defined, 1:95
Central Americans and Mexicans, diets of, **1:113–117**
  changes in dietary practices, 1:116
  cooking methods, 1:114–115
  dishes, 1:115
  fruits and vegetables, 1:114
  influence of Central American and Mexican culture, 1:116
  nutritional benefits, 1:115
  nutritional limitations, 1:115–116
  traditional dietary habits, 1:113–114, *114*
  See also Hispanics and Latinos, diet of; South Americans, diet of
Central Europeans and Russians, diets of, **1:117–121,** 1:120t
  Central Europe, 1:117–118
  former Soviet Union (Russian Federation), 1:118, *119*
  lifestyle and nutrition, 1:118–120, *119*
  See also Northern Europeans, diet of; Southern Europeans, diet of
Ceramic cookware, and lead poisoning, 2:25
Cereal
  Battle Creek Sanitarium, 1:60–61, *61*
  marketing strategies, 2:37, *39*
  Mediterranean diet, 1:257
Cerebrovascular accident (CVA), 1:100, 147
Certification
  nutritionists, 1:105, 266, 2:105
  organic foods, 2:114
Certified Diabetes Educator (CDE), 1:105
Certified health education specialist (CHES), 1:266
Certified in Nutrition Support (CNS), 1:105
CFNI (Caribbean Food and Nutrition Institute), 1:111

CFNP (Community Food and Nutrition Program), 1:285
Champagne, 2:87
Channel One, 2:191
Chasteberry, 2:148
CHD (congenital heart disease), 1:272, 2:48, *49*
Check Out for Children program, 2:227
Chelating agents, as food additive, 1:2
Chelation therapy, for lead poisoning, 2:26–27
CHES (certified health education specialist), 1:266
Chewing difficulties, 1:21, 2:110, 111
Child and Adult Care Food Program (CACFP), 1:129, 284
Child Nutrition Act (1972), 2:255–256
Childhood obesity, **1:121–123,** 1:*122*, 2:153, 192–193
  See also Obesity
Children
  African-American, 2:166–167
  and caffeine, 1:82
  calcium requirements, 1:84–85, 86
  dental caries, 2:110, 111–112
  diarrhea, 1:149–151
  fiber requirements, 1:221–222
  food insecurity, 1:*229*, 229–230
  homeless, 1:283–284
  iron requirements, 1:39
  kwashiorkor, 2:21
  lead poisoning, 2:24, 25, *25*, 26
  malnutrition, 2:33–34, *34*, 35, *36*
  marasmus, 2:35–36
  marketing strategies aimed at, 2:38, *38*
  Mexican-American, 2:168
  nutritional deficiency, 2:*103*
  obesity, 2:153
  overweight, 2:153, 192–193
  protein requirement, 2:159
  and vegetarianism, 2:230
  white American, 2:166–167
  See also Adolescent nutrition; Preschoolers and toddlers, diet of; School-aged children, diet of
Chile, 2:201, 202, 203
China
  food-borne illness, 2:118
  functional foods, 1:241
Chinese, diet of, 1:50t, 53, 221
Chinese Americans, diet of, 1:50
Chiropractic, defined, 1:30
Chitin, as ergogenic aid, 1:192
Chloride, 2:60, 61

Chocolate
  caffeine in, 1:81*t*
  effect on mood, 2:*65*, 66
Cholecystokinin (CCK), 1:170, 216
Cholera, 2:75
  defined, 2:73
Cholesterol
  and cardiovascular disease, 1:103
  defined, 1:33
  and fat intake, 1:217
  Healthy Eating Index, 1:268
  metabolism, 2:57–58, 77
  optimal, borderline, and high levels, 2:29*t*, 30
  and rice, 2:181–182
  and saturated fatty acids, 2:93
Cholesterol, bad. *See* Low-density lipoprotein (LDL)
Cholesterol, good. *See* High-density lipoprotein (HDL)
Cholesterol to HDL ratio, 2:29*t*, 30
Choline, 2:244
Christmas, 2:189
Chromium, 1:191, 2:62
Chronic, defined, 1:6
Chronic diarrhea, 1:149
Chronic diseases
  Asian Americans, 1:51
  women's nutritional issues, 2:260–261, *261*
Chronic rheumatic heart disease, 1:272
Church World Service (CWS), 1:175*t*
Chylomicrons, 1:216, 2:29
Chyme, 1:169–170, *171*
Chymosin, 1:65
Cigarettes. *See* Smoking
Circadian rhythms, 2:65–66
Cirrhosis of the liver, 1:24, *25*
Citric acid cycle, 1:96–97, 2:55
Clinical, defined, 1:62
Clinical dietitians, 1:104–105, 168
Cloning, defined, 1:66
Clostridium botulinum, 2:1, 120*t*
Clostridium perfringens, 2:1, 119, 120*t*
CNS (Certified in Nutrition Support), 1:105
Cobalamin, 1:40
Coca-Cola, 2:136, *136*
Coconuts, 1:53, 110
Code of Federal Regulations, 1:232, 233
Cod-liver oil, 2:46, *47*, 234–235
Coenzyme A, 2:241
Coffee
  caffeine, 1:81, 81*t*
  South America, 2:201, 202, 203

Cognitive restructuring, and weight management, 2:251
Colcannon, 2:86
Cold, common
  and hand washing, 2:3
  and vitamin C, 2:134, 244
Collagen, 2:244
College students, diets of, **1:123–127**, 1:*124*, *126*
  alcohol use, 1:25, 124
  eating patterns and serving sizes, 1:123
  female students, 1:124–125
  food and nutrient intake, 1:123–125
  male students, 1:124
  recommendations for improvement, 1:125–126
Colombia, 2:201, 202, *202*
Colon cancer, 1:91, *92*
Color Additives Amendment (1960), 1:2–3
Color food additives, 1:2–4
Colostrum, 1:76
Columbus, Christopher, 2:78, *79*
Combs, Sean "P. Diddy," 2:*217*
Comfort foods, 1:137
Commission on Accreditation for Dietetics Education (CADE), 1:105, 2:44, 105
Commission on Dietetic Registration (CDR), 1:106, 168, 2:44, 105
Commodity foods, **1:127–130**, 1:*129*
  Commodity Supplemental Food Program, 1:127, 2:97
  for disaster relief, 1:128
  Emergency Food Assistance Program, 1:128
  Food and Nutrition Service (FNS), 1:127, 128
  Food Distribution Program on Indian Reservations, 1:128
  other programs, 1:128–129
  See also Nutrition programs in the community; WIC program
Commodity Supplemental Food Program (CSFP), 1:127, 2:97
Common cold
  and hand washing, 2:3
  and vitamin C, 2:134, 244
Communion, 2:176, *176*
Community Food and Nutrition Program (CFNP), 1:285
Community gardens, 2:222
Community nutrition programs, 2:96–99, *98*
Community Nutritionists, 1:105
Community-based organizations (CBOs), 2:83

Community-supported agriculture (CSA), 2:222
Complementary and alternative medicine (CAM), 1:30, 2:148–149
  See also Alternative medicines and therapies
Complete proteins, 2:156
Complex carbohydrates, 1:94–96, *95*, 2:91
Comprehensive School Health Program (CSHP), **1:130–132**, 1:*131*
Compulsive overeating. *See* Binge eating
Congenital, defined, 1:40
Congenital heart disease (CHD), 1:272, 2:48, *49*
Congenital lactose intolerance, 2:22
Congregate Dining, defined, 1:22
Constipation
  and calcium, 1:84
  defined, 1:8
Consumerism, defined, 2:139
Contaminated water, 1:150, 173, 174–175, 2:*228*
Continuing Survey of Food Intakes by Individuals (CSFII), 1:160, 269, 2:72
Contraindicated, defined, 1:192
Convenience foods, **1:132–133**
  American dietary trend, 1:160
  defined, 1:51
  popular culture, 2:141
  See also Fast foods
Convention on the Rights of the Child, 2:226, 227–228
Cooking difficulties, 1:22
Cool down, in exercise, 1:201
Cooperative for Assistance and Relief Everywhere (CARE), 1:175*t*
Copper, 2:62, *63*
Corn, genetically modified, 1:245, 246–247, *248*
Corn flakes cereal, 2:16, *17*
Corn- or maize-based diets, 1:*133*, **1:133–136**
  maize varieties, 1:133–134
  Native Americans, 2:79
  protein quality, 1:134
  vitamins, 1:134–136, *135*
  See also Rice-based diets
Cornaro, Luigi, 1:255
Coronary artery disease (CAD), 1:272–274
  as cardiovascular disease, 1:100, *101*
  and fat intake, 1:217
  and omega-6 fatty acids, 2:109

Coronary artery disease *(continued)*
  prevention, 1:274, *274*
  risk factors, 1:274
  See also Cardiovascular disease (CVD)
Coronary heart disease
  defined, 1:99
  and estrogen, 2:48
Coumadin, 2:88t, 236, 237
Cous-cous, 1:17
Cows, in Hinduism, 2:176–177, *177*
Cravings, **1:136–139**, 1:*138*
  causes, 1:136–138
  conquering, 1:138–139
  as eating disturbance, 1:184
  during pregnancy, 1:136, 2:146
  See also Eating disorders
Creatine, as ergogenic aid, 1:190, 2:218
Creole cooking, 1:12–13
Cretinism, defined, 1:252
Creutzfeldt-Jakob disease, 2:118–119
Crossbreeding, 1:65, 245
  defined, 1:65
Cruveilhier, Jean, 1:79
Cruveilhier's disease, 1:79, 172
CSA (community-supported agriculture), 2:222
CSFII (Continuing Survey of Food Intakes by Individuals), 1:160, 269, 2:72
CSFP (Commodity Supplemental Food Program), 1:127, 2:97
CSHP (Comprehensive School Health Program), 1:130–132, *131*
Cuban Americans. *See* Hispanics and Latinos, diet of
Cuisine, defined, 1:12
Cultural competence, **1:139–142**
  attaining, 1:140, *140*, 141
  and healthcare, 1:139–140
  organizational responsibilities, 1:140–142
Curry, 1:109
Cuy, 2:*202*
CVA (cerebrovascular accident), 1:100, 147
CVD. *See* Cardiovascular disease (CVD)
CWS (Church World Service), 1:175t
Cyclamate, 1:48
Cyclospora cayetanensis, 2:1, 120
Cysteine, 2:156t
Cytoplasm, defined, 1:96
Cytotoxic testing, for food allergies, 1:29

D

Dairy products
  as functional food, 1:242t
  glycemic index, 1:251t
  Mediterranean diet, 1:257
  with probiotics, 1:242t
  See also Milk
DALE (Disability Adjusted Life Expectancy), 2:28
DASH (Dietary Approach to Stop Hypertension), 1:100, 290–291
Deamination, 2:157
  defined, 2:56
Defibrillators, 1:*273*
Deficiencies
  calcium, 1:84, 2:61
  fluoride, 2:63
  iodine, 1:56, 2:35, 63, 159–160
  iron, 1:38–40, 56, 2:24, 26, 62–63, 153
  magnesium, 2:61
  minerals, 2:61, 62–63
  niacin (vitamin B_3), 2:103
  nutritional, 1:38, 2:102–104, *103*
  potassium, 2:61
  selenium, 2:63
  sodium, 2:61
  thiamine (vitamin B_1), 1:62, 2:103, 181
  vitamin A, 1:56, 2:233t, 234, 264
  vitamin C, 1:119, 120, 2:219–220, *220*
  vitamin E, 2:233t, 237
  vitamin K, 2:94, 233t, 236
  zinc, 2:63
  See also Vitamin D deficiency
Dehydration, **1:142–143**
  defined, 1:142
  and fasting, 2:175
  and food-borne illness, 2:3, 4
  occurrence, 2:247
  sports nutrition, 2:217, *217*
  See also Oral rehydration therapy
Delaney Clause, 1:3
Dementia, defined, 1:135
Denaturation, of proteins, 1:37
Dent corn, 1:133
Dental caries, 2:110, 111–112, 153
  See also see Baby bottle tooth decay
Deoxyribonucleic acid (DNA)
  and cancer, 1:90, 91
  defined, 1:245
  Human Genome Project, 2:75
Dependence, defined, 1:24
Depression
  defined, 1:22
  and eating disorders, 1:178
  and serotonin, 2:66–67, 75
DERA (Disaster Preparedness and Emergency Response Association), 1:175t
Dermatitis, 2:135, *135*
DETERMINE, defined, 1:21
Developing countries
  breastfeeding, 2:146
  diarrhea, 1:149–151
  fast food, 1:*165*
  food insecurity, 1:228, 229–230
  food-borne illness, 2:118
  hunger, 1:287
  kwashiorkor, 2:20
  lead poisoning, 2:24, 26
  malnutrition, 2:34, *34*
  maternal mortality rate, 2:42
  oral health, 2:111
  undernutrition, 2:111, 141
  underweight, 2:35
  vitamin A deficiency, 2:234
  water pasteurization, 2:133
Development, defined, 1:272
DEXA (dual energy X-ray absorbitometry) scans, 2:124
DHS (U.S. Department of Homeland Security), 2:172
Diabetes, defined, 1:5
Diabetes mellitus, **1:143–148**
  adolescents, 1:6
  African Americans, 1:14, 14t
  and carbohydrates, 1:98, 2:54
  complications, 1:146
  exchange system, 1:98
  gestational diabetes, 1:145, 2:146, 259
  glycemic index, 1:250, 251
  and heart disease, 1:147, 274
  Hispanic Americans, 1:277
  and hyperglycemia, 1:287–288
  and hypoglycemia, 1:292
  men, 2:51
  Native Americans, 2:81
  Pacific Islander Americans, 2:126
  prevalence, 1:143–144, 164
  and socioeconomic status, 2:167
  and stroke, 1:147
  treatment, 1:*144*, 145, 147–148, 2:77
  types, 1:144–146
  women, 2:260
  See also Exchange system; Hyperglycemia; Insulin
Diabetic ketoacidosis (DKA), 1:146
Diabetic retinopathy, 1:146
Diarrhea, 1:*149*, **1:149–151**
  acute, 1:149, 150

causes, 1:149, 150*t*
chronic, 1:149
developing countries, 1:149–151
HIV/AIDS patients, 1:280
traveler's, 1:149
treatment, 1:151, 2:113
See also Oral rehydration therapy
Diastolic pressure, 1:99, *100*, 288
Diet, **1:151–152**
defined, 1:7
high-fiber, 1:222, 2:37
high-protein, 2:249
influence on health, 1:*163*, 164
low-carb, 1:97
macrobiotic, 2:31–33, *32*
whole foods, 1:242*t*, 2:255
See also Eating habits
Diet and Health, 1:154
Dietary Approach to Stop Hypertension (DASH), 1:100, 290–291
Dietary assessment, **1:152**, 2:214
See also Nutritional assessment
Dietary directors, 1:168
Dietary Goals for the United States, 1:153–154
Dietary Guidelines, **1:153–154**
early dietary advice, 1:153
evolution, 1:153–154
versus food guides, 1:153
and Healthy Eating Index, 1:267
and Howard Johnson's restaurants, 2:16
and hypertension, 1:290
school food service, 2:194
school-aged children, 2:191
See also Food Guide Pyramid
Dietary Reference Intakes (DRIs), **1:155**
defined, 1:20
elderly, 1:20
National Academy of Sciences, 2:67
preschoolers and toddlers, 2:151
See also Recommended Dietary Allowances (RDAs)
Dietary Supplement Health and Education Act (DSHEA) (1994), 1:31–32, 33, 156, 157–158, 241–243, 2:74
Dietary supplements, **1:155–159**
American dietary trend, 1:159
baby boomers, 1:156
as biologically-based treatment, 1:31
controversies, 1:157–158
dangerous ergogenic aids, 1:193
Food and Drug Administration, 1:33, 156, 158, 2:59–60
and medical nutrition therapy, 2:43
minerals, 2:59–60, *60*
and popular culture, 2:141
preschoolers and toddlers, 2:153
and quackery, 2:161–162, 163–164
regulation, 1:156–157
selecting, 1:33–34
supplement facts label, 1:32–33
See also Alternative medicines and therapies; Vitamins, fat-soluble; Vitamins, water-soluble
Dietary trends, American, **1:159–162**
away-from-home foods, 1:163–164
by decade, 1:161*t*
dietary patterns, 1:159
nutritional adequacy, 1:161–162
obesity, 1:164
portion sizes, caloric intake, and obesity, 1:160
sweet, quick, and easy, 1:160, *160*
Dietary trends, international, **1:162–165**
food safety, 1:164–165
influence of diet on health, 1:*163*, 164
Westernization of dietary patterns, 1:163–164, *165*
Dietetic technician, registered (DTR), 1:104, 106, **1:166**
See also Careers in dietetics
Dietetics, **1:166–167**
See also Careers in dietetics
Dieting, **1:167–168**
chronic, 1:185
and eating disorders, 1:179
and eating disturbances, 1:184–185
and popular culture, 2:141
and weight cycling, 1:184–185
Dietitian, 1:106, *168*, **1:168–169**
See also Careers in dietetics; Nutritionist
Diets, corn- or maize-based. *See* Corn- or maize-based diets
Diets, fad. *See* Fad diets
Diets, rice-based. *See* Rice-based diets
Digestion and absorption, **1:169–173**, 1:*171*
absorption, 1:172
difficulties, 1:22
factors affecting, 1:250
fat-soluble vitamins, 2:232
fiber, 1:221, 222
GI tract physiology, 1:169
nutrients into blood or to heart, 1:172
protective factors, 1:170–171
protein, 2:157
from stomach to small intestine, 1:169–170
See also Glycemic index (GI)
Dilantin, 2:88*t*
Dipeptides, 1:37
Diphtheria, defined, 2:132
Direct additives, 1:1
Direct Relief International (DRI), 1:175*t*
Disability Adjusted Life Expectancy (DALE), 2:28
Disaccharide carbohydrate, defined, 2:21
Disaccharides, 1:93–94, 94*t*
Disaster Preparedness and Emergency Response Association (DERA), 1:175*t*
Disaster relief organizations, **1:173–176**, 1:175*t*
commodity foods, 1:128
disease risks, 1:174–176
health risks, 1:173–174, *174*
needs assessment, 1:173
See also Emergency Nutrition Network; Famine
Discourse on a Sober and Temperate Life (Cornaro), 1:255
Disease
and exercise, 1:199–200
infectious, 1:35, 2:234
and minerals, 2:60–61, *62*
and obesity, 1:217
risks after disasters, 1:174–176
vector-borne, 1:176
Disease-risk reduction claims. *See* Health claims
The Diseases of Children and Their Remedies (Rosenstein), 2:186, *186*
Dispensable amino acids, 1:36, 36*t*, 2:155–156
Diuretics, 1:291
defined, 1:142
Diversity, defined, 1:10
Diverticulosis, defined, 1:8
DKA (diabetic ketoacidosis), 1:146
DNA
and cancer, 1:90, *91*
defined, 1:40
Human Genome Project, 2:75
Dominica
popular dishes, 1:110
public health initiative, 1:111
Dopamine, effect on mood, 2:64, 66*t*
Double-blind, placebo-controlled food challenge, 1:28
Dowager's hump, 2:124, *124*
Dr. Atkins' New Diet Revolution, 1:97, 203*t*, 204, *204*, 206

DRI (Direct Relief International), 1:175t
Drinking water. *See* Water
DRIs. *See* Dietary Reference Intakes (DRIs)
Drug-nutrient interactions. *See* Nutrient-drug interactions
Drugs
 defined, 1:3
 function, 2:88
DSHEA. *See* Dietary Supplement Health and Education Act (DSHEA) (1994)
DTR (dietetic technician, registered), 1:104, 106, 166
Dual energy X-ray absorbitometry (DEXA scans), 2:124
Duodenum, 1:170
Dyazide, 2:88t
Dysentery, 1:149, 2:3
Dyslipidemia, defined, 1:122
Dysmorphia, 1:70, 71
 defined, 1:70

E

E. coli. *See* Escherichia coli
EAR (Estimated Average Requirement), 1:155
Earthquake (Bam, Iran), 2:226
East Africans, diet of, 1:18
East Asians, diet of, 1:53–54
Eastern Orthodox Christianity food practices, 2:176, 178t
Eating disorder not otherwise specified (EDNOS), 1:178
Eating disorders, **1:176–182,** 1:*179, 180*
 adolescents, 1:6, 2:193
 athletes, 1:125
 body image, 1:69–71, *70*
 causes, 1:179
 college students, 1:124–125
 defined, 1:41
 diagnosis, 1:176–178
 in female athlete triad, 1:219, 2:218
 Fiji, 2:131
 history, 1:181
 and malnutrition, 2:140
 outcomes, 1:181
 prevalence, 1:178, 184
 risk factors, 1:178–179
 treatment modalities, 1:179–181
 See also Anorexia nervosa; Bulimia nervosa
Eating disturbances, **1:182–185,** 1:*183*
 binge eating, 1:63–64, 177–178, 181, 182, 184, 2:140

 chronic dieting, 1:185
 cravings, 1:136–139, *138*, 184
 excessive exercising, 1:184
 weight cycling, 1:184–185, 2:250, 264–265
 See also Eating disorders
Eating habits, **1:186–188**
 exposure to foods, 1:187, *187*
 food choice influences, 1:*186*, 187–188
 obtaining, storing, using, and discarding food, 1:187
 what people eat, 1:187
 why and how people eat, 1:186
 See also Popular culture, and food
Ebola vaccine, 2:75
Eclampsia, 1:289
Ecological, defined, 1:188
Ecuador, 2:201, *202*, 203
Eczema, defined, 2:5
Edamame, 2:208, 210
Edema, 2:158, 248
 defined, 1:289
EDNOS (eating disorder not otherwise specified), 1:178
Efficacy, defined, 1:156
EFNEP (Expanded Food Nutrition and Education Program), 1:202–203
Eggs, 1:*241*, 242t, 2:242
El Salvador, 1:113
Elderly. *See* Aging and nutrition
Electrolytes
 defined, 1:37
 for dehydration, 2:4
 HIV/AIDS patients, 1:280
Electronic pasteurization, 2:13–14
Elemental, defined, 1:84
Elimination diet, defined, 1:28
The Emergency Food Assistance Program (TEFAP), 1:128, 284–285
Emergency Health Kits, 1:174
Emergency Nutrition Network (ENN), **1:189**
 See also Disaster relief organizations
Emergency Prevention System for Transboundary Animal and Plant Pests and Diseases (EMPRES), 1:225
EMPRES (Emergency Prevention System for Transboundary Animal and Plant Pests and Diseases), 1:225
Endorphins, effect on mood, 2:*65*, 66
Endotoxins
 defined, 1:245

 in genetically modified foods, 1:246–247
Enema, defined, 2:61
Energy, defined, 1:5
Energy boosters (ergogenic aids), 1:192
Energy needs. *See* Calories
Energy therapies, 1:31, 31t
England, 2:84, *85*
Enhanced foods, as functional food type, 1:242t
ENN (Emergency Nutrition Network), 1:189
Enriched foods, as functional food type, 1:242t
Enrichment, 1:239
 defined, 1:2
Enteral nutrition, 1:281
Enteric, defined, 2:35
Entrepreneur, defined, 1:61
Environment, defined, 1:22
Environmental illness, defined, 1:29
Enzymatic, defined, 1:65
Enzymes
 and biotechnology, 1:65
 brush border, 2:157
 defined, 1:24
 and protein, 2:158
 role, 1:37
EPA (U.S. Environmental Protection Agency), 2:172
Ephedra, 1:192, 2:218
Epiglottis, 1:169, 170
Epinephrine, defined, 2:244
Epithelial cells, defined, 1:88
Erectile dysfunction, 2:53
Ergogenic aids, **1:189–193**
 anabolic agents, 1:190–192, *191*
 dangerous supplements, 1:193
 energy boosters, 1:192
 weight loss agents, 1:192
 See also Dietary supplements; Sports nutrition
Errors of metabolism, inborn. *See* Inborn errors of metabolism
ERT. *See* Estrogen replacement therapy (ERT)
Erythrocyte, 1:38, 2:212
Erythrosine, 1:3–4
Escherichia coli, 2:1–2, 3, 118, 119, 120t
 defined, 2:1
Essential amino acids, 1:36, 36t, 38, 2:155–156
Essential fatty acids, 2:94, 108–109
 defined, 1:210
Essential hypertension, 1:289

Estimated Average Requirement (EAR), 1:155
Estradiol, defined, 1:191
Estrogen
  and coronary heart disease, 2:48
  defined, 1:92
  female athletes, 2:218–219
  versus isoflavones, 2:14
Estrogen replacement therapy (ERT), 2:48, 49, 124, 208
Ethiopian refugees, 2:*165*
Ethnicity, and body mass index, 1:73
Etiology, defined, 2:33
Etiquette, and eating habits, 1:186
Europe, food additive and preservative regulation, 1:4
European Union
  artificial sweeteners, 1:48
  genetically modified foods, 1:248
  organic foods, 2:115
European Union Scientific Committee for Food, 1:4, 47
Europeans, Central. *See* Central Europeans and Russians, diets of
Europeans, Northern. *See* Northern Europeans, diet of
Europeans, Southern. *See* Southern Europeans, diet of
Evaporated milk, 2:10
Exchange system, 1:147, **1:193–197**, 1:287
  advantages and disadvantages, 1:194–196
  definition, 1:194
  history, 1:196–197, 196t, 197t
  using, 1:195
  See also Diabetes
Exercise, **1:198–201**
  aerobic, 1:198
  anaerobic, 1:198
  benefits, 1:198–199, *199*
  and cancer, 1:91
  and cardiovascular disease, 1:100–101, 103
  childhood obesity, 1:122
  defined, 1:198
  and dehydration, 1:143
  and diabetes, 1:147, 287–288
  and disease prevention, 1:199–200
  and endorphins, 2:66
  excessive, 1:184
  and heart disease, 1:274
  and insulin, 2:13
  and menopause, 2:48, 50
  and obesity, 2:106
  physical fitness components, 1:200
  and pregnancy, 2:144–145

  for premenstrual syndrome, 2:148
  recommended, 1:201
  and space travel, 2:211–212
  strategies, 2:251
  trends, 1:161
  and weight management, 1:205–206, 2:107, 249, 251, *252*
  See also Sports nutrition
Exercise addiction, **1:201–202**, 1:*202*
Expanded Food Nutrition and Education Program (EFNEP), **1:202–203**
"Extra lean," as nutrient content claim, 1:265t
Extracellular fluid compartment, 1:37

F

Fad diets, 1:167, **1:203–206**, 1:203t, *204*, 2:141, 250
  See also Dieting; Weight loss diets
FAE (fetal alcohol effects), 1:25, 220
Failure to thrive, **1:206–207**
  defined, 1:167
  See also Infant nutrition
Famine, **1:207–208**, 1:*208*
  defined, 1:19
  See also Food insecurity
FAO (Food and Agriculture Organization), 1:118, 224–225, 248
Farmers markets, 2:97, 222, 256–257
FAS (fetal alcohol syndrome), 1:25, *220*, 220–221
Fast foods, 1:*209*, **1:209–210**
  American dietary trend, 1:160
  Caribbean Islands, 1:110
  defined, 1:111
  developing countries, 1:*165*
  and health, 2:52
  popular culture, 2:139–140, *140*
  Saudi Arabia, 1:*165*
  school-aged children, 2:192
  See also Convenience foods
Fasting, **1:210**
  and dehydration, 2:175
  and gastric acidity, 2:175
  and lipid profile, 2:29–30
  religion and dietary practices, 2:174–175, 176, 177, 178–179
  See also Dieting; Religion and dietary practices
Fasting hypoglycemia, 1:292
Fat substitutes, **1:210–214**, 1:217–219
  carbohydrate-based, 1:212, 212t, 217–218
  categories, 1:*211*, 212–213, 212t
  described, 1:211–212

  effectiveness, 1:213–214, 213t
  fat-based, 1:212t, 213, 218–219
  protein-based, 1:212, 212t, 218
  safety, 1:213
  See also Artificial sweeteners; Fats
Fat-free products, 1:219
Fatigue, defined, 1:5
Fats, **1:214–219**, 1:*217*
  absorption, 1:172
  actual and recommended intake, 1:216–217, *218*
  adolescents, 2:192
  and cancer, 1:91
  and cardiovascular disease, 1:101–102
  defined, 1:7
  fat-replacement strategies, 1:217–219
  function, metabolism, and storage, 1:215–216
  Healthy Eating Index, 1:267–268
  Mediterranean diet, 1:259, 260
  metabolism, 1:216, 2:56–57
  as nutrient, 1:210–211, 216, 2:92–94
  sports nutrition, 2:216
  See also Fat substitutes; Lipid profile
Fat-soluble vitamins. *See* Vitamins, fat-soluble
Fatty acids
  defined, 1:31
  metabolism disorders, 2:7
FDA. *See* U.S. Food and Drug Administration (FDA)
FDAMA (Food and Drug Administration Modernization Act) (1997), 1:264–265
FD&C Red No. 3, 1:3–4
FD&C Yellow No. 3, 1:4
FDPIR (Food Distribution Program on Indian Reservations), 1:128
Federal Food, Drug, and Cosmetic Act (1938), 1:241–243
  Color Additives Amendment (1960), 1:2–3
  Food Additives Amendment (1958), 1:2
Federal Register, 1:232
Federation Internationale de Football Association (FIFA), 2:227–228
Feijoda completa, 2:202
Female athlete triad, 1:125, **1:219–220**, 2:218–219
  See also Eating disorders; Osteoporosis; Sports nutrition
Females. *See* Women's nutritional issues

293

Fermentation
    as biotechnology technique, 1:65
    defined, 1:4
Fertilizers, 2:221
Fetal alcohol effects (FAE), 1:25, 220
Fetal alcohol syndrome (FAS), 1:25, 220, **1:220–221**
    See also Alcohol and health; Pregnancy
Fetus, 2:*145*
FH (Food for the Hungry), 1:175*t*
Fiber, **1:221–223**
    actual and recommended intake, 1:221–222
    and cancer, 1:91
    and cardiovascular disease, 1:103
    as complex carbohydrate, 1:94–96, 2:91
    defined, 1:8
    food content, 1:222*t*
    as functional food, 1:242*t*
    high-fiber diets, 1:222
    insoluble, 1:221
    intake during menopause, 2:50
    in juices, 1:242*t*
    recommended intake, 1:97
    soluble, 1:221
    types, 1:221
FIFA (Federation Internationale de Football Association), 2:227–228
Fight-or-flight response, 1:138
Fiji, 2:131
Filipinos, diet of, 1:50*t*, 54–55
Finland, vitamin C deficiency in, 1:120
Fish
    as functional food, 1:242*t*
    and omega-3 fatty acids, 2:108, 109, *109*
    Pacific Islanders, 2:130
    Scandinavia, 2:188, *188*
Fish stew, 2:204
FITT (Frequency, Intensity, Time, Type) principle, 1:200–201
Flavonoids, and heart disease, 1:240
Flaxseed, as functional food, 1:242*t*
Flexibility, as physical fitness component, 1:200
Flint corn, 1:133
Flower corn, 1:133
Fluids
    compartments for, 1:37
    pregnancy, 2:144
    and protein, 2:158
    space travel, 2:214
    sports nutrition, 2:*217*, 217–218, 218*t*

Fluoride
    deficiency, 2:63
    disease prevention and treatment, 2:62
    infant nutrition, 2:8
    and oral health, 2:112
    toxicity, 2:63
Fluorosis, 2:63
FMNV (foods of minimum nutritional value), 2:195, 196
FNS. *See* U.S. Food and Nutrition Service (FNS)
Folate, 2:240*t*, 242–243
    and anemia, 1:40
    defined, 1:38
    fortification of food, 1:242*t*, 2:72
    and pregnancy, 1:40, 2:142–143
    women, 2:259
Folic acid. *See* Folate
Folk remedies
    African Americans, 1:13
    lead poisoning, 2:26
Follicular hyperkeratosis, 2:234
Food additives
    defined, 1:2
    See also Additives and preservatives
Food Additives Amendment (1958), 1:2
Food Aid for Development and the World Food Programme, 1:223–224, *224*
    See also Famine; Food insecurity; United Nations
Food and Agriculture Organization (FAO), 1:118, **1:224–225**, 1:248
    See also Famine; Food insecurity; United Nations
Food and Agriculture Organization Joint Expert Committee on Food Additives, 1:4
Food and Drug Administration Modernization Act (FDAMA) (1997), 1:264–265
Food *Code,* 1:235–236
Food Distribution Program on Indian Reservations (FDPIR), 1:128
Food for the Hungry (FH), 1:175*t*
Food Guide Pyramid, **1:225–228**, 1:*227*
    alternative pyramids, 1:226–227
    and DASH eating plan, 1:291
    design and recommendations, 1:225–226
    and Dietary Guidelines, 1:153, 154
    elderly, 1:20
    and Healthy Eating Index, 1:267
    nutrients, 2:93

    school-aged children, 2:191
    uses, 1:226
    Vegetarian Food Guide Pyramid, 2:231
    See also Dietary Guidelines
Food Guide Pyramid for Young Children, 2:151, 191
Food habits. *See* Eating habits
Food insecurity, **1:228–231**, 1:*229*
    Africa, 1:19
    after disasters, 1:173–174, *174*
    Asia, 1:55
    and hunger, 1:287
    See also Famine; Hunger; Malnutrition
Food jags, 2:153
Food labels, **1:231–235**
    dietary supplements, 1:156
    fat content, 1:216, *217*, 219
    Food and Drug Administration, 1:232–233, 234, 237, 241–243, 2:161
    functional foods, 1:241–243
    genetically modified foods, 1:67–68, 248
    ingredient list, 1:232
    and marketing strategies, 2:39
    net quantity of contents, 1:232
    Nutrition Facts statement, 1:233, *234*
    nutrition labeling, 1:232–234, 233*t*
    organic foods, 1:237, 2:114
    overview, 1:231–232
    Percent Daily Value, 1:233*t*, 234
    Product Identity statement, 1:232
    required nutrients, 1:233–234
    serving size, 1:234
    See also Health claims; Regulatory agencies
Food poisoning
    defined, 1:164
    See also Illnesses, food-borne
Food safety, **1:235–239**
    additives and preservatives, 1:2–4
    biotechnology, 1:67–68, 237
    bioterrorism, 1:237–238, 2:172
    control and oversight, 1:235–236
    fat substitutes, 1:213
    food-borne illness, 1:236, *237*
    genetically modified foods, 1:246–248
    international dietary trends, 1:164–165
    organic foods, 2:116–117
    pesticides, 1:236–237
    regulation history and purpose, 1:238–239, 238*t*

World Health Organization, 2:172–173, 262–263
See also Biotechnology; Genetically modified foods; Irradiation; Pesticides
Food Safety Initiative Activity, 2:172
Food security. *See* Food insecurity
Food Stamp Program, 1:127, 128, 284, 2:97, 256t
Food-based dietary guidelines, 2:205
Food-borne illness. *See* Illnesses, food-borne
Food-borne organisms. *See* Organisms, food-borne
Food-for-Growth program, 1:223
Food-for-Life program, 1:223
Food-for-Work program, 1:223–224, 224
Foods of minimum nutritional value (FMNV), 2:195, 196
Formula feeding, 1:242t, 2:9–10, 38–39
See also Breastfeeding; Infant nutrition
Fortification, **1:239**, 1:242t, 2:72
defined, 1:2
See also Functional foods
Fortified, defined, 1:2
Fractures, and osteoporosis, 2:124, 125
Framingham Heart Study, 1:103
France
diet, 2:86–87
food-borne illness, 2:118, 119
life expectancy, 2:28
organic foods, 2:115
See also French paradox
Franchising, 2:15, 15
"Free," as nutrient content claim, 1:265t
Free food, in exchange system, 1:195
Free radicals
and antioxidants, 1:42, 43–44
and carotenoids, 2:234
and cigarette smoke, 1:43
defined, 1:42
French Guiana, 2:203
French paradox, **1:239–240**, 2:84
See also France; Heart disease
French Wine Coca, 2:135–136
Frequency, Intensity, Time, Type (FITT) principle, 1:200–201
Fructose, 1:93, 94t
Fruit juice
glycemic index, 1:251t
nutrient-drug interaction, 2:89
and oral health, 2:111–112

Fruits
Asia, 1:52–53, 54
and cancer prevention, 1:91
Caribbean Islands, 1:108–109, 110
Central America and Mexico, 1:114
as functional food, 1:242t
glycemic index, 1:251t
Mediterranean diet, 1:257
FTC (U.S. Federal Trade Commission), 2:164
Functional foods, **1:240–243**, 1:241
antioxidants, 1:43–44
defined, 1:43
future, 1:243
popular culture, 2:141
regulations, 1:241–243
types, 1:242t
See also Antioxidants; Phytochemicals
Fungal, defined, 1:279
Funk, Casimir, 1:244, **1:244–245**
See also Vitamins, fat-soluble; Vitamins, water-soluble

G

Galactose, 1:93, 2:6, 21
Galactosemia, 2:6
defined, 1:75
Gallbladder, 1:170
Gamma butyrolactone and gamma hydroxy butyric acid (GBL/GHB), 1:193
Gamma rays, defined, 2:13
Garlic, 1:242t, 2:161
Gasoline, leaded, 2:24, 25
Gastric, defined, 1:79
Gastric acidity, 2:175
Gastric ulcer, 1:79, 172
Gastrointestinal, defined, 1:27
Gastrointestinal tract physiology, 1:169
GAVI (Global Alliance for Vaccines and Immunizations), 2:227
GBL/GHB (gamma butyrolactone and gamma hydroxy butyric acid), 1:193
GDNNPP (Global Database on National Nutrition Policies and Programmes), 1:249–250
Gemini space program, 2:212
Gene expression, defined, 2:55
Generally Recognized as Safe (GRAS), **1:245**
artificial sweeteners, 1:46–47
fat substitutes, 1:212, 213
sugar alcohols, 1:47
See also Food safety

Genes
and cancer, 1:90
defined, 1:24
and obesity, 2:106
Genetic, defined, 1:38
Genetic engineering, 1:65, 66
Genetically modified foods, **1:245–248**
acceptance, 1:247, 248
examples, 1:245–246
labeling, 1:248
potatoes, 1:245, 246–247
rice, 1:66, 68, 245, 246–247, 2:182, 264
safety, 1:237, 246–248
soybeans, 1:245
tomatoes, 1:65, 245–246
See also Biotechnology; Food safety
Genetics, defined, 2:47
Genistein, 2:208
Germany
herbal therapy, 1:157
organic foods, 2:115
Gestational diabetes, 1:145, 2:146, 259
GI (glycemic index), 1:250–252, 251t, 2:13
See also Carbohydrates; Diabetes mellitus
GI tract physiology, 1:169
Giardia lamblia, 2:120, 120t
Ginger, for seasickness, 1:33
Gingivitis, 2:112
Ginseng, as ergogenic aid, 1:192
Give Me Five program, 2:227
Glandular fever, 2:12
Glickman, Dan, 2:151
Glisson, Francis, 1:249, **1:249**
Global Alliance for Vaccines and Immunizations (GAVI), 2:227
Global Database on National Nutrition Policies and Programmes (GDNNPP), **1:249–250**
Global Movement for Children program, 2:228
Global Outbreak Alert and Response Network (GORAN), 2:262
Global Polio Eradication Initiative, 2:227
Global Public Health Intelligence Network (GPHIN), 2:262
Globalization, defined, 1:116
Glossitis, 2:111
Glucagon, 1:170
Gluconeogenesis, 2:55, 57
Glucose
defined, 1:28

Glucose *(continued)*
  and diabetes, 1:*144*, 147
  as energy source, 2:91–92
  and inborn errors of metabolism, 2:6, 7
  and insulin, 1:37, *37*
  and lactose intolerance, 2:21
  metabolism, 2:54
  and pregnancy, 2:144
  as simple carbohydrate, 1:93, 94*t*
Glutamine, 2:156*t*
Gluten, defined, 2:42
Glycemic index (GI), **1:250–252**, 1:251*t*, 2:13
  See also Carbohydrates; Diabetes mellitus
Glycerol, 2:57
  defined, 2:29
Glycine, 2:155, 156*t*
Glycogen
  as complex carbohydrate, 1:94
  defined, 1:94
  and sports nutrition, 2:216
  storage diseases, 2:6–7
Glycogenesis, 2:55
Glycogenolysis, 2:55
Glycolysis, 1:96–97, 2:55, 57, 157
  defined, 1:93
GMP (Good Manufacturing Practice), 1:158
GnRH (gonadotropin-releasing hormone) agonists, 2:149
Goiter, 1:*252*, **1:252–253**
Goldberger, Joseph, 1:*253*, **1:253–254**, 2:73
  See also Pellagra
Golden rice, 1:*66*, 68, 245, 246–247, 2:182, 264
Gonadotropin-releasing hormone (GnRH) agonists, 2:149
Good cholesterol. *See* High-density lipoprotein (HDL)
Good Manufacturing Practice (GMP), 1:158
"Good source," as nutrient content claim, 1:265*t*
GORAN (Global Outbreak Alert and Response Network), 2:262
"Got Milk?" advertisements, 2:37–38
GPHIN (Global Public Health Intelligence Network), 2:262
GR (Green Revolution), 1:261–262, 2:182
Graham, Sylvester, **1:254–255**
Grains, as functional food, 1:242*t*
Grapefruit, glycemic index, 1:251*t*
Grapes/grape juice, 1:240, 242*t*

GRAS. *See* Generally Recognized as Safe (GRAS)
Grazing, **1:255–256**
  See also Eating habits; Snacking
Greece, life expectancy in, 2:28
Greeks and Middle Easterners, diet of, **1:256–261**, 1:*257*
  culture, 1:259
  food preparation and storage, 1:258, 259*t*
  Mediterranean Basin, 1:256
  nutrition and disease, 1:259–260
  present day, 1:258
  traditional, 1:256–258
Green Revolution (GR), **1:261–262**, 2:182
Grenada
  popular dishes, 1:110
  public health initiative, 1:112
Growth charts, **1:262**, 2:72
Growth factor, defined, 1:91
Growth hormone, 1:246, **1:262–263**
  See also Ergogenic aids
Growth spurts, defined, 1:86
Guadeloupe, 1:110
Guar gum, defined, 1:212
Guatemala, 1:113
Guinea pigs, 2:*202*
Gumbo, 1:11, *11*, 13
Gums, as dietary fiber, 1:96
Guthrie test, 2:5
Guyana, 1:110, 2:203
Gynoid fat distribution, 1:68

H

HACCP (Hazard Analysis Critical Control Point) system, 1:236, 2:121, 172
Haggis, 2:85
Halal foods, 1:258, 259*t*, 2:177
Hand washing, 2:3, 12, 120, 121
Hardening of the arteries. *See* Atherosclerosis
Harris-Benedict equation, 2:101, 102
  defined, 2:101
Harvey, William, 1:205
Hawaiians. *See* Pacific Islander Americans, diet of; Pacific Islanders, diet of
Hazard Analysis Critical Control Point (HACCP) system, 1:236, 2:121, 172
HDL
  defined, 1:191
  See also High-density lipoprotein (HDL)
Head Start program, 2:98

Health, **1:263**
  See also Health promotion
Health, or How to Live (Graham), 1:255
Health claims, **1:263–266**
  dietary supplements, 1:156
  food labels, 1:232
  functional foods, 1:242, 243
  general requirements, 1:265
  "healthy," 1:264
  and marketing strategies, 2:37–38
  nutrient content claims, 1:264, 265*t*
  soy protein, 1:243, 2:207
  types, 1:265–266
  See also Food labels; Regulatory agencies
Health communication, **1:266**
Health education, 1:131, **1:266–267**
Health promotion, **1:267**
  defined, 1:106
"Healthy," on food labels, 1:264
Healthy Eating Index (HEI), **1:267–269**, 1:*268*
Healthy People (1979), 1:269
Healthy People 2000 report, 1:210, 270, 271
Healthy People 2010 report, **1:269–271**, 1:*270*
  African Americans, 1:14
  childhood obesity, 1:121
  dental caries, 2:110
  exercise, 1:198, 201
Heart attack, 1:*272, 273*, 2:75
  defined, 1:59
Heart disease, **1:271–275**, 1:*273, 274*
  adolescent risk, 1:6
  congenital, 1:272
  coronary artery disease, 1:272–274
  defined, 1:5
  and diabetes, 1:147
  French paradox, 1:239–240
  and hypertension, 1:*289*
  men, 2:51–53, *52*
  myocardial infarction, 1:272, 2:75
  Native Americans, 2:81
  and omega-3 fatty acids, 2:108–109
  Pacific Islander Americans, 2:126–127
  rheumatic, 1:272
  and soy, 2:207–208
  women, 2:260–261
  See also Atherosclerosis; Cardiovascular disease (CVD)
Heartburn, during pregnancy, 2:146
Heavy metal, defined, 2:23
HEI (Healthy Eating Index), 1:267–269, *268*

Height and weight tables, 2:99–100, 100t
Hemicellulose, 1:95
Hemoglobin, defined, 1:38
Hemorrhoids, defined, 1:8
Henrich, Christy, 1:*180*
Hepatitis, defined, 1:24
Hepatitis A, 2:118, 119, 120t
Hepatitis C, and breastfeeding, 2:146
Herbal, defined, 1:54
Herbicide-resistant weeds, 1:246
Herbs
    as dietary supplement, 1:156, 157, 2:49
    in food and beverages, as functional food, 1:242t
    in menopause, 2:49
HGH (human growth hormone), 1:262–263
HHANES (Hispanic Health and Nutrition Examination Survey), 2:69
HHS. *See* U.S. Department of Health and Human Services (HHS)
HHS (hyperosmolar hyperglycemia state), 1:146
"High," as nutrient content claim, 1:265t
High blood pressure
    defined, 1:14
    See also Hypertension
High potency, defined, 1:33
High density lipoprotein (HDL)
    and cardiovascular disease, 1:103
    cholesterol/HDL ratio, 2:29t, 30
    HDL/LDL ratio values, 2:30t
    in lipid profile, 2:29, 30
    optimal, borderline, and high levels, 2:29t
    and soy, 2:207
High-fiber diets, 1:222, 2:37
High-protein diets, 2:249
High-quality proteins, 2:156
High-yield variety (HYV) seeds, 1:261–262
Hindu food practices, 2:175, 176–177, 177, 178t
Hispanic Health and Nutrition Examination Survey (HHANES), 2:69
Hispanics and Latinos, diet of, **1:275–279**, 1:278t
    acculturation, 1:276–278, 2:169
    characteristics, 1:275–276, *277*
    childhood obesity, 1:121
    diet-related disease, 1:14t
    regional diet, 2:168–169
    socioeconomic status, 2:168, 169

See also Central Americans and Mexicans, diets of
Histidine, 2:156t
HIV/AIDS, **1:279–282**, 1:*281*
    antiretroviral drugs, 2:76
    breastfeeding, 2:146
    complications, 1:280
    cures as quackery, 2:163
    ethical considerations for care, 1:281–282
    nutrition, 1:279–280
    oral nutrition alternatives, 1:280–281
    statistics, 1:280
    United Nations Children's Fund (UNICEF), 2:226
    See also Immune system
HMB (beta-hydroxy beta-methylbutyrate), 1:190
Hmongs, diet of, 1:50t
Homelessness, **1:282–287**, 1:*283*
    diet deficits, 1:285–286
    government programs, 1:284–285
    organizations, 1:285
    poverty and undernutrition, 1:283
    undernutrition among children, 1:283–284
    See also Food insecurity
Homeostasis, 2:245, 246
    defined, 2:144
Hong Kong, organic foods in, 2:115
Hookworm, defined, 1:40
Hoppin' John, 1:11, 12
Hormiga, 2:202, *202*
Hormone replacement therapy. *See* Estrogen replacement therapy (ERT)
Hormones
    and cravings, 1:137
    defined, 1:31
    production, 2:158
    regulatory functions, 1:37
Howard Johnson's restaurants, 2:15, *15*, 16
HRT (hormone replacement therapy). *See* Estrogen replacement therapy (ERT)
Human Genome Project, 2:75
Human growth hormone (HGH), 1:262–263
Human immunodeficiency virus. *See* HIV/AIDS
Human subjects, 2:75–76
Hungary, 1:118
Hunger, 1:44–45, **1:287**
    See also Appetite; Food insecurity
Hydration, defined, 1:72
Hydrochloric acid, 2:157

Hydrogen breath test, 2:22
Hydrolysis, 2:157
Hydrolyze, defined, 2:157
Hygiene, defined, 1:236
Hygienic Laboratory, 2:73
Hype, defined, 1:33
Hyperactivity, 1:29
Hypercalcemia, 1:84
Hypercarotenemia, 2:234
Hypercholesterolemia, defined, 1:117
Hyperglycemia, 1:146, 148, **1:287–288**
    defined, 1:143
    See also Diabetes mellitus; Insulin
Hyperinsulinemia, 1:145
Hyperlipidemia, defined, 1:164
Hyperosmolar hyperglycemia state (HHS), 1:146
Hypertension, **1:288–291**, 1:*289*
    African Americans, 1:14, 14t, 290, 2:167
    Asia, 1:56–57
    as cardiovascular disease, 1:99–100, *100*, 103
    causes, 1:289–290
    DASH eating plan, 1:290–291
    defined, 1:10
    described, 1:288
    and diet, 1:290
    and exercise, 1:199
    lifestyle treatment, 1:291, 2:76–77
    men, 2:53
    pharmacological treatment, 1:291
    and potassium, 2:167
    and pregnancy, 1:289, 2:223
    primary, 1:289
    and rice, 2:181
    secondary, 1:289, 291
    types, 1:289
    women, 2:261
    See also Cardiovascular disease (CVD)
Hypertrophy, defined, 1:190
Hypervitaminosis A, 2:233t, 234
Hypochromic anemia, 1:38, 39t
Hypoglycemia, 1:24, **1:292**
    defined, 1:24
    See also Diabetes mellitus
HYV (high-yield variety) seeds, 1:261–262

I

IBIDS (International Bibliographic Information on Dietary Supplements), 1:156
Ice cream, glycemic index, 1:251t

IFG (impaired fasting glucose), 1:145
IGT (impaired glucose tolerance), 1:145
Ileum, 1:170
Illnesses, food-borne, 1:236, *237*, **2:1–4**
  causes, 2:1–3, *2*
  historical outbreaks, 2:118–119
  international dietary trends, 1:164–165
  intoxication and infection, 2:1, 120*t*
  magnitude, 2:118
  and organic foods, 2:116
  Pacific Islands, 2:132
  prevention, 2:3, 121
  Scandinavia, 2:187
  South America, 2:203–204
  symptoms, 2:3
  treatment, 2:3–4
  See also Food safety; Organisms, food-borne
The Immune Advantage (Mazo and Berndtson), 1:279–280
Immune system, 2:1, 3, **2:4**, 2:34, 232
  defined, 1:26
  See also Infection
Immunocomprised, defined, 2:117
Immunoglobulins, 1:37
Immunologic, defined, 1:75
Immunoproteins, 1:37
Impaired fasting glucose (IFG), 1:145
Impaired glucose tolerance (IGT), 1:145
Impotence, 2:53
Inborn errors of metabolism, **2:4–7**, *2:5*
  amino acid metabolism disorders, 2:5–6
  carbohydrate metabolism disorders, 2:6–7
  See also Phenylketonuria (PKU)
Incidence, defined, 1:41
Incisor, defined, 2:153
Incomplete proteins, 2:156
India, oral cancer in, 1:88
Indian corn, 1:134
Indians, American. *See* Native Americans
Indians, Asian, diet of, 1:50*t*, 55
Indigestion, defined, 1:256
Indirect additives, 1:1
  See also Additives and preservatives
Indispensable amino acids, 1:36, 36*t*, 38, 2:155–156
Infant mortality rate, **2:7–8**
  See also Maternal mortality rate

Infant nutrition, **2:8–12**
  beikost (solid food), 1:62, 2:*9*, 10–11
  breastfeeding, 2:8–9, 11
  calcium, 1:84–85
  formula feeding, 2:9–10
  nutrient requirements, 2:8
  protein, 2:159
  self-feeding, 2:11
  South, 2:258, *258*
  vegetarianism, 2:230
  vitamin D, 2:235
  vitamin E, 2:237
  WIC program, 2:255, 256, 257, *257*
  See also Beikost; Breastfeeding
Infection, 2:*12*, **2:12**
  and diarrhea, 1:149, 150
  as food-borne illness, 2:1, 120*t*
  and malnutrition, 2:34
  mastitis, 2:41, *41*
  See also Immune system
Infectious agents, and cancer, 1:89–90, 91
Infectious diseases
  defined, 1:35
  and vitamin A deficiency, 2:234
Informed consent, defined, 2:75
Insoluble, defined, 1:63
Insoluble fiber, 1:221
Institute of Food Technologists, 1:248
Institutional Review Board (IRB), 2:75
Insulin, **2:12–13**
  defined, 1:37
  and diabetes, 1:143, 144, *145*, 147
  in digestion, 1:170
  and genetic engineering, 1:65
  regulating blood glucose levels, 1:37, *37*
  See also Diabetes mellitus; Glycemic index
Insulin injections, 1:*145*, 147, 2:12–13
Insulin pens, 2:12–13
Insulin pumps, 1:*145*, 2:12–13
Integrative medicine, 1:30
  See also Alternative medicines and therapies
International Bibliographic Information on Dietary Supplements (IBIDS), 1:156
International Children's Day of Broadcasting, 2:226
International Conference on Child Labour, 2:227
International Conference on Health Promotion (1986), 1:263

International Conference on Nutrition, 2:205
International dietary trends. *See* Dietary trends, international
International disaster relief organizations. *See* Disaster relief organizations
International nongovernmental organizations, 2:83
International Space Station, 2:210, 212, *213*, 214, 215
Internships, 1:105–106
  defined, 1:105
Interstitial, defined, 2:246
Intestines, defined, 1:64
Intolerances. *See* Allergies and intolerances
Intoxication, as food-borne illness, 2:1, 120*t*
Intracellular fluids, 1:37, 2:246
Intrauterine growth retardation, 2:197–198
  See also Low birth weight infant
Intravascular fluid compartment, 1:37
Intravenous, defined, 1:84
Intrinsic factor, 1:40, 2:243
Iodine
  Asia, 1:56
  deficiency, 1:56, 2:35, 63, 159–160
  functions, 2:62
  poisoning, 1:253
Iodism, 1:253
Iran
  eating habits, 1:*186*
  United Nations Children's Fund (UNICEF), 2:226
Iraq, disaster relief in, 1:*174*
IRB (Institutional Review Board), 2:75
Ireland, 2:86
Iron
  adolescents, 1:5
  Asia, 1:56
  children, 1:39
  deficiency, 1:38–40, 56, 2:24, 26, 62–63, 153
  defined, 1:5
  disease prevention and treatment, 2:62
  fortification of food, 2:72
  as functional food, 1:242*t*
  functions, 2:62
  infant nutrition, 1:242*t*, 2:9, 10
  and lead poisoning, 2:24, 26
  and menopause, 2:50
  and pregnancy, 1:40, 2:145
  preschoolers and toddlers, 2:152, 153

and space travel, 2:212, 215
sports nutrition, 2:217
supplements, 2:59
toxicity, 2:63
vegetarians, 2:230
women, 2:259
Iron-deficiency anemia, 1:38–40, 2:153
Irradiation, **2:13–14**
See also Biotechnology; Food safety
Irritability, defined, 1:249
Islam. See Muslims
Isoflavones, **2:14**, 2:207, 208
defined, 2:14
Isoleucine, 2:6, 156t
Italy
cuisine, 2:204, 205, 206
life expectancy, 2:28
organic foods, 2:115

J

Jamaica, 1:110
Japan
diet, 1:53–54
food-borne illness, 2:118
life expectancy, 2:28
organic foods, 2:115
postmenopausal symptoms, 2:208
stomach cancer, 1:88
Japanese Americans, diet of, 1:50
Jefferson, Thomas, 2:79
Jejunum, 1:170
Jerk meat, 1:108, 109
Jewish food practices, 1:259, 2:176, 177–178, 178t
Job sharing, defined, 1:77
Johnson, Howard, **2:14–16**, 2:15
Joint Centre for Bioethics, University of Toronto, 1:67, 68
Joint United Nations Programme on HIV/AIDS, 1:280
Judaism. See Jewish food practices
Juices, as functional food, 1:242t, 243
Junk food
defined, 2:191
in schools, 2:191, 192

K

Kashrut, 1:259, 2:177–178
Kava, 2:131
Kcalorie, 1:87, 216
See also Calories
Kellogg, John Harvey, 1:60, 61, 255, **2:16–18**, 2:17, 254
See also Battle Creek Sanitarium
Kellogg, Will Keith, 2:16, 17, 17

Kempner, Walter, 2:181–182
Keto-acid, defined, 2:157
Ketoacidosis, defined, 1:146
Ketones, 1:210
defined, 1:146
Ketosis, 1:97, 2:56
defined, 1:97
Kidney
and diabetes, 1:146
and hypertension, 1:289, 289
and mineral toxicity, 2:61
Kidney stones, defined, 1:84
Killer-cell, defined, 1:43
Kilocalorie, 1:87, 216
See also Calories
Kimchi, 1:50, 54
Kinetic, defined, 2:158
Kiwanis Worldwide Service Project, 2:227
Korean Americans, diet of, 1:50
Koreans, diet of, 1:54
Kosher, 1:259, 2:177
Krebs Cycle, 1:96–97, 2:55
defined, 1:96
Kroc, Ray, **2:18–20**, 2:19
See also Fast foods
Kwanzaa, 1:13
Kwashiorkor, 1:40, **2:20–21**, 2:35, 92, 160
defined, 1:40
See also Malnutrition; Protein

L

Lactase, 1:26, 28, 172, 2:21, 22
Lactation. See Breastfeeding
Lacteals, 1:216
Lactic acid, defined, 1:96
Lacto vegetarians, 2:229
Lacto-ovo vegetarians, 2:179, 229
Lactose, 1:93, 94, 94t, 2:6, 21
Lactose intolerance, 1:26, 28, **2:21–23**
and absorption, 1:172
Asia, 1:56
clinical diagnosis, 2:22
congenital, 2:22
defined, 1:18
nutrition for, 2:22–23
prevalence, 2:21–22, 22
secondary, 2:22
structure and functions of lactose, 2:21
treatment, 1:29
types, 2:22
Lactose tolerance test, 2:22
Laotians, diet of, 1:50t

Lasix, 2:88t
Latin America, underweight in, 2:35
Latinos. See Hispanics and Latinos, diet of
Latvia, cardiovascular disease mortality in, 1:118
Laws
Biologics Control Act (1902), 2:73
Child Nutrition Act (1972), 2:255–256
Color Additives Amendment (1960), 1:2–3
Dietary Supplement Health and Education Act (DSHEA) (1994), 1:31–32, 33, 156, 157–158, 241–243, 2:74
Federal Food, Drug, and Cosmetic Act (1938), 1:241–243
Food Additives Amendment (1958), 1:2
Food and Drug Administration Modernization Act (FDAMA) (1997), 1:264–265
National Consumer Health Information and Health Promotion Act (1970), 1:269
National Health Survey Act (1956), 2:68–69
Nutrition Labeling and Education Act (NLEA) (1990), 1:232–233, 263–264, 266
Older Americans Act (1965), 2:42
Organic Foods Production Act (1990), 2:113–114
Pure Food and Drug Act (1906), 2:162, 171
Lay health advisor (LHA), **2:23**
LDL. See Low-density lipoprotein (LDL)
Lead poisoning, **2:23–27**, 2:72
definition, 2:24
educational interventions, 2:26
medical treatment, 2:26–27
nutritional interventions, 2:26
populations at risk, 2:24
prevalence, 2:26
sources of lead, 2:25, 25–26
symptoms, 2:24
Leading health indicator (LHI), 1:270
League of Red Cross and Red Crescent Societies (LICROSS), 1:175t
"Lean," as nutrient content claim, 1:265t
Learned behaviors, defined, 1:186
Leavening, defined, 1:2
Leeks, 2:85–86

Legumes, 1:109, 2:27, **2:27–28**
  defined, 1:5
  See also Vegetarianism
Leptin, 2:77
"Less," as nutrient content claim, 1:265t
Letrozol, 2:75
Letter on Corpulence (Banting), 1:205
Leucine, 2:6, 156t
Leukemia, 1:88
LHA (lay health advisor), 2:23
LHI (leading health indicator), 1:270
Licensing, of nutritionists, 1:106, 2:104
LICROSS (League of Red Cross and Red Crescent Societies), 1:175t
Life expectancy, 1:120t, **2:28**
  See also Infant mortality rate
Lifestyle, defined, 1:24
"Light"
  as marketing strategy, 2:39
  as nutrient content claim, 1:265t
"Light in sodium," as nutrient content claim, 1:265t
Light therapy, 2:149, *149*
Lignin, 1:95
Lind, James, 2:197, *220*, 244
Linoleic acids. *See* Omega-3 and omega-6 fatty acids
Linolenic acids. *See* Omega-3 and omega-6 fatty acids
Lipase, 1:170, 172, 2:29
Lipid
  defined, 1:36
  See also Fats
Lipid profile, **2:28–31**, 2:29t, 30t
  blood lipids and lipid transport, 2:29
  and exercise, 1:199–200
  treating abnormal blood lipids, 2:30
  See also Cardiovascular disease (CVD)
Lipitor, 2:88t
Lipogenesis, 2:57
Lipolysis, 2:56
Lipoprotein, 1:37
  defined, 1:103
Listeria monocytogenes, 2:2, 116, 119, 120t
Listeriosis, defined, 2:118
Lithuania
  obesity, 2:105
  vitamin C deficiency, 1:120
Liver
  and alcohol, 1:24, *25*
  in digestion, 1:170, 171
Lobsters, 1:*187*

Long-term care facilities, defined, 1:105
"Low," as nutrient content claim, 1:265t
Low birth weight infant, **2:31**, 2:197
  See also Pregnancy
Low-carb diet, 1:97
Low-density lipoprotein (LDL)
  and cardiovascular disease, 1:103
  and carotenoids, 1:112
  drug treatment, 2:30
  HDL/LDL ratio values, 2:30t
  in lipid profile, 2:29
  and Mediterranean diet, 1:259, 260
  optimal, borderline, and high levels, 2:29t
  and soy, 2:207
Lower-quality proteins, 2:156
Low-fat products, 1:219
Luau, 2:131
Lunch Program, National School, 1:284, 2:96–97, 190–191, 194
Lung cancer, 2:234
Lutefisk, 2:189–190
Lutein, 1:113, 2:234
Lutheran World Federation (LWF), 1:175t
Lycopene, 1:91, 113, 2:53, 234
Lymph node, defined, 1:90
Lymph system, defined, 1:88
Lymphatic system, defined, 1:88
Lymphoma, 1:88
Lysine, 1:134, 2:156t

M

Macaroni and cheese, glycemic index, 1:251t
Macrobiotic, defined, 1:31
Macrobiotic diet, **2:31–33**, 2:*32*
Macrocytic anemia, 1:38, 39t, 2:243
Macrominerals, 2:95
Macronutrient, defined, 1:113
Macrophage, 2:29
Macrovascular disease. *See* Atherosclerosis
Macular degeneration, 2:234
  defined, 1:112
Mad cow disease, 2:118–119, *119*, 187
Magnesium
  deficiency, 2:61
  disease prevention and treatment, 2:61
  functions, 2:60
  premenstrual syndrome, 2:148
  toxicity, 2:61

Maize
  Central America and Mexico, 1:113, 114–115
  varieties, 1:133–134
Maize-based diets. *See* Corn- or maize-based diets
Major minerals, 2:60–61
Malabsorption
  defined, 2:101
  in HIV/AIDS patients, 1:280
Malaria, defined, 1:40
Malaysians, diet of, 1:55
Males. *See* Men's nutritional issues
Malignant, defined, 1:88
Malignant tumors, 1:88, 90
Malnourished, defined, 1:39
Malnutrition, **2:33–36**, 2:*36*
  and alcohol, 1:24–25
  Caribbean Islands, 1:110
  defined, 1:22
  and diarrhea, 1:150
  and growth, 2:35–36
  and infection, 2:34
  necessary nutrients, 2:35
  people at risk, 2:33–35, *34*
  and popular culture, 2:140–141
Maltose, 1:94, 94t
Manganese toxicity, 2:63
Mangoes, 1:108
Maple sugar, 2:80
Maple syrup urine disease (MSUD), 2:6
Marasmus, **2:36–37**
  defined, 1:40
  malnutrition, 2:35, 92
  vitamin deficiencies, 1:40
March of Dimes, 2:143
Marijuana, 2:176
Marine Hospital Service (MHS), 1:253, 2:73
Marker genes, 1:246
Marketing strategies, **2:37–41**
  impact and influence, 2:37–38, *38*
  inappropriate advertisements, 2:38–40, *39*
  recommendations for responsible food marketing, 2:40
  See also Health claims
Martinique, 1:110
Masa, 1:114–115
Mastitis, 2:*41*, **2:41–42**
  See also Breastfeeding
Matambre, 2:203
Maté;, 2:201
Maternal Child Health Program Title V, 2:98
Maternal mortality rate, 2:36, **2:42**

See also Infant mortality rate
Maturity onset diabetes of the young (MODY), 1:145
Mazo, Ellen, 1:279–280
McDonald, Maurice (Mac), 2:18–19
McDonald, Richard, 2:18–19
McDonald's restaurants, 2:18–19, *19*, *20*, *38*
McGwire, Mark, 1:*191*
Meals On Wheels, 1:*23*, 129, **2:42**
    See also Nutrition programs in the community
Measurements, anthropometric. *See* Anthropometric measurements
Meat
    Africa, 1:16, 18
    Central America and Mexico, 1:115
    Mediterranean diet, 1:257
    Scandinavia, 2:188–189
Meat analogs, **2:42–43**
    See also Vegetarianism
Medical nutrition therapists, 1:104–105, 168
Medical nutrition therapy (MNT), **2:43–46**
    assessment components, 2:43–44
    for diabetes, 1:147
    insurance coverage, 2:45–46
    therapy provision, 2:44–45
    See also Nutritional assessment
Medicare, medical nutrition therapy coverage, 2:45
Meditation, defined, 1:30
Mediterranean diet. *See* Greeks and Middle Easterners, diet of
Mediterranean Pyramid, 1:226–227
Megaloblastic anemia, 1:40
Melatonin, and premenstrual syndrome, 2:*149*
Mellanby, Edward, **2:46–47**, *2:47*
    See also Rickets
Melo Palheta, Francisco de, 2:201
Menaquinones, 2:236
Menopausal, defined, 2:47
Menopause, **2:47–50**, 2:260
    defined, 1:10
    dietary and lifestyle changes, 2:50
    physiological changes, 2:47–48
    and soy, 2:48–49, 208, 260
    stages, 2:47
    treatments and remedies, 2:48–49, *49*
    See also Women's nutritional issues
Men's nutritional issues, **2:51–54**
    body image, 1:69, 70, 71
    cancer, 2:51, *52*
    college students, 1:124
    cravings, 1:137–138, *138*

diabetes mellitus, 2:51
eating disorders, 1:177, 178, 184
heart disease, 2:51–53, *52*
hypertension, 2:53
impotence, 2:53
life expectancy in Europe, 1:120*t*
prostate health, 1:91, 2:53, 208, 234
Menstrual cycles, defined, 2:47
Metabolic, defined, 1:46
Metabolic disorders. *See* Inborn errors of metabolism
Metabolism, **2:54–58**, 2:*57*
    carbohydrates, 2:6–7, 54–55
    cholesterol, 2:57–58, 77
    defined, 1:42
    fats, 1:216, 2:56–57
    during menopause, 2:260
    protein, 2:55–56, 157
Metabolism, inborn errors of. *See* Inborn errors of metabolism
Metabolite, defined, 1:31
Metabolize, defined, 1:24
Metastasis, 1:88
Methionine, 2:156*t*
Metropolitan Life Insurance Company height and weight tables, 2:99, 100*t*
Mexican Americans
    children, 2:168
    diabetes, 1:277
    diet, 1:276–277, 278*t*
    See also Hispanics and Latinos, diet of
Mexicans. *See* Central Americans and Mexicans, diets of
Mexico
    fruits and vegetables, 1:114
    traditional dietary habits, 1:113
MHS (Marine Hospital Service), 1:253, 2:73
Micelles, 1:216
Microbial fermentation, 1:65
Microcytic anemia, 1:38, 39*t*
Microflora, defined, 2:154
Microminerals, 2:95
Micronutrients
    deficiency in Asia, 1:55–56
    defined, 1:19
Microorganisms, defined, 1:2
Middle Easterners. *See* Greeks and Middle Easterners, diet of
Midsummer's Day, 2:190
Mid-upper arm circumference (MUAC), 1:74
Midwest cooking, 2:167
Milk
    and bovine somatotropin, 1:262

evaporated, 2:10
as functional food, 1:242*t*
glycemic index, 1:251*t*
health claims, 2:37–38
and infants, 2:9, *197*
pasteurization, 2:133
and scurvy, 2:*197*
with vitamin D, 1:242*t*, 2:122, 235
Milk sugar. *See* Lactose
Mind-body interventions, 1:31, 31*t*
Minerals, **2:58–64**
    bioavailability, 2:59
    deficiency, 2:61, 62–63
    defined, 1:2
    disease prevention and treatment, 2:60–61, 62
    functions, 2:60, 62
    major, 2:60–61
    as nutrient, 2:94–95
    pregnancy requirements, 2:145, *145*
    sports nutrition, 2:217
    supplementation, 2:59–60, *60*
    toxicity, 2:61, 63
    trace, 2:61–63
    See also Dietary supplements; Vitamins, fat-soluble; Vitamins, water-soluble
Miscarriage, defined, 1:82
Mitochondria, defined, 2:55
MNT. *See* Medical nutrition therapy (MNT)
Models, fashion, 1:69
MODY (maturity onset diabetes of the young), 1:145
Molar, defined, 2:153
Mold, and food poisoning, 2:3
Molecule, defined, 1:36
Monaco, life expectancy in, 2:28
Monckeberg's arteriosclerosis, 1:45
Monocultural, defined, 1:140
Monoglycerides, 1:216
    defined, 1:170
Mononucleosis, 2:12
Monosaccharides, 1:93, 94*t*, 2:54
Monosodium glutamate (MSG), 1:2, 4, 28
Monounsaturated fat, 1:102, 215, 217, 260
Montserrat, 1:110
Mood-food relationships, **2:64–67**, 2:66*t*
    circadian rhythms, 2:65–66
    meal size, 2:65
    neurotransmitter effects, 2:64–65, 66*t*
    positive moods and stress reduction, 2:*65*, 66–67

Mood-food relationships *(continued)*
  See also Cravings
Moore, Mary Tyler, 2:76
Morbidity, defined, 1:73
"More," as nutrient content claim, 1:265t
Mormon food practices, 2:176, 178, 178t
Motor proteins, 1:37
MSG (monosodium glutamate), 1:2, 4, 28
MSUD (maple syrup urine disease), 2:6
MUAC (mid-upper arm circumference), 1:74
Mucilages, 1:96
Mucosa, defined, 1:159
Multiple cropping, 1:261–262
Muscle wasting
  defined, 1:202
  during space travel, 2:211–212
Muscular endurance and strength, 1:200, 2:216
Muslims
  alcohol, 1:259
  food practices, 1:16–17, 259, 2:177, 178t
  Halal foods, 1:258, 259t, 2:177
  southern Europe, 2:204
Mycotoxins, 2:120–121
  defined, 2:3
Myocardial infarction, 1:272, 273, 2:75
Myoglobin, defined, 2:62
Myristicin intolerance, 1:28

N

Nandrolone, defined, 1:191
National Academy of Sciences (NAS), **2:67**
  diet, 1:97
  food additives, 1:4
  health claims, 1:264–265
  Recommended Dietary Allowances, 2:164
  See also Dietary Reference Intakes (DRIs); Recommended Dietary Allowances (RDAs)
National Center for Complementary and Alternative Medicine, 1:30–31, 31t, 2:161
National Center for Health Statistics (NCHS), 2:68
National Cholesterol Education Program, 2:29–30
National Consumer Health Information and Health Promotion Act (1970), 1:269
National Diabetes Education Program, 1:147
National Food Processors Association, 1:238
National Health and Nutrition Examination Survey (NHANES), 1:72, 73, **2:68–73**
  caloric intake, 1:161
  childhood obesity, 1:121, 122
  data collection procedures, 2:71
  future, 2:72
  and Healthy Eating Index, 1:268–269
  history, 2:68–70, *70*
  procedures, 2:70–71
  results, 2:71–72
  sampling, 2:70
National Health Examination Survey (NHES), 1:121, 2:68–69
National Health Interview Survey (NHIS), 2:72
National Health Survey Act (1956), 2:68–69
National Immunization Days, 2:227
National Institute of Mental Health, 1:184
National Institute on Alcohol Abuse and Alcoholism, 1:24
National Institutes of Health (NIH), **2:73–78**
  accomplishments, 2:75
  Atkins Diet, 1:97
  childhood obesity, 1:122
  diarrhea, 1:149
  funding, 2:76, *76*, *77*
  history, 2:73–74
  human subjects, 2:75–76
  impotence, 2:53
  institutes and centers, 2:74–75
  mission, 2:74
  Office of Dietary Supplements, 1:156, 2:74
  Office of Legislative Policy and Analysis, 2:74
  Office of Science Policy, 2:75–76
  research and biomedical advances, 2:76–78
  Trans-NIH Bioethics Committee, 2:76
National nongovernmental organizations, 2:83
National Nutrition Surveillance System, 2:69
National Osteoporosis Foundation, 2:123, 124
National Research Council, 1:154
National School Lunch Program (NSLP), 1:284, 2:96–97, 190–191, 194
Native Americans, diet of, **2:78–82**
  alcohol use, 1:25
  childhood obesity, 1:122
  before colonial period, 2:79–80
  current food practices, 2:80, *81*
  diet-related health issues, 2:79t, 81
  Food Distribution Program on Indian Reservations, 1:128
  homelessness, 1:*283*
  overweight and obesity, 2:79t, 81
  sacred and ceremonial foods, 2:80
  settlement hardships, 2:78–79
  See also Corn- or maize-based diets
Nausea
  defined, 1:27
  during pregnancy, 2:146
NBI (nitrogen balance index), 2:159–160
NCHS (National Center for Health Statistics), 2:68
Needs assessment, defined, 1:173
Needy Family Program, 1:127
Negative nitrogen balance, 2:160
Neoplasm, 1:88, 90
Neotame, 1:46–47
Nervous system, defined, 1:38
Neural, defined, 1:40
Neural tube defects (NTDs), 2:142–143, 243
Neurological, defined, 1:184
Neuropathy, defined, 2:181
Neurotransmitters
  defined, 1:137
  mood-food relationships, 2:64–65, 66t
Nevis, 1:110
New England cooking, 2:167
NGOs (nongovernmental organizations), 2:82–83
NHANES. *See* National Health and Nutrition Examination Survey (NHANES)
NHES (National Health Examination Survey), 1:121, 2:68–69
NHIS (National Health Interview Survey), 2:72
Niacin (vitamin B_3), 2:239–241, 240t
  in corn- or maize-based diets, 1:134–136, *135*
  deficiency, 2:103
  defined, 1:2
  and pellagra, 2:135
Nicotinamide, 2:239
Nicotine. *See* Smoking
Nicotinic acid, 1:244, 254, 2:239
Night blindness, 2:234

NIH. *See* National Institutes of Health (NIH)
Nitrite, defined, 1:4
Nitrogen
  defined, 1:134
  and inborn errors of metabolism, 2:7
Nitrogen balance index (NBI), 2:159–160
Nitrosamines, and cancer, 1:4
Nixtamalizacion, 2:79
NLEA (Nutrition Labeling and Education Act) (1990), 1:232–233, 263–264, 266
NLM (U.S. National Library of Medicine), 2:74
Nonessential amino acids, 1:36, 36t, 2:155–156
Nongovernmental organizations (NGOs), **2:82–83**
  See also Disaster relief organizations
Nonpathogenic, defined, 2:154
Nonpolar, defined, 2:155
Noodles, glycemic index, 1:251t
Norepinephrine, effect on mood, 2:64, 66t
Normochronic anemia, 1:38, 39t
North Africans, diet of, 1:16–17, *17*
Northern Europeans, diet of, **2:83–87**
  eating habits and meal patterns, 2:84
  England, 2:84, *85*
  France, 2:86–87
  Ireland, 2:86
  nutritional status, 2:84
  Scotland, 2:84–85
  Wales, 2:85–86
  See also Central Europeans and Russians, diets of; Southern Europeans, diet of
Norvasc, 2:88t
Norwalk-type viruses, 2:119, 120t
NOSB (U.S. National Organic Standards Board), 2:113–114
NSLP. *See* National School Lunch Program (NSLP)
NTDs (neural tube defects), 2:142–143, 243
Nursing bottle mouth syndrome. *See* Baby bottle tooth decay
NutraSweet, 1:46
Nutrient additives, 1:2
  See also Additives and preservatives
Nutrient content claims, 1:156, 232
Nutrient density, **2:87**
Nutrient-drug interactions, **2:88–90**, 2:88t, *89*
  adverse effects, 2:88–89

avoiding, 2:90
drug functions, 2:88
elderly, 2:89
impact, 2:89
Nutrients, **2:90–95**, *2:93*
  carbohydrates, 2:91–92
  defined, 1:2
  functions, 2:91t
  lipids, 2:92–94
  minerals, 2:94–95
  proteins, 2:92
  vitamins, 2:94
  water, 2:95
  See also specific nutrients by name
Nutrition, **2:95**
  defined, 1:7
Nutrition education, **2:96**
Nutrition Educators, 1:105
Nutrition Facts statement, 1:233, *234*
Nutrition Labeling and Education Act (NLEA) (1990), 1:232–233, 263–264, 266
Nutrition managers, 1:104–105, 168
Nutrition Program for Older Americans, 2:98
Nutrition programs in the community, **2:96–99**
  Food and Nutrition Service programs, 2:96–98, *98*
  Health and Human Services Department programs, 2:98
  See also Meals On Wheels
Nutrition Screening Initiative, 1:20–21
Nutritional assessment, **2:99–102**
  anthropometrics, 2:99–101, 100t
  biochemical data, 2:101
  clinical data, 2:101
  dietary data, 2:101–102
  elements, 2:99–102
  evaluation, 2:102
  See also Dietary assessment
Nutritional deficiency, **2:102–104**, *2:103*
  defined, 1:38
Nutritional requirements, defined, 1:7
Nutritional transition
  Asia, 1:56–57
  Central America and Mexico, 1:116
  Hispanics and Latinos, 1:276–278, 2:169
  Pacific Islander Americans, 2:128
  Pacific Islanders, 2:131–132
Nutritionist, 1:106, 2:44, *104*, **2:104–105**
  See also Careers in dietetics; Dietitian

Nutrition-support-team dietitians, 1:168
Nuts, 1:53, 242t, 2:108

O

Oats, as functional food, 1:242t
Obese, defined, 1:64
Obesity, **2:105–108**
  adolescents, 1:6, 2:192–193
  adults, 1:8
  African Americans, 1:14, 14t
  Asia, 1:56, 57, *163*
  body mass index, 2:105, 125, 140
  causes, 2:106
  costs, 2:106
  defined, 1:6
  and disease, 1:217
  as health risk, 2:105–106
  international dietary trends, 1:164
  and leptin, 2:77
  Native Americans, 2:79t, 81
  and oral health, 2:111–112
  versus overweight, 2:125
  Pacific Islander Americans, 2:126
  Pacific Islanders, 2:129, 131
  and popular culture, 2:140
  and portion sizes, 1:160
  prevalence, 1:203, 2:105
  treatment, 2:106–107, *107*
  water in body, 2:245–246
  See also Body mass index; Childhood obesity; Overweight
Observationes Medicae (Tulp), *2:224*
Ohsawa, George, 2:31
Okra, 1:11, *11*, 12, 13
Older adults. *See* Aging and nutrition
Older Americans Act (1965), 2:42
Olestra, 1:*211*, 212, 213, 218–219
Oligosaccharides, 1:93
Olive oil, 1:256, 258, 259, 260
Olives, 2:204
Omega-3 and omega-6 fatty acids, **2:108–110**, *2:109*
  benefits, 2:108–109
  and cardiovascular disease, 1:102–103
  in eggs, 1:*241*, 242t
  Mediterranean diet, 1:260
  types, 2:108
  See also Heart disease
Oncogenes, and cancer, 1:91
Oneworld Alliance for UNICEF, 2:227
Opacity, defined, 2:264
Operational nongovernmental organizations, 2:83

Opportunistic infections, defined, 1:279
Opsin, 2:232
Oral contraceptives, 2:88t
Oral health, **2:110–112**
  factors affecting, 2:110
  and fluoride, 2:112
  and overnutrition, 2:111–112, *112*
  and undernutrition, 2:111
  See also Baby bottle tooth decay
Oral rehydration therapy (ORT), 1:151, **2:113**, 2:226, 247
  See also Dehydration; Diarrhea
Oral-pharyngeal, defined, 1:280
Orange juice
  calcium-fortified, 1:242t, 243
  glycemic index, 1:251t
Organic foods, **2:113–117**
  advantages and disadvantages, 2:114, *115*
  certification and labeling, 1:237, 2:114
  market, 2:115, *116*
  nutrition quackery, 2:162
  safety and nutritional value, 2:116–117
  sustainable food systems, 2:222
  See also Food safety
Organic Foods Production Act (1990), 2:113–114
Organisms, food-borne, **2:117–122**
  mad cow and Creutzfeldt-Jakob, 2:118–119, *119*
  magnitude of food-borne illness, 2:118
  outbreaks, 2:118–119
  prevention of food-borne illness, 2:121
  types, 2:119–121, 120t
  See also Food safety; Illnesses, food-borne
ORT. *See* Oral rehydration therapy (ORT)
Osteoarthritis, defined, 1:217
Osteoblast, defined, 2:123
Osteomalacia, 1:84, **2:122**, 2:183, 235
  defined, 1:84
  See also Rickets
Osteopathic, defined, 1:30
Osteopenia, **2:122–123**
Osteoporosis, **2:123–125**, *2:124*
  and calcium, 1:85, *85*, 2:61, 124
  defined, 1:5
  in female athlete triad, 1:219, 2:219
  and nutritional deficiency, 2:103
  prevalence, 2:124–125

  risk factors, 2:123–124
  and soy, 2:208
  and spaceflight bone loss, 2:211
  and vitamin D deficiency, 2:235
  women, 1:10, 219, 2:123, *124*, 125, 219, 260
  See also Calcium; Women's nutritional issues
Outcrossing, 1:248
Overnutrition, and oral health, 2:111–112, *112*
Over-the-counter, defined, 1:31
Overweight, **2:125–126**
  body mass index, 2:125, 140
  children, 2:153, 192–193
  defined, 1:64
  international dietary trends, 1:164
  Native Americans, 2:79t, 81
  versus obesity, 2:125
  prevalence, 1:203, 2:105
  southern Europe, 2:206
  See also Obesity
OXFAM International, 1:175t
Oxidative, defined, 2:56
Oxygen, defined, 1:2
Oxytocin, 1:76

P

Pabellón caraqueño, 2:203
Pacific Islander Americans, diet of, **2:126–128**, *2:127t*
  eating habits and meal patterns, 2:127
  nutrition and health status, 2:126–127
  nutritional transition, 2:128
Pacific Islanders, diet of, **2:128–132**
  childhood obesity, 1:122
  eating habits and meal patterns, 2:129–130
  nutritional status, 2:129
  nutritional transition, 2:131–132
  traditional cooking methods and food habits, *2:130*, 130–131
  See also Asians, diet of
Pacific Northwest cooking, 2:167
Pacifier caries, 2:111
Paella, 2:*205*, 206
Pain, and endorphins, 2:66
Paint, lead-based, 2:24, 25, 26
Palestinian refugees, 2:*165*
Pancreas, 1:170, 171
Pantothenic acid (vitamin B$_5$), 2:240t, 241
Papain, 1:65
Papayas, 1:108
Paraguay, 2:201, 203

Paralysis
  and bone loss, 2:211
  defined, 1:236
Parasites
  defined, 1:41
  and food-borne illness, 2:120
Parasitic, defined, 1:40
Parathyroid hormone (PTH), 1:83–84
Parenteral nutrition, 1:280
Parkinson's disease, 2:75
Pasta, glycemic index, 1:251t
Pasteur, Louis, **2:132–133**, *2:133*
Pasteurization, **2:133**
  defined, 1:65
  electronic, 2:13–14
  invention of, 2:132–133
  See also Food safety
Patent medicines, 2:161, *162*
Pathogen, defined, 1:235
A Pattern for Daily Food Choices, 1:225
Pauling, Linus, **2:133–134**, *2:134*
PCM (protein-calorie malnutrition), 2:35, 159–160
PDD (premenstrual dysphoric disorder), 2:147
Peanut allergies, 1:29
Peas, glycemic index, 1:251t
Pectin, 1:96
Pediatric Nutrition Surveillance System, 2:153
Pellagra, *2:135*, **2:135**
  corn- or maize-based diets, 1:134–136, *135*
  Funk, Casimir, 1:244
  Goldberger, Joseph, 1:*253*, 253–254, 2:73
  and nutritional deficiency, 2:103, 240–241
PEM (protein-energy malnutrition), 2:35, 36, 141
Pemberton, John S., **2:135–136**, *2:136*
Penicillin, 2:89
Pepsinogen, 2:157
Percent Daily Value, 1:233t, 234
Perimenopausal period, 2:47
Periodontitis, 2:*112*
Peristalsis, 1:169
Pernicious anemia, 1:40, 2:243
Persistent diarrhea, 1:149
Peru
  food habits, 2:202, 203
  food-borne illness, 2:118
Pesticides, **2:137**
  food safety, 1:236–237, 2:116–117
  genetically modified foods, 1:247

nutrition quackery, 2:162
organic foods, 2:116
sustainable food systems, 2:221
See also Food safety; Organic foods
Petechiae, 2:111
pH, 1:37
  defined, 1:1
Phenylalanine, 1:46, 2:5–6, 137–138, 156*t*
Phenylethylamine, 2:66
Phenylketonuria (PKU), 1:46, 2:5–6, **2:137–138**
  defined, 1:46
  See also Amino acids
Phosphate toxicity, 2:61
Phospholipids, 1:215–216
  defined, 2:29
Phosphorus
  defined, 2:58
  functions, 2:60
  and osteomalacia, 2:122
  and vitamin D, 2:235
PHS (U.S. Public Health Service), 1:238–239, 253, 2:73
Phylloquinone, 2:236
Physical activity. *See* Exercise
Physical education, 1:*131*, 131–132
Physical fitness, 1:200
Physicians Committee for Responsible Medicine, 2:37–38
Physiological, defined, 1:8
Physiology, defined, 1:168
Physiology of Taste, or Meditations on Transcendental Gastronomy (Brillat-Savarin), 1:78
Phytate, defined, 2:59
Phytochemicals, 1:91, **2:138**, 2:207
  defined, 1:91
Phytoestrogens, 2:48–49
  defined, 2:48
Pica, **2:138**, 2:146
  See also Cravings
Pickling, as preservative, 1:1
Pick-your-own farms, 2:222
Pigs, in Pacific Islander diet, 2:130
PIH (pregnancy-induced hypertension), 1:289
Pipes, lead-soldered, 2:24, 25, 26
Pituitary gland, defined, 1:244
PKU. *See* Phenylketonuria (PKU)
Plant proteins, 2:156
Plantains, 1:18
Plant-based diets, **2:138–139**
  See also Vegetarianism
Plaque, 1:59, 60
  defined, 1:60
Plasma, defined, 1:120

PLP (pyridoxal phosphate), 2:242
Plumbism. *See* Lead poisoning
Pluralistic, defined, 1:140
PMS. *See* Premenstrual syndrome (PMS)
Pneumonia, defined, 1:146
Pod corn, 1:134
Poi, 2:127, 130
Poland, 1:118
Polar, defined, 2:155
Polydextrose, as fat substitute, 1:211–212
Polypeptides, 2:155
Polyphenols, and heart disease, 1:240
Polysaccharides, 1:94–96, *95*, 2:91
Polyunsaturated, defined, 1:101
Polyunsaturated fat, 1:102, 215, 217
Popcorn, 1:133
Popular culture, and food, **2:139–142**
  adolescents, 2:192
  convenience foods, 2:141
  current trends, 2:139
  dieting, 2:141
  eating away from home, 2:139–140, *140*
  ethnic foods, 2:142
  functional foods, 2:141
  obesity and malnutrition, 2:140–141
  supplements, 2:141
Population, world, 1:230
Pork, folk beliefs about, 1:13
Porridge, 2:84–85, 189
Portion sizes, 1:123, 160, 234, 2:65, 106, 140
Portugal, cuisine of, 2:204, 205
Positive nitrogen balance, 2:160
Post, C. W., 2:17
Postmenopausal period, 2:47
Potable, defined, 1:173
Potassium
  and cardiovascular disease, 1:103
  deficiency, 2:61
  disease prevention and treatment, 2:60–61
  functions, 2:60
  and hypertension, 1:290, 2:167
  toxicity, 2:61
Potassium iodide, 2:62
Potatoes
  genetically modified, 1:245, 246–247
  glycemic index, 1:251*t*
  Ireland, 2:86
Poverty
  and WIC program, 2:255, 256
  worldwide, 1:230
Prednisone, 2:88*t*

Preeclampsia, 1:289, 2:146, 223
  See also Pregnancy
Preformed retinoids, 2:232, 234
  See also Vitamin A
Pregnancy, **2:142–147**
  alcohol use, 1:25
  aspartame, 1:46
  beta-carotene, 2:36
  caffeine, 1:82
  calcium, 1:85
  cravings, 1:136, 2:146
  folate, 1:40, 2:243
  iron, 1:40
  nutrition requirements, 2:144–145, 144*t*, *145*, 146, 259
  pica, 2:138, 146
  protein, 2:159
  smoking, 2:198
  teens, 1:7
  vegetarians, 2:230
  vitamin A, 2:36, 234
  vitamin and mineral requirements, 2:145, *145*
  weight gain, 2:143–144, 143*t*
  WIC program, 2:146–147, 255, 256, 257
  See also Breastfeeding; Low birth weight infant
Pregnancy-induced hypertension (PIH), 1:289
Premenstrual dysphoric disorder (PDD), 2:147
Premenstrual syndrome (PMS), **2:147–150**, 2:*148*, 259
  symptoms, 2:148
  treatments, 2:148–149, *149*
  See also Women's nutritional issues
Pre-renal, defined, 2:45
Preschoolers and toddlers, diet of, **2:150–154**
  energy and protein needs, 2:151–152, 152*t*
  nutritional requirements, 2:150–153
  potential feeding problems, 2:153–154
  vitamin and mineral needs, 2:152–153
  WIC program, 2:255, 256, 257–258
  See also Baby bottle tooth decay
Preservatives. *See* Additives and preservatives
Pressure cuffs, 1:99, *100*
Prevalence, defined, 1:14
Preventive medicine, defined, 1:253
Primary hypertension, 1:289
Primary lactose intolerance, 2:22

305

Primary sampling unit (PSU), 2:70
Probiotics, 1:242t, **2:154–155**
    See also Functional foods
Problem solving, and weight management, 2:253
Processed foods
    Central America, 1:113
    defined, 1:12
    and food allergens, 1:27
    Mexico, 1:113
    and vitamin C, 2:197
    versus whole foods, 2:255
Product Identity statement, 1:232
Proenzymes, 1:37
Progesterone, and premenstrual syndrome, 2:149
Prolactin, 1:76
Proline, 2:156t
Proscription, defined, 1:188
Prostaglandin, defined, 2:108
Prostate, defined, 1:88
Prostate cancer, 1:91, 2:208, 234
Prostate health, 2:53
Protein, **2:155–160**
    absorption, 1:172, 2:157
    adolescents, 1:5
    amino acids, 2:155–156, 156t
    animal, 2:156
    blood, 2:158
    cancer patients, 1:92
    and cardiovascular disease, 1:103
    Caribbean Islands, 1:108
    corn- or maize-based diets, 1:134
    cravings, 1:137–138
    defined, 1:5
    denaturation, 1:37
    digestion, 2:157
    effect on mood, 2:66, 66t
    functions, 1:37, 2:158–159
    high-quality, 2:156
    infants, 2:8
    and kwashiorkor, 2:20, 21
    in legumes, 2:27–28
    lower-quality proteins, 2:156
    metabolism, 2:55–56, 157
    motor, 1:37
    as nutrient, 2:92
    plant, 2:156
    preschoolers and toddlers, 2:151–152, 152t
    protein-calorie malnutrition, 2:35, 159–160
    protein-energy malnutrition, 2:35, 36, 141
    quality, 1:134, 2:156
    requirement, 2:159

    sources, 2:159, 159t
    soy, 1:243, 2:207, 207t, 208
    sports nutrition, 1:192, 2:216, 218
    structural, 1:37
    supplements, 1:192, 2:218
    See also Amino acids
Protein Power, 1:203t, 204
Protein-based fat substitutes, 1:212, 212t, 218
Protein-calorie malnutrition (PCM), 2:35, 159–160
Protein-energy malnutrition (PEM), 2:35, 36, 141
Protestant food practices, 2:176, 178t
Psoriasis, defined, 2:108
PSU (primary sampling unit), 2:70
Psychological, defined, 1:1
Psyllium, defined, 1:240
PTH (parathyroid hormone), 1:83–84
Puberty
    defined, 1:4
    See also Adolescent nutrition
Public Health Nutritionists, 1:105
Pubs, 2:84, *85*, 86
Puerto Rican Americans. *See* Hispanics and Latinos, diet of
Pure Food and Drug Act (1906), 2:162, 171
Pyridoxal phosphate (PLP), 2:242
Pyruvate, 2:55
Pyruvic acid, 1:96

Q

QPM (quality protein maize), 1:134
Quackery, **2:160–164**
    claims and promises, 2:161, *161*, *163*
    nutrition quackery, 2:161–162
    patent medicines, 2:161, 162
    victims, 2:162–164
    See also Fad diets
Quality protein maize (QPM), 1:134
Quinoa, 2:202
Quinones, 2:236

R

RACC (Reference Amounts Customarily Consumed Per Eating Occasion), 1:234
Radiation, and cancer, 1:89
Radio programming, for children, 2:226
Radura, 2:14
Ramadan, 2:175, 177
Rastafarian food practices, 2:175, 176, 178, 178t

Ravioli, glycemic index, 1:251t
RD. *See* Registered dietitian (RD)
Reactive hypoglycemia, 1:292
Reactivity, defined, 1:275
Recombinant bovine growth hormone, 1:246
Recombinant DNA technology. *See* Biotechnology
Recombinant human growth hormone, 1:262
Recommended Dietary Allowances (RDAs), **2:164**
    during breastfeeding, 1:76
    defined, 1:20
    and Dietary Reference Intakes, 1:155, 2:164
    dietary trends, 1:161
    elderly, 1:20
    National Academy of Sciences, 2:67
    preschoolers and toddlers, 2:151, 152, 152t
    school food service, 2:194, 196t
    school-aged children, 2:190–191
    See also Dietary Reference Intakes (DRIs)
Recommended Nutrient Intakes for Canadians, 1:155
Red blood cell, 1:38, 2:212
"Reduced," as nutrient content claim, 1:265t
Reduced-fat products, 1:219
Reeve, Christopher, 2:76
Reference Amounts Customarily Consumed Per Eating Occasion (RACC), 1:234
Refugee Nutrition Information System (RNIS), **2:164–166**, 2:*165*
    See also Disaster relief organizations
Regional diet, American, **2:166–170**
    African Americans, 1:12, 2:166–168
    Hispanics, 2:168–169
    regional cooking, 2:167
    See also Dietary trends, American
Regional diet, South American, 2:202, 202–203
Registered dietetic technician. *See* Dietetic technician, registered (DTR)
Registered dietitian (RD)
    careers in dietetics, 1:105, 106, *106*
    as dietitian, 1:168, 169
    as medical nutrition therapy provider, 2:44–45, *45*
    as nutritionist, 2:104
Registration Examination, 1:105, 106

Regulations
  additives and preservatives, 1:2–4
  dietary supplements, 1:156–157
  drugs and food additives, 1:158
  food safety, 1:238–239, 238t
  functional foods, 1:241–243
Regulatory agencies, **2:170–174**
  United States, 2:170–172, *171*
  worldwide, 2:172–173
  See also Food safety; *specific agencies by name*
Relief organizations. *See* Disaster relief organizations
Religion and dietary practices, **2:174–179**
  fasting, 2:174–175, 176, 177, 178–179
  food customs, 2:174, *176*
  food proscriptions, 2:176–179, *177*, 178t
  health benefits and risks, 2:175–176
  stimulants, 2:176, *177*
  See also Eating habits; Fasting; *specific religions by name*
Rembrandt, 2:224, *224*
Renal failure, defined, 2:21
Renaud, Serge, 1:240
Rennin, 2:248
Report on the Nutrition Situation of Refugees and Displaced Populations, 2:165
Respiratory system, defined, 1:27
Retinoids, 2:232, 234
Rewards, and weight management, 2:253
R-group, 2:155
Rheumatic heart disease, 1:272
Rhodopsin, 2:232
Riboflavin (vitamin B$_2$), 2:238, 240t
Rice
  in African-American diet, 1:11, 13
  genetically modified (golden rice), 1:*66*, 68, 245, 246–247, 2:182, 264
Rice porridge, 2:189
Rice-based diets, **2:179–183**, 2:*180*
  Asia, 1:52, *53*
  genetically modified rice, 1:*66*, 68, 245, 246–247, 2:182, 264
  for medical therapy and prevention, 2:181–182
  nutritional properties, 2:180–181, 181t
  and thiamine deficiency, 2:181
  See also Asians, diet of; Corn- or maize-based diets
Rickets, **2:183–186**, 2:*184*
  defined, 1:84

Glisson, Francis, 1:249, *249*
Mellanby, Edward, 2:46, *47*
nutritional deficiency, 2:104
vitamin D deficiency, 1:84, 2:46, *47*, 104, 183, 184, *184*, 185, 235
See also Osteomalacia
Ritual, defined, 1:11
RNA, defined, 1:40
RNIS (Refugee Nutrition Information System), 2:164–166, *165*
Roadside stands, 2:222
Roman Catholic food practices, 2:176, *176*, 178–179, 178t
Romania, 1:118
Ronald McDonald (fictional character), 2:*38*
Rosenstein, Nils Rosén von, 2:*186*, **2:186**
Rotary International, 2:227
Roti, 2:203
Roughage. *See* Fiber
Rugby, 1:*199*
Runner's high, 2:66
Russia
  cardiovascular disease mortality in, 1:118
  vitamin C deficiency, 1:120
  See also Central Europeans and Russians, diets of

S
Saccharin, 1:47
Saffron, 2:204, *205*
Salmonella
  food-borne illness, 1:236, 2:2, 119, 120t
  hand washing, 2:3
  organic foods, 2:116
  photographs, 1:*237*, 2:*2*
  Scandinavia, 2:187
Salmonellosis, defined, 2:118
Salt. *See* Sodium
Salvation Army World Service Office (SAWSO), 1:175t
Sanitarium Food Company, 2:17
Sarcoma, 1:88
SARS (Severe Acute Respiratory Syndrome), 2:262
Satiety, **2:187**
  See also Appetite; Weight management
Saturated fat
  actual and recommended intake, 1:217, *218*
  and cardiovascular disease, 1:101
  chemical structure, 1:214–215
  defined, 1:51

Healthy Eating Index, 1:268
Mediterranean diet, 1:260
  as nutrient, 2:93
Saudi Arabia, fast food in, 1:*165*
SAWSO (Salvation Army World Service Office), 1:175t
Say Yes for Children program, 2:227
SBP (School Breakfast Program), 1:284, 2:97, 190–191, 194
Scandinavians, diet of, **2:187–190**
  eating habits and dietary patterns, 2:187–189, *188*, *189*
  nutrition and health status, 2:187
  special meals, 2:189–190
  See also Central Europeans and Russians, diets of; Northern Europeans, diet of
Scavenger cell, 2:29
School Breakfast Program (SBP), 1:284, 2:97, 190–191, 194
School dietitians, 1:168
School food service, **2:194–197**, 2:*195*, 196t
  competitive foods, 2:195–197
  plate waste, 2:195
School gardens, 2:222
School health services, 1:110, 131
School-aged children, diet of, **2:190–194**
  dietary patterns, 2:191–192
  junk food in schools, 2:191, *192*
  nutritional needs, 2:190–191
  obesity, 2:192–193
  snacking, 2:192
  See also Adolescent nutrition; Preschoolers and toddlers, diet of
Schools/Child Nutrition Commodity Programs, 1:129
Scotland, 2:84–85
Scurvy, 2:*197*, **2:197**
  defined, 1:156
  Glisson, Francis, 1:249, *249*
  Stark, William, 2:219–220, *220*
  and vitamin C, 2:219–220, *220*
SDR (standardized death rate), 1:117
Seasickness, ginger for, 1:33
Secondary hypertension, 1:289, 291
Secondary lactose intolerance, 2:22
Second-hand smoke, 2:198
Secretin, 1:170
Sedentary, defined, 1:51
Selective serotonin reuptake inhibitor (SSRI), 1:180–181, 2:149
  See also Serotonin

307

Selenium
- as antioxidant, 1:43, 44t
- deficiency, 2:63
- disease prevention and treatment, 2:62
- functions, 2:62

Self-monitoring, and weight management, 2:251
Self-starvation, 1:181, 2:140
See also Anorexia nervosa
Semi-vegetarians, 2:229
Sen, Amartya, 1:207–208
Serine, 2:156t
Serotonin
- cravings, 1:137
- defined, 1:137
- depression, 2:75
- eating disorders, 1:178
- effect on mood, 2:64, 65, 66–67, 66t
- premenstrual syndrome, 2:149
- selective serotonin reuptake inhibitor (SSRI), 1:180–181, 2:149

Serum, defined, 1:103
Service-systems paradox, 1:282
Seventh-day Adventist Church, 2:17, 175, 178t, 179
Severe Acute Respiratory Syndrome (SARS), 2:262
Shigella, 2:2, 119, 120t
Shock, defined, 1:149
Shuttle space program, 2:212, 213, 214
Shuttle-Mir program, 2:213, 214
Sickle-cell anemia, 1:39
Sideroblastosis, defined, 1:38
Sierra Leone, life expectancy in, 2:28
Siesta, 2:201, 206
Simple sugars, 1:93–94, 94t, 2:91
Simplesse, 1:218
Singapore, 1:55, 2:115
Skinfold calipers, 2:101, 102, 253
Skylab space program, 2:212, 214
Slavery
- and African-American diet, 1:10–11
- and Caribbean Islanders diet, 1:107, 108

Sleep apnea, defined, 1:122
Small for gestational age, **2:197–198**
See also Low birth weight infant
Smog, defined, 2:183
Smoking, **2:198–200**, 2:199
- and atherosclerosis, 1:59
- and cancer, 1:89, 90, 91, 2:51
- and cardiovascular disease, 1:101
- and free radicals, 1:43
- and heart disease, 1:274
- and hypertension, 1:290
- and pregnancy, 2:198
- religious proscriptions, 2:176

Smorgasbords, 2:188
Snacking
- adolescents, 1:5–6
- American dietary trends, 1:159
- college students, 1:123
- eating habits, 1:186
- school-aged children, 2:192
See also Grazing

SNE (Society for Nutrition Education), 2:200
Social group, defined, 1:143
Social support, and weight management, 2:252–253
Society for Nutrition Education (SNE), **2:200**
Socioeconomic status
- defined, 1:20
- and diabetes, 2:167
- Hispanics and Latinos, 2:168, 169
- and maternal mortality rate, 2:42

Sodium
- and cardiovascular disease, 1:103
- deficiency, 2:61
- disease prevention and treatment, 2:60, 61
- as food additive, 1:1, 2
- functions, 2:60
- Healthy Eating Index, 1:268
- and hypertension, 1:290, 2:53
- nutrient content claims, 1:265t
- and space travel, 2:211, 215
- toxicity, 2:61

Sodium-sensitive individuals, 1:290, 2:53
Soft drinks
- American dietary trends, 1:160, 160
- caffeine, 1:81, 81t
- glycemic index, 1:251t
- and oral health, 2:111–112
- school-aged children, 2:192

Solder, lead, 2:24, 25, 26
Soluble fiber, 1:221
Somalia, 1:224
Soul food, 1:11–12
Soursop, 1:109
South Americans, diet of, **2:200–204**
- eating habits and meal patterns, 2:201
- nutritional status, 2:201
- regional food habits, 2:202, 202–203
- traditional cooking methods and food habits, 2:201–202

See also Central Americans and Mexicans, diets of
South Asians, diet of, 1:55
South Beach diet, 1:97
Southeast Asians, diet of, 1:54–55
Southern Africans, diet of, 1:18
Southern cooking, 1:11–12, 2:167
Southern Europeans, diet of, **2:204–207**, 2:205
- dietary benefits, deficits, and changes, 2:205–206
- influences on American diet, 2:206
- traditional foods, 2:204–205

See also Central Europeans and Russians, diets of; Northern Europeans, diet of
Southwest cooking, 2:167
Soy, **2:207–210**, 2:209
- and cancer, 2:208
- as functional food, 1:242t
- genetically modified, 1:245
- and heart, 2:207–208
- and menopause, 2:48–49, 208, 260
- and osteoporosis, 2:208
- protein, 1:243, 2:207, 207t, 208
- sources, 2:207t

See also Legumes; Meat analogs
Space travel and nutrition, **2:210–215**
- dietary intake during spaceflight, 2:214–215
- space food systems, 2:212–214, 213
- space physiology, 2:210–212

Spaghetti, glycemic index, 1:251t
Spain, 2:204, 205, 205, 206
Special Milk Program, 2:97
Special Supplemental Program for Women, Infants, and Children (WIC). *See* WIC program
Sphygmomanometers, 1:99, 100
Spices, 1:108, 2:204, 205
Splenda, 1:47
Spores, and food-borne illness, 2:119
Sports bars, as functional food, 1:242t
Sports drinks, 2:4, 217–218
Sports nutrition, **2:215–219**
- caffeine, 1:83
- calories, 2:216
- carbohydrates, 2:216
- eating disorders, 1:125
- fat, 2:216
- female athlete triad, 2:218–219
- fluids, 2:217, 217–218, 218t
- glycemic index, 1:251–252
- human growth hormone, 1:262–263
- nutritional needs, 1:7

protein, 2:216
sports supplements, 2:218
timing of meals, 2:218
vitamins and minerals, 2:217
water, 2:245, 246, 247, *247*
See also Ergogenic aids; Female athlete triad
Sri Lankans, diet of, 1:55, 2:*180*
SSRI (selective serotonin reuptake inhibitor), 1:180–181, 2:149
See also Serotonin
St. Vincent and the Grenadines, 1:110
Stabilizing agents, 1:2
Stacking, 1:190
Standardized death rate (SDR), 1:117
Stanol esters, 1:242*t*
Staphylococcus aureus, 2:3, 119, 120*t*
Staples, defined, 1:16
Starch, 1:94
Stark, William, **2:219–220**, 2:*220*
See also Scurvy
Starvation, self-imposed, 1:181, 2:140
See also Anorexia nervosa
Steam doctors, 2:135
Stem cell research, 2:74–75
Steroid hormones, 1:215
Steroids, defined, 1:190
Sterol, defined, 2:30
Stevioside, 1:48
Still birth, defined, 1:252
Stimulants, religion and dietary practices, 2:176, 177
Stimulus control, and weight management, 2:251
Stool acidity test, 2:22
Stress, defined, 1:44
Stress management
mood-food relationships, 2:*65*, 66–67
and weight management, 2:251–252
Stress response, 1:138
Stroke, 1:100, 147
defined, 1:24
See also Cardiovascular disease (CVD)
Structural proteins, 1:37
Structure and function claims
for dietary supplements, 1:33, 156
for functional foods, 1:241–243
Subcutaneous, defined, 2:37
Sucralose, 1:47
Sucrose, 1:93–94, 94*t*
defined, 1:46
Sudan refugees, 2:*165*

Sugar
Caribbean Islands, 1:107
comparison, 1:94*t*
maple, 2:80
and oral health, 2:110
and pregnancy, 2:144
simple, 1:93–94, 94*t*, 2:91
Sugar alcohols, 1:47, 242*t*
Sugar Busters!, 1:203*t*, 204
Sulfite intolerance, 1:28
Summer Food Service Program for Children, 1:284, 2:97
Sun exposure, and vitamin D, 2:183, *184*, 184–185, *235*, 235–236
Sunette, 1:46
Sunscreens, 2:235, *235*
Superweeds, 1:246
Supplements, dietary. *See* Dietary supplements
Surgeon General's Report on Nutrition and Health, 1:154
Suriname, 2:203
Sustainable food systems, **2:220–223**, 2:*222*
importance, 2:221
promoting, 2:221–222
See also Organic foods; Pesticides
Swallowing difficulties, 1:21, 2:110, 111
Swanson TV Dinner, 2:141
Sweden
life expectancy, 2:28
obesity, 2:105
vitamin C deficiency, 1:120
Sweet corn, 1:133–134
Sweeteners, artificial. *See* Artificial sweeteners
Sweet'n Low, 1:47
Switzerland
food-borne illness, 2:118
life expectancy, 2:28
Systolic pressure, 1:99, *100*, 288

T

Tacos, 1:115, 116, 2:*81*
Taiwan, organic foods in, 2:115
Tajines, 1:17, *17*
Tamales, 1:115
Tartrazine, 1:4
Tea
caffeine, 1:81, 81*t*
England, Wales, and Scotland, 2:84
Ireland, 2:86
South America, 2:201
Teenagers. *See* Adolescent nutrition

TEFAP (The Emergency Food Assistance Program), 1:128, 284–285
Television
African Americans, 2:167–168
body image, 2:131
International Children's Day of Broadcasting, 2:226
obesity, 2:106
TV Dinners, 2:141
Temperance, 1:254, 255, 2:254
Temperate zone, defined, 1:18
Ten Steps to Successful Breastfeeding program, 2:226
Testosterone, defined, 1:137
Tetracycline, 2:88*t*, 89
Tex-Mex cuisine, 1:116
Thailand, food insecurity, 1:*229*, 230
Thalassemia, defined, 1:38
Thermoregulate, defined, 2:225
Thiamine (vitamin B_1), 2:238, 240*t*
and beriberi, 1:62
Casimir, Funk, 1:244
deficiency, 1:62, 2:103, 181
and rice, 2:181
Thiazide, 2:88*t*
Thickening agents, 1:2
Thirst, 2:217, *217*, 247
Threonine, 2:156*t*
Thrifty Food Plan, 1:153
Thrifty gene, 1:145, 2:126
Title V Maternal Child Health Program, 2:98
Tobacco. *See* Smoking
Tocopherol. *See* Vitamin E
Toddlers. *See* Preschoolers and toddlers, diet of
Tofu, 2:*207*, *209*, 230, *231*
defined, 1:5
Tolerable Upper Intake Level, 1:155
Tolerance, defined, 1:24
Tomatoes
carotenoids, 1:113, 2:234
genetically modified, 1:65, 245–246
and prostate cancer, 1:91, 2:234
Tortillas, 1:113, *114*, 114–115, 116
Total vegetarians, 2:229, 243
Toxemia, 1:289, 2:146, **2:223**
See also Pregnancy
Toxicant, defined, 1:4
Toxicity
calcium, 1:84, 2:61
fluoride, 2:63
iron, 2:63
magnesium, 2:61
manganese, 2:63
minerals, 2:61, 63

Toxicity *(continued)*
   phosphate, 2:61
   potassium, 2:61
   sodium, 2:61
   vitamin A, 2:233*t*, 234
   vitamin D, 2:233*t*, 236
   vitamin E, 2:233*t*, 237
   vitamin K, 2:233*t*, 236
Toxins
   defined, 1:77
   in genetically modified foods, 1:246
Trace, defined, 1:43
Trace minerals, 2:61–63
Traditional Healthy Mediterranean Diet Pyramid, 1:226–227
Trall, Russell, 2:17
Trans-fatty acids
   defined, 1:100
   on food labels, 1:*217*
   Mediterranean diet, 1:260
Traveler's diarrhea, 1:149
A Treatise of the Rickets, 1:249, *249*
Treatise on Bread and Bread Making (Graham), 1:255
Trichinella spiralis, 2:3, 120*t*
Trick or Treat for UNICEF, 2:228
Triglycerides
   as basic fat unit, 1:215, 216, 2:92–93
   defined, 1:68
   in fat metabolism, 2:56
   optimal, borderline, and high levels, 2:29*t*
Trinidad and Tobago, 1:110
Tripeptides, 1:37
Tryptophan, 2:156*t*
   in maize, 1:134
   and niacin, 2:239, 240–241
   and pellagra, 2:135, 240–241
   as precursor of serotonin, 2:64
   and pyridoxal phosphate, 2:242
Tuber, defined, 1:108
Tuberculosis
   and breastfeeding, 2:146
   defined, 1:51
Tularemia, defined, 2:187
Tulp, Nicolaas, **2:223–225,** 2:*224*
   See also Beriberi
Tumor, 1:88, 90
Tumor suppressor gene, 1:91
TV. *See* Television
Type I diabetes, 1:144, *145*, 146
Type II diabetes, 1:144–145, 146, 147
   defined, 1:14
   and exercise, 1:288
   Native Americans, 2:81
   prevalence, 1:164
Typhoid, defined, 1:253
Typhus, defined, 1:253
Tyramine, 1:28, 2:89
Tyrosine, 2:66, 137, 156*t*
Tzotzil, 1:*114*

U

Ulcer, defined, 1:79
Ulcer, gastric, 1:79, 172
Ultraviolet radiation
   and space travel, 2:211
   and vitamin D, 2:183, *184*, 184–185, *235*, 235–236
UN. *See* United Nations
Uncharged, defined, 2:155
Undernutrition
   defined, 1:113
   developing countries, 2:111, 141
   homelessness, 1:283–285
   oral health, 2:111
   prevalence, 2:33
Underweight, 2:35, **2:225**
   See also Body mass index
UNHCR (United Nations High Commissioner for Refugees), 1:189
UNICEF. *See* United Nations Children's Fund (UNICEF)
United Kingdom
   mad cow disease, 2:118
   organic foods, 2:115
United Nations
   Administration Committee on Coordination Sub Committee on Nutrition (ACC/SCN), 2:165
   Economic and Social Council, 2:198
   food insecurity, 1:228
   Food Safety Agency, 1:246
   homelessness, 1:282
   nongovernmental organizations, 2:82–83
   Office for the Coordination of Humanitarian Affairs (OCHA), 1:175*t*
   Universal Declaration of Human Rights, 2:35–36
   urban population, 2:221
   world population, 1:230
   See also Food and Agriculture Organization (FAO)
United Nations Children's Fund (UNICEF), 1:175*t*, **2:225–228,** 2:*228*
   accomplishments, 2:226–227
   administration, 2:226
   in Bam (Iran), 2:226
   mission, 2:226
   oral rehydration therapy, 2:113, 226
   programs and operations, 2:227–228
   resources, 2:226
United Nations High Commissioner for Refugees (UNHCR), 1:189
Universal Declaration of Human Rights, 2:35–36
University of Toronto Joint Centre for Bioethics, 1:67, 68
Unsaturated fatty acids, 1:215, 2:93, 94
Urban growth, and sustainable food systems, 2:221
Urban Institute, 1:282
Urea cycle disorders, 2:7
Uric, defined, 2:6
Uruguay, 2:201, 203
U.S. Agency for Healthcare Research and Quality, 2:198
U.S. Agency for International Development (USAID), 1:175*t*
U.S. Census Bureau, 1:275, 284
U.S. Centers for Disease Control and Prevention (CDC)
   bioterrorism, 1:237
   body mass index, 1:121
   fetal alcohol syndrome, 1:*220*
   food-borne illnesses, 1:236, 2:4
   Global Polio Eradication Initiative, 2:227
   growth charts, 1:262
   high school students, 2:191–192
   hypertension, 2:53
   National Immunization Days, 2:227
   physical activity, 1:161
   prostate cancer, 2:53
   as regulatory agency, 2:172
U.S. Department of Agriculture (USDA)
   Center for Nutrition and Public Policy, 1:269
   commodity foods, 1:127–129, *129*, 284–285
   Continuing Survey of Food Intakes by Individuals, 1:160
   Dietary Guidelines, 1:153–154
   Economic Research Service, 2:116
   Emergency Food Assistance Program, 1:128, 284–285
   Food and Nutrition Information Center, 2:171
   Food and Nutrition Service (FNS), 1:127, 128, 2:96–98, *98*, 194, 255

Food Guide Pyramid for Young Children, 2:151
food insecurity, 1:228
food labels, 1:232, 233
food safety, 1:164
Food Safety and Inspection Service, 2:171
food-borne organisms, 2:118
genetically modified foods, 1:247–248
health claims, 1:263, 264, 266, 2:37–38
Healthy Eating Index, 1:267–269, 268
junk food in schools, 2:191
mad cow disease, 2:119
organic foods, 2:114, 116, 162
as regulatory agency, 2:171, 171
school food service, 2:194, 195
See also Food Guide Pyramid
U.S. Department of Health and Human Services (HHS)
community nutrition programs, 2:98
cultural competence, 1:141–142
Dietary Guidelines, 1:154
nutrition programs for elderly, 1:129
U.S. Department of Homeland Security (DHS), 2:172
U.S. Environmental Protection Agency (EPA), 2:172
U.S. Federal Trade Commission (FTC), 2:164
U.S. Food and Drug Administration (FDA)
additive definition, 1:1
additive regulation, 1:2–4, 158
approved artificial sweeteners, 1:46–47
artificial sweeteners pending approval, 1:48
bioterrorism, 1:238, 2:172
dietary supplements, 1:33, 156, 158, 2:59–60
drug regulation, 1:158
fat intake, 1:217
fat substitutes, 1:211–212, 213
food labels, 1:232–233, 234, 237, 241–243, 2:161
food safety, 1:164, 235–236, 238
functional foods, 1:241–243
Generally Recognized as Safe (GRAS), 1:245
genetic engineering, 1:66–67, 68
Hazard Analysis Critical Control Point program, 1:236
health claims, 1:263, 264, 266
nutrition quackery, 2:161

organic food, 1:237
as regulatory agency, 2:171–172
soy, 2:207
U.S. Food and Nutrition Board, 2:59
U.S. Food and Nutrition Service (FNS)
commodity foods, 1:127, 128
community nutrition programs, 2:96–98, 98
school food service, 2:194
WIC program, 2:255
U.S. Institute of Medicine
beta-carotene, 1:63
homelessness, 1:283
pregnancy weight gain, 2:143
U.S. National Center for Environmental Health, 2:26
U.S. National Library of Medicine (NLM), 2:74
U.S. National Organic Standards Board (NOSB), 2:113–114
U.S. Office of Minority Health, 1:141–142
U.S. Public Health Service (PHS), 1:238–239, 253, 2:73
U.S. Senate Select Committee on Nutrition and Human Needs, 1:153–154
U.S. Surgeon General
college binge drinking, 1:25
dental caries, 2:110
diabetes, 1:164
nutrition and health report, 1:154
USAID (U.S. Agency for International Development), 1:175t
USDA. See U.S. Department of Agriculture

V

Vaccine, defined, 1:91
Valine, 2:6, 156t
Vector-borne diseases, 1:176
Vegan, **2:229**, 2:243
defined, 1:7
See also Plant-based diets; Vegetarianism
Vegetable oils, 2:108
Vegetables
and cancer prevention, 1:91
Caribbean Islands, 1:108
Central America and Mexico, 1:114
as functional food, 1:242t
glycemic index, 1:251t
Mediterranean diet, 1:258
Vegetarian Food Guide Pyramid, 2:231

Vegetarianism, **2:229–232**, 2:231
Battle Creek Sanitarium, 1:60, 61
benefits, 2:229–230
at different ages, 2:230–231
legumes, 2:27–28
nutritional adequacy, 1:7, 2:230
and osteomalacia, 2:122
and religion, 2:175–176, 176, 177, 179
types, 2:229
and vitamin D, 2:236
See also Meat analogs
Vegetative bacteria, and food-borne illness, 2:119
Veins, 1:99
Venezuela, 2:202–203
"Very low," as nutrient content claim, 1:265t
Very low-density lipoprotein (VLDL), 2:29
Vietnamese, diet of, 1:50t, 54
Viral disease, defined, 2:262
Virus
defined, 1:37
and food-borne illness, 2:119–120
Vitamin A, 2:232, 233t, 234
Asia, 1:56
and beta-carotene, 1:62–63
from carotenoids, 1:112, 113
daily recommended intakes, 2:233t
deficiency, 1:56, 2:233t, 234, 264
functions, 2:232, 233t
and golden rice, 2:182
people at risk, 2:233t
sources, 2:233t
supplements during pregnancy, 2:36
toxicity, 2:233t, 234
and vitamin E, 2:232
and vitamin K, 2:236
and xerophthalmia, 2:264
Vitamin B_1. See Thiamine (vitamin B_1)
Vitamin B_2 (riboflavin), 2:238, 240t
Vitamin B_3. See Niacin (vitamin B_3)
Vitamin B_5 (pantothenic acid), 2:240t, 241
Vitamin B_6, 2:240t, 242
Vitamin B_8. See Biotin (vitamin B_8)
Vitamin B_9. See Folate
Vitamin B_{12}, 1:40, 2:230–231, 241t, 243
Vitamin C, 2:241t, 244
as antioxidant, 1:42, 44t
and cancer, 2:167
Central Europe and Russia, 1:119, 120

Vitamin C (continued)
  deficiency, 1:119, 120, 2:219–220, *220*
  and illness, 2:134
  and oral health, 2:111
  processed foods, 2:197
  and scurvy, 2:197, 219–220, *220*
Vitamin D, 2:233t, 234–236
  and calcium, 1:84, 86, 2:235
  daily recommended intakes, 2:233t
  defined, 1:2
  functions, 2:233t, 235
  infant nutrition, 2:8
  in milk, as functional food, 1:242t
  and osteomalacia, 2:122
  and osteoporosis, 2:124
  people at risk, 2:233t
  and phosphorus, 2:235
  preschoolers and toddlers, 2:152
  sources, 2:233t
  during space travel, 2:211
  and sun exposure, 2:183, *184*, 184–185, *235*, 235–236
  toxicity, 2:233t, 236
  and vegetarianism, 2:230–231
Vitamin D deficiency, 2:235–236
  and cod liver oil, 2:234–235
  and osteomalacia, 1:84, 2:183, 235
  and osteoporosis, 2:235
  and rickets, 1:84, 2:46, *47*, 104, 183, 184, *184*, 185, 235
  symptoms, 2:233t
Vitamin E, 2:233t, 236–237
  as antioxidant, 1:43, 44t, 2:237
  daily recommended intakes, 2:233t
  deficiency, 2:233t, 237
  functions, 2:233t
  people at risk, 2:233t
  sources, 2:233t
  toxicity, 2:233t, 237
  and vitamin A, 2:232
  and vitamin K, 2:236, 237
Vitamin K, 2:233t, 236
  daily recommended intakes, 2:233t
  deficiency, 2:94, 233t, 236
  functions, 2:233t, 236
  people at risk, 2:233t
  sources, 2:233t
  toxicity, 2:233t, 236
  and vitamin A, 2:236
  and vitamin E, 2:236, 237
Vitamins
  in corn- or maize-based diets, 1:134–136

  defined, 1:2
  discovery, 1:244, *244*
  as nutrient, 2:94
  pregnancy, 2:145
  sports nutrition, 2:217
Vitamins, fat-soluble, 2:94, 153, **2:232–237**, 2:233t, *235*
  See also Vitamin A; Vitamin D; Vitamin E; Vitamin K
Vitamins, water-soluble, 2:94, **2:230–244**, 2:*239*, 240–241t
  See also Choline; Vitamin C; *specific B vitamins by name*
VLDL (very low-density lipoprotein), 2:29

W

Waist circumference, 1:73–74
Waist-to-hip ratio, 1:68–69, **2:245**
  See also Anthropometric measurements
Wales, 2:85–86
Warfarin, 2:88t, 236, 237
Warm-up, in exercise, 1:201
Wasting
  defined, 1:73
  HIV/AIDS patients, 1:280
  and malnutrition, 2:35
Water, **2:245–248**, 2:*246*
  contaminated, 1:150, 173, 174–175, 2:228
  functions, 2:245
  in human body, 245–246
  as nutrient, 2:95
  older women and men, 2:50
  pasteurization, 2:133
  recommendations, 2:246
  sports nutrition, 2:217
  water balance, 2:246
  water excretion regulation, 2:*247*, 247–248
  water intake regulation, 2:247
  water intoxication, 2:248
  See also Dehydration; Oral rehydration therapy (ORT)
Waterhouse, Debra, 1:137
Water-soluble, defined, 1:42
Water-soluble vitamins. *See* Vitamins, water-soluble
Wean, defined, 1:76
Weight and height tables, 2:99–100, 100t
Weight cycling, 1:184–185, 2:250, 264–265
Weight gain
  menopause, 2:50
  pregnancy, 2:143–144, 143t

Weight loss
  diarrhea, 1:149
  HIV/AIDS patients, 1:280
Weight loss agents, as ergogenic aids, 1:192
Weight loss diets, 1:167, 2:106–107, **2:248–250**, 2:*249*
  See also Dieting; Fad diets; Yo-yo dieting
Weight loss soap, 2:*163*
Weight management, **2:250–253**, 2:*252*, *253*
  adults, 1:7–8
  and caffeine, 1:83
  methods, 2:106–107, *107*, 251–253
  See also Eating habits; Exercise; Fad diets; Weight loss diets
Weight Watchers, 1:167
Wellness, **2:253**
  defined, 1:7
  See also Health
Wernicke-Korsakoff syndrome, 1:62, 2:238
West Africans, diet of, 1:17–18
West Indies, 1:11
West Nile Virus vaccine, 2:75
Western Health Reform Institute, 1:60, 2:254
  See also Battle Creek Sanitarium
Westernization of dietary patterns, 1:163–164, *165*
  See also Nutritional transition
WFP (World Food Programme). *See* Food Aid for Development and the World Food Programme
White, Ellen G., 1:60, 2:17, *254*, **2:254–255**
  See also Battle Creek Sanitarium
White blood cell, defined, 2:4
Whites
  childhood obesity, 1:121
  diet-related disease, 1:14t
  specific food consumption, 1:278t
WHO. *See* World Health Organization (WHO)
Whole foods diet, 1:242t, **2:255**
WIC program, 2:97, **2:255–258**, 2:256t, *257*
  and Commodity Supplemental Food Program, 1:127
  history, 2:255–256
  and homelessness, 1:284
  new directions, 2:258
  outcomes and evaluation, 2:257–258
  and pregnancy, 2:146–147, 255, 256, 257
  rules, 2:256–257

See also Infant nutrition; Pregnancy; Preschoolers and toddlers, diet of
Wilson, Owen, 2:*258*, **2:258**
   See also Infant nutrition
Wine, as functional food, 1:240, 242*t*
Women, Infants, and Children (WIC) program. *See* WIC program
Women's Health Initiative, 2:48, *49*
Women's nutritional issues, **2:259–261**
   anemia, 2:259
   body image, 1:69, *70*, 71
   breast cancer, 2:260
   calcium, 2:259, 260
   chronic diseases, 2:260–261, *261*
   college students, 1:124–125
   cravings, 1:137, *138*
   diabetes, 2:260
   eating disorders, 1:177, 178, 184
   folic acid, 2:259
   heart attack symptoms, 2:75
   heart disease, 2:260–261
   hypertension, 2:261
   iron, 2:259
   life expectancy in Europe, 1:120*t*
   menopause, 2:260
   osteoporosis, 1:10, 2:123, *124*, 125, 260
   pregnancy and breastfeeding, 2:259
   premenstrual syndrome, 2:259
   serotonin, 2:64
   See also Menopause; Pregnancy; Premenstrual syndrome (PMS)
World Bank, 1:230
World Declaration and Plan of Action for Nutrition (1992), 1:250
World Food Programme (WFP). *See* Food Aid for Development and the World Food Programme

World Food Summit, 1:225, 230
World Health Organization (WHO), **2:262–264**, 2:*263*
   Applied Nutrition Program, 2:262
   artificial sweeteners, 1:48
   biotechnology, 1:67, 68
   breastfeeding, 1:75, 2:226, 263
   Department of Nutrition for Health and Development, 2:35
   diabetes, 1:143
   diarrhea, 1:149, 151
   dietary supplements, 1:156
   food insecurity, 1:229
   Food Safety Department, 2:172–173
   Food Safety Program, 2:262–263
   food-borne illness prevention, 2:121
   Global Database on National Nutrition Policies and Programmes, 1:249–250
   Global Outbreak Alert and Response Network, 2:262
   Global Public Health Intelligence Network, 2:262
   health definition, 1:263
   Health for All Database, 1:117
   history and mission, 2:262
   HIV/AIDS, 1:280
   hunger, 1:287
   irradiation, 2:13
   lead poisoning, 2:26
   life expectancy, 2:28
   malaria prevention, 2:227
   malnutrition, 2:34, 35
   marasmus, 2:36
   nutritional deficiency, 2:*103*
   obesity, 1:164
   oral rehydration therapy, 2:113
   osteoporosis, 2:122
   programs, 2:262–264

   Severe Acute Respiratory Syndrome (SARS), 2:262
   smoking, 2:198
   See also Food Aid for Development and the World Food Programme
World Health Organization (WHO) Joint Expert Committee on Food Additives, 1:4, 46, 47
Wurtman, Judith, 2:64

X

Xerophthalmia, 2:234, **2:264**
   See also Beta-carotene; Vitamin A

Y

Yeast allergy, defined, 1:29
Yellow root, 1:13
Yerba maté;, 2:201
Yin and yang, in macrobiotic diet, 2:31
Yogurt, 2:22–23, 154
Yohimbe, as ergogenic aid, 1:190–191, 2:218
Yo-yo dieting, 1:184–185, 2:250, **2:264–265**
   See also Dieting; Weight loss diets

Z

Zeaxanthin, 1:113, 2:234
Zein, in maize, 1:134
Zeisel, Steven H., 1:157–158
Zinc
   deficiency, 2:63
   defined, 1:41
   disease prevention and treatment, 2:62
   functions, 2:62
   preschoolers and toddlers, 2:152
Zocor, 2:88*t*
The Zone (diet), 1:203*t*, 204